SURGICAL MANAGEMENT of Soft Tissue Sarcomas

Myron Arlen, M.D.
Attending in Neoplastic Surgery
North Shore University Hospital
Affiliate of Cornell University
Manhasset, N.Y.

Ralph C. Marcove, M.D.
Associate Attending Surgeon
Memorial Sloan-Kettering Cancer Center
New York, N.Y.

1987

W. B. SAUNDERS COMPANY
Philadelphia London Toronto Sydney Tokyo Hong Kong

W. B. Saunders Company: West Washington Square
Philadelphia, PA 19105

Library of Congress Cataloging-in-Publication Data

Arlen, Myron.

Surgical management of soft tissue sarcomas.

1. Sarcoma—Surgery. I. Marcove, Ralph C. II. Title.
[DNLM: 1. Soft Tissue Neoplasms—surgery. 2. Sarcoma—surgery. WD 375 A723s]

RD651.A75 1987 616.99'4 86–26155

ISBN 0–7216–1399–3

Editor: Dean Manke
Designer: Terri Siegel
Production Manager: Carolyn Naylor
Manuscript Editor: Cynthia Fazzini
Illustration Coordinator: Walt Verbitski
Indexer: David Harvey/Mary Anne Folcher

Surgical Management of Soft Tissue Sarcomas ISBN 0–7216–1399–3

Last digit is the print number: 9 8 7 6 5 4 3 2 1

To SUSAN AND CHRIS,
for their encouragement and support

and to
THEODORE MILLER, M.D.,
our former Chief
at Memorial–Sloan Kettering Cancer Center

CONTRIBUTORS

JULES HARRIS, M.D.: Professor of Medicine and Professor of Immunology; Director, Section of Medical Oncology, Rush Medical College, Chicago, Illinois.

PATRICIA A. JOHNSON, M.D., Ph.D.: Medical Oncologist, Carle Clinic Association, Urbana, Illinois.

K. PARIKH, M.D.: Clinical Instructor, State University of New York Health Science Center, Brooklyn, New York; Assistant Attending, Radiation Oncology, Methodist Hospital, Lutheran Medical Center, and Maimonides Medical Center, New York, New York.

S. RAFLA, M.D., Ph.D.: Clinical Professor, Radiation Oncology, State University of New York Health Science Center, Brooklyn, New York; Director, Department of Radiation Oncology, Methodist Hospital, Lutheran Medical Center, Maimonides Medical Center, New York, New York; Chief, Department of Radiation Oncology, New York Infirmary, New York, New York.

H. SELIM, M.D.: Clinical Assistant Professor in Radiation Oncology, State University of New York Health Science Center, Brooklyn, New York; Attending, Radiation Oncology, Methodist Hospital and Lutheran Medical Center, New York, New York.

E. YOUSSEF, M.D.: Instructor, State University of New York Health Science Center, Brooklyn, New York; Attending, Radiation Oncology, Methodist Hospital, New York, New York; Associate Attending, Radiation Oncology, Lutheran Medical Center; and Assistant Attending, Radiation Oncology, Maimonides Medical Center, New York, New York.

PREFACE

Soft tissue sarcomas present as a unique group of tumors; they are ubiquitous, arising in essentially every known structure of the body and may produce a variety of signs and symptoms ranging from extremity lesions to abdominal masses that may even suggest that they are of visceral origin. For the most part, however, the sarcomas are known to present as relatively asymptomatic lesions during their initial growth phase, producing few if any warning signs to alert one to their potential hazards. Since many of these tumors have a benign counterpart that may be hard to differentiate from the malignant lesion, many patients have been and are still occasionally cautioned to ignore their presence until they are symptomatic. A false sense of security may therefore be given even in the absence of a biopsy.

The management of these soft part sarcomas offered little interest and had minimal impact on the overall management of neoplastic disease until the last decade. The more recent improvements in pathologic diagnosis as well as imaging techniques, coupled with better surgical procedures, has led to a major change in the philosophy of their management. In the early 1960s, when we were residents at Memorial–Sloan Kettering, many of the lesions that were commonly encountered and not recognized were lumped into a rhabdomyosarcoma category. Stout's and Enzinger's contributions to sarcoma pathology were not yet fully appreciated by many clinical pathologists. Pack and Ariel's text, *Tumors of the Soft Somatic Tissues*, had only recently been published, and few training programs with enough experience in managing these tumors existed. Having an extremity sarcoma at that time was tantamount to requiring amputation. Retroperitoneal sarcomas had a low resection rate because they were usually diagnosed at a time when they were virtually unresectable.

In the past two decades careful reevaluation of the soft part sarcomas by light as well as electron microscopy coupled with immunohistochemical staining techniques have led to an appreciation of tumors such as malignant fibrous histiocytoma, malignant mesenchymoma, monophasic synovioma, epithelioid sarcoma, alveolar soft part sarcoma, etc. This has allowed us to extricate these lesions from the more general classification of muscle, fat, fascial, nerve and blood vessel tumors, and develop a concept of behavior patterns. Imaging techniques such as CT scan and MRI have defined the groups of muscles that might require muscle group resection and newer drugs coupled with radiation have all added to our view of what we consider to be the modern-day approach to the surgery of soft part sarcomas.

This text was conceived as a means of helping our house staff understand the basics of sarcoma surgery. It became readily apparent that understanding how a liposarcoma of the shoulder girdle should be handled could not be appreciated by reviewing the natural history of liposarcoma. Rather an understanding of how lesions presented on the shoulder girdle in contrast to the thigh, pelvis, or retroperitoneum was of primary importance; this was followed by the need to understand behavioral patterns based on the grade of the tumor. Histologic classification was only of secondary importance. The format of the text, therefore, is a regional one, covering topics such as head and neck, chest and abdominal wall, retroperitoneum, and then the extremity lesions. For the sake of completeness, we have also defined the visceral sarcomas, extraskeletal osseous sarcomas, and management of metastatic lesions. Concepts such as perineal approach to the retroperitoneum, the "one-bone forearm," and total femoral replacement are also discussed. Although we wrote the chapters on surgical oncology and orthopedic oncology, we are most appreciative of the help given by Drs. Jules Harris and Sameer Rafla, who were extremely helpful in supplying chapters on the medical oncology and radiation oncology of soft part sarcomas. We also appreciate the efforts of Elizabeth Arlen for her drawings, Dr. Barbara Atkinson for the pathology material supplied from North Shore University Hospital, and Frances Silverman, Barbara Kayne, and Diana Paganelli's work in preparing the manuscripts.

MYRON ARLEN, M.D.
RALPH C. MARCOVE, M.D.

CONTENTS

CHAPTER 1

The Classification and Behavior of Soft Tissue Sarcomas

PRINCIPLES OF MANAGEMENT

Sarcomas of soft tissue origin represent a ubiquitous group of neoplasms that can arise from any of the supportive structures of the body. What has become quite apparent to us is that the more soft tissue sarcomas we treat, the more variations we see in their clinical appearance and patterns of distribution. One begins to realize, however, that there is a certain degree of similarity in these neoplasms and that a liposarcomatous tumor arising in the leg really does not behave differently from one arising under the sternocleidomastoid muscle of the neck or in the region of the trapezius muscle of the back. What we have had to learn in managing these tumors is how to handle the varied patterns of distribution so that the surgical techniques for removal of these sarcomas can be tailored to their anatomic location.

Of importance to our house staff has been "surgical decision-making" based on specific location and size, rather than pathologic diagnoses per se, as the initial step in determining the procedure to be employed. Next in importance has been the tumor grade, followed by the histologic classification. We have used this approach to help in deciding on the management of a wide array of tumors—e.g., a 5-cm sarcomatous lesion near the supraspinatous muscle approximating the glenoid compared with a similar lesion of retroperitoneal origin near the area of the psoas muscle and ureter or one arising in the gluteus maximus near the sciatic notch. In our opinion an appreciation of the regional approach to these tumors supersedes any decision as to whether the lesion is a liposarcoma or a malignant fibrous histiocytoma. The histologic type and grade play a role in fine-tuning our decisions, which now are concerned with the potential for a tumor to recur locally or spread to distant sites. Figure 1–1 shows the characteristic appearance of a recurrent epithelioid sarcoma that began on the wrist, was incompletely resected because the pattern of spread was not appreciated, and further recurred even though the patient underwent forequarter amputation. For such an aggressive and highly malignant tumor, although it first appeared in the region of the hand, high amputation was thought to be essential in any initial attempt at cure. Few tumors are as aggressive and able to disseminate through subcutaneous and lymphatic spaces as epithelioid sarcoma; its potential for such permeation into distant planes must be understood.[37]

The recognition of sarcomas as a distinct tumor type, in terms of clinical behavior, occurred early in the history of medicine. Microscopic definition occurred later and has still not been fully realized for all lesions. In 1838 Miller attempted cytologic assessment of various tumor types, which led to the recognition of different architectural arrangements not readily appreciated by microscopists of his time. This descriptive analysis of a wide array of tumors represented an early step in the differentiation of the carcinomas from the sarcomas. Miller's pupils Schwann and Virchow were able to distinguish these tumors further and to classify larger groups of sarcomas on a his-

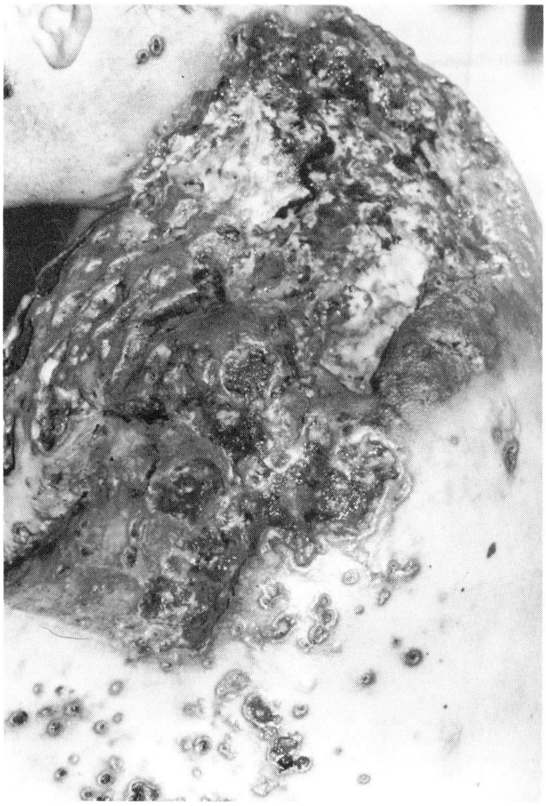

FIGURE 1–1. Extensive spread of epithelioid sarcoma at the site of forequarter amputation.

tologic basis. Eventually, major contributions were offered by Ewing and Stout, bringing the analysis and differentiation of sarcomas to the forefront of present-day oncologic evaluation and management.

Neoplastic transformation that takes place in bone and cartilaginous tissue results in the formation of a group of tumors known to us as the osteosarcomas; those tumors arising from other mesodermal structures such as muscle, fascia, fat, nerves, and blood vessels are known collectively as the soft part or soft tissue sarcomas. The largest number of soft tissue tumors clinically defined are those that are most frequently encountered in the extremities, followed by the retroperitoneum, the abdominal and chest walls, and the head and neck regions. A review of the cases at Memorial Hospital, as well as other institutions having large experiences in the treatment of soft part sarcomas, indicates that the majority of these neoplasms are found in the lower extremity followed by the upper extremity. The trunk is usually next in frequency; a fair percentage of these tumors often appear in the retroperitoneum.

Although the sarcomas with which we are concerned are considered to be primarily soft tissue in origin, there are gray zones for which identification of sites of development may not be clearly established. It is not uncommon to find large primary soft tissue masses invading the cortex and medullary cavity of bone or instances in which bone sarcomas have large soft tissue components. More difficult to assess are those situations in which common soft tissue tumors such as desmoid, hemangiopericytoma, malignant fibrous histiocytoma, or fibrosarcoma appear to arise primarily in bone. The occasional failure of clear-cut separation among the osseous and soft tissue lesions is further exemplified by the appearance of soft tissue osteosarcomas that have no known osseous origin. These situations are discussed in Chapter 14 in terms of their nature and the clinical approach used in their management.

TUMOR INDUCTION

Causative factors are not well defined but are believed to be related to the activation of viral oncogenes. The ability or inability of a virus to transform cultured cells is connected with its mechanism of oncogenesis. Some viruses have a single gene that is primarily responsible for the capacity to induce tumors; in some cases several oncogenes are necessary for such viral induction to take place. The action of viral oncogenesis occurs rapidly and dominates over all other activities in the cell. Other viruses lack oncogenes and induce tumors by more subtle means. The Rous virus oncogene was the first to be studied and has been termed the "src" (sarcoma) oncogene. A number of such oncogenes have been defined in human tumors. The mechanism by which they alter the amino acid components of proteins that affect cell behavior is being studied. Radiation-induced sarcomas are well defined[2] and may represent the activation of viral oncogenes by the radiation or resultant DNA damage. At times patients have described traumatic episodes thought to be associated with the initiation of sarcoma growth. Ewing[20] postulated that any traumatic relationship depends on the following factors: (1) the authenticity and adequacy of the trauma, (2) previous integrity of the wounded part, (3) a reasonable time relationship, (4) continuity of symptoms of the injury within the time of tumor appearance, (5) microscopic proof of tumor, and (6) location of tumor at the site of injury. Most of the evidence that trauma causes malignancy is circumstantial, but there are cases that do satisfy Ewing's postulates. Pack cited the case of a 34-year-old woman who was injured by a mule. The imprint of the animal's foot with an associated laceration was found on the woman's thigh. A tender subcutaneous hematoma persisted for about 2 months, after which time a small nodule was found in the scarred area. Six months after the injury, a tumor appeared, which on biopsy was found to be a myxoliposarcoma. The woman died of metastatic disease within 1 year from the time of injury.

CLINICAL PRESENTATION

The soft tissue sarcomas clinically present in a variety of ways,[3, 8, 11, 22] depending on how superficial or deep they are as they develop within the limb, chest, abdominal wall, or retroperitoneum. Cutaneous and subcutaneous lesions may be diffuse, nodular, or exophytic. Figure 1–2 demonstrates the appearance of diffuse Kaposi's sarcoma of the upper thigh, where all normal skin has been replaced by tumor. The surface of the leg is markedly keratinized and the underlying lymphatics are completely infiltrated by tumor. Here, the extremity presents with elephantiasis. The leg is not only edematous but is also markedly keratinized by the infiltrative process, which has involved cutaneous and subcutaneous planes, eventually occluding all superficial lymphatic channels. On initial examination the patient's lesions involved both legs and extended to the lower abdominal wall. Management at this stage of the disease is exceedingly difficult, and progression to the retroperitoneal nodes with further dissemination can be predicted.

Figure 1–3 shows the appearance of a superficial sarcoma arising in the head and neck area. The large nodular mass developed on the left cheek of the patient. Biopsy revealed the presence of an alveolar soft part sarcoma arising from underlying structures in the cheek. Among the original 12 cases reviewed and later updated by Lieberman,[31] only one appeared on the face, most having been found in the lower extremity.

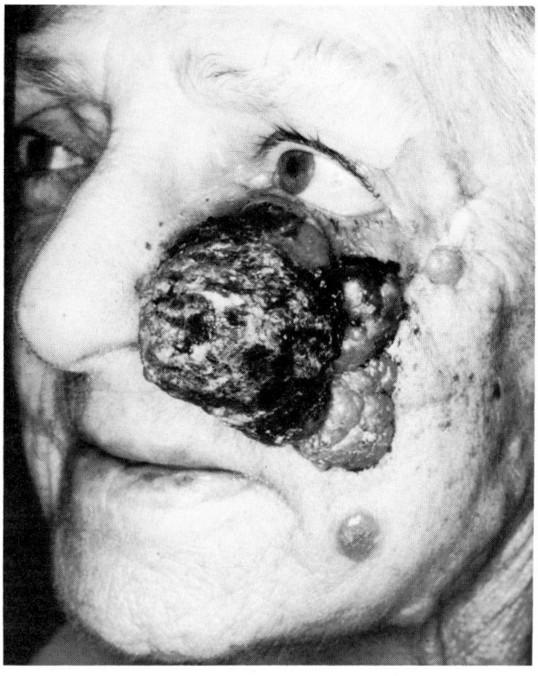

FIGURE 1–3. Alveolar soft-part sarcoma presenting as a nodular mass of the cheek.

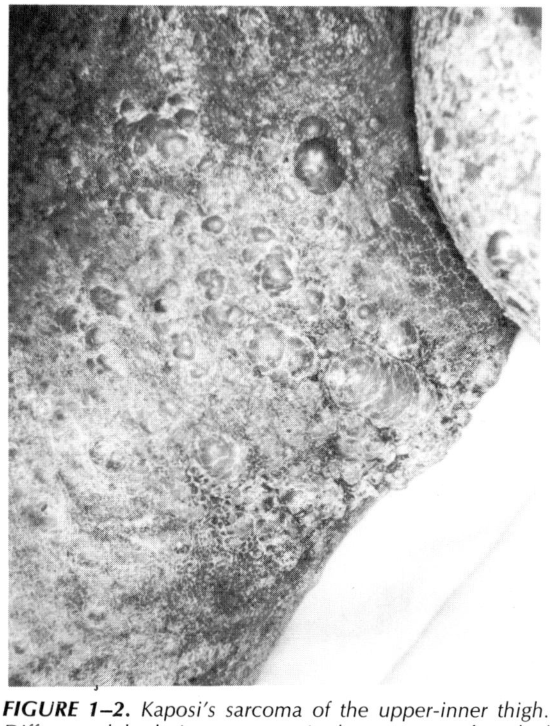

FIGURE 1–2. Kaposi's sarcoma of the upper-inner thigh. Diffuse nodular lesions are seen in the presence of marked keratosis of the skin.

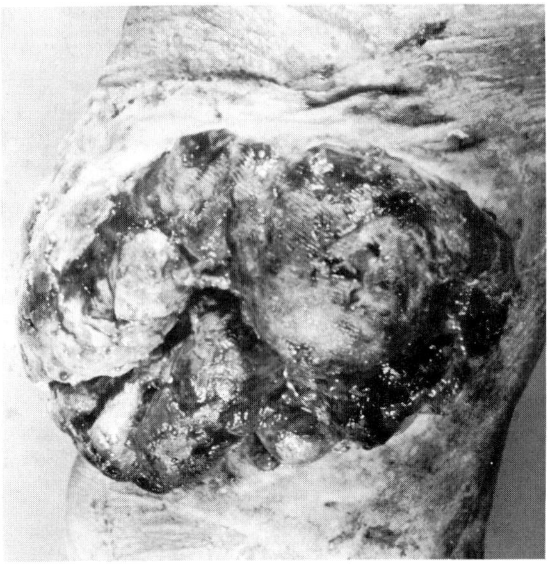

FIGURE 1–4. *Large exophytic necrotic rhabdomyosarcoma of the posterior thigh.*

Figure 1–4 shows the exophytic appearance of rhabdomyosarcoma of the posterior leg above the popliteal space. Such lesions are usually the result of the incomplete resection of masses which rapidly outgrow their blood supply, ulcerating through the skin and presenting in the later stages of the clinical course with the exophytic apearance illustrated by this case. Exophytic lesions, while not uncommon, are usually found among the more superficial tumors that are present for long periods of time, such as dermatofibrosarcoma protuberans, or in cases of rapidly growing tumors that ulcerate skin and begin to fungate.

Multiple cutaneous lesions are unusual for sarcomas and characteristically appear in only a few situations, for example, as the sequela of Recklinghausen's disease. Multiple cutaneous lesions can also be found with cutaneous angiosarcomas and the lymphangioendotheliomas. Figure 1–5*A* shows the appearance of a patient with the diffuse skin nodules, café au lait spots, and sessile polypoid lesions characteristic of cutaneous neurofibromatosis. The marked swelling in her right thigh, which was of recent onset, should make one suspicious for the malignant transformation that can be seen with a deeply seated neurofibromatous lesion. Rapid growth in a neurogenic lesion or sudden development of pain in this type of tumorous growth should lead one to consider that malignant transformation is underway or has already occurred. A biopsy of the mass proved that the patient had devel-

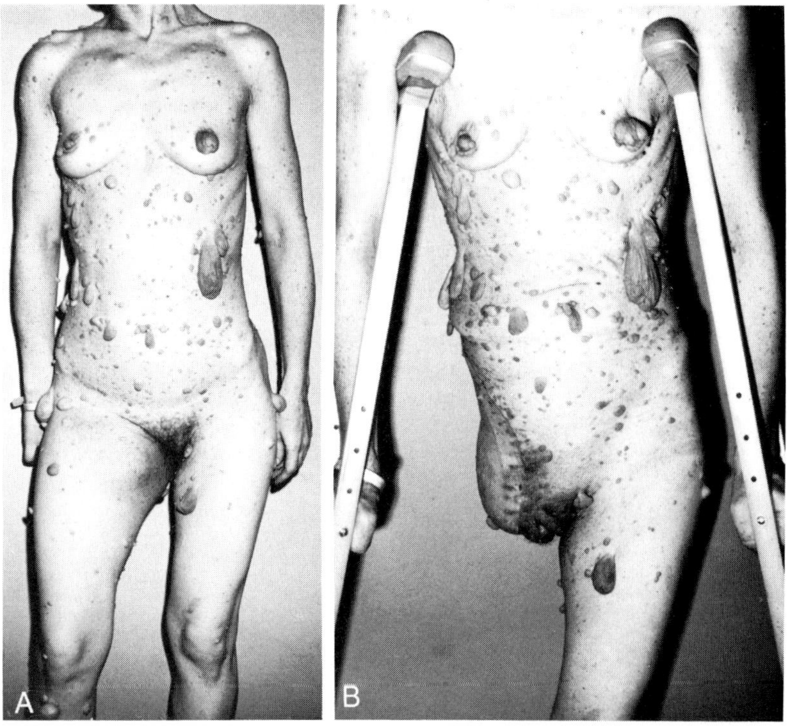

FIGURE 1–5. *Diffuse cutaneous neurofibromatosis. A, Swelling in the upper right thigh resulted from malignant transformation of one of the lesions. B, Appearance of the patient after hemipelvectomy for neurogenic sarcoma of the upper thigh.*

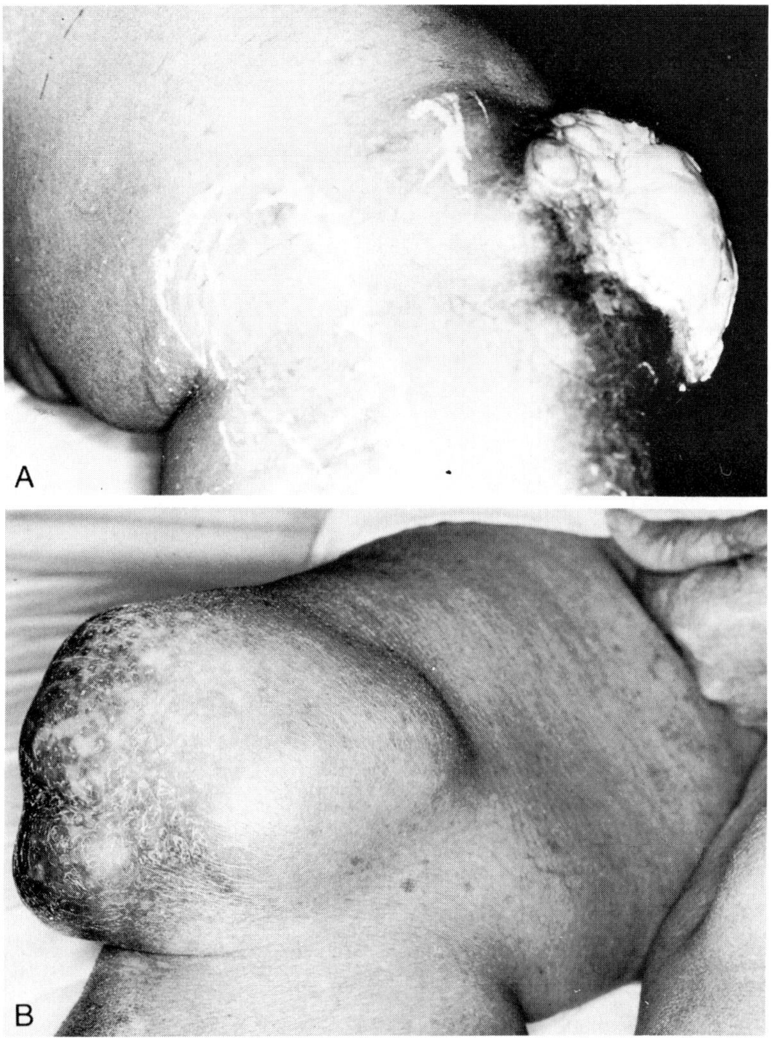

FIGURE 1–6. *A, Giant cell tumor of tendon sheath in region of the knee. B, Large cavernous hemangioma arising over the patella.*

oped a neurogenic sarcoma within the lesion. Hemipelvectomy was the only treatment that we were able to offer for control of such a malignant growth in proximity to the groin (Fig. 1–5*B*).

Large nodular masses can be seen on the extremity as a result of the growth of both benign and malignant soft tissue tumors. Figure 1–6 shows large masses near the knee, one the result of growth of a cavernous hemangioma (Fig. 1–6*B*) and another, a giant cell tumor of the tendon sheath (Fig. 1–6*A*). Hemangiomas of this type, uncommon in adults, are more frequently seen in young children. For example, an atypical, extremely large cavernous hemangioma was seen in a newborn infant (Fig. 1–7). The infant also had thrombocytopenia secondary to platelet sequestration due to the benign hemangioma: the Kasabach-Merritt syndrome.

The thrombocytopenia seen with this condition is believed to result from the intratumoral entrapment of platelets, since removal or obliteration of the lesion by surgical or radiation therapy allows the platelet count to return to normal. Warrel et al.,[44] using autologous platelets labeled with indium-111, confirmed that platelets were locally consumed within certain tumors but that when multiple lesions appeared in the same individual considerable heterogeneity existed among these lesions with respect to their platelet-trapping ability. By means of gamma camera imaging, the increase in platelet-associated radioactivity observed over time confirmed that the platelets were locally consumed in certain of the tumors

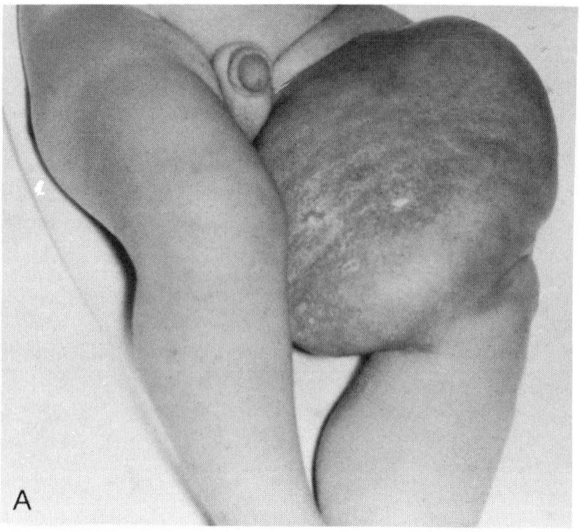

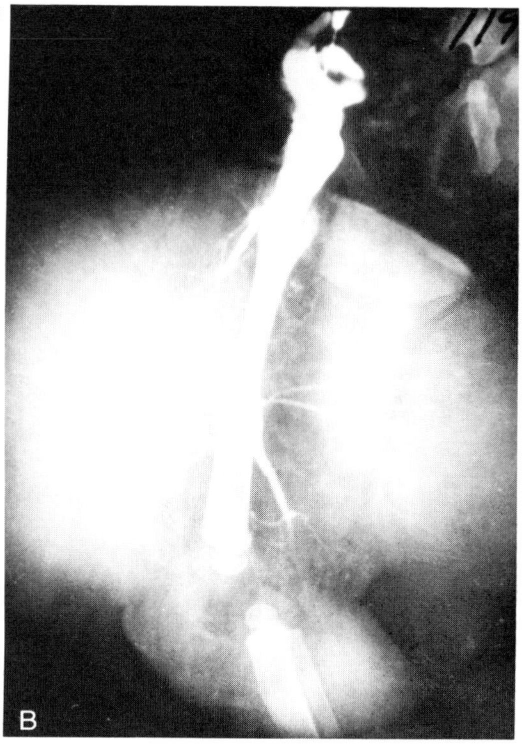

FIGURE 1–7. A, Large cavernous hemangioma of the newborn occupying the entire left thigh. B, Angiogram of the cavernous hemangioma of the thigh.

and not in others. Possible mechanisms for destruction of the platelets may be the shedding of platelet-aggregating substances from tumor cells, or the defective synthesis or release of prostaglandin I_2 (PGI_2) by the neovascular endothelium.

Among other benign tumors of the extremity, the giant cell tumor of tendon (see Fig. 1–6*B*) usually has a growth pattern that is determined by its location. When such tumors occur on the fingers and hands, they usually remain relatively small compared with an expansile growth pattern that may be seen in sites more proximal to the hip or shoulder girdle. In the lesion in Figure 1–6*A*, resection was employed for functional and cosmetic appearances.

Sometimes the largest extremity masses can be seen secondary to the development of fully malignant sarcomatous tumors that have a rapid doubling time, such as rhabdomyosarcoma arising within the superficial muscle groups of the extremity. As these tumors spread along the fascial planes, they tend to assume enormous proportions, expanding within the overlying cutaneous structures to exert pressure on the deeper musculature and vascular structures. This type of expansile tumor growth may also be seen with liposarcomas of low-grade malignancy. Figure 1–8 shows a rhabdomyosarcoma of the quadriceps developing diffuse venous collaterals as a result of deep vein

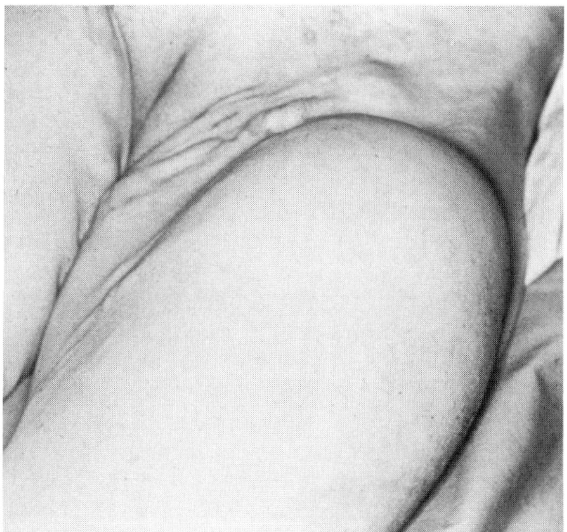

FIGURE 1–8. Large rhabdomyosarcoma of the thigh obstructing venous return, producing dilated varices in the region of the groin.

compression. This pattern of venous collateralization may be seen with any deeply placed tumor that slowly compresses points of major venous return, e.g., larger retroperitoneal sarcomas that totally obstruct the vena cava. In such instances the entire retroperitoneal venous return occurs via extensive shunting through veins in the gutters of the colon along the psoas muscle, while the return from the lower extremities is accomplished through the abdominal wall (caput medusae). The deeper the sarcoma develops within an extremity, the more difficult it becomes to define it early in its clinical course. A good rule to remember is that deeply situated tumors usually do not present as large distinct masses. Rather, such lesions are seen as poorly defined swellings similar to what may be seen in the initial growth phase of an expansile soft part rhabdomyosarcoma (Fig. 1–9*A*) or osteosarcoma (Fig. 1–9*B*) of the femur. Frequently, the patient with such a tumor has consulted the physician on several occasions with vague complaints and the presence of a questionable swelling that was initially dismissed as inconsequential, or possibly diagnosed as phlebitis. When these sarcomas arise deep within the large muscle groups of an extremity, the dimensions of the lesion are not clearly noted since the overlying structures are usually draped over the tumor, obscuring its surface features and borders. This holds true for large retroperitoneal sarcomas as well. The finding of a poorly defined swelling, therefore, is usually indicative of a deeply placed tumor and, if persistent, should be investigated.

CLASSIFICATION

Sarcomas are classified according to the tissue type from which they originate.[18, 19, 39] Table 1–1 provides a standard outline of the more frequently encountered soft part tumors. There are more extensive subclassifications but, in general, benign and malignant soft part tumors have their origin in the fibrous, tendosynovial, adipose, muscular, vascular, and peripheral nerve structures. Hajdu[24] provides a detailed classification, which represents an interpretation with regard to what he believes to be the tissue of origin of a number of more recently defined tumors. For many poorly defined sarcomas that cause confusion in terms of their histologic classification, a more thorough understanding of the antigenic make-up of membrane markers will be necessary before we fully understand the interrelationship of many of these tumors and the anatomic structures from which they are derived. Immunoperoxidase techniques are now being developed to define many of the sarcomas. The gradation of tumors is gradually becom-

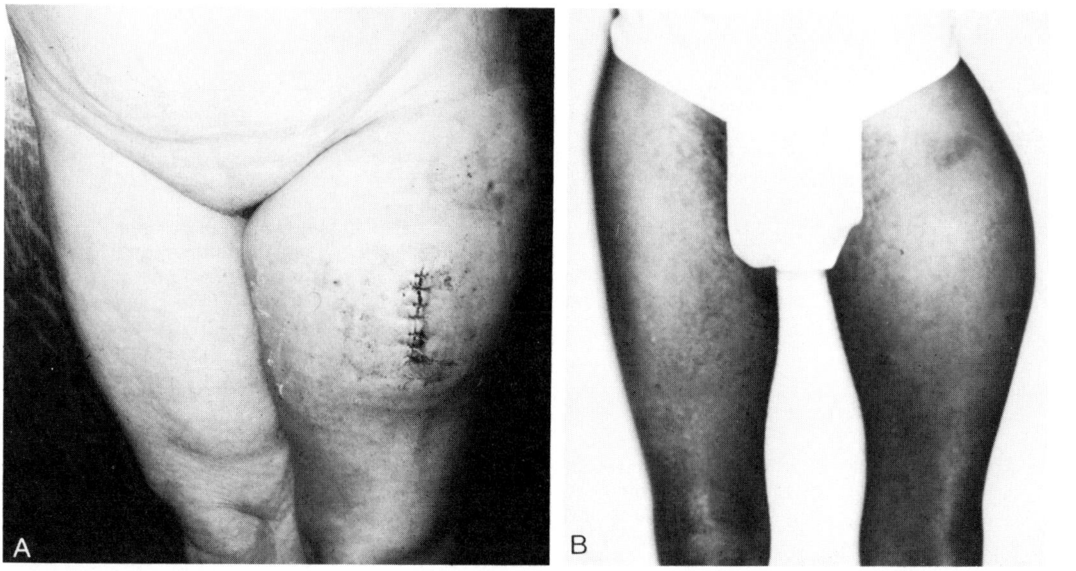

FIGURE 1–9. *A, Diffuse swelling of the thigh secondary to long-standing deeply placed rhabdomyosarcoma. B, Diffuse swelling of the thigh secondary to osteosarcoma of the femur.*

TABLE 1–1. Classification of Somatic Soft Tissue Tumors

	Benign Tumors	Malignant Tumors
Fibrous Tissue	Fibroma Keloid Dupuytren's contracture; palmar and plantar fibromatosis Peyronie's disease of penis; chronic fibrosing cavernitis Desmoid tumor of abdominal wall (desmoma) Progressive fibrosing myositis (Meyenburg's disease) Dermatofibrosarcoma protuberans	Fibrosarcoma Myxosarcoma
Undifferentiated Mesenchyme	Myxoma Mesenchymoma (hamartoma)	Myxoma Malignant mesenchymoma
Heterotopic Bone and Cartilage	Myositis ossificans	Osteogenic sarcoma Chondrosarcoma
Adipose Tissue	Lipoma (solitary and multiple) Congenital diffuse lipomatosis	Liposarcoma (well differentiated; myxoid) Pleomorphic (anaplastic)
Blood and Lymph Vessels	Hemangioma Systemic angiomatosis Rendu-Osler-Weber's disease Lymphangioma Cystic hygroma Glomus tumor Hemangiopericytoma	Angiosarcoma Lymphangiosarcoma Angioendothelioma Kaposi's idiopathic sarcoma Hemangiopericytoma
Histiocytes	Fibrous histiocytoma xanthoma Giant cell tumor (soft tissue)	Dermatofibrosarcoma protuberans; fibroxanthosarcoma Malignant fibrous histiocytoma; malignant giant cell tumor
Synovial Tissue	Giant cell tumor of tendon sheath Synovial xanthoma Hypertrophic arborescent synovitis of joints	Malignant synovioma (synovial sarcoma)
Smooth Muscle	Leiomyoma Leiomyoblastoma	Leiomyosarcoma
Striated Muscle	Rhabdomyoma	Rhabdomyosarcoma
Peripheral Nervous System		
Non-neoplastic neurectodermal tumors	Traumatic and amputation neuroma	
Peripheral nerve		
Supportive tissues	Neurilemmoma Neurofibroma Multiple neurofibromatosis (Recklinghausen's disease)	Malignant schwannoma (malignant neurilemmoma; malignant neuroepithelioma)
Secondary neoplasms		Direct invasion into nerve sheath Intraneural metastasis Tumors of ganglia lying within nerves
Sympathetic ganglia	Ganglioneuroma (differentiated)	Partly differentiated ganglioneuroma; sympathicoblastoma (neuroblastoma)
Paraganglionic cells	Pheochromocytoma Paraganglioma Carotid bodies Ganglion nodosum of vagus nerve	Malignant pheochromocytoma Malignant paraganglioma
Granular cell myoblastoma		Alveolar soft part sarcoma
Miscellaneous		

ing the task of cell biologists, who are utilizing cell sorters to determine DNA diploidy-aneuploidy patterns.

Thirteen of the more common soft tissue sarcomas have been fully evaluated by the American Joint Committee Task Force on Soft Tissue Sarcomas. Table 1–2 has served as a guide for further grading of these tumors by the degree of differentiation: G-1 represents the well-differentiated lesion; G-2, the moderately well-differentiated; and G-3, the poorly differentiated tumor. Grading is based on the degree of cellularity, cellular pleomorphism, and mitotic activity. The presence of large amounts of intercellular material, such as collagen and mucoid material, decreases the accuracy of grading. For the surgical oncologist the ability to have a tumor graded is of the utmost importance, since low-grade tumors unquestionably have a better prognosis. In such instances, while adequate surgical resection is important, greater risks in terms of limb preservation can be attempted. We do, under such circumstances, employ ancillary modalities such as hyperthermia with chemotherapy, arterial infusion, and cryosurgery to lend support to our surgical methods. With fully malignant sarcomas, proximity to bone and vessels suggests the need for more radical approaches and the possible use of adjuvant therapy before and after surgery, or the use of radiation and chemotherapy.[7, 21, 26, 36, 38, 43] A TNM classification has been proposed by the Joint Committee (Table 1–3) and has been the basis for the staging of the sarcomas. All grade I tumors are considered to represent stage I disease; grade II tumors, stage II; and grade III tumors, stage III. Subclassification A or B is based on whether the tumor is smaller (A) or larger (B) than 5 cm in diameter. Once nodes or distant metastasis is present, the lesion is automatically classified as a stage III-C tumor. We are just beginning to realize that most of the tumors

TABLE 1–2. Soft Tissue Sarcomas Evaluated by the American Joint Committee Task Force

Alveolar soft part sarcoma
Angiosarcoma
Extraskeletal chondrosarcoma
Extraskeletal osteosarcoma
Fibrosarcoma
Leiomyosarcoma
Liposarcoma
Malignant fibrohistiocytoma
Malignant mesenchymoma
Malignant schwannoma
Rhabdomyosarcoma
Synovial sarcoma

TABLE 1–3. TNM Classification and Staging of Soft Tissue Sarcoma

Primary Tumor (T)	
T_x	Minimum requirements cannot be met
T_0	No demonstrable tumor
T_1	Tumor < 5 cm in diameter
T_2	Tumor ≥ 5 cm in diameter
T_3	Tumor that grossly invades bone, major vessel, or major nerve
Nodal Involvement (N)	
N_x	Minimum requirements cannot be met
N_0	No histologically verified metastases to lymph nodes
N_1	Histologically verified regional lymph node metastases
Distant Metastasis (M)	
M_x	Not assessed
M_0	No (known) distant metastasis
M_1	Distant metastasis present
Stage Grouping	
Stage I	
IA	$G_1\ T_1\ N_0\ M_0$ Grade 1 tumor, < 5 cm in diameter, no regional lymph node or distant metastases
IB	$G_1\ G_2\ N_0\ M_0$ Grade 1 tumor, ≥ 5 cm in diameter, no regional lymph node or distant metastases
Stage II	
IIA	$G_2\ T_1\ N_0\ M_0$ Grade 2 tumor, < 5 cm in diameter, no regional lymph node or distant metastases
IIB	$G_2\ T_2\ N_0\ M_0$ Grade 2 tumor, ≥ 5 cm in diameter, no regional lymph node or distant metastases
Stage III	
IIIA	$G_3\ T_1\ N_0\ M_0$ Grade 3 tumor, < 5 cm in diameter, no regional lymph node or distant metastases
IIIB	$G_3\ T_2\ N_0\ M_0$ Grade 3 tumor, ≥ 5 cm in diameter, no regional lymph node or distant metastases
IIIC	Any G $T_{1,2}\ N_1\ M_0$ Tumor of any histologic grade or size, (no invasion) with regional lymph node metastases but without distant metastases
Stage IV	
IVA	Any G T_3 Any N M_0 Tumor of any histologic grade of malignancy that grossly invades bone, major vessels, or major nerves, with or without regional lymph node metastases, but without distant metastases
IVB	Any G Any T Any N M_1 Tumor with distant metastases

that we are dealing with are heterogeneous in terms of cell population, and that after surgical resection, additional forms of therapy may affect residual cells in an unpredictable fashion.

PROGNOSTIC CONSIDERATIONS

The need to separate tumors by size as a means of predicting their behavior is recognized by many authors. In evaluating the treatment of lower extremity sarcomas at Memorial Hospital, Shiu compared small tumors (less than 5 cm) with the larger tumors (greater than 5 cm).[40] The large tumors had an overall survival rate of 46% compared with 63% for the smaller lesions. The grade is also an important characteristic of many types of tumors. A comparison of medullary fibrosarcoma of bone with respect to similar lesions arising primarily in soft tissue[14] found that large primary osseous tumors extending into and replacing muscle mass had a survival rate that was relatively higher if they were of low grade, when compared with the more anaplastic tumors, regardless of how small these anaplastic tumors were (Table 1–4). One of the major considerations in our approach to managing a sarcoma is based, to a degree, on its grade on biopsy.

In a review of the survival rate for lower extremity neoplasms seen at Memorial Hospital (Table 1–5), fibrosarcoma was associated with the best prognosis, with a 5-year survival rate of 70%. The experience of other investigators in the management of fibrosarcoma is summarized in Table 1–6. In the Memorial series, surprisingly, malignant schwannoma had a 63% survival followed by liposarcoma, with a survival of 56% at 5 years. Grading in this particular study had not been taken into consideration. Survival among the 1215 cases reviewed by the Joint Committee Task Force on Soft Tissue Sarcoma is summarized in Table 1–7. Here, the difference between stage I and stage IV sarcomas is quite obvious, with stage I having a 75% overall survival compared with 29% for the more anaplastic lesions. It has been noted by most investigators that low-grade fibrosarcomas have a better survival (65%) when compared with liposarcoma (57%).

TABLE 1–4. Histologic Differentiation of Medullary Fibrosarcoma of Bone Related to Survival

	No. of Cases	No. of Survivors at 5 Yr with No Evidence of Disease	Per Cent Survivors at 5 Yr with No Evidence of Disease
Low-grade tumors*	2	2†	100
Intermediate tumors	12	4	33
Anaplastic tumors	12	2	19
TOTAL	26*	8*	31

*Not included: one patient with low-grade tumor, alive, free of disease for 4 years at the time of this study.

†One patient dead of disease at 8 years.

RADIOLOGIC EVALUATION

Whereas plain roentgenograms are quite limited in their ability to evaluate soft tissue lesions, in selected instances they can be of value in demonstrating the presence of fat

TABLE 1–5. Distribution and Survival of Lower Extremity Sarcomas, 1949–1968 (Memorial Sloan-Kettering Cancer Center)

	Thigh	Leg	Foot	5-Yr Survival Rate (%)
Liposarcoma	67	14	1	56
Fibrosarcoma	37	23	—	70
Rhabdomyosarcoma	39	12	1	48
Synovial sarcoma	28	5	9	45
Malignant schwannoma	14	2	—	63
Leiomyosarcoma	7	—	—	(3/7)
Angiosarcoma	6	—	—	(2/6)
Undifferentiated sarcoma	13	4	4	57
Miscellaneous sarcomas	10	—	1	45
TOTAL	221	60	16	55

TABLE 1–6. Review of Studies on Medullary Fibrosarcoma of Bone

	Local Recurrences (%)	Distant Metastases (%)	Lymph Node Metastases (%)	5 Yr Survival (%)
Stout (1948)	60	8	—	—
Ivins et al. (1950)	—	—	6	38
Pack and Ariel (1952)	56	21	5.1	59
Brindley et al. (1955)	49	—	—	63
Mackenzie (1964)	68	47	—	54
Vanderwerf (1965)	55	—	8.6	57

and calcium deposits. The radiographic density of the tumor being studied depends on the effective atomic number, thickness, geometric density, and quality of radiation employed. The ability to attenuate radiation occurs to the maximum degree in bone, followed by water and soft tissue, fat, and finally air. While relatively low kilovoltages are useful in soft tissue imaging, bone is poorly visualized. Fine-grained film should be employed when attempting to get high-resolution anatomic detail.

With angiographic imaging a high level of confidence is possible in differentiating benign from malignant tumors. Contrast between hypovascular inflammatory masses and malignancies may be more difficult. A differential response of normal and tumor

TABLE 1–7. Histologic Types of Lower Extremity Sarcomas

	All Stages	Stage I	Stage II	Stage III	Stage IV
All Types*					
No. of cases	1215	177	86	329	110
Survival rate† (%)	41	75	(55)	29	7
Fibrosarcoma					
No. of cases	231	65	15	36	12
Survival rate (%)	48	(73)	5/15	(43)	1/12
Malignant Fibrohistiocytoma					
No. of cases	128	15	29	45	7
Survival rate (%)	46	11/13	(72)	(22)	1/7
Liposarcoma					
No. of cases	221	57	18	48	13
Survival rate (%)	55	(78)	10/17	(35)	0/12
Angiosarcoma					
No. of cases	33	2	2	9	4
Survival rate (%)	24	2/2	1/2	0/9	1/4
Synovial Sarcoma					
No. of cases	84	5	6	25	6
Survival rate (%)	(43)	4/5	4/6	(16)	2/5
Rhabdomyosarcoma					
No. of cases	234	1	0	97	35
Survival rate (%)	23	0/1	0/0	(30)	0
Leiomyosarcoma					
No. of cases	79	14	5	12	11
Survival rate (%)	(32)	8/14	1/5	3/11	1/11
Malignant Schwannoma					
No. of cases	60	11	7	7	1
Survival rate (%)	(45)	8/10	1/6	—	0/1
Unclassified					
No. of cases	121	4	4	41	18
Survival rate (%)	36	4/4	2/4	(31)	0/17

*There were 24 cases of nine other types, each of which occurred too infrequently to warrant a separate listing. The specific diagnoses for these types were as follows: extraskeletal osteosarcoma (6 cases), alveolar soft part sarcoma (5), extraskeletal chondrosarcoma (4), malignant mesenchymoma (4), malignant embryonal mesenchymal tumor (1), epithelioid sarcoma (1), fibrosarcoma with areas of chondrosarcoma (1), mesothelioma (1), and malignant hemangiopericytoma.

†Rates in parentheses have standard errors between 5% and 10%. When there were too few cases to calculate a reliable rate, a fraction is given with respect to the status of the group at the end of the 5 years. The numerator equals the denominator (the total number of cases in the group) minus losses to follow-up and/or patients diagnosed too recently to be observed for 5 years.

vessels is noted after injection of agents such as epinephrine into the major vessels supplying the tumor. Subtraction angiography clearly allows better delineation of angiographic detail where soft tissue lesions are partially calcified or where skeletal structures obscure the area of interest. The bridging of intramuscular compartments on angiography suggests malignancy.

Tumors that appear radiolucent because of fat content include lipomas, hematomas, and teratomas. Only well-differentiated liposarcomas have sufficient fat to be identified as such radiographically. The interface between a benign tumor and adjacent subcutaneous or intramuscular fat may be displaced but is characteristically preserved. Distortion at the interface suggests proximity to the tumor and, in the case of malignancy, is generally associated with blurring.

Smooth subperiosteal surface resorption near a tumor without reactive bone formation is suggestive, but not diagnostic, of malignancy. Irregular cortical destruction with adjacent permeated lytic zones is more indicative of malignancy. We routinely employ computed tomography (CT) for any sizable lesion more than 5 cm in diameter. Additional details may be noted with the use of magnetic resonance imaging (MRI). Figure 1–10*A* illustrates a large lipomatous tumor of the right thigh. MRI T1 weighted images show fatty tumors as whitish images (Fig. 1–10*B* and *C*). The fine trabeculation within the stroma suggests low-grade malignancy.

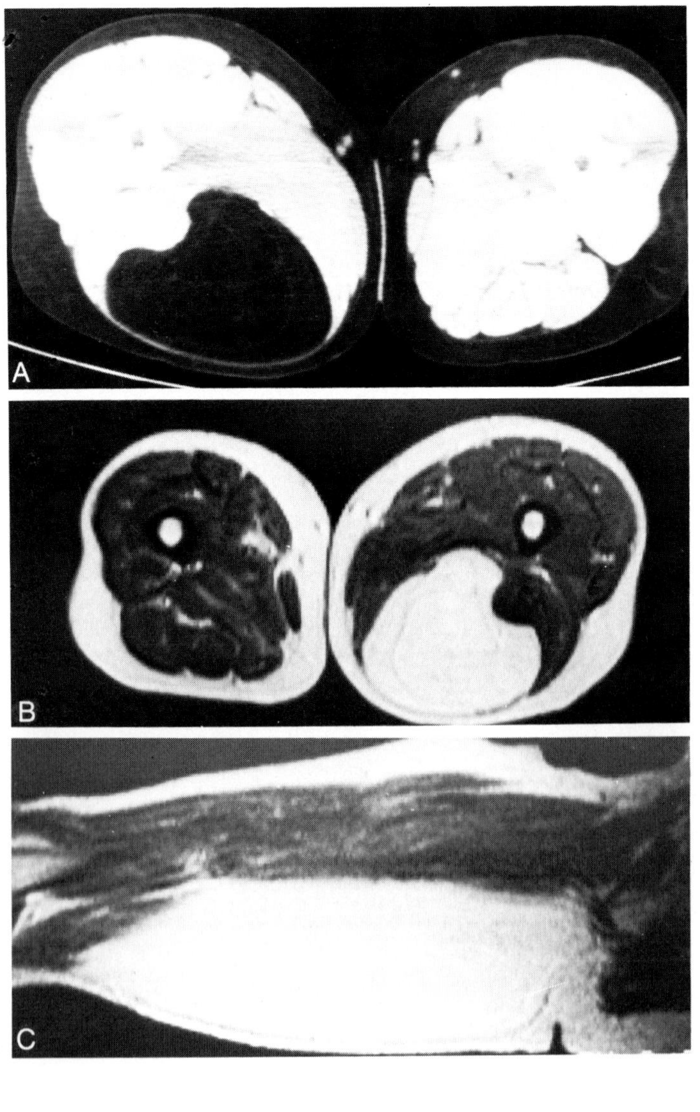

FIGURE 1–10. *A, CT scan of the thigh showing a large tumor of the posterior thigh. The radiolucent appearance suggested a primary lipomatous tumor, probably low-grade liposarcoma. B, MRI appearance of the same lesion. C, Longitudinal view of the lipomatous tumor with MRI.*

TABLE 1–8. Distribution of the More Common Sarcomas

	Shoulder	*Abdomen*	*Chest*	*Back*	*Head and Neck*	*Arm*	*Thigh, Buttock, and Groin*	*Leg*	*Hands*	*Feet*
Dermatofibrosarcoma	15	19	17	17	11	7	20	6	—	2
Desmoid tumor	9	13	20	22	29	14	30	18	2	3
Fibrosarcoma	6	4	10	6	11	28	51	10	3	—
Fibrous histiocytoma	5	7	7	6	10	16	28	14	1	3
Liposarcoma	4	3	8	35	7	119	—	29	1	1
Pleomorphic rhabdomyosarcoma	11	6	8	5	8	9	58	10	1	2
Synovioma	11	1	—	3	5	12	49	14	10	25
Neurogenic sarcoma	2	3	9	13	17	8	21	2	1	1
Angiosarcoma	1	2	4	2	12	4	9	1	—	—

PATTERNS OF DISTRIBUTION

The soft tissue sarcomas are ubiquitous, being found in all cutaneous, subcutaneous, muscular, retroperitoneal, and visceral structures from head to foot. For instance, although synoviomas are commonly found in the feet, they may also be encountered as a primary tumor in the head and neck region. Table 1–8 summarizes the distribution of the more common sarcomas seen at Memorial Hospital. The lower extremity proved to be the most common site for most of these sarcomas, with liposarcoma the predominant lesion, followed by the fibrosarcomas and pleomorphic rhabdomyosarcomas. The liposarcomas were most frequently seen in the lower extremity but were also found, to a lesser degree, to arise from the arms, back, chest wall, and head and neck regions. For the more deeply placed noncutaneous lesions, certain characteristics helped in identifying the origin of the tumor clinically. When a tumor was found to be rapidly growing with an extensive vascular supply and potentially ulcerating through skin, then rhabdomyosarcoma was the most likely lesion. Figure 1–11 shows the appearance of a rhabdomyosarcoma developing in the groin of a 20-year-old man. The lesion began to break down spontaneously and hemorrhage. The presenting mass was thought initially to represent a hematoma since it was fluctuant, highly vascular, and when drained by his local physician yielded a large quantity of blood. The tumor began to ulcerate through the skin, and on careful examination it became apparent that we were dealing with a sarcoma. The clinical diagnosis of rhabdomyosarcoma was confirmed on histologic examination of the resected tumor.

Among the relatively avascular tumors seen on angiography are the neurogenic sarcomas, fibrosarcomas, and malignant fibrous histiocytomas. Figure 1–12*A* shows the CT scan of a male patient in his forties who presented with an asymptomatic swelling in the right flank. There was no weight loss or pain. The scan showed a well-defined right lower pelvic mass sitting on the psoas muscle. Angiography showed minimal tumor vascularity (Fig. 1–12*B*). The lesion was ex-

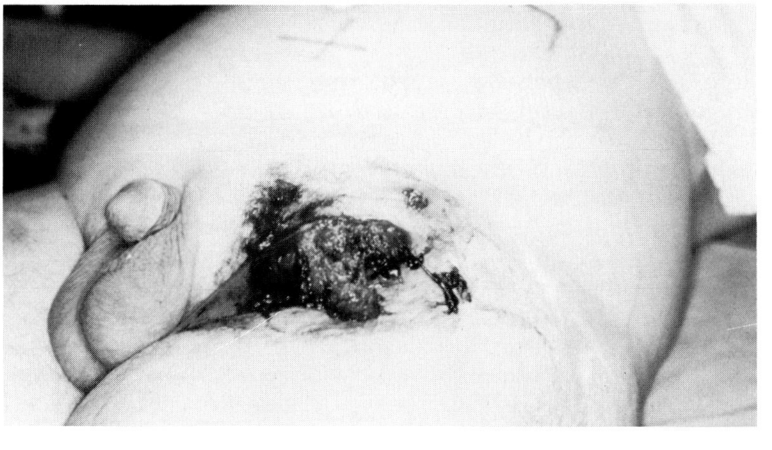

FIGURE 1–11. *Ulcerating rhabdomyosarcoma of the groin. The original appearance of the tumor was that of a hematoma.*

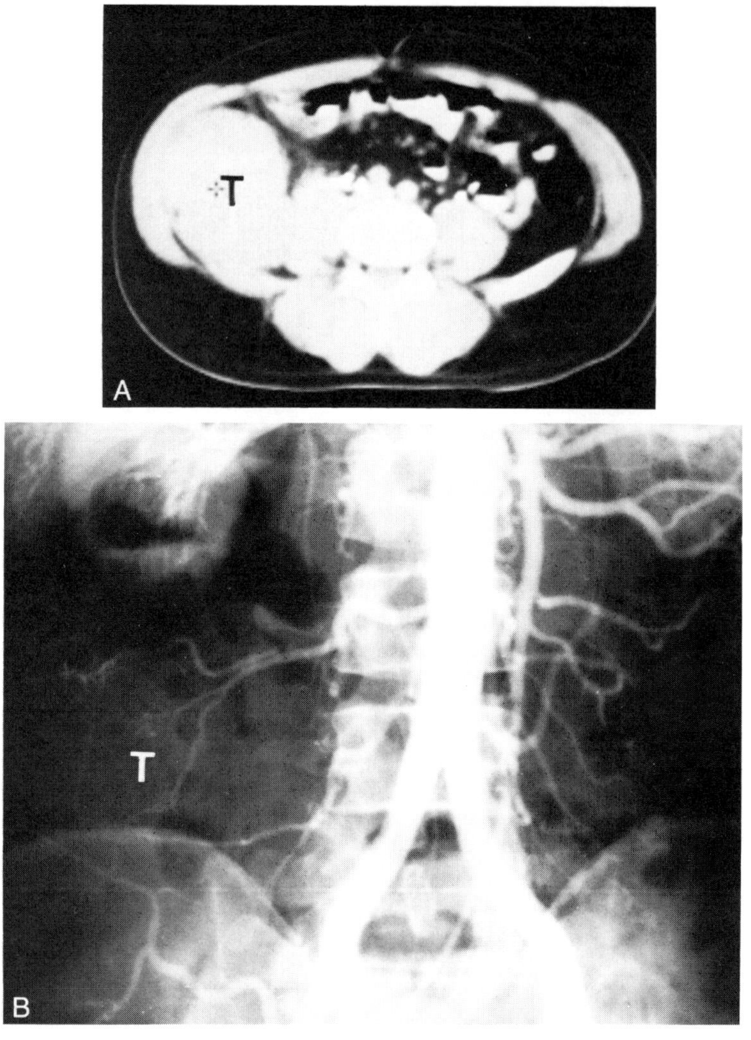

FIGURE 1–12. A, CT scan of a large flank mass (T) situated over the psoas muscle. B, Angiogram of the tumor, revealing the relatively hypovascular pattern of the lesion.

cised and clinically was believed to be a low-grade liposarcoma or myxoliposarcoma. Review of the slides suggested, however, that the tumor was a myxomatous presentation of malignant fibrous histiocytoma. On angiography liposarcomas tend to be moderately vascular and may have a relatively large fatty component surrounding them. Many of these tumors parasitize the local blood supply from surrounding vascular structures, particularly in the retroperitoneum, where the mesentery and renal vessels may lead to a major source of their blood supply. Clinically, the lipogenic variety of liposarcoma may be difficult to distinguish from the benign lipoma. We are all familiar with the possible variations in the appearance of sarcomas and still tend to call the small innocuous lesion benign. The CT scan in Figure 1–13 shows a small nontender subcutaneous lesion in the posterior upper thigh adjacent to buttock, clinically thought to represent a lipoma. When the scan suggested a denser lesion, we considered that it might be a benign schwannoma. Biopsy proved it to be an intermediate-grade liposarcoma, but it just as well could have been a malignant fibrous histiocytoma or subcutaneous leiomyosarcoma.

Clinically the presence of fibrous nodular masses usually suggests fibrosarcoma or dermatofibrosarcoma. Figure 1–14 illustrates the appearance of a multinodular mass that developed on the patella after trauma. Clinically we thought the lesion was fibrous in origin, possibly dermatofibrosarcoma protuberans. A diagnosis of a fibrous tumor was entertained on biopsy. The lesion was so

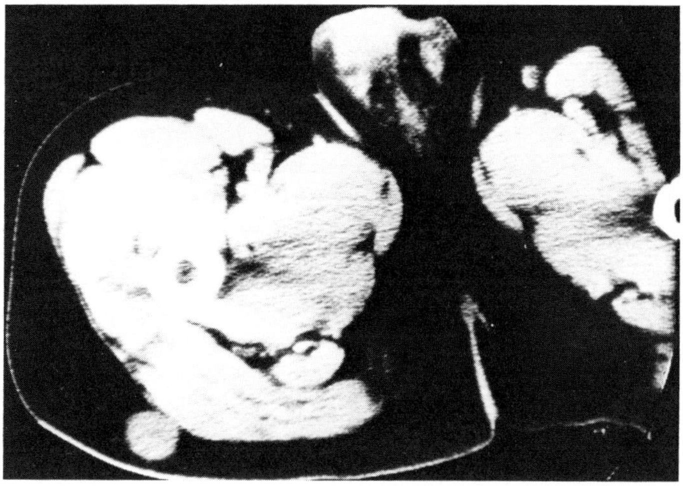

FIGURE 1–13. *Small nodular subcutaneous mass at the junction of the buttock and upper thigh that proved to be an intermediate-grade liposarcoma on histologic examination.*

low grade on microscopic examination that the initial interpretation of malignancy was questioned. In addition to the lesion on the knee, there was a small cluster of nodes in the groin which was biopsied at this time. Microscopic examination of the nodes revealed metastasis from an anaplastic tumor. On the basis of this finding, a groin dissection en-bloc with the patella was performed. A graft was applied to the area about the knee. Two months later the graft site was replaced with recurrent nodular lesions, which were biopsied and proved to be malignant melanoma. In essence, we were dealing with the fibroblastic phase of malignant melanoma, which we have encountered on several occasions on the lower extremity and in the head and neck region.

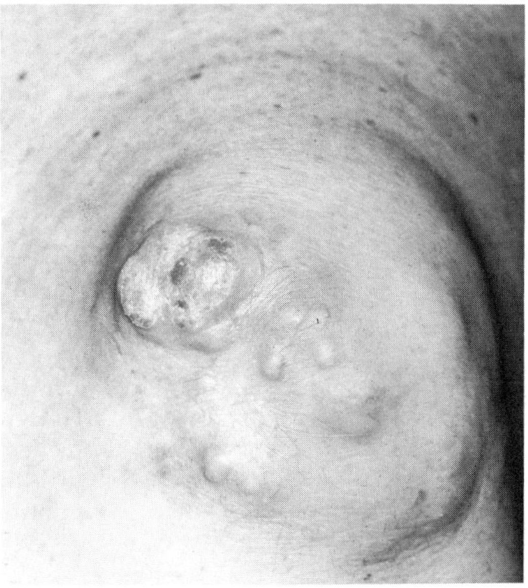

FIGURE 1–14. *Multinodular lesion of the patella which clinically appeared after trauma and was thought to be dermatofibrosarcoma. This fibrous lesion recurred and proved to be the fibrous phase of malignant melanoma.*

In a review of sarcomas by Krementz and Muchmore[29] at Charity Hospital, the lower limb, as anticipated, represented the most frequent site of sarcoma development (35%), followed by the trunk (18%), upper extremity (15%), head and neck (12.5%), and abdomen and pelvis (10.5%). Table 1–9 shows the relative type and distribution of sarcomas (extremity, nonextremity) that were encountered in the series from Charity Hospital.

The majority of tumors that we have seen arising from the supportive structures of the

TABLE 1–9. Distribution of Sarcomas at Charity Hospital, 1948–1980

		Location	
	No. of Patients	EXTREMITY	NON-EXTREMITY
Fibrosarcoma	60	34	26
Synovial sarcoma	22	19	3
Liposarcoma	57	35	22
Rhabdomyosarcoma	40	16	24
Leiomyosarcoma	36	10	26
Mesenchymoma	4	2	2
Hemangiosarcoma	26	8	18
Neurofibrosarcoma	34	13	21
Dermatofibrosarcoma protuberans	33	10	23
Kaposi's sarcoma	35	30	5
Sarcoma (miscellaneous)	53	29	24

extremities are usually benign, as most of the subcutaneous nodular masses that the patients present with are small lipomas or fibromas. In the case of tumors larger than 5 cm, the majority have the potential for being sarcomatous. In such instances muscle group dissection should be performed. Figure 1–15 illustrates the approach to be used in widely resecting sarcomas of the extremities. These principles will be covered in detail in later chapters.

For tumors arising in the retroperitoneal region, the rule to be followed is that a tumor mass is malignant until proven otherwise. In a review of several series appearing in the literature, it was noted that 75 to 85% of the retroperitoneal tumors were malignant (Table 1–10). While lymphomas, including lymphosarcomas, are the most frequent retroperitoneal tumors, the fibrosarcomas, followed by liposarcomas, are the next most commonly encountered lesions. In general, the pathologic evaluation of sarcomas has become more sophisticated, suggesting that the classification of unusual lesions made by many pathology services over the previous decade should be reviewed and reanalyzed.

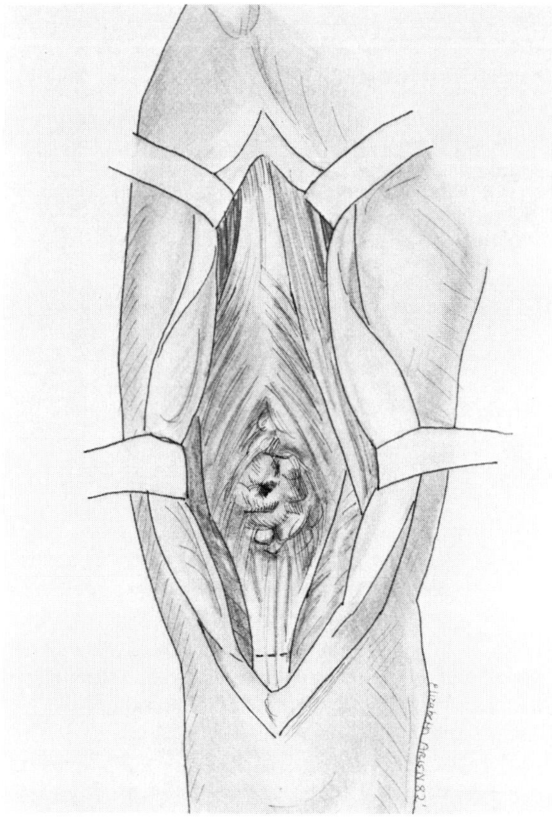

FIGURE 1–15. Schematic representation of the classic approach to sarcoma of the extremity by means of muscle group dissection.

BIOCHEMICAL EVALUATION

A number of tumors still defy proper assessment and require additional analytical modalities for clarification. A better understanding of the biochemical behavior of these tumors can offer assistance in clarifying the type of malignancy under study as well as indicate something of their potential behavior. Newer immunologic and enzymatic techniques are being introduced so that more precise diagnosis of the mesenchymal tumors can be made. The preparation of antisera for specific cell types such as muscle, associated with the introduction of fluorescein labeling, has made it possible to demonstrate the presence of actinomycin in leiomyosarcoma and myosin in embryonal rhabdomyosarcoma.[1] Enzyme studies of biopsies of Kaposi's sarcoma have demonstrated the presence of acid phosphatase and ATPase and the absence of alkaline phosphatase in the spindle cells from the tumor, distinguishing its cellular components from those of endothelial cells. The analysis of substances secreted from the surface of the tumors[45] has provided data on chemohistologic properties useful in describing specific characteristics of the sarcomas.[15–17] Mucosubstances shown to be sensitive to hyaluronidase have been demonstrated in myxoid liposarcoma, whereas extraskeletal myxoid chondrosarcoma has been found to have hyaluronidase-resistant mucosubstances.[27]

The nature of calcium deposition in tissues is also important.[23, 41] When soft tissue calcification occurs with an elevated serum calcium-phosphorus ion product, the term "metastatic calcification" is employed. Amorphous calcium phosphate and calcium hydroxyapatite crystals are deposited in the tissue. Calcium deposits can also occur in lung, stomach, and kidney and appear as large periarticular soft tissue masses. Should soft tissue calcification occur in altered, necrotic, or dead tissue where serum calcium and phosphorus levels are normal, the process is called "dystrophic calcification" and is related to soft tissue injury, tissue pH, and vascular supply.

Metastatic calcification usually results with calcium-phosphorus ion products

TABLE 1–10. Retroperitoneal Tumors

	Donnelly	Newman and Pinck	Melicow	Pack and Ariel	Johnson et al.	Donhauser and Bigelow	Braasch and Mon	Das Gupta
No. of cases	91	33	162	120	72	48	101	48
Per cent benign	10	16	23	14	22	23	13	25
Per cent malignant	90	84	77	86	78	77	87	75
Lymphoma and lymphosarcoma	1	10	48	28	27	17	31	—
Fibrosarcoma	19	—	11	6	16	2	16	2
Liposarcoma	2	2	14	17	—	3	6	10
Leiomyosarcoma	—	1	15	5	1	3	2	7
Neurosarcoma	2	5	13	8	7	5	2	3
Hemangiopericytoma	—	—	1	1	—	—	—	5
Rhabdomyosarcoma	—	—	1	22	—	—	1	4
Urogenital tumors	13	1	5	1	3	1	3	—
Undifferentiated sarcoma	37	4	3	8	1	6	7	—
Undifferentiated carcinoma	7	5	10	6	1	—	6	—
Mesenchymal tumors	1	—	3	2	—	—	3	—
Mesothelial tumors	—	—	—	2	—	—	—	—
Synovial tumors	—	—	—	1	—	—	—	1
Other	—	—	—	—	—	—	11	—

greater than 70 mg/dl. Large amorphous masses are frequently present in periarticular regions. The process is rarely identified in primary hyperparathyroidism but may be seen with secondary hyperparathyroidism. While calcium deposits can be seen in patients undergoing long-term renal dialysis, it is rarely a complication of the hypercalcemia of malignancy.

The term "tumoral calcinosis" refers to the presence of large periarticular calcific masses usually characterized biochemically by hyperphosphatemia, normal serum calcium levels, and reduced fractional phosphate excretion. Other forms of calcium deposition are observed in collagen vascular disease.

Calcinosis circumscripta is characterized by small, well-defined, localized calcium deposits most commonly in the hands, particularly around the distal phalangeal tufts in scleroderma. Calcinosis universalis is the diffuse sheet-like deposition of calcium involving muscles, subcutaneous tissue, and focal planes commonly noted in dermatomyositis.

Specific enzyme determinations such as diastase have been used to separate PAS-positive glycogen in rhabdomyosarcoma from other vic-glycoles and to demonstrate particulate or needle-like PAS-positive and diastase-stable material in alveolar soft part sarcoma and Ewing's sarcoma. Mucosubstances constitute an important fraction of ground substance in the connective tissue of many sarcomas.[16, 29] Different tissues normally contain various forms of mucosubstances, and their comparable sarcomas (those arising from the various tissues) retain characteristic mucosubstances, offering another aid to diagnosis.

The term "heteroglycan" applies to all biochemically identified mucopolysaccharides. Because of the presence of sulfate groups in their molecular structure, heteroglycans are negatively charged and may be precipitated by cationic dyes. Separation is achieved by "critical electrolyte concentration (CEC)," which is defined as the salt concentration needed to dissolve the heteroglycan into solution. By means of this technique, it has been shown that intramuscular myxomas and myxoid liposarcomas showed a CEC that indicated the presence of hyaluronic acid. Extraskeletal chondrosarcomas and chondroid lesions have shown a pattern similar to that of moderately differentiated chondrosarcomas, clarifying that these soft part lesions are closely related to their osseous counterparts. Chordomas, on the other hand, have histochemical patterns of notochordal remnants. Hyaluronic acid, but not sulfated mucosubstances, can be demonstrated in myxoid liposarcoma and may be used for differentiation of this lesion from soft tissue myxoid chondrosarcoma.

BEHAVIOR RELATED TO CHEMICAL RESPONSE

In attempting to understand the behavior of sarcomas[34] and their influence on host reactivity, there has been increasing evidence showing the existence of effective immunity aimed at escaping surface antigens. Moore's studies have provided additional evidence of an anti-inflammatory effect found in progressive tumor growth reflected by a reduction in the histamine-forming enzyme activity of the growing "SV-40 virus-induced and transplanted syngeneic nonmetastasizing fibrosarcoma" in hamsters. When repeated intratumor injections of bradykinin were given, histamine levels increased out of proportion to levels expected for comparably sized growing tumors. In this group of bradykinin-injected animals, significantly greater tumor growth inhibition was found.

A preoperative clinical appraisal of fatty soft part sarcomas may be possible with radionuclide imaging. Chew et al.[10] reported that this technique demonstrated disparate scintigraphic characteristics. Soft tissue technetium radionuclide accumulation in 2 of 13 lipomas corresponded to radiographically evident calcification. All liposarcomas that were studied were uncalcified and demonstrated intense radionuclide activity.

Steroid receptors have been evaluated in a diverse group of human sarcomas. Cytosol receptors were measured for androgens, estrogens, glucocorticoid, and progesterone.[9] Nineteen of 26 lesions (66%) were found to have at least one steroid present on the cell surface. Density gradient analysis suggested that androgen and estrogen receptors were located predominantly in the 6S and 7-8S regions; glucocorticoid receptors sedimented in the 8S region. The existence of estrogen receptors may have some correlation with the clinical observation that women have a better prognosis for most soft part sarcomas, with any improvement inversely proportional to menopausal status. Benign metastasizing leiomyomas and desmoids[28, 30] also seem to be affected by hormones: regression has been observed following administration of various hormonal agents. A significant correlation between receptor distribution and the histology of the sarcoma was demonstrated by the complete absence of estrogen receptors in fully malignant fibrous tumors compared with the high incidence of these receptors in adipose tissue tumors.[9]

The potential stimulation of certain fibrous tumors by hormones is seen in the desmoid tumor and the benign metastasizing leiomyoma.[5, 12] The predilection for desmoid tumors in women of childbearing age suggests the possibility of their control by hormone manipulation. Kinzbrunner[28] reported a case of a 29-year-old woman with Gardner's syndrome and multiple recurrent painful desmoids complicated by metastatic adenocarcinoma of the colon. Antiestrogens were given, 20 mg four times a day. By the second week of therapy there was symptomatic relief of pain and regression of the desmoid lesions. The association of desmoids with Gardner's syndrome is well known. McAdam and Goligher[32a] reviewed 89 cases in which this association was identified. Forty-four had abdominal lesions, 26 extra-abdominal, and 19 the combination. Experimental production of such tumors has been described. It has been possible to induce these tumors in animals implanted with high-dose estrogen pellets and to suppress tumor formation by the addition of the 9-α-fluoro derivative of progesterone.

In certain tumor systems an association with hypoglycemia can be defined. This hypoglycemia may represent the predominant symptomatology defining the clinical course of disease and the major problem that must be dealt with aside from the possibility of tumor resection, should such be possible. The existence of the hypoglycemia must, therefore, be part of the therapeutic evaluation and possible treatment.[4] Crocker and Veith[13] have reviewed the problems of mesodermal tumors associated with hypoglycemia. In one series with nonpancreatic tumors, four patients were reported to have such symptoms. Two had pleural mesotheliomas, one had primary fibrosarcoma of the liver, and one had pheochromocytoma metastatic to the liver. Concomitant hypoglycemia is well recognized, especially with large sarcomas. Four mechanisms for this syndrome have been proposed: there is (1) insulin or insulin-like activity produced by the tumor; (2) decreased neogluconeogenesis; (3) disruption of glucagon metabolism; or (4) increased utilization of glucose by the tumor.[25]

Insulin-like substances have been described in a variety of tumors.[32, 33] Radioimmunoassays have shown that in addition to the presence of insulin, an insulin-like peptide called "nonsuppressible insulin-like activity" (NSILA) may also be present in a number of the patients. Elevated concentrations of NSILA were found to be present in five of seven patients. Other instances of suppression of gluconeogenesis have been demonstrated in hepatoma, leiomyosarcoma, and mesothelioma and are generally believed to be caused by factors possibly mediated through metabolites of tryptophan. Decreased glucagon secretion resulting in reduction of gluconeogenesis has been reported by Lindakaer et al.,[32] who showed that an extract from a liver tumor composed of fibroblasts in a patient with normal insulin levels greatly decreased the secretion of glucagon in an isolated perfused porcine pancreas.

Although some mesenchymal tumors associated with hypoglycemia do not involve the liver, most do. As the liver is invaded, functioning hepatic parenchyma, and thus liver function is compromised. In dogs it has been shown that approximately 85% of the liver must be destroyed before hypoglycemia becomes apparent. For the larger tumors one must rule out production of NSILA and then consider these factors for hypoglycemia: (1) depletion of the substrate necessary for gluconeogenesis, (2) the possibility of impaired liver function when associated with parenchymal damage, and (3) increased utilization of glucose by the tumor.

Because of the improving therapeutic responses that have been attained in the treatment of certain sarcomas such as rhabdomyosarcoma, the correct diagnosis of this tumor is important.[42] Errors in reporting these neoplasms are common, with the diagnosis confirmed in only 27% of the cases referred to the Eastern Cooperative Oncology Group. With this in mind, researchers have investigated the use of tumor markers such as immunoreactive myoglobin to enhance diagnostic capabilities. An immunoperoxidase procedure was performed according to Steinberger using the chromogen of Graham and Karnofsky. Cardiac and skeletal muscle demonstrated increased staining of gross striations, and skeletal muscle demonstrated decreased staining in the periphery of muscle fibers adjacent to sarcolemma. All carcinomas tested were negative regardless of the primary lesion. Sarcomas other than rhabdomyosarcoma, such as liposarcoma, synovioma, and malignant fibrohistiocytoma, were negative. Positive reactions were elicited from 89% of rhabdomyosarcomas, as well as from tumors that contained rhabdomyosarcomatous differentiation, such as mixed müllerian tumors and in some instances neurogenic sarcoma. It appears that further development of these techniques may be extremely useful in differentiating tumors that may be difficult for the pathologist to diagnose, especially in those instances in which the tumor is largely undifferentiated.

THE SPREAD OF SARCOMAS

The majority of sarcomas spread along fascial planes, especially when arising within the extremity. Many lesions may be multifocal—e.g., epithelioid sarcoma and lymphangiosarcoma—so that wide muscle group dissection is important. This is especially true in the fully malignant (high-grade) T_3 sarcomas. Failure to achieve adequate margins of resection results in rapid local recurrence. Liposarcoma high in the thigh region, especially in proximity to the femoral triangle, can rapidly recur in the retroperitoneum, spreading along fascial planes adjacent to the psoas muscle and through the obturator membrane into the pelvis. In one patient in whom total control was achieved in the extremity, the patient became hypertensive; angiography showed renal artery stenosis and arterial repair was attempted. At the time of retroperitoneal exploration, a large retroperitoneal tumor was noted to have spread up the psoas muscle to encroach on the renal vascular supply. The lungs are also a common site for parenchymal metastasis, and the use of posteroanterior and lateral chest views is indicated routinely in follow-up examination of such patients, as well as in those who are being prepared for surgery. CT scan of the chest or tomography of the lung is a necessary preoperative procedure for large lesions. Malignant fibrous histiocytoma and synovioma frequently produce "cannonball" lesions in the lung fields. Liposarcoma, while capable of producing large metastatic foci within the lungs, can also produce multiple micronodules in the parenchyma, making resection of the lung tumor unfeasible. Liposarcoma, leiomyosarcoma, and embryonal rhabdomyosarcoma are also frequently found to metastasize to the liver. The management of such metastatic lesions is discussed in Chapter 16.

METHODS OF MANAGEMENT

The principles and techniques for resection of extremity neoplasms were clearly defined in 1958 by Bowden and Booher:[6] "Herewith submit a method of surgical treatment which is consistent with the natural behavior of these tumors, which satisfies good tenets of cancer surgery and which obviates in selected instances a loss of an extremity." These principles were described earlier by Pack and associates at Memorial Sloan-Kettering and were based on an understanding of the patterns of spread of sarcomas initially described by Ewing and Stout. In general, the concept of muscle group dissection holds true where normal tissue planes are removed around the tumor to include, in many of the larger lesions, origin and insertion of the muscles (see Fig. 1–15).

Lymph node involvement should be taken into consideration when performing muscle group dissection for tumors that have the potential for lymphatic metastasis. Under such circumstances en-bloc lymph node dissection should be performed where feasible.

The failure to cure sarcomas has been investigated by almost everyone who manages soft tissue lesions, and most have theorized that this failure should not be the result of local recurrence, which can be avoided by adequate resection or, if necessary, amputation. Essentially those tumors that fail to be controlled by proper resection are those that readily metastasize by transgressing beyond the margins of resection. For the following reasons, one cannot obtain good statistical analysis of newer modalities that have been described as adjuvant therapy in any single study: (1) the diversity of tumor populations treated, (2) the few numbers of each specific type of sarcoma seen, (3) their site of location within a given extremity, (4) the stage of the particular tumor (size, degree of undifferentiation, invasion of vessels, nerves, and bones), and (5) the fact that surgical resection was performed by physicians of different skills and experience. Morton and Eilber et al.[36] have reviewed their experience in attempting limb salvage for skeletal and soft tissue sarcomas. In a group of 183 patients, 100 had soft tissue sarcomas. All patients received identical preoperative treatment with intra-arterially administered doxorubicin (Adriamycin), 30 mg/day for three consecutive days. The catheter was then removed, and radiation therapy begun on the following day. A total dose of 3500 rad was delivered through the posteroanterior and anteroposterior parallel opposed ports, at a dose fraction of 350 rad/day over ten treatments. After 1 to 2 weeks of preoperative therapy, en-bloc resection of all gross tumor was performed. In this study there was no statistical difference in survival rates between a group of patients who had amputation and adjuvant therapy and another group treated by limb salvage and adjuvant therapy. This has been our philosophy even though we have not utilized preoperative arterial infusions. We have even gone to the extent of replacing femur when indicated at the time of muscle group resection for soft part tumors.

Local Reappearance of Disease

Cantin (see Chapter 16) investigated the problem of whether local recurrence alters prognosis following resection of primary sarcomas. In his review of Memorial Hospital data he noted that distant metastases were present on admission in 11% of patients previously untreated as well as 22% of patients with recurrent tumors. Such figures will probably be altered with the use of more sophisticated scanning devices and earlier detection due to a better understanding of the nature of soft tissue sarcomas. Between 1935 and 1959 (Memorial Hospital study), there were 187 cases of local recurrences among 653 patients treated with the objective of cure. Of the 466 patients who did not show local recurrence, 138 (30%) died of disease. In each extremity, lesions that were situated distal to the major joint (elbow, knee) recurred slightly more frequently than those lesions situated proximally. On the trunk, abdominal wall tumors were controlled less frequently than those on the thoracic wall. The highest recurrence rates occurred in those tumors near the joints. A number of studies have addressed the problem of managing advanced soft tissue sarcoma with chemotherapy and whole body hyperthermia. Thermotherapy was found to be feasible for selected patients with advanced soft tissue sarcoma and especially for the subset of liposarcomas and leiomyosarcomas.

Nodal Involvement

When performing muscle group dissection, it is often important to define the major vascular structures in proximity to the site of dissection and those blood vessels that may be sacrificed. At this time, the prime node-bearing area may be entered to define the vascular supply, and if clinical nodal disease is palpable or if there is a high likelihood of micronodal disease, then node dissection should be performed as part of the operative procedure. Kearney (see Chapter 16) found that 5 of 11 of his patients with malignant fibrous histiocytoma and clinically involved nodes had prolonged survival after the use of lymphadenectomy. Others have reported therapeutic benefits from node dissection as part of sarcoma surgery. In general, however, the presence of nodal disease is frequently accompanied by distant metastasis, obviating any benefits to resection. Russell,[39] in evaluating 1105 sarcoma cases, found only a 4% incidence of nodal disease without more distal tumor spread. The presence of nodal disease is usually equivalent to clinical stage III or IV disease. In patients with embryonal rhabdomyosarcoma, node involvement is an important part of the disease picture and an area that must be taken into consideration in offering prophylactic therapy. For this particular tumor and for patients with synoviomas there are reports of nodal involvement as high as 20%. The other tumors that are occasionally seen to metastasize to the regional nodes are the leiomyosarcoma with a 10% incidence of metastasis, fibrosarcoma with 5%, and liposarcoma with 5%. In general, the overall incidence for nodal involvement by sarcomas is quoted as approximately 8% to 10% of cases.

Neural Involvement

Another pathway for spread of sarcomas within an extremity is along the peripheral nerves. The spread of other tumors, such as carcinomas, along nerve trunks has been described and extensively reviewed. In 1905 Ernst had postulated that neural spaces served as channels for tumor metastasis. These spaces were believed to be preexistent and a mechanism whereby tumor invaded the nerve. One of the concomitant findings was a frequent degenerative effect on the medullary sheath caused by tumor growth. In 1917 Peet described a spindle cell sarcoma that completely engulfed the radial nerve. In 1936 Meyerding et al. found neural symptoms including referred pain, numbness, and partial and complete palsy secondary to peripheral neuritis resulting from pressure on nerves or actual nerve involvement. In patients with sacral chordoma, it is not unusual to find sciatic nerve root invasion by the lesion, such that decompression of the nerve by tumor removal frequently alleviates the sciatic nerve symptoms. The encroachment of peripheral nerves by tumor does not always become symptomatic. Willis, in 1952, noted that in some cases large nerve trunks pass directly through the tumor mass without becoming involved, so that they are identified throughout their course of dissection. In a review of patterns of nerve invasion by sarcoma seen at the Mayo Clinic, 30 patients were evaluated. In four instances, the nerve trunks were markedly displaced by tumor. Thirteen instances of tumor adherence to nerves were identified but in each instance the tumor was able to be separated. In 11 cases, the lesion was firmly adherent to the nerve, requiring stripping or separation. Six patients demonstrated localized nerve involvement suggestive of tumor invasion. In four instances, there was diffuse enlargement of the nerve, suggesting that the tumor had spread within the nerve itself.

It was believed that sarcomas frequently invaded peripheral nerves but that the invasion occurred mainly within the perineural connective tissue. The perineurium apparently resists invasion. Once invasion does occur, spread of tumor then develops along the tissue planes. Tumor dissected free of the major nerve trunks and roots left as part of the dissection should be treated with the possibility that recurrence will develop frequently. Only low-grade tumors—e.g., desmoids and low-grade liposarcomas—should be dissected away from the nerve tissue. Otherwise, amputation or high-dose chemotherapy plus radiation therapy should be employed to control the potential spread.

SUMMARY

Survival for sarcomas has been far from optimal. Stage I lesions have a survival rate of approximately 75%, dropping to 55% for stage II disease. Patients in clinical stage III are poor responders, with maximal survival rates of 30% and 7%, respectively. Surgery and radiation therapy have probably reached the levels of sophistication that we can anticipate in the near future. Therefore, a better understanding of immune mechanisms of tumor control and the development of more effective drug therapy are believed to be essential in our attempts to cure this type of tumor.

References

1. Archer F. L., Kao, V. C. Y.: Immunohistochemical identification of actomyosin in myoepithelium of human tissues. Lab. Invest. 18:669–674, 1968
2. Arlen M., Higinbotham N., Huvos A. G., et al.: Radiation: induced sarcoma of bone. Cancer 28:1087–1099, 1971
3. Atkinson L., Garuam J.M., Newton N.C.: Behavior and management of soft connective tissue sarcomas. Cancer 16:1552–1562, 1963
4. August J.T., Hiatt H.H.: Severe hypoglycemia secondary to a non-pancreatic fibrosarcoma with insulin activity. N. Engl. J. Med. 258:17–20, 1958
5. Banner A.S., Carrington C.B., Emory W.B., et al. Efficacy of oophorectomy in lymphangiomyomatosis and benign metastasizing leiomyoma. N. Engl. J. Med. 305:204–209, 1981
6. Bowden L., Booher R.J.: The principles and technique of resection of soft parts for sarcoma. Surgery 44:963–977, 1958
7. Brennhoud I.O.: The treatment of soft tissue sarcomas: A plea for a more urgent and aggressive approach. Acta Chir. Scand. 131:438–442, 1966
8. Cade S.: Soft tissue tumors and their natural history and treatment. Proc. Roy. Soc. Med. 44:19–36, 1951
9. Chaudhuri P.K., Wilson M.J., Beatti C.W.: Presence of steroid receptors in human soft tissue sarcomas of diverse histologic origin. Cancer Res. 40:861–865, 1980
10. Chew F.S., et al.: Radionuclide imaging of lipoma and liposarcoma. Radiology 136:741–745, 1980
11. Clark R.L., Martin R.G., White E.C., Old J.W.: Clinical aspects of soft tissue tumors. Arch. Surg. 74:859–870, 1957
12. Cramer S.F., Meyer J.S., Kraner J.F., et al.: Metastasizing leiomyoma of the uterus: S-phase fraction, estrogen receptor and ultrastructure. Cancer 45:932–937, 1980
13. Crocker D.W., Veith F.: Mesodermal tumors associated with hypoglycemia: Review of literature and report of a case. Ann. Surg. 161:418, 1965
14. Cunningham M.P., Arlen M.: Medullary fibrosarcoma of bone. Cancer 21:31–37, 1968
15. Dempsey E.W., Bunting J., Singer M., Wislock G.B.: The dye-binding capacity and other chemohistological properties of mammalian mucopolysaccharides. Anat. Rec. 98:417–429, 1947
16. Dobrogorski O.J., Braunstein H.: Histochemical study of staining lipid, glycogen and mucin in human neoplasms. Am. J. Clin. Pathol. 40:435–443, 1963
17. Dorfman A.: Polysaccharides of connective tissue. J. Histochem. Cytochem. 11:2–13, 1963
18. Enterline H.T.: Histopathology of sarcoma. Semin. Oncol. 8:133–155, 1981
19. Enzinger F.M., Lattes R., Torloni H.: Histologic Typing of Soft Tissue Tumors. International Histologic Classification of Tumors, No. 3, Geneva, WHO, 1969
20. Ewing J.: Neoplastic Diseases. 4th ed. Philadelphia, W.B. Saunders, 1940
21. Exelby P. R.: Soft Part Sarcomas in Children—1972. Seventh National Conference Proceedings. Philadelphia, J.B. Lippincott Co., 1973, pp. 619–625
22. Fine C., Horn R.D.: Soft tissue tumors: Aids in differential diagnosis. Pathol. Annu. 4:227, 1967
23. Goldman A.B.: Myositis ossificans circumscripta: A benign lesion with a malignant differential diagnosis. A.J.R. 126:32–40, 1976
24. Hadju S.I.: Pathology of Soft Tissue Tumors. Philadelphia, Lea & Febiger, 1979
25. Immerman S.C., Sener S.F., Khandekar J.D.: Causes and evaluation of tumor-induced hypoglycemia. Arch. Surg. 117:905–908, 1982
26. Kilman J.W., Clatworthy H.W., Jr., Newton W.A., Jr., Grosfeld J.L.: Reasonable surgery for rhabdomyosarcoma: A study of 67 cases. Ann. Surg. 178:346–351, 1973
27. Kindblom L.G., Angervall L.: Histochemical characterization of mucosubstances in bone and soft tissue tumors. Cancer 36:985–994, 1975
28. Kinzbrunner B., Ritter S., Domingo J., Rosenthal C.J.: Remission of rapidly growing desmoid tumors after tamoxifen therapy. Cancer 52:2201–2204, 1983
29. Krementz E.T., Muchmore, J.H.: Soft tissue sarcomas: Behavior and management. Adv. Surg. 16:147–196, 1983
30. Lanari A.: Effect of progesterone on desmoid tumors. N. Engl. J. Med. 309:1523, 1983
31. Lieberman P.H., Foote F.W., Stewart F.W., Berg J.W.: Alveolar soft part sarcoma. J.A.M.A. 198: 121–125, 1966
32. Lindakaer S., Kuhl C., Lauritsen K.B., et al.: Mesenchymal tumor hypoglycemia: The effect of a tumor tissue extract on the insulin and glucagon secretion from the isolated perfused porcine pancreas. Am. J. Surg. 135:192–195, 1978

32a. McAdam W.A., Goligher J.C.: The occurrence of desmoids in patients with familial polyposis coli. Br. J. Surg. 57:618–631, 1970

33. Millard P.R., Jerrome D.W., Millard-Sadler G.H.: Spindle cell tumors and hypoglycemia. J. Clin. Pathol. 20:520–529, 1976
34. Moore T.C., Koppelmann L.E., Lemmi C.A.E.: Decreases in histamine-forming enzyme activity of non-metastasizing fibrosarcomas in hamsters with progressive tumor growth. Ann. Surg. 188:175–180, 1978
35. Morgan R.T., Quinn L.A., Moore G.E., et al.: A human liposarcoma cell time producing hyaluronic acid. Cancer 45:1400–1407, 1980
36. Morton D.L., Eilber F.R., Townsend C.M., et al.: Limb salvage from a multidisciplinary treatment approach for skeletal and soft tissue sarcomas of the extremity. Ann. Surg. 184:268–278, 1976
37. Prat J., Woodruff J.M., Marcove R.C.: Epithelioid sarcoma. Cancer 41:1472–1487, 1978
38. Rosenberg S.A., Kent H., Costa J.: Prospective randomized evaluation of the role of limb-sparing surgery, radiation therapy and adjuvant chemo-

immunotherapy in the treatment of adult soft tissue sarcoma. Surgery 84:62–69, 1978
39. Russel W.O., Cohen J., Enzinger F., et al.: A clinical and pathological staging system for soft tissue sarcomas. Cancer 40:1562–1570, 1977
40. Shiu M.H., Casteo E.B., Hadju S.I., et al.: Surgical treatment of 247 soft tissue sarcomas of the lower extremity. Ann. Surg. 182:597–602, 1975
41. Stewart V.L., Herling, P., Dalinka M.K.: Calcification in soft tissues. J.A.M.A. 250:73–81, 1983
42. Suit H.D., Fussell W.O., Martin R.G.: Sarcoma of soft tissue: Clinical and histopathological parameters and response to treatment. Cancer 35:1478–1483, 1975
43. Suit H.D., Proppe K.H., Mankin H.J., Wood W.C.: Preoperative radiation therapy for sarcoma of soft tissue. Cancer 47:2269–2274, 1981
44. Warrel R.P., Jr., Kempin S.J., Benua R.S., et al.: Intratumoral consumption of indium-111-labelled platelets in a patient with hemangiomatosis and intravascular coagulation (Kasabach-Merritt syndrome). Cancer 52:2256–2260, 1983
45. Wood W.C., Morton D.L.: Host immune response to common cell surface antigen in human sarcoma. N. Engl. J. Med. 284:569, 1971

CHAPTER 2

Sarcomas of the Head and Neck

GENERAL PRINCIPLES

Sarcomas of the head and neck are uncommon and represent only a small percentage of tumors arising in this area. As with the epithelial tumors of head and neck origin, the sites for development of sarcomatous lesions are the face, orbit, and paranasal sinuses. Most of the sarcomas that are encountered here do not have characteristic ulcerating lesions that one commonly sees with carcinomas of the floor of the mouth or the tongue, a feature that might characterize them as epithelial. Rather, when these particular tumors are discovered, one should be able to identify them as nonepithelial in origin.

When these tumors are finally identified histologically, some modifications are required in those principles that are usually employed in treating sarcomas elsewhere in the body. These techniques can be incorporated into the operative procedures that are considered standard for head and neck tumors. The surgery for sarcomas of head and neck origin entails resection of surrounding muscle and fascial structures in combination with operations such as maxillectomy, the commando resection, and radical neck dissection. The concept of muscle group dissection, however, continues to be predominant, as most of these lesions do begin within the muscular or fascial structures of the face and neck.

Eighty percent of the neoplasms that normally arise in the head and neck are usually squamous (epithelial) in origin, with lymphoma occurring next in frequency. Soft part sarcomas are relegated to the small remaining group of lesions that may occasionally be encountered. Most reports are limited by the number of cases, and many of the reviews are necessarily cumulative studies that span a long interval of time. During a period of 28 years (1949 to 1977) Memorial Sloan-Kettering Cancer Center admitted 285 patients who were treated for various sarcomatous lesions arising in the head and neck. This represents one of the larger series available for evaluation. The determinate group contained 242 patients who were followed for 5 years.[13] This group is relatively large when compared with other reports and essentially represents a referral pattern to specialty institutions. At M.D. Anderson Hospital, from a group of 449 patients with sarcomas noted at all sites in the body, only 70 patients (15%) had representative lesions arising in the head and neck (Table 2–1).[29] The distribution of tumors in this report from M.D. Anderson is typical of the pattern observed for most sarcomas arising in the head and neck region.

CLINICAL PRESENTATION

Most of the tumors that have been reported have presented as innocuous nodular lesions free from underlying structures. Figure 2–1 illustrates such a case, in which a 3-year-old male child had a 2- to 3-cm nodular lesion just below the medial canthus of the left eye. The lesion was excised and was found to be a well-defined low-grade fibrosarcoma. Wide excision of the surrounding tissue appeared to be adequate therapy for preventing recurrence. He has been followed for more than 10 years and has remained clinically free of recurrence. The sarcomas listed in Table 2–1

TABLE 2–1. Sarcomas of the Head and Neck in 449 Patients (M. D. Anderson Hospital)[29]

	No. of Cases	Percent
Rhabdomyosarcoma	48	69%
Dermatofibrosarcoma protuberans	8	11%
Fibrosarcoma	4	6%
Unclassified (synovioma, etc.)	4	6%
Hemangiosarcoma	3	4%
Kaposi's sarcoma	2	3%
Liposarcoma	1	1%

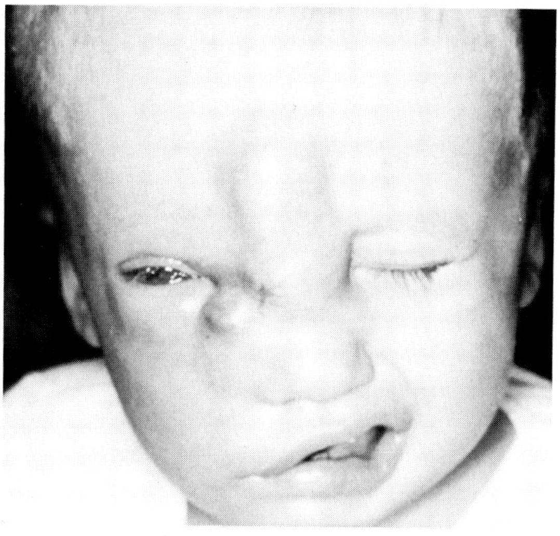

FIGURE 2–2. *Embryonal rhabdomyosarcoma of the paranasal sinuses presenting as an expansile multinodular mass in the frontal and paranasal regions of the face.*

were essentially described as nontender and were frequently recognized as sarcoma only at the time of biopsy. In this group of cases, rhabdomyosarcoma was the most common tumor to be found, particularly in the younger patient.

The distribution of tumors arising in the head and neck of children is somewhat different from that for adults and is noted in reviewing cases reported by Stout:[39] rhabdomyosarcoma, 92 cases; fibromatosis, 75; hemangioendothelioma, 62; angiofibroma, 29; benign fibrous histiocytoma, 25; and lymphangioma, 21.

EMBRYONAL RHABDOMYOSARCOMA

Embryonal rhabdomyosarcoma of head and neck origin is a common lesion of childhood and in its mature form is also encountered in adults. As indicated by the distribution of cases in Stout's review, rhabdomyosarcoma should be considered the prime lesion of the head and neck from the period of infancy to adolescence. It may present in several different ways: as a primary neck mass, present on the face or cheek (Fig. 2–2), bulge, from the parotid gland, arise within the maxillary sinus with its growth producing orbital proptosis (Fig. 2–3*A*), or grow and expand within the paranasal sinuses to invade the nasopharynx and base of the skull. In the sinuses, it develops an expansile grape-like pattern of growth similar to what is seen in sarcoma botryoides of the vagina (Fig. 2–3*B*). The patient in Figure 2–3*A*, a 12-year-old girl, had presented with orbital proptosis. A sinus study identified the presence of a tumor of the maxillary antrum invading the orbit. Exploration of the sinuses through a Weber-Fergusson approach revealed a primary rhabdomyosarcoma, which infiltrated through the floor of the orbit to invade the intrinsic muscles. An orbital exenteration was performed, followed by radiation therapy and chemotherapy. An aggressive multidisciplinary approach must be employed when these tumors are first identified. More recently, with the effectiveness of many of the newer chemotherapy protocols, we have attempted to limit the extent of surgical resection for this particular group of tumors.[12, 26, 45] Because neck node metastasis occurs in more than 20% of these patients, neck dissection should be contemplated when palpable disease is present. For large bulky lesions, prophylactic neck dissection may be

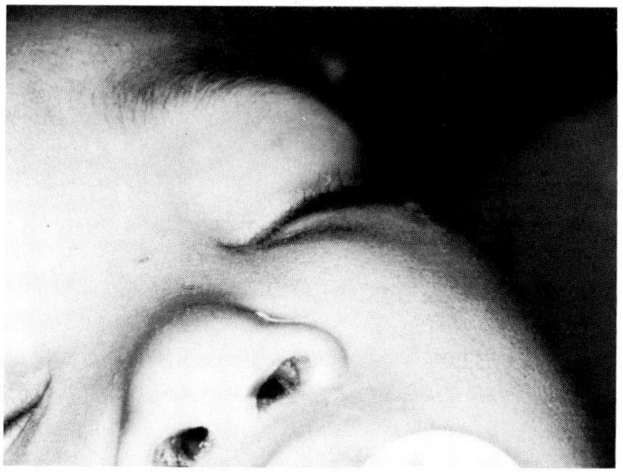

FIGURE 2–1. *Low-grade fibrosarcoma situated under the medial canthus of the left eye.*

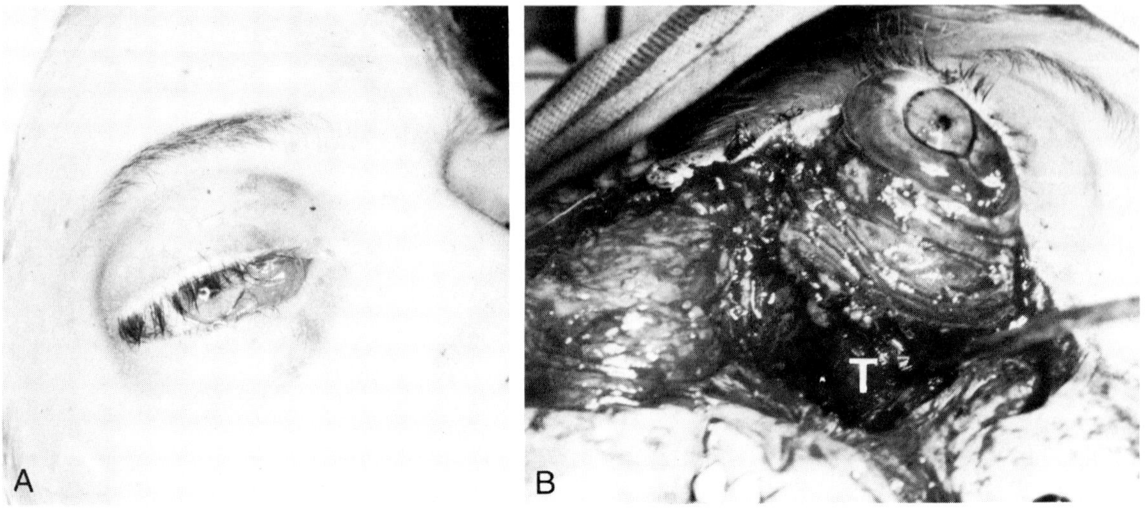

FIGURE 2–3. A, *Proptosis of the right orbit secondary to embryonal rhabdomyosarcoma.* B, *Exposure of the maxillary antral tumor (T) that invaded the floor of the orbit to cause orbital proptosis.*

in order, followed by radiation therapy. If the lesion occurs on the face below a line drawn between the mouth and the parotid gland, and there is a question of cervical node involvement, then neck dissection should be performed. If there is no palpable cervical adenopathy, then prophylactic radiation therapy to the neck nodes should be considered. For lesions above this line, somewhat higher on the face, patterns of spread are not clearly defined. In these cases, chemotherapy should be used. If possible, wide excision of the primary lesion is advantageous, followed by a short course of chemotherapy usually containing doxorubicin (Adriamycin). Radiation therapy, usually 5000 to 6000 rad, delivered to the site of the primary lesion, follows priming with chemotherapy. The patient should then be placed on maintenance chemotherapy after the use of radiation.

Figure 2–4 shows the presence of a small nodular lesion arising in the buccinator muscle of a 19-year-old woman. This facial lesion had ulcerated through the mucous membrane near the left upper gingiva to protrude into the cheek. A nodular mass could be palpated as outlined (Fig. 2–4*A*),

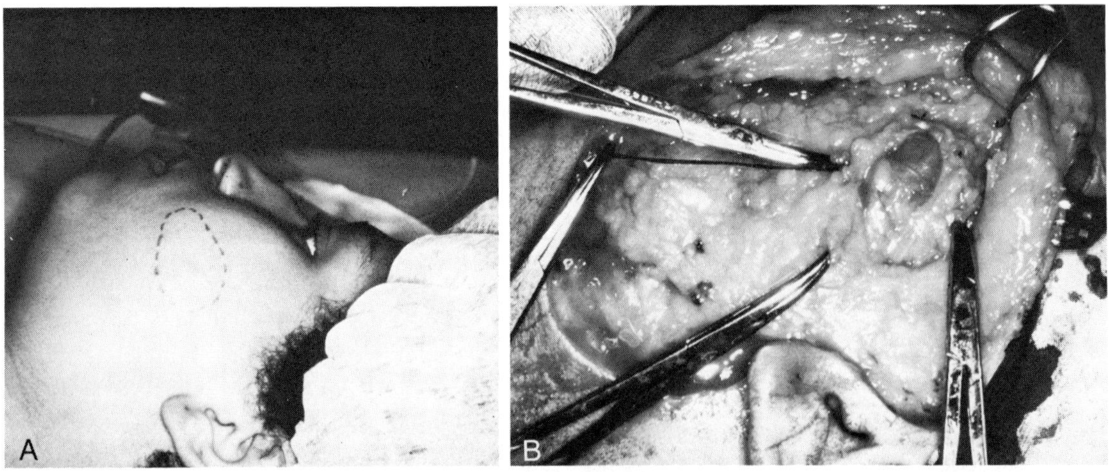

FIGURE 2–4. A, *Patient with embryonal rhabdomyosarcoma of the cheek. The circle defines the limit of the tumor palpable through the cheek. It rose in the buccinator muscle and invaded the bucco-gingival gutter.* B, *Exposure of the tumor after raising a large parotid flap to the angle of the mouth.*

and biopsy revealed embryonal rhabdomyosarcoma. While results in the treatment of this tumor have improved over the past decade using combination surgery, radiation, and chemotherapy, the best results are still obtained when the tumor can be widely resected or debulked. Areas of necrosis that may be present in such a lesion prevent adequate delivery of chemotherapeutic agents and minimize the effectiveness of radiation therapy, thus necessitating resection of the lesion whenever possible.

Two surgical approaches can be used for excision. The first is to make an elliptical transverse incision over the mass, extending from the buccal commissure to the temporomandibular joint, raising a superior and inferior skin flap, and incising through buccinator muscle above and below the tumor into the oral cavity, so that complete resection is accomplished. Any major defect in the mucosal surface can be surfaced with the use of a lateral tongue pedicle flap. Skin flaps are resutured and derive support and blood supply from the underlying tongue pedicle. On repairing the defect in the skin right to the corner of the mouth, complete healing of the commissure will occur, contrary to what has usually been taught. What is not advisable in removal of a tumor near the angle of the mouth is resection of a portion of the commissure with approximation of the upper and lower lateral vermilion borders without the use of a cheiloplasty.

In this particular case of rhabdomyosarcoma of the buccal membrane, because of the anterior position of the tumor, an extended parotid incision was employed. The incision was carried behind the ear and then anteroinferiorly to cross over the hyoid bone, almost reaching midline neck. A flap was raised anteriorly to the buccal commissure to expose the tumor (Fig. 2–4*B*). Branches of the facial nerve were defined with a nerve stimulator, and buccal fascia was incised between them to expose the tumor. The entire tumor was resected through the buccal membrane, and the oral defect was then repaired using a primary mucosa-to-mucosa repair. The cheek flap was then returned to its normal position and resutured. Postoperative healing was normal. Two courses of chemotherapy were given prior to radiation therapy to the cheek and neck nodes. Postoperative maintenance chemotherapy was begun 1 month after completion of radiation therapy.

Variants of Rhabdomyosarcoma

The diagnosis of rhabdomyosarcoma has been refined over the past two decades with the reclassification of tumors that previously had been lumped into the rhabdomyosarcoma classification, e.g., malignant fibrous histiocytoma. With improvement in chemotherapy protocols, this refinement in histologic interpretation has become important for the proper development of treatment protocols.

The most common variant of the muscle tumors observed in the head and neck is the embryonal rhabdomyosarcoma. It arises in the head and neck, genitourinary tract, retroperitoneum and, less frequently, in the extremities. It is composed mainly of rhabdomyoblasts with identifiable cross-striations. When this tumor appears within a cavity, such as the vagina or the maxillary sinus, it develops into a nodular or grape-like cluster, the so-called sarcoma botryoides. This tumor is usually aggressive and stands in contrast to fibrous tumors such as the angiofibromas and the fibrous dysplasias, which tend to expand within the sinuses (Fig. 2–5); orbital contents are easily displaced by such tumors without direct invasion. When muscles of the orbit are clinically free, then salvage of the globe is attempted, even when a portion of the oribtal floor must be removed. One can gain an impression of orbital invasion at the time of surgery when raising the cheek flap of the Weber-Fergusson incision, which extends just under the eyelid. The orbital fat

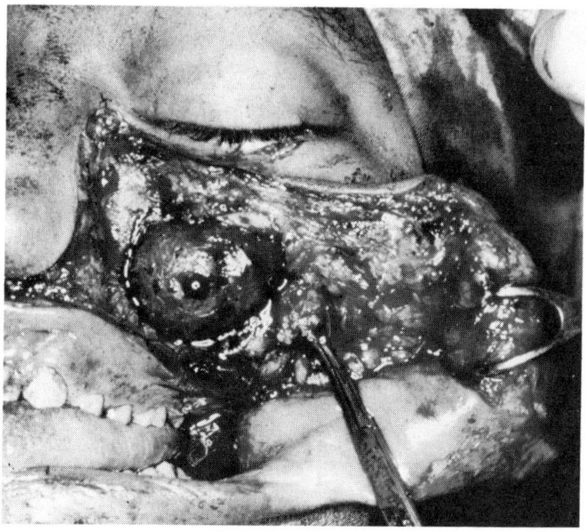

FIGURE 2–5. Fibrous dysplasia of the maxillary antrum.

pad is dissected and the orbital floor palpated for signs of invasion.

Four types of embryonal sarcomas have been described: pleomorphic, embryonal, alveolar, and sarcoma botryoides.

In this group, the alveolar tumor has the worst prognosis. The sarcoma botryoides is usually found within cavities so that it expands in a grape-like cluster. This tumor, first described in infants, arises within the vaginal cavity or, more rarely, in the larynx. When the tumor grows within the maxilla it has the opportunity to present with the nodular clusters of tumor that characterize it. The nasopharynx is probably the most common site of spread from tumors arising in the orbit.

In a review of 170 cases of embryonal rhabdomyosarcomas of the head and neck by Dito and Batsakis,[11] 54 (31.8%) appeared in the orbit and 49 (28.8%) in the nasopharynx, nasal and oral cavities. As these tumors grow, they can present as expansile masses, especially when they have originated in a relatively closed space. When attempts to control the tumor fail, the local growth with which the patient presents can be overwhelming. An 11-year-old boy was referred to us after having received radiation therapy and conservative chemotherapy for 1 year in an attempt to control a primary tumor of the paranasal sinus. The entire oral cavity was filled by tumor (Fig. 2–6*A*), which extended into the maxillary sinus, the frontal sinus, the masseter and pterygoid muscles, the orbit, and the base of the skull. For palliative purposes, the tumor was removed using a Weber-Fergusson approach (Fig. 2–6*B*). The base of the tumor was treated cryosurgically (Fig. 2–6*C*), and satisfactory reconstruction was accomplished (Fig. 2–6*D*). Postoperative chemotherapy was initiated 1 week after surgery, but the patient died 4 months after discharge as a result of complications due to neoplastic invasion of the brain.

Among the cases of embryonal rhabdo-

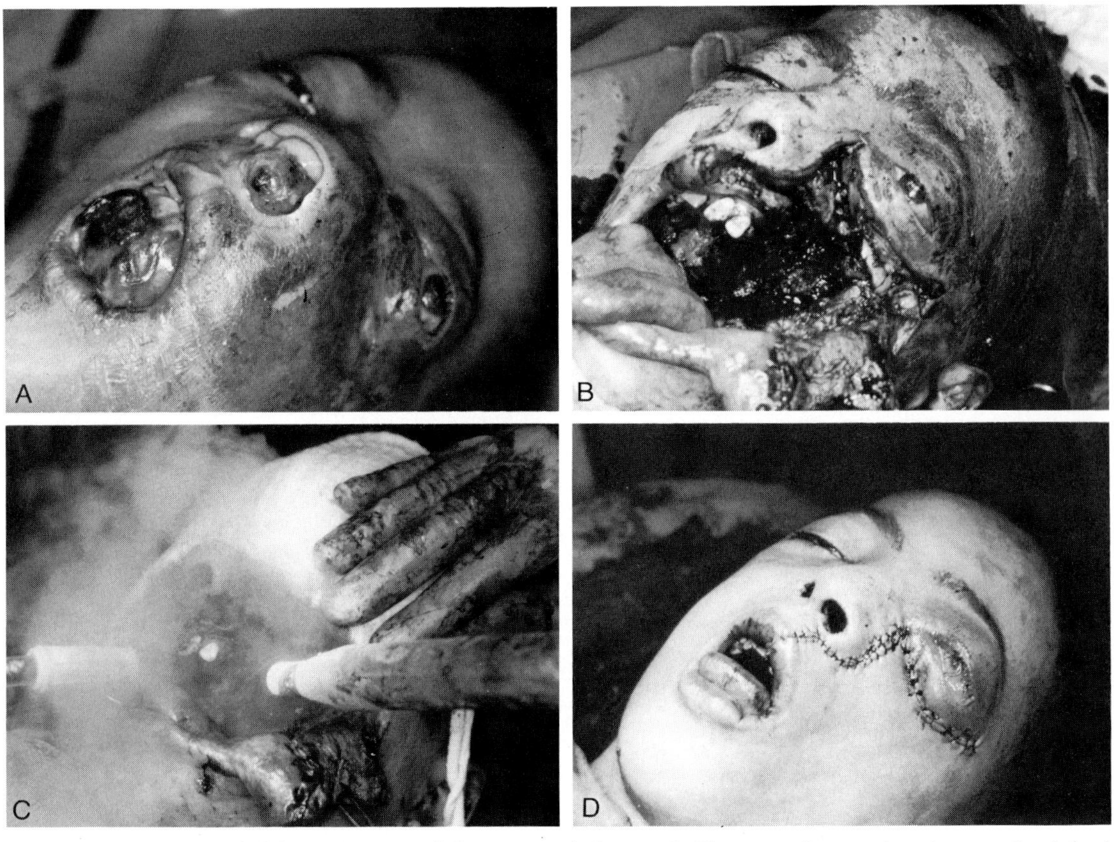

FIGURE 2–6. *Embryonal rhabdomyosarcoma of the paranasal sinuses. A, The tumor has produced proptosis of the left orbit, fills the nasal cavity, and is protruding from the mouth. B, Appearance of the operative defect after radical maxillectomy. All gross tumor was resected to base of the brain. C, Cryosurgery of the operative defect using liquid nitrogen spray. D, Appearance of the patient at the time of closure of the operative defect.*

myosarcoma reviewed by Stout,[39] 10 arose in the orbit (a frequent site for this tumor), 9 in the nasopharynx, 7 in the oral cavity, 6 in the maxilla, 5 in the soft parts of the face, 4 in the temple, 3 in the nasal cavity and in the neck, and 1 each in the ethmoid sinus and the larynx. In these tumors, both the stellate and the spindle cells have scanty rings of cytoplasm usually set in a matrix stroma containing round cells with vacuolated and eosinophilic cytoplasm. Strap-like cells are also seen with eosinophilic cytoplasm, and tube-like fibers with multicentric nuclei appear in a relatively clear cytoplasm. In such tumors arising adjacent to the cranial vault, extension can occur intracranially by direct invasion through the skull as well as by retrograde extension along the cranial nerves similar to the pattern seen with squamous cell carcinoma. Nodal metastases may be noted in as many as 20% of patients, with distant metastases to lung and bone also common.

In general, embryonal rhabdomyosarcoma grows rapidly, tends to infiltrate the surrounding structures, and may invade bone and brain if initiation of therapy is delayed. CT scans of the skull are important for detection of any invasion. When the orbit is infiltrated by tumor, there is usually blurring of vision and diplopia, followed by proptosis in a downward or temporal direction. The eyelids may be invaded, causing edema of the lids and the conjunctivae. Erosion of the paranasal sinuses tends to follow, with subsequent extension to the meninges.

PARANASAL SINUS INVOLVEMENT

Lesions of the paranasal sinuses in children are almost invariably sarcomatous; however, they rarely reach the proportions seen in the case described. Early symptoms of any tumor arising in this region are similar to those seen in inflammatory processes and, as such, are usually dismissed. In the region of the ethmoids and superior maxillary sinus, the patient may present with nosebleed. Progression of tumor within the posterior nasal wall can result in infiltration, with the tumor extending to nasopharynx with subsequent obstruction of the eustachian orifices. Disease frequently continues along the infraorbital ridge. Late in the clinical course, the infraorbital nerve becomes involved, causing the upper lip to become anesthetic. External swelling in the ethmoid region can become prominent, with widening of the space between the nasal midline and medial canthus (Fig. 2–6*A*). Another important symptom is anesthesia of the palate, which is caused by posterior extension of the tumor through the nerve of the pterygoid canal (vidian nerve) and the sphenopalatine ganglion. Lymphatic drainage from the antrum and the ethmoid sinuses spreads the tumor to the retropharyngeal nodes. Involvement of the cervical nodes, however, appears late in the course of the disease.

Liebner, in 1976, reviewed 19 consecutive cases of rhabdomyosarcoma of the head and neck in children from 13 months to 17 years of age (mean, 6 to 7 years).[28] The two most frequent sites of involvement were the orbit and facial soft tissue. Management was predominantly accompanied by radiation therapy, especially if the paranasal sinuses or the orbit were part of the site of tumor invasion. At times, it was necessary to debulk the tumor along with necrotic sites, since radiation therapy could not produce the required results in an anoxic field. Whether or not the sequela of overzealous radiation therapy to the orbit of children has been retardation of osseous growth, there is always the potential for cataract formation and even the development of radiation sarcoma.

If tumor growth cannot be brought under control by radiation therapy and chemotherapy, then orbital exenteration must be considered at the proper time. Radiation therapy can be increased in selected patients, but they will be at risk for developing secondary neoplasms. Arlen et al.[2] had the opportunity of reviewing the bone sarcomas arising secondary to radiation therapy for retinoblastomas. Many of the patients had received a booster dose of radiation to the orbit to control residual disease.

Wharam et al.,[45] representing the IRS Committee of the Pediatric Oncology Group, reported on 72 patients with embryonal rhabdomyosarcoma, extraosseous Ewing's sarcoma, and undifferentiated small round cell mesenchymal sarcoma. Protocols utilizing vincristine, dactinomycin, and cyclophosphamide were used. Sixty-three (88%) of those treated attained complete remission, but 13 subsequently relapsed. The patients with primary tumor arising in sites other than the neck had a complete response rate in excess of 90%. In contrast, 11 relapses occurred in the 26 patients with primary tumors in the neck.

LIPOMAS AND LIPOSARCOMAS

Some sarcomatous lesions of the head and neck can demonstrate characteristic features seen with epithelial tumors. They can present with membrane ulceration or as nodular masses on the face, suggesting minor or major salivary gland origin. Even benign lesions, such as the head and neck lipomas, can give the illusion of firmness, especially when they arise in subfascial planes. We have seen such tumors in the parotid region, arising deep to the facial nerve, appear to mimic deep lobe parotid tumors (Fig. 2–7); they can arise under the sternomastoid muscle or adjacent to the carotid sheath, suggesting the presence of metastatic nodal disease. When these lesions are exposed, however, they tend to pop into the wound and are easily recognized as deep subfascial lipomas. Other benign forms of lipomas—e.g., lipoblastoma in the cheek—have also been noted.[37]

On occasion, the malignant form of these benign tumors, the liposarcomas, can be encountered. They are rare in this part of the body, occurring more frequently in the extremities. We have seen one patient with liposarcoma of posterior neck. In this instance, wide muscle group dissection, including the erector spinae muscle, was performed. This procedure appears to have been curative, as the patient was alive and free of disease at 10 years. When liposarcomas are found in the head and neck region, they present as relatively substantial lesions. The benign forms are not uncommon in the subfascial planes of the head and neck; malignancy is usually ruled out by the protracted clinical course, with little, if any, evidence for displaying any growth potential. Forty cases of malignant liposarcoma, including two oral liposarcomas, have been reported. The skull, scalp, orbit, and pharynx were the sites most commonly involved;[34, 35] the cheek (buccal surface) and the floor of the mouth were the preferred intraoral sites. Of the 35 cases that were available for analysis, 71.4% were myxoid liposarcomas, 14.2% were round cell liposarcomas, and 8.5% were of the mixed type. The highest survivals were expected among the well-differentiated myxoid liposarcomas, and the lowest, among the round cell type. Baden et al.[3] presented the two cases that arose in the oropharynx: the first, a well-differentiated liposarcoma of the floor of the left side of the mouth in a 55-year-old black woman; and the second a soft, smooth mass in the right parapharyngeal space, displacing the right tonsil inferomedially and the right half of the soft palate downward in a 37-year-old black man. The location of the second tumor is a more common site for presentation of minor salivary gland tumors, which may develop in the roof of the mouth. In the first patient, a clinical diagnosis of ranula had been made; under local anesthesia the lesion was found to be lipomatous and to infiltrate the myelohyoid muscle. The tumor was grossly removed. Signet cells with large hyperchromatic nuclei and occasional nuclear pleomorphism and the presence of giant cells were noted. The diagnosis of a well-differentiated lipomyxosarcoma was made. The patient was followed for 3 years without evidence of recurrence. Should the tumor have been more aggressive histologically and clinically, mandibular resection with a suprahyoid neck dissection may have been indicated. However, such a lesion might then have responded favorably to postoperative radiation therapy at the time of the original surgery. The second patient underwent primary resection of a

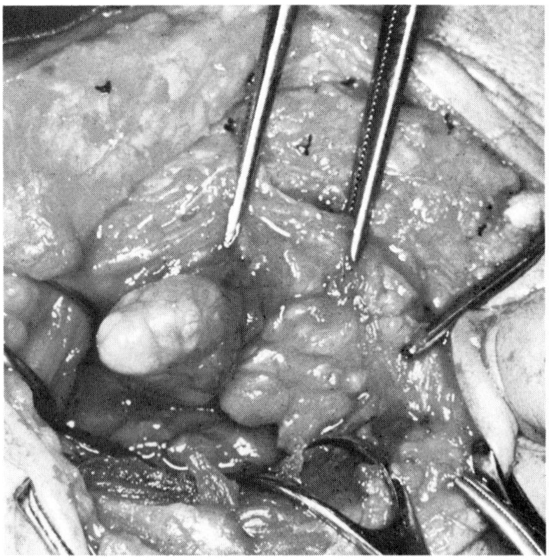

FIGURE 2–7. Lipoma appearing from under the tail of the right parotid.

well-encapsulated mass. Once again, local resection of a well-differentiated myxoliposarcoma was performed, without evidence of recurrence at 30 months.

NASOPHARYNGEAL ANGIOFIBROMA

In the young patient, juvenile nasopharyngeal angiofibroma is a highly vascular, essentially benign neoplasm arising from the basilar fibrocartilage area and occurring in the nasopharynx or posterior nasal cavity of pubescent boys.[1] Approximately 15% occur in patients over 20 years of age. There is a 25% incidence of local recurrence and an overall mortality rate of 30%. Histologically, the tumor is composed of large vascular spaces with varying amounts of fibrous stroma. A malignant counterpart of either sarcomatous or carcinomatous nature has been reported by Gisselsson.[18] The tumors are locally invasive and erode adjacent sinuses. Angiograms are characterized by enlargement and displacement of the internal maxillary artery, with opacification of numerous dilated vessels, homogeneous blush, and absence of venous filling. When extension occurs in the orbit and cranial vault, feeding vessels can be derived from the ophthalmic and internal carotid arteries.

TUMORS OF FIBROUS TISSUE ORIGIN

Tumors of fibrous tissue origin are not infrequent in this area, probably representing the second most common tumor requiring treatment. Fu and Perzin[16] reviewed 256 nonepithelioid tumors arising in the nasal cavity, paranasal sinuses, and nasopharynx: 156 benign and 100 malignant tumors. In reviewing those tumors that proved to be fibrous in origin, 23 were classified as fibrous tissue tumors, 4 as fibromas, 6 as fibromatoses, and 13 as fibrosarcomas.

Fibromas of head and neck origin presented as polypoid lesions usually in the nasal cavity, pharynx, and larynx. No recurrences were seen following simple local excisions of any of the lesions. These tumors probably represented a reparative process rather than true neoplastic change.

The fibromatoses that occur in this region are usually aggressive and generally do not metastasize. Considerable morbidity may be seen owing to infiltration of surrounding structures that are uncontrollable surgically. In six patients a second lesion of the turbinates with cloudiness of the sinuses was characteristic. On resection, the abnormalities were found to be fibrous masses that infiltrated the adjacent tissue. Microscopically, these lesions were composed of relatively mature fibrous tissue with abundant collagenous stroma. Within the sinuses, especially where maxillary antral invasion has occurred, maxillectomy is usually necessary. Three of the six patients had clinical recurrence 6 months to 11 years following limited, incomplete resection. Surgical resection is the only treatment that appears to control this disease. Neither the primary nor the recurrent tumors appear to be permanently arrested by radiotherapy. If tumors are identified as arising from bone, they will invariably recur, even as late as 11 years later. These tumors may be confused with fibrous dysplasia and ossifying fibromas, myxomas, and even neurofibromas. If vascular, they may even be confused with angiofibromas. An angiofibroma should consist of stellate stromal cells that do not grow in bundles, as may be seen with fibromatoses. When fibromatosis and desmoid lesions become aggressive, chemotherapy may have some role.[19]

Fu and Perzin reported on 13 fibrosarcomas in patients ranging in age from 10 to 77 years. Ten had masses growing into the nasal passage. In the maxillary sinus, swelling and tenderness was noted. Four patients had destruction of adjacent bone. The lesions were composed of elongated spindle-shaped cells arranged in bundles of 10 with a herringbone pattern. In some cases, areas of new bone formation or regeneration were seen at the interface of the tumor and adjacent bone. This could occasionally be confused with malignant osteoid, suggesting osteosarcoma.

Figure 2–1 shows a fibrosarcoma of the face in a 3-year-old boy. This tumor was considered clinically to represent a minor salivary gland neoplasm or even a subcutaneous cystic structure. Biopsy was necesary to obtain histologic verification of the sarcomatous nature of this lesion. When such lesions are fully malignant, they have the same aggressive potential as adult fibrosarcomas arising in the extremity. It is essential that treatment be aggressive and early in order to be curative. In this particular case, wide resection of the fibrosarcoma was accomplished by extending the incision to the lacrimal apparatus. The use of wide resection here resulted in a 10-year survival free of disease.

In Fu and Perzin's series, five patients with fibrosarcoma were treated with limited local resection and all subsequently developed recurrence. The patients who responded best were initially treated by en-bloc resection that usually necessitated radical maxillectomy with or without orbital exenteration, as was necessary. Some recurrences were small enough and could be controlled with the second resection. We recently treated a 14-year-old boy with a well-defined nodular mass on the forehead that proved to be fibrosarcoma. Following wide resection, a hair flap was turned into the defect to establish a new hairline on the forehead and the donor site was skin-grafted.

Fibrosarcoma is more easily managed than other tumors of the head and neck, including lesions such as leiomyosarcoma and rhabdomyosarcoma. Many have recommended the importance of examining multiple sections of tumors in order to rule out other pathologic diagnoses. While reactive new bone formation and osteoid may be seen in the margins, such changes should not be seen within their central regions. In a review of fibrosarcomas, it was possible to assign a different diagnosis to as many as 15% of the cases studied. In reviewing fibroblastic tumors involving the head and neck, Conley[8] reported a 5-year survival rate of 69%; 79% of the cases were fibromatoses and 3% were fibrosarcomas. Recurrence was seen in 52% of the fibromatoses treated by local excision and in 49% treated by wide resection.

Although fibromatoses are considered benign, a rare case may metastasize to the viscera. In adults, one must rule out the fibrous phase of malignant melanoma. The tumor masses may occur anywhere on the head and neck, even arising within the paranasal sinuses. When suspected recurrent tumors are found at distant sites and present as nodular subcutaneous lesions, this should suggest that the primary mass is an aggressive lesion and probably a melanoma. If nodular lesions are present during the first month of life, a fibromatous process will probably resolve by maturation. Occasionally, nodular lesions of the neck that are seen in the neonate are part of the process of cystic hygroma. These lesions are a result of obstructed lymphatics and usually have a large intraoral component (Fig. 2–8) or may fill the whole neck.[5, 36] Early resection of these lesions is not in the best interest of the patient. Rather, the initial approach should be to establish an airway. The associated neck masses that appear to be firm fibrous lesions are usually fibrous and lymphatic lesions in a swiss-cheese pattern or honeycomb matrix, making easy removal impossible. Neck dissection in these patients can lead to injury of structures such as the hypoglossal and superior laryngeal nerves, which can be devastating to the child. As the patient gets older, residual lesions can always be removed with more ease in accomplishing the neck dissection. A one-stage resection for massive hygromas has been described by Grosfeld et al.[21] In the young child and adolescent the fibrous tumor that proves to be well-differentiated fibrosarcoma is usually well controlled by wide local resection. Among the fibrosarcomas of the head and neck mentioned in several series, none had metastasized even though the potential existed.[40] These tumors have a high degree of persistence at the site of surgery. Local recurrence does, however, double the probability that the patient will die of the disease.

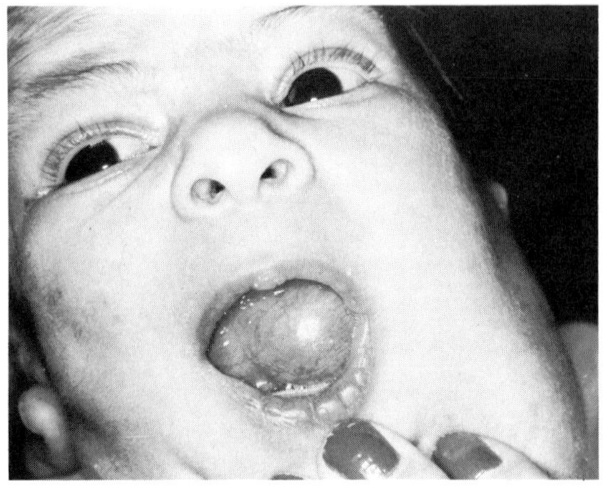

FIGURE 2–8. *Large lymphangiomatous hygroma filling the floor of the mouth and neck. The resultant obstructed airway required tracheostomy. In such cases the tracheostomy site should be marsupialized to skin.*

Connolly[8] presented data on the methods of managing recurrent fibrosarcoma of the face, most of which occurred in the region of the cheek. Melanoma of head and neck region, which can present as a fibrous tumor, is difficult to distinguish from fibrosarcoma but must be ruled out. Many of the low-grade desmoids were characterized by scar tissue that replaced the antral contents to invade the sphenoids and base of the brain. Biopsies of multiple sites, including the sphenoids, have been interpreted by pathologists to represent benign scar tissue. Failure to treat at this point has only resulted in progression of disease to the brain. Depending on their site of occurrence, the desmoid tumors can present major problems with regard to the extent of resection needed for control. Figure 2–9*A* illustrates the appearance of a long-standing desmoid tumor arising in the region of the floor of the mouth to invade the mandible and the appearance of the specimen after complete removal by classic commando resection (Fig. 2–9*B*).

In the cheek area, resection of the desmoid tumor inevitably results in large defects that have to be replaced by pedicle flaps derived from forehead, neck, and pectoral regions. Forehead flaps have been used to line the buccal cavity, and neck flaps to surface the skin of the face. In recent years the forehead flap has lost importance, and other sites substituted. These other flaps have yielded good, if not better, cosmetic results and similarly effective coverage. McGregor et al.[30] have described the extended role of the deltopectoral flap in such cases. One of us (Arlen) has employed the tongue pedicle flap in numerous instances to line mucosal defects. The tongue flap can also be used to provide a base for neck flaps to cover large defects resulting from major full-thickness resections of the cheek.

The surgical approach to tumors in this region is an important consideration. Well-defined surgical procedures are available for the common squamous cell and salivary neoplasms. For the sarcomas, variations of the head and neck dissection techniques, as well as the commando resection and maxillectomy, may be necessary. A 26-year-old man presented with orbital invasion secondary to fibrosarcoma of the ethmoid sinuses. A classic maxillectomy was considered, but because of the size of the tumor, the craniofacial technique as described by Ketcham, Wilkens, and Van Buren[25] was used. This technique allows complete control of the tumor, especially when the superior orbital plate is invaded by the lesion. No local recurrence was noted over an 8-year period of follow-up. At 3 years, however, the patient developed pulmonary metastasis, which was resected. Later, a metastatic lesion to the rib was removed, and the patient continues to remain free of disease.

Among the fibrous tissue tumors seen at Memorial Hospital, two dermatofibrosarcomas occurred in the region of the face, four on the neck, four in the clavicular area, four

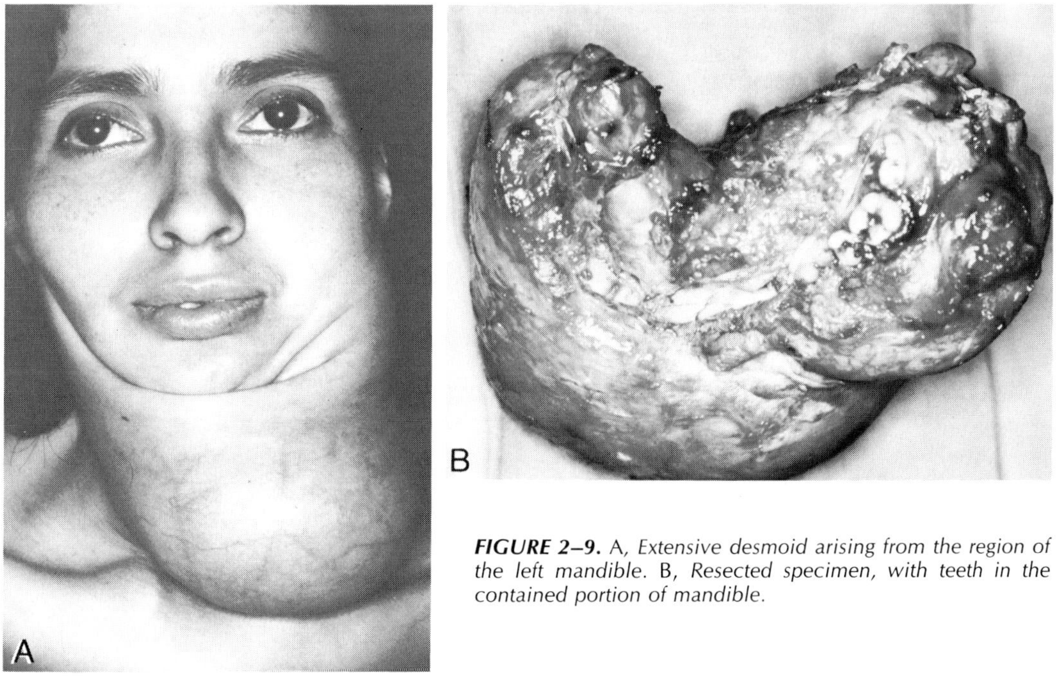

FIGURE 2–9. *A, Extensive desmoid arising from the region of the left mandible. B, Resected specimen, with teeth in the contained portion of mandible.*

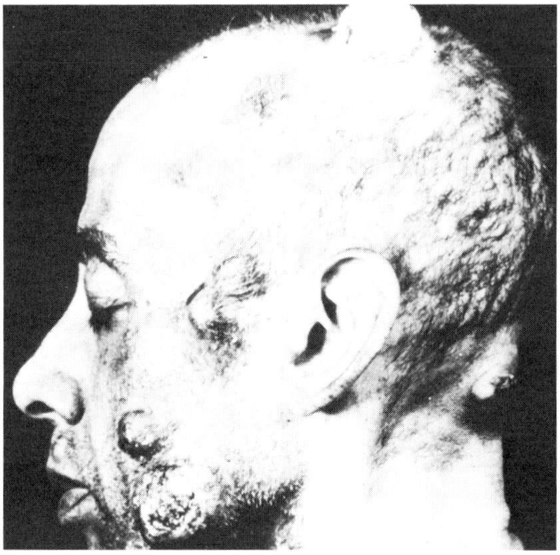

FIGURE 2–10. Multiple lesions of dermatofibrosarcoma protuberans.

in the posterior neck, and four in the region of the skull (Fig. 2–10). In our personal experience, one large dermatofibrosarcoma was seen at the base of the skull, having recurred after local excision of a small nodular lesion in the region (Fig. 2–11). At the time of recurrence, the lesion occupied a major portion of the posterior scalp but was completely resected. The base of the skull was grafted, as a rotation pedicle flap could not be obtained easily from the anterior chest wall sites where such flaps are usually raised. In Figure 2–12 a large sarcomatous lesion (dermatofibrosarcoma) is seen to fill the entire supraclavicular fossa. Metastasis is rare[31] and occurs only in the late stages of disease.

CRYOSURGERY FOR SCALP LESIONS

The presence of a large scalp mass representing a solid primary tumor is uncommon among the sarcomas. We have, however, treated two patients with malignant fibrous histiocytoma of the scalp. In both, local recurrence was the major problem. One of us (Arlen) has seen several metastatic carcinomas, usually of renal or pulmonary origin, presenting in this fashion. The patient in Figure 2–13 presented with an extensive mass over the occiput of at least 1 year's duration. After wide resection to the galea, liquid nitrogen was applied three times using a Brymill spray unit. In many instances, the application of liquid nitrogen, freezing the tumor site to below −50°C, is an effective method of control without the consequences of repeated radiation therapy to the area. When a similar type of tumor en-

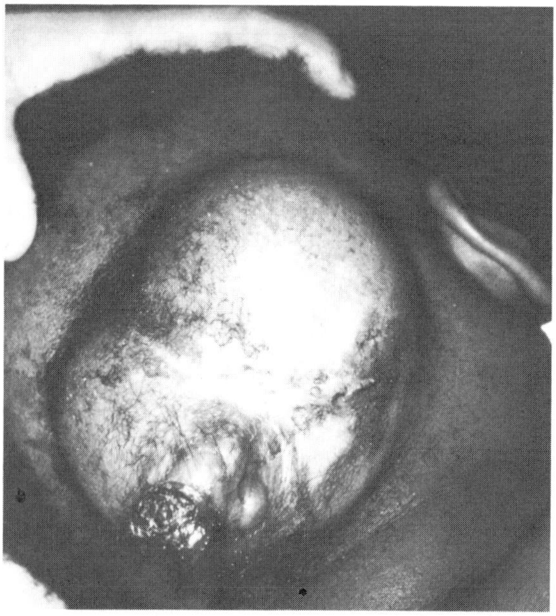

FIGURE 2–11. Dermatofibrosarcoma arising in the region of the occiput.

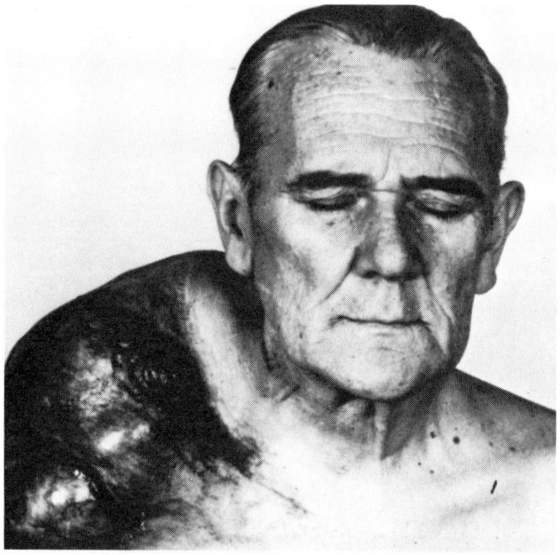

FIGURE 2–12. Dermatofibrosarcoma arising in the right supraclavicular fossa.

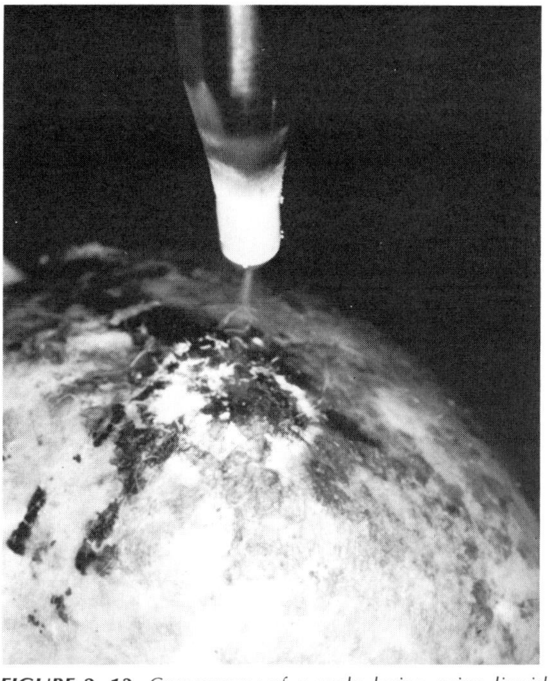

FIGURE 2–13. Cryosurgery of a scalp lesion using liquid nitrogen spray.

croaches the forehead hairline anteriorly, a hair pedicle can be rotated to create a new hairline and the donor site skin-grafted.

We have used cryosurgical techniques to control tumors that appear to involve the periosteum of the skull. This seems to bring under local control most lesions that have occurred in the area of the outer table of the skull; grafting can then usually be performed without difficulty. When cryosurgery is applied to the skull, one must be careful not to destroy the periosteum, as skin grafts may not take at the site of application. The pouring of liquid nitrogen into bone cavities has been used successfully by Marcove to control many tumors. In the head and neck region, however, pouring is difficult since the liquid nitrogen cannot stay in direct contact with the tumor bed site. Spraying, then, is an effective approach. In other instances, a probe with short teeth for direct insertion into the tumor can be used for applying the cryogen to the tumor. Freezing produces a spherical nidus within the tumor. When the zone of freezing extends 0.5 to 1 cm beyond the border of the tumor, the process is discontinued, the lesion warmed with heated saline, and the process repeated twice.

DERMATOFIBROSARCOMA AND THE DESMOID TUMORS

Although dermatofibrosarcomas are essentially low-grade fibrous tissue tumors and metastasize only rarely, a number of cases of dissemination from such tumors have been reported.[31] One of our patients presented with a supraclavicular mass that had undergone excisional biopsy and which was diagnosed as dermatofibrosarcoma.

A wide resection was then performed and closure carried out by rotation pedicle flap from the chest. The patient remained free of disease for 4 years, at which time a pulmonary nodular lesion was seen. The lesion proved to arise from the pleural surface. Radiation therapy with chemotherapy initially appeared to offer some control of tumor growth, but the lesion continued to enlarge. Chest wall resection included removal of the diaphragm and a portion of the lung that contained the tumor. The patient remained free of disease for more than 1 year; after the first year he suffered a convulsive episode, and CT scan revealed metastatic tumor to the brain.

The fibrous tumors, in general, are fairly resistant to many forms of nonsurgical treatment and, as their complexity increases (such as with the fully malignant fibrohistiocytomas and synoviomas), the response markedly diminishes. We have seen desmoid tumors and other variations of extra-abdominal desmoid lesions in the region of the shoulder. These desmoid tumors are most frequently found arising from the abdominal wall but also can be found at distant sites such as the shoulder girdle, chest wall, and thigh. In the region of the head and neck, the tumor comprises less than 2% of the spectrum of lesions that appear extra-abdominally. The tumor appears microscopically to be benign. Its behavior, however, is that of a low-grade fibrosarcoma, and it should be completely resected. We have seen recurrent desmoids in the neck infiltrating to the spinous process of the cervical vertebrae; these were widely resected without attempting to dissect into the neural foramina and have not reappeared. Should such lesions reappear, laser surgery may be an effective way to destroy invasion by tumor into small nerve roots, possibly in combination with a laminectomy. When possible, these tumors are treated conservatively by wide resection; amputation or techniques that involve major nerve loss should be reserved for the fully malignant fibrosarcomas. Radiation, with a median dose range of approximately 5000 R, has been suggested in selected cases. There have, however, been occasional reports of malignant transformation of a fibromatous tumor to a fibrosarcoma, a situation that may have resulted from early use of radiation therapy. Osseous sarcomas in the head and neck have been known to arise following use of radiation therapy to primary lesions.[2]

In the series reported by Memorial Hospital, there were 4 dermatofibrosarcomas, 11 extra-abdominal desmoids, 32 fibrosarcomas, 4 synoviomas, and 14 spindle cell sarcomas. One patient had congenital fibrosarcoma of the tongue. The average age of the patients with the fibrosarcomas of the head and neck was 50. The most common site of the fibrous tumors was maxilla (in 16 patients), followed by the neck (8), palate (4), and lip (4). Eleven patients underwent radical maxillectomy, six requiring orbital exenteration.

SYNOVIOMAS

Synoviomas, which typically occur as tumors of the lower extremity and shoulder region, may also be found in the head and neck.[4, 22, 38] Roth et al.[33] found this disease occurred most frequently in young men. Presenting symptoms were hoarseness as well as respiratory and swallowing disturbances. The primary sites were almost always the retropharyngeal and hypopharyngeal regions. Pulmonary metastasis was the cause of death in 57% of the patients. Peripherally placed synovial sarcomas have a 20% incidence of metastasis to the lymph nodes. Such metastases, however, have not been reported in any case of synovial sarcoma of the head and neck region. In several cases histologic appearance was similar enough to papillary carcinoma of the thyroid to consider thyroidectomy. In each instance, the thyroid was free of neoplasm and subsequent review of the original specimen confirmed the diagnosis of synovial sarcoma. Cadman et al.[6] reported that recurrence developed in 91.5% of patients treated by excision alone, compared with a 50% recurrence rate in those who underwent postoperative irradiation.

NEURAL TUMORS, INCLUDING CHEMODECTOMAS

Among the nodular lesions appearing in the head and neck, one must consider those of nerve origin. Chemodectomas (nonchromaffin paragangliomas) can arise in such sites as the bifurcation of the common carotid, adjacent to ganglion nodosum of the vagus nerve, and in the region of the jugular bulb and in relation to the arch of the aorta. By anatomic location, these tumors are referred to as carotid body tumors. Glomus jugulare tumors and vagus body tumors are other terms that are employed. A cervical mass is the most typical finding in patients with this type of lesion, followed by a hypopharyngeal mass and hoarseness due to laryngeal nerve impingement. Patients with glomus jugulare tumors note hoarseness, conduction deafness, oral pain, vertigo, and tinnitus. All tumors are characterized microscopically by cells arranged in nests surrounded by vascular fibrous septa. The distribution of reticulum in the septa, which does not engulf the tumor cells, proves to be a distinguishing feature. Nuclear and cytoplasmic hypertrophy further substantiate the diagnosis of a malignant tumor. Occasionally tumors metastasize to cervical nodes. Excision of carotid body tumors has been facilitated by hypothermia and temporary ligation of the carotid artery.[27] Because of the relative inaccessibility, glomus jugulare tumors were rarely totally excised and as such had a high incidence of recurrence, with approximately 50% reappearing after the first operation. In many instances these tumors have been misdiagnosed, on examination of biopsy material, as squamous cell carcinoma, hemangioma, hemangiosarcoma, and hemangiopericytoma. Cummings et al.[9] reviewed 45 patients with glomus jugulare tumors of the temporal bone treated by radiation therapy. Only three patients had recurrence or progression of tumor during the follow-up period that ranged from 3 to 23 years (mean, 10 years). No patient died from uncontrolled glomus tumor. The majority noted symptomatic relief after radiation, but objective neurologic deficits usually remained unchanged or improved only partially. Sarcomas have been known to arise in the larynx.[20, 44] Among such tumors, there have been occasional reports of paraganglionic tissue arising from laryngeal tissue.[44] While paraganglionic tissue is most often associated with the carotid bifurcation (carotid body tumor), other common sites also include the inferior ganglion, the cervical portion of the vagus nerve (vagal body tumor), and the temporal bone (jugular body tumor). In the head and neck this tissue can also be found to occur in such areas as orbit, mandible, trachea, nasal cavity, and larynx. Seventeen cases involving the larynx have been reported. Tomography, laryngography, and CT scanning have been useful in defining the extent of tumor involvement. Partial laryngectomy has been employed most frequently in the treatment of this particular laryngeal tumor. Radical neck dissection was necessary in four patients.

Malignancy in paraganglionic tissue has been reported: for carotid body tumors, the incidence is 6% to 9%; for vagal body, 16%; for aortic arch, 13%; and for glomus jugulare, 4%. There is some suggestion that laryngeal paragangliomas have the highest incidence of malignancy.

When tumors are found to arise in proximity to, or directly from cranial nerves or their branches, a likely diagnosis is primary neurogenic tumor arising from branches of the facial nerve, the vagus nerve, or the cervical plexus. After radical neck dissection the presence of a firm mass in the neck may represent recurrent tumor or the appearance of an amputation neuroma. Katz et al.[24] described 15 extracranial solitary neurogenic tumors of the face and neck. The vagus nerve was involved in four instances, cervical sympathetic plexus in three, brachial plexus and facial nerve each in two, and trigeminal nerve, spinal accessory nerve, hypoglossal nerve, and cervical plexus each in one. Origins of tumor from the neural sheaths, Schwann cells, neurogenic sites, or mixtures of these may be seen, although tumors of Schwann cell origin appear to be the most common. Occasionally, such tumors may have intrathecal extensions, requiring laminectomy.

These tumors are essentially benign, and preservation of the nerve should be attempted in most instances. A high degree of suspicion for neurogenic tumor should exist when a sharply demarcated, seemingly encapsulated, pale pink-white, uniformly firm, rubbery tumor is observed. At this point, one should preserve all or most of the eccentrically placed nerves of those fibers entering or leaving the neoplasm, or both. Depending on which nerve is involved, careless resection could produce motor and sensory loss resulting in severe disfigurement. Metastatically involved lymph nodes, inflammatory masses, and congenital cystic lesions could simulate primary nerve masses. Occasionally, after neck dissection, firm neck lesions consistent with recurrent tumor may develop. In such cases, tender lesions of 3 to 4 cm have proved to be neuromas of the transected branches of the cervical plexus.

The commonest neoplasm has been schwannoma, followed by neurofibroma. Ultrastructural studies of schwannomas and neurofibromas[43] support the concept that these neoplasms are derived from Schwann cells. In our own series, two schwannomas have arisen from branches of the facial nerve within parotid tissue. Many reports have noted these tumors to be in proximity to major salivary glands. In each instance a deficit in the ramus mandibularis was noted on completion of a superficial parotidectomy. Examination of the specimen by frozen section suggested a neurogenic tumor, a diagnosis that was later confirmed on permanent section. The nerve defect was repaired primarily by graft and resulted in the complete return of function.

In a review of neurogenic tumors at Memorial Hospital,[10] 45% of solitary schwannomas occurred in the head and neck region, most in the lateral neck. The incidence for intraoral schwannoma was 6.5%, with the tongue the most common site. The tongue was also a major site for granular cell myoblastoma, which is also considered to be of neural origin. These tumors have been reported in the larynx, arising from the area of the glottic fold and the false cord.

In another series from Memorial Hospital,[13] 40% of patients who had neurofibrosarcoma as another form of neurogenic tumor had associated von Recklinghausen's disease. Half of all cases involved children. The tumors were more aggressive and anaplastic in this age group. Neural sarcomas, in general, present as slowly expanding encapsulated tumors that may exhibit rapid growth. At Memorial Hospital, there were 22 malignant schwannomas, 5 malignant carotid body tumors, 30 neuroblastomas, and 18 esthesioneuroblastomas. Thirteen of these tumors occurred in the neck, and four involved vagus nerve. There were five cases of liposarcoma and four of leiomyosarcoma. We have treated two patients with leiomyosarcoma, one of whom presented with a massive lesion that began in the posterior neck and eventually involved a major portion of the chest wall and shoulder girdle, extending from the anterior to the posterior neck and base of the skull. The tumor was considered unresectable. Metastases developed in a short period and resulted in the patient's death. The second patient presented with a small nodular mass that was removed and diagnosed as leiomyosarcoma. The neck was re-explored and wide resection carried out. After 3 years, the patient shows no signs of recurrence. Mandibular involvement by neurofibrosarcoma has been reported by Upton.[41] Commando resection of the mandible is usually required to encompass such tumors.

Esthesioneuroblastoma is an uncommon neurogenic tumor arising from the olfactory epithelium of the nasal vault. As it expands, it grows downward into the nasal cavity, eventually involving the nasopharynx and ethmoid sinuses. This vascular lesion bleeds easily, causing the patient to present with nasal obstruction and epistaxis. One of the common patterns of extension is into the cranial vault; distant metastases to lungs and cervical nodes occur in 20 to 30% of cases. Because of the high failure rate in controlling a disease that usually cannot be detected in the early stages, various therapies have been attempted. Wade et al.[42] reported 13 cases treated with chemotherapy either at the time of diagnosis or at the time of recurrence after surgery and radiation. The tumor appears sensitive to several chemotherapeutic agents including cyclophosphamide, vincristine, nitrogen mustard, and thiotepa.

TUMORS OF VASCULAR ORIGIN

The presence of a nodular lesion on the back of the neck most frequently represents a chronic sebaceous cyst or long-standing lipoma. Rarely, resection may prove the lesion to be a liposarcoma, in which case cure can usually be achieved by muscle group dissection, excising all muscles clinically adherent to the bed of the locally excised lesion. Figure 2–14*A* shows a typical lesion of the back of the neck, suggestive of a large lipoma but which proved to be a hemangiopericytoma. Wide resection was performed; and a section taken through the tumor mass is seen in Figure 2–14*B*. The hemangiopericytomas that arise from vascular pericytes show a richly vascular pattern of thin-walled vessels lined by a single layer of flattened endothelium. The angiogram, an especially useful method for diagnosing extremity and retroperitoneal lesions, will show a significant vascular pattern with a diffuse capillary blush or opacification in the arterial phase and dilatation of the draining veins during the venous phase. Among several series, the head and neck lesions comprise 15 to 20% of the tumors defined at surgery, the majority appearing in the lower extremity. Hemangiopericytoma-like tumors in nasal passages and paranasal sinuses and parotid region have been reported and are

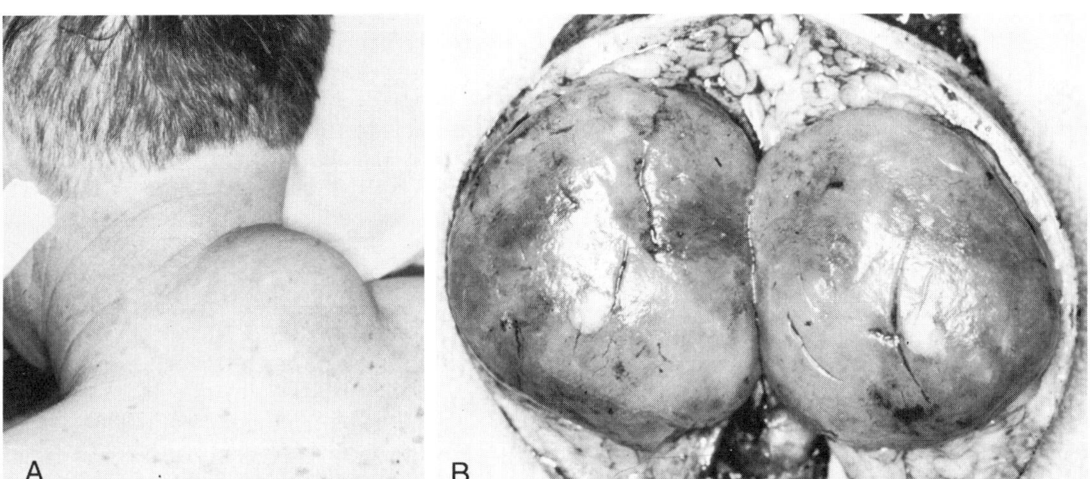

FIGURE 2–14. *A, Hemangiopericytoma of the back of the neck. B, Cross-sectional appearance of the resected hemangiopericytoma.*

relatively benign in their clinical course.[15] Pulmonary metastases from these tumors have had slow growth patterns, extending over 10 to 20 years. While surgical resection is the prime treatment of choice and ligation of afferent vessels is of value in controlling hemostasis, mitotic activity and cellular pleomorphism may serve as guides to the extent to which radical removal should be performed. The metastatic rate varies from 11 to 56%, depending on the series, which in turn relates to the site of origin, histologic pattern, and surgical approach used. Mira, Chu, and Fortner[32] have reported complete remission in 47% of the patients treated with radiation therapy. An unusual case of hemangiopericytoma of the maxillary sinus was reported by Caldarelli and Sperling.[7] Because of the high possibility of local recurrence of this lesion, a radical excision was performed.

Vascular tumors comprise a moderate percentage of patients with head and neck sarcomas. At Memorial Hospital, hemangiopericytoma was diagnosed in 11 patients, 30% of whom had regional node involvement. There were 19 patients with angiosarcoma. With these vascular neoplasms, a wide array of patterns may be seen: from discrete lesions to the more frequently seen multiple tumor nodules, as noted on the lower extremity.

A 20-year-old woman presented with diffuse superficial nodularity around the left ear. The initial biopsies were considered to show pyogenic granuloma. As the lesions became more diffuse and began involving the outer ear (Fig. 2–15*A* and *B*) repeat biopsies were taken, and angiosarcoma was diagnosed (Fig. 2–15*C* and *D*). In discussing management it became apparent that surgical resection would offer no possibility of totally encompassing the multiple lesions. Various attempts at radiation therapy and chemotherapy were made without any response. Progression of the tumor led to a final effort that employed cryosurgery before any attempt at radical resection was made (Fig. 2–15*E*). This method of using cryosurgical spray led to rapid necrosis and involution of the tumor (Fig. 2–15*F*) within 2 weeks of therapy. The patient presented 2 years later with metastasis to the parotid gland. Following parotidectomy, cryosurgery was again used, at the site of the nerve dissection. Nerve impairment did not result. The patient has remained free of disease for 10 years (Fig. 2–15*G*). We have used cryosurgery in several instances in which resection of a vascular tumor was considered

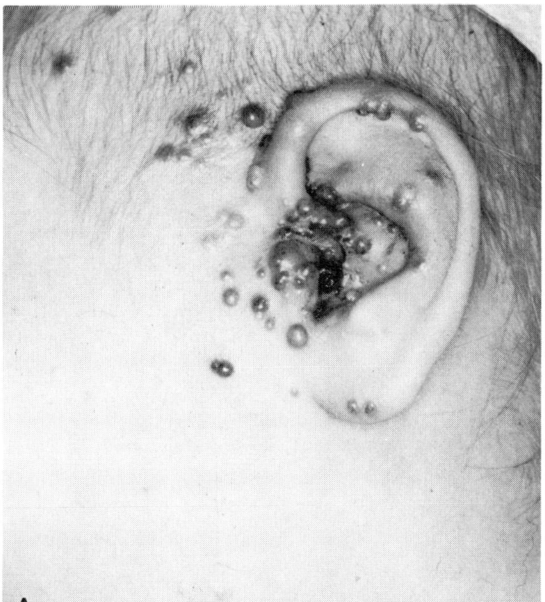

A

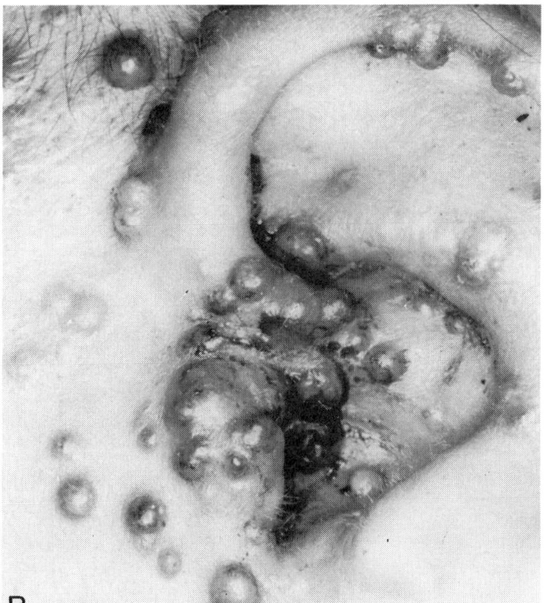

B

FIGURE 2–15. *A, Angiosarcoma arising in the region of the external auditory canal and spreading over the temporal region. B, Close-up view. C, Microscopic view (× 100) of the cutaneous lesion of the ear. A typical vascular cleft is seen, suggesting its vascular origin. D, High-power view (× 430) shows malignant cells lining the vascular cleft. E, Cryosurgical spraying of tumor in the ear canal. F, Appearance 2 weeks after cryosurgery. G, One year after parotidectomy and cryosurgery, there is no evidence of any residual or recurrent tumor.*

Illustration continued on following page

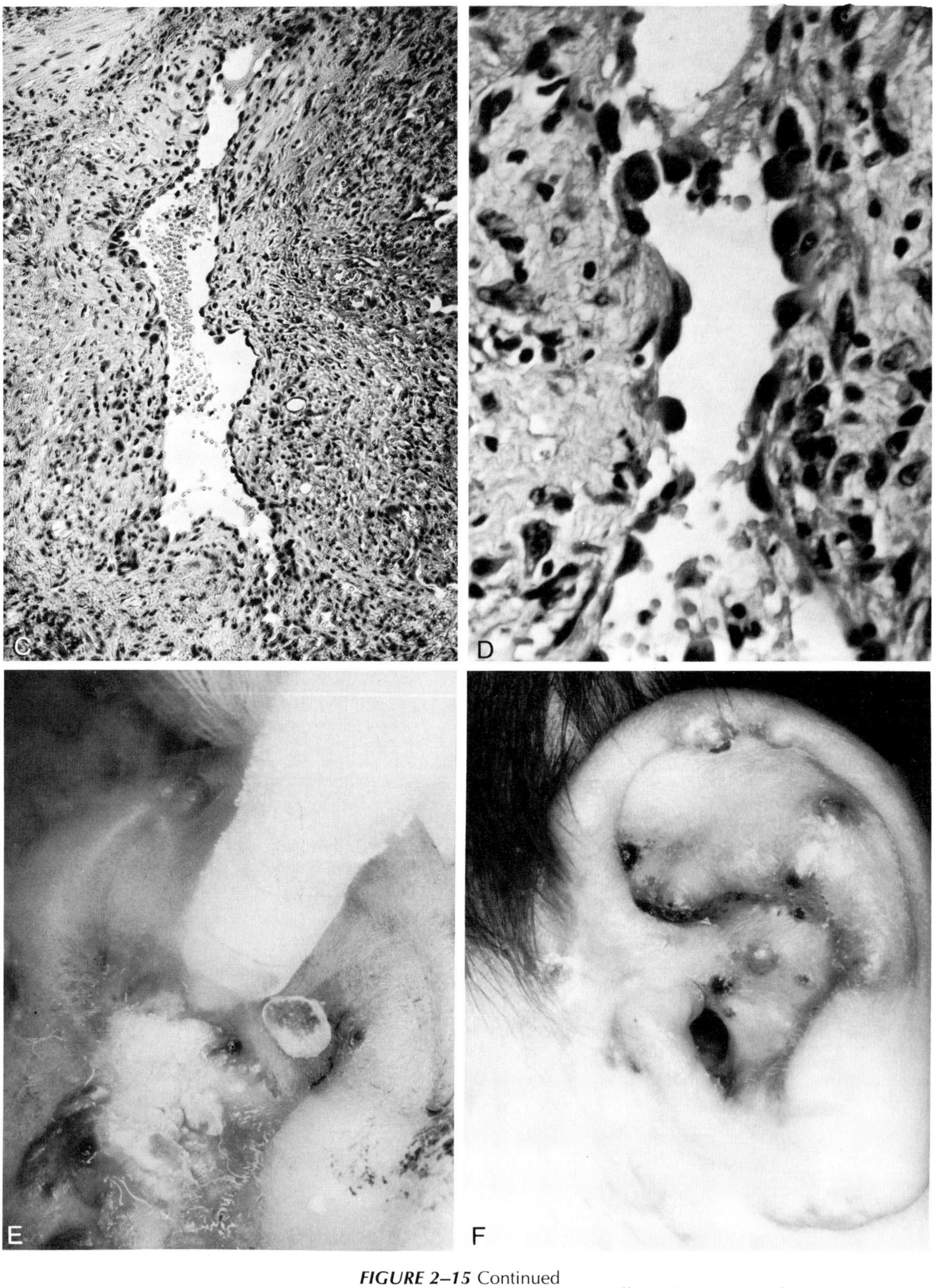

FIGURE 2–15 Continued

Illustration continued on opposite page

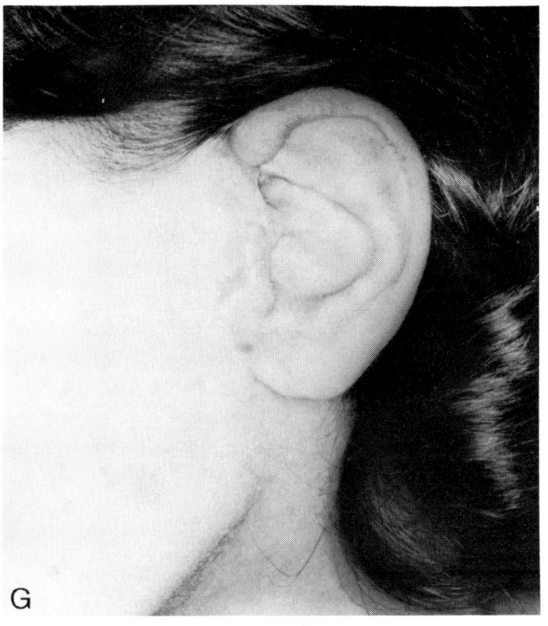

FIGURE 2–15 Continued

impossible. In each instance, complete involution of the angiosarcoma was noted.

Angiosarcomas arise both as cutaneous neoplasms and as soft tissue masses.[17] The cutaneous appearance of the tumor is not uncommon in the head and neck area. Many of these tumors tend to be aggressive, with a high potential for regional node metastasis. Metastasis to the parotid gland, as in the above case, probably represented parotid nodal spread. In reviewing angiosarcomas reported in the literature between 1934 and 1949, Kinkade[26] advanced the concept of regional node dissection for this group of tumors, since nodal spread occurred in 45% of the cases that he noted. Stout described the tumors as demonstrating "first the formation of atypical endothelial cells in greater numbers than are required to line the vessels with a simple endothelial membrane, and then the formation of vascular tubes with a delicate framework of reticular fibers and marked tendency for their lumens to anastomose." In the head and neck region, angiosarcomas are usually seen in elderly men. When they are localized, attempts at surgical resection should include reconstruction of the area with a split-thickness skin graft. About 75% of these tumors tend to recur, and about one third metastasize to cervical nodes and lungs.

RARE TUMORS

Other tumors that should be considered in the head and neck region are those related to expansile masses in the skull of patients with Paget's disease. Occasionally these convert to osteogenic sarcoma (Fig. 2–16). At times these lesions can expand as soft tissue masses with direct extension into the brain. We have had patients in whom removal of the tumor has been attempted neurosurgically; however, the end results have been uniformly poor. Another unusual tumor is the alveolar soft part sarcoma (see Fig. 1–3). Figure 2–17 shows another pattern of presentation of this tumor arising in the base of the tongue of a young child. Radiation therapy produced no response. Intraoral cryosurgery resulted in some temporary regression of tumor, but eventual regrowth caused the tumor to fill the major portion of the oral cavity. Resection was then reattempted, this time through a transhyoid-pharyngotomy approach. Figure 2–17 shows the appearance through the pharyngotomy site, where the epiglottis is retracted inferiorly with an Allis clamp and the base of the tongue appears in the upper field. The tumor appears as a large nodular mass in this region. In

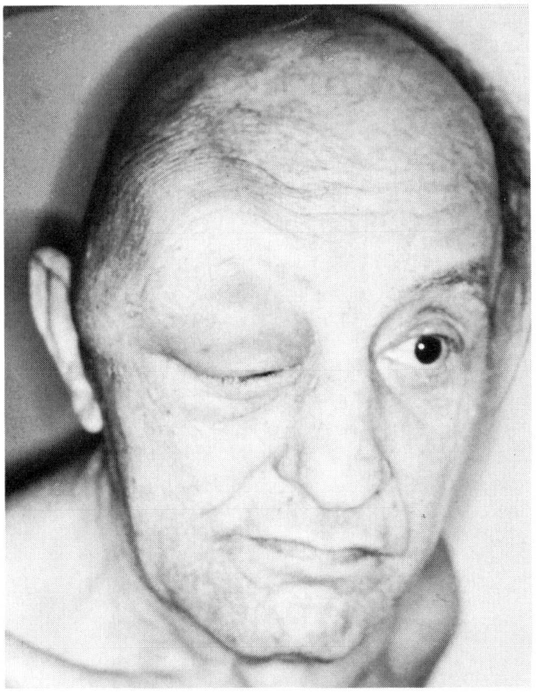

FIGURE 2–16. *Malignant transformation in Paget's disease of the skull.*

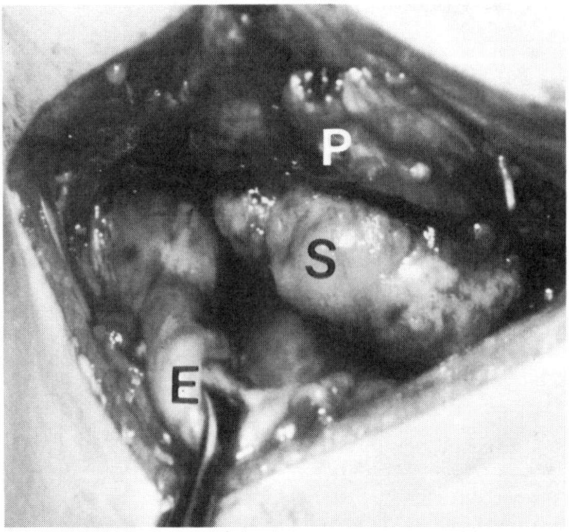

FIGURE 2–17. Transhyoid pharyngotomy showing sarcoma (S) arising from the posterior tongue (P). The epiglottis (E) is being retracted inferiorly with an Allis clamp.

using the transhyoid pharyngotomy to expose lesions of the pharynx and the base of the tongue, a transverse incision is made over the hyoid bone. The cornu of the hyoid is carefully dissected to avoid injury to the superior laryngeal nerves that enter the larynx between the wing of the hyoid and thyroid cartilages. After mobilizing the hyoid bone and retracting it inferiorly, the vallecula is divided transversely and the pharyngeal mucosa is opened transversely. Resection and reconstruction were easily accomplished, but the tumor recurred in the submental and suprahyoid regions despite radiation therapy and chemotherapy. Diffuse pulmonary metastases eventually developed 1 year after the resection of this lesion in the base of the tongue.

Figure 2–18*A* shows the intraoral appearance of a large mass invading the base of the tongue. Biopsy proved the lesion to be sarcomatous, with tumor osteoid throughout the lesion. It was believed that complete resection should be attempted. Several approaches to this lesion could be used. Median labial glossotomy has been tried, dividing the mandible and the tongue at the midline posteriorly, until the lesion is approached. Another approach has been the use of the mandibular swing operation, in which the mandible is divided at the midline and the floor of the mouth incised along the median mandible. This incision is continued toward the posterior tongue, swinging the mandible outward to achieve the required exposure. As in the case of the alveolar soft part sarcoma, we chose to do a transhyoid pharyngotomy. Figure 2–18*B* shows the lesion at the base of the prolapsed tongue in the pharyngotomy incision. Resection was easily accomplished and the remaining base of tongue was reapproximated to the region of the hyoid bone.

SUMMARY

In general, the overall outlook for sarcomas arising in the head and neck is not

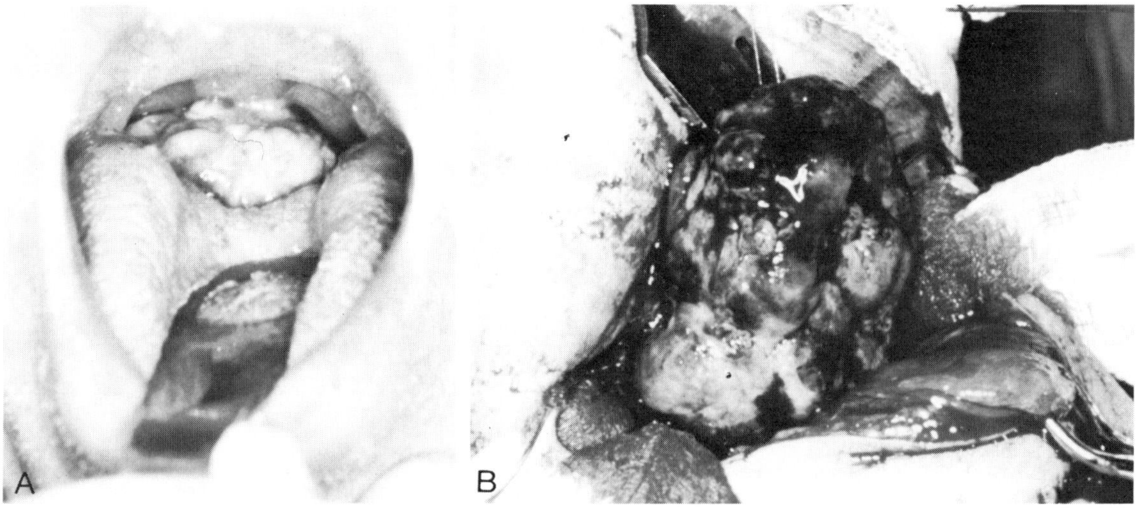

FIGURE 2–18. A, Sarcomatous lesion of the base of the tongue filling the vallecula. B, Exposure of the sarcomatous mass through a transverse pharyngotomy. The epiglottis is being retracted inferiorly with a towel clip.

bright. In the series reported by Farr, 30% of patients had biopsies prior to referral. Of these, 41% had undergone one or more attempts at resection and 15% had undergone one or more courses of radiation therapy prior to referral. Twenty-five percent of this group of previously treated patients survived for 5 years. The 5-year free-of-disease period for the entire group of tumors was 32%, attesting to a relatively aggressive pattern of behavior for sarcomas of the head and neck. Early recognition and prompt adequate surgical resection are the treatments of choice, with adjuvant chemotherapy and radiation therapy employed in the appropriate situations.

REFERENCES

1. Apostle J. V., Frazel E. L.: Juvenile nasopharyngeal angiofibroma: A clinical study. Cancer 18:869, 1965
2. Arlen M., Shah I. C., Higinbotham N., Huvos A. J.: Osteogenic sarcoma of the head and neck induced by radiation therapy. N.Y. State J. Med. 72: 929–934, 1972
3. Baden E., Newman R.: Liposarcoma of the oropharyngeal region. Oral Surg. 44:889–902, 1977
4. Batsakis J. G., Nishiyana R. H., Sullinger G. D.: Synovial sarcomas of the neck. Arch. Otolaryngol. 85:113–117, 1967
5. Bill A. H., Jr., Summer D. J.: A unified concept of lymphangioma and cystic hygroma. Surg. Gynecol. Obstet. 120:79–86, 1965
6. Cadman N. L., Soule E. H., Kelly P.: Synovial sarcoma: An analysis of 134 tumors. Cancer 18:613, 1965
7. Calderelli D. D., Sperling R. L.: Hemangiopericytoma of the maxilla. Arch. Otolaryngol. 102:49–50, 1976
8. Conley J., Stout A. P., Healey W. V.: Clinicopathologic analysis of eighty-four patients with an original diagnosis of fibrosarcoma of the head and neck. Am. J. Surg. 114:564–569, 1967
9. Cummings B. J., Beale F. A., Garrett P. G., Harwood A. R., et al.: The treatment of glomus tumors in the temporal bone by megavoltage radiation. Cancer 53:2635–2640, 1984
10. Das Gupta T. K., Brasfield R. D.: Solitary malignant schwannoma. Ann. Surg. 171:419–428, 1970
11. Dito W. R., Batsakis J. G.: Rhabdomyosarcoma of the head and neck. Arch. Surg. 84:582, 1962
12. Donaldson S. S., Castro J. R., Wilber J. R., Jessee R. H.: Rhabdomyosarcoma of head and neck in children: Combination treatment by surgery, irradiation and chemotherapy. Cancer 31:26–35, 1973
13. Farr H.: Soft part sarcomas of the head and neck. Semin. Oncol. 8:185–190, 1981
14. Farr H. W., Caracang C. M., Huvos A. G.: Malignant vascular tumors of the head and neck. Am. J. Surg. 120:501, 1970
15. Fisher J. H.: Hemangiopericytoma: Review of 20 cases. Can. Med. Assoc. J. 83:1136, 1960
16. Fu Y., Perzin K. H.: Nonepithelial tumors of the nasal cavity, paranasal sinuses and nasopharynx. VI. Fibrous tumors. Cancer 37:2912–2928, 1976
17. Girard C., Johnson W. C., Graham J. H.: Cutaneous angiosarcoma. Cancer 26:865, 1970
18. Gisselsson L., Lindgren A., Stenram V.: Sarcomatous transformation of a juvenile nasopharyngeal angiofibroma. Acta Pathol. Microbiol. Scand. 42:305, 1958
19. Goepfort H., Cangir A., Ayala A., Eftekhari F.: Chemotherapy of locally aggressive head and neck tumors in the pediatric age: Desmoid, fibromatosis and nasopharyngeal angiofibroma. Am. J. Surg. 144:437–444, 1982
20. Gorenstein A.: Sarcoma of the larynx. Arch. Otolaryngol. 106:8–12, 1980
21. Grosfeld J. L., Weber T. R., Vane D. W.: One-stage resection for massive cervico-mediastinal hygroma. Surgery 92:693–699, 1982
22. Harrison E. G., Blach B. M., Divien K. D.: Synovial sarcoma primary in the neck. Arch. Pathol. 71: 137–141, 1961
23. Hermann S. F.: Liposarcoma involving the neck. Northwest Med. 53:1014–1016, 1954
24. Katz A. D., Passy V., Kaplan L.: Neurogenous neoplasms of major nerves of the face and neck. Arch. Surg. 103:51–56, 1971
25. Ketcham A. S., Wilkens R. H., Van Buren J. M., Smith R. R.: A combined intracranial facial approach to the paranasal sinuses. Am. J. Surg. 106:698–703, 1963
26. Kinkade J. M.: Angiosarcoma: A review of the literature. Ann. Otol. Rhinol. 58:159, 1949
27. Lees C. D., Levine H. L., Beven E. G., Tucker H. M.: Tumors of the carotid body: Experience with 41 operative cases. Am. J. Surg. 142:360–361, 1981
28. Liebner E. J.: Embryonal rhabdomyosarcoma of the head and neck in children. Cancer 37:2777–2788, 1976
29. MacCombs W. S., Fletcher, G. H.: Cancer of the Head and Neck. Baltimore, Williams and Wilkins, 1967
30. McGregor I. A., Jackson I. T.: The extended role of the delto-pectoral flap. Br. J. Plast. Surg. 23: 173–185, 1970
31. McPeak C. J., Cruz T., Nicastri A. D.: Dermatofibrosarcoma protuberans: An analysis of 86 cases, five with metastasis. Ann. Surg. 166:803–816, 1967
32. Mira J. G., Chu F. C., Fortner J. G.: The role of radiotherapy in the management of malignant hemangiopericytoma. Cancer 39:1254, 1977
33. Roth J. A., Enzinger F. M., Tannenbaum M.: Synovial sarcoma of the neck: A follow-up study of 24 cases. Cancer 35:1243–1253, 1975
34. Sauk J. J., Jr.: Liposarcoma of the head and neck. J. Oral Surg. 29:38–40, 1971
35. Saunders J. R., Jagnes D. A., Caterline P. F., et al.: Liposarcoma of the head and neck. Cancer 43: 162–168, 1979
36. Seashore J. H., Gardener L. J., Ariyan S.: Management of giant cystic hygromas in infants. Am. J. Surg. 149:459–465, 1985
37. Shear M.: Lipoblastomatosis of the cheek. Br. J. Oral Surg. 5:173–179, 1967
38. Smookler B. M., Enzinger F. M., Brannon R. B.: Orofacial synovial sarcoma—a clinicopathologic study of 11 new cases and review of the literature. Cancer 50:269–276, 1982

39. Stout A. P.: Rhabdomyosarcoma of skeletal muscles. Ann. Surg. 123:447, 1946
40. Stout A. P.: Hemangioendothelioma: A tumor of blood vessels featuring vascular endothelial cells. Ann. Surg. 118:445, 1943
40a. Stout A. P.: Fibrosarcoma in infants and children. Cancer 18:1028, 1968
41. Upton L. G., Hayward J. R., Kerr D. A.: Neurofibrosarcoma of the mandible. J. Oral Surg. 35:504–506, 1977
42. Wade P. M. Jr., Smith R. E., Johns M. E.: Response of esthesioneuroblastoma to chemotherapy. Cancer 53:1036–1041, 1934
43. Waggener J. D.: Ultrastructure of benign peripheral nerve sheath tumors. Cancer 19:699, 1966
44. Wetmore R. F., Tronzo R. D., Lane R. J., Lowry L. D.: Nonfunctional paraganglioma of the larynx. Cancer 48:2717–2723, 1981
45. Wharam M. D., Foulkes M. A., Lawrence W. Jr., Lindberg R. D., et al.: Soft tissue sarcoma of the head and neck in childhood. Cancer 53:1016–1019, 1984

CHAPTER 3

Tumors of the Shoulder Girdle

A wide spectrum of benign soft tissue tumors and sarcomatous lesions can develop on or about the shoulder girdle. They arise from the superficial tissues as well as deeper soft tissue structures in this region. In the subcutaneous planes, extra-abdominal desmoids, dermatofibrosarcoma protuberans, fibrosarcoma, malignant fibrous histiocytoma, and angiosarcomas of the lymphadematous extremity are known to occur. The deeper structures give rise to tumors such as rhabdomyosarcomas, fibrosarcomas, and synoviomas. These shoulder lesions can approximate the clavicle and sternum anteromedially, involve humeral head and glenoid laterally, and arise off the posterior surface of the scapula or chest wall. Figure 3–1*A* shows the radiographic appearance of a sarcomatous lesion of the right scapula. The therapeutic goals in such cases include not only curative resection but also preservation of as much function of the shoulder girdle and arm as possible. In this patient, a forequarter amputation had been suggested. An angiogram showed no significant vascular displacement (Fig. 3–1*B*). A Tikhoff-Lindberg resection (scapulectomy with en-bloc removal of a portion of the humerus and preservation of the neurovascular pedicle to the arm) was performed, and the proximal residual humerus was sewn into the pectoralis major and latissimus dorsi (Fig. 3–1*C*).

An understanding of the natural history of the tumors that arise in this region usually allows for proper decision-making in terms of therapy. The distribution of the major tumors arising in this region is listed in Table 3–1. The cases, treated at Memorial Hospital, are listed in decreasing frequency as a percentage of the total number of cases of that particular type of tumor. Dermatofibrosarcoma, in most series, has been the most common lesion treated, followed by neurogenic sarcoma, synovioma, rhabdomyosarcoma, and desmoid tumor. The neurogenic sarcomas frequently arise in the subscapular fossa from branches of the brachial plexus where neurofibromas that have been present had undergone malignant transformation as part of von Recklinghausen's disease.

CLINICAL PRESENTATION

Clinically, most nodular lesions and diffuse swellings that arise on and about the shoulder girdle must be considered to be suspicious until defined by biopsy. These tumors appear either as small nodular lesions that can be mistaken for sebaceous cysts, as superficial infiltrating masses, e.g., angiomatous malformation in muscle (Fig. 3–2), or as large bulky tumors that essentially destroy the entire shoulder girdle and the scapula (Fig. 3–3). The extensive sarcoma of the upper humerus in Figure 3–3, resected by the Tikhoff-Lindberg procedure, illustrates the extent of tumor growth that can be successfully removed. On microscopic examination, the edge of tumor was less than 2 mm from the preserved vascular supply to the arm. Figure 3–4*A* shows the clinical appearance of an early dermatofibrosarcoma of the shoulder with pedicle flap reconstruction of the operative defect. In this particular case, the patient presented with a small nodular lesion that had been locally resected. Six months later the patient was referred for local recurrence in the biopsy site. Wide resection was carried out and

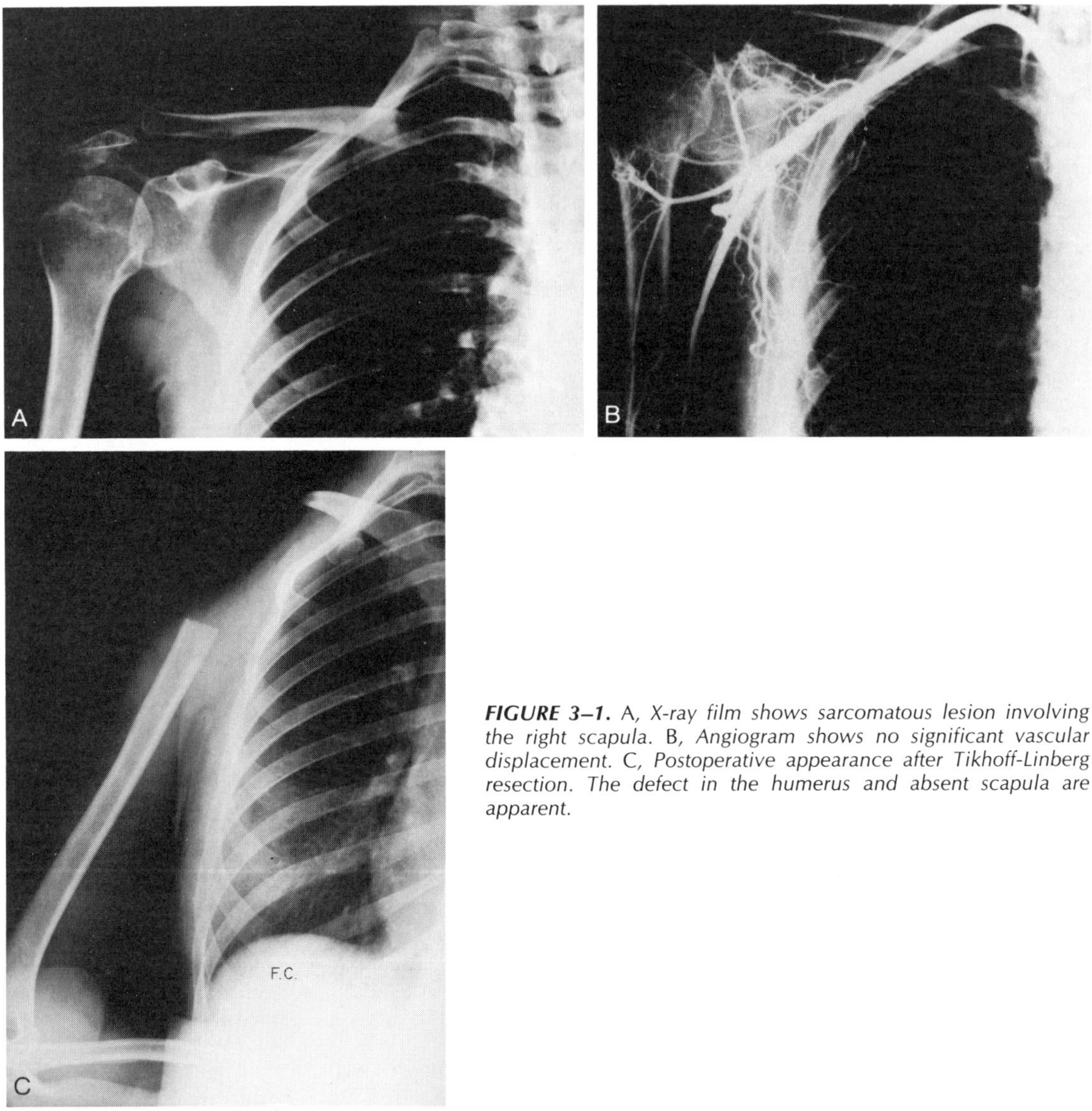

FIGURE 3–1. *A, X-ray film shows sarcomatous lesion involving the right scapula. B, Angiogram shows no significant vascular displacement. C, Postoperative appearance after Tikhoff-Linberg resection. The defect in the humerus and absent scapula are apparent.*

TABLE 3–1. Tumors of the Shoulder Girdle (Memorial Sloan-Kettering Cancer Center)

	No. of Cases in Shoulder Girdle	*Total No. of Cases in All Body Regions*	*Percent of Total*
Dermatofibrosarcoma	15	119	12.6
Neurogenic sarcoma	12	91	13.1
Synovioma	11	136	8.0
Rhabdomyosarcoma	11	121	9.0
Desmoid	9	162	5.5
Liposarcoma	7	173	4.0
Fibrosarcoma	5	124	4.0
Malignant fibrous histiocytoma	5	133	3.0
Hemangiosarcoma	1	32	3.1

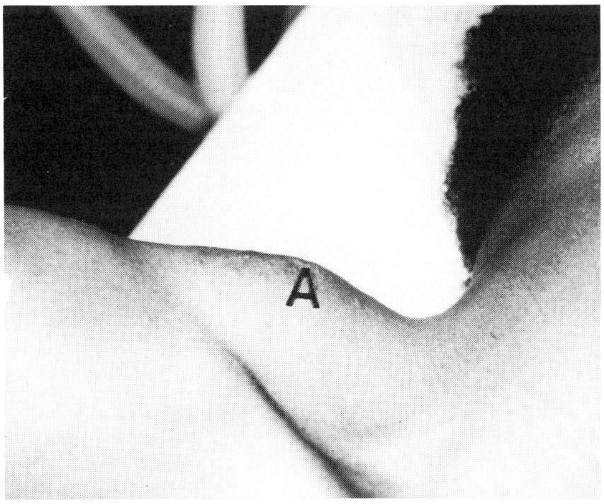

FIGURE 3–2. *Angiomatous malformation (A) in the trapezius muscle adjacent to the suprascapular fossa.*

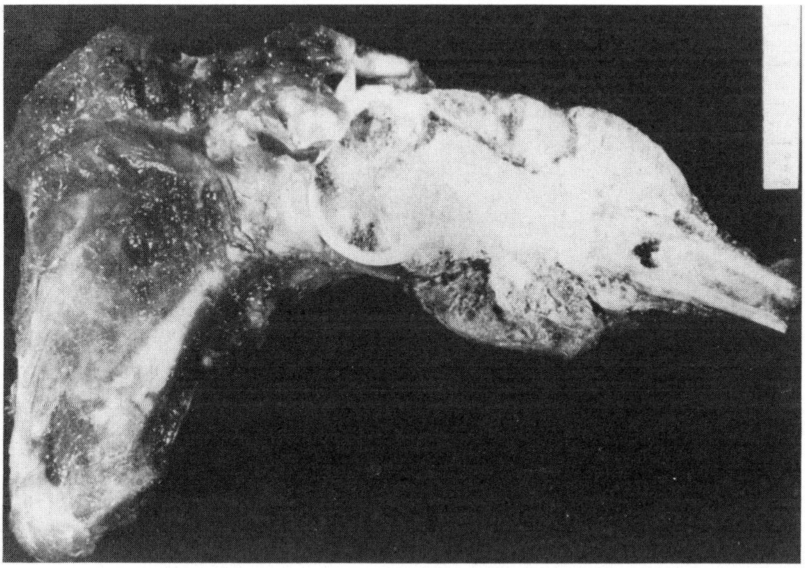

FIGURE 3–3. *Extensive sarcoma involving the scapula and upper humerus.*

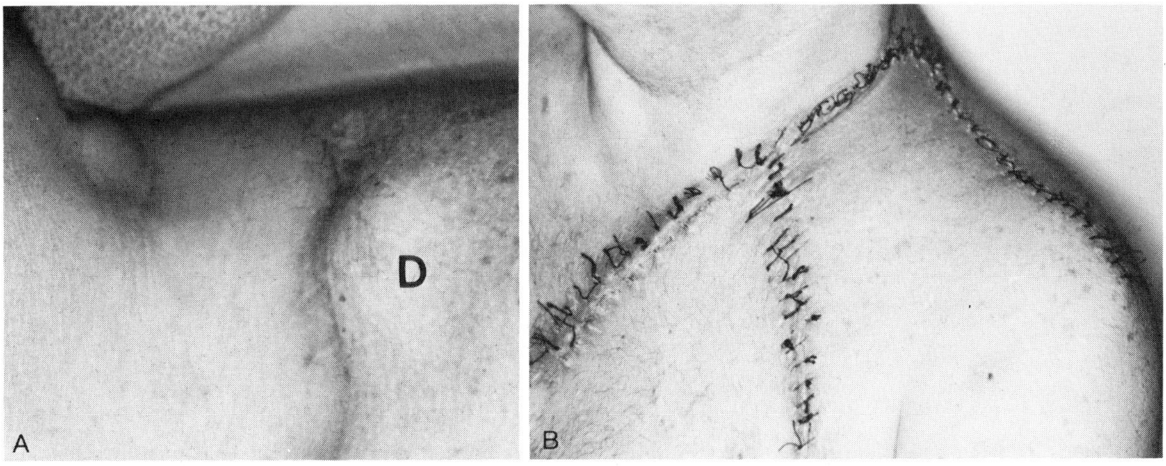

FIGURE 3–4. A, *Dermatofibrosarcoma (D) involving the left shoulder.* B, *Operative site with reconstruction using a chest pedicle flap.*

because it was impossible to close the defect primarily, a full-thickness rotation pedicle flap was utilized (Fig. 3–4*B*). The patient did well until 2 years after surgery, when pleural metastases were noted. He underwent chest wall resection with a partial pneumonectomy. The disease eventually progressed to the brain.

RADIOGRAPHIC PRESENTATION

Most lesions of the shoulder girdle are considered innocuous and do not require radiographic evaluation, as they are usually small and do not compromise underlying structures. Even in the case of a histologic diagnosis of a fully malignant tumor and findings suggesting that residual tumor persists after biopsy, local radiographic evaluation would offer little additional information about the clinical behavior of the superficial lesion. Except for chest films, which are routine, a definitive operative procedure that serves to establish the diagnosis as well as ablate the lesion is in order. Should the histologic nature of the lesion have been underestimated, there would still be ample time for deciding on the need for further resection and possible adjuvant therapies. In the case of somewhat larger tumors, it is important to define how smaller resections with surrounding normal muscle and fascial planes can be employed and to consider whether one needs to resort to en-bloc resections (including underlying bone), if not amputation, to achieve a cure.

CLINICAL EVALUATION

When clinically studying extensive tumorous lesions that encroach on or arise from underlying bone, a number of diagnostic tests are required: posteroanterior and lateral films of the area of involvement, as well as CT scans and angiograms.

The type of biopsy we employ for a suspicious lesion is based both on whether the lesion is thought to be primary bone or soft tissue in origin and on anticipated therapy (the definitive surgical procedure), so that contamination of the neurovascular bundle and planned incision sites will not occur. The incisional approach should be flexible, depending on the presentation of the tumor mass. Stress tests for coracoacromial ligaments should be performed routinely in the case of any tumor around the shoulder joint. The region under the scapula should be palpated for lesions arising on or near the chest wall, e.g., fibrosarcoma, chondrosarcoma, and grating scapula syndromes. X-ray films should be taken in a neutral position as well as in internal and external rotation. Tangential scapular and axillary scapular views may be required to clarify the site of origin of any ill-defined lesion. Shoulder arthrography may also prove useful. Special x-ray films are almost always necessary in defining extraosseous growths and extensions of these tumors into surrounding muscle and neurovascular structures. Newer generation scanners have increased our ability to define subtle features, but in many instances they only confirm what can be noted by the clinician at the time of complete physical examination. Vascular invasion, for instance, usually produces arm edema. Paresthesia of the hand is an important sign of nerve infiltration by tumor. Resection of the tumor with preservation of the extremity is impossible under such circumstances; forequarter amputation must be considered. It is especially important to define the possible extension of tumor to the nerve roots at the base of the neck. Should tumor be found in the suprascapular or supraclavicular fossa fixed against the neck structures, the CT scan may help to define the extent of operability. CT scanning may also be used to define infections and in many instances to suggest the presence of lymphoma. Where necessary, venography may prove helpful. Sonography in this area has been of variable quality and has not offered additional information.

A complete physical examination is an essential part of any diagnostic work-up prior to tumor sampling. For examination of the shoulder, the patient should be stripped to the waist. Metastatic lesions with referred pain, or cervical disks producing similar complaints, may have to be ruled out. Range of motion and scapulothoracic rhythm as well as muscle strength should be noted. The patient should be examined in all positions, particularly from behind while leaning forward. This allows relaxation of the deltoids and proper evaluation of the humeral head, bicipital groove, and rotator cuff.

BIOPSY

Sampling of lesions should be based on impressions gathered from the work-up as to whether the tumor is thought to be a primary lesion or a metastatic focus, e.g., colon carcinoma metastatic to the scapula. In the latter instance, needle aspiration biopsy may be more than adequate for diagnosis. At times, the deeper-placed lesion can more effectively be sampled under CT scan localization. Here, a smear on a slide, a clot in formalin, or a small amount of aspirated tissue may be an adequate sample for analysis. If the tumor appears extensive and radical resection is believed to be necessary for cure, as with the moderate-grade and high-grade sarcomas, then a larger tissue sample may be necessary for analysis. Multiple sites of biopsy may also be needed when heterogeneity is present. Liposarcomas, for instance, may have variable patterns ranging from myxomatous, to well-differentiated, to anaplastic regions at different areas that may be sampled. The discovery of a low-grade sarcoma may influence us to use a more conservative approach, especially when a potential failure may only result in local recurrence of the tumor. Architectural patterns are also important with fibrous tumors, such as fibrosarcoma and synoviomas. Open biopsies may be the only practical way to establish the diagnosis, thereby avoiding inadequate random sampling that can occur with needle biopsy. We usually obtain frozen sections to assure that representative tumor samples free of extensive necrosis have been obtained. All slides are reviewed with the pathologist and all diagnostic procedural information is carefully analyzed in planning for a definitive surgical approach.

We have found that when a lesion is 2.5 cm or smaller, radical local resections (essentially wide excisional biopsies) can be performed with a fair degree of safety. Under most circumstances, the resulting skin defect can be covered with a rotational pedicle flap, as motion over an underlying joint prevents adequate healing of split-thickness grafts. This technique is also easier to use than a free skin graft, since the skin graft may be dislodged even when the extremity is adequately immobilized. In some instances we have found that if a skin graft is used and takes only partially over an area of motion, granulation tissue and further healing by ingrowth from the periphery will occur. Large defects are easily covered by myocutaneous, deltopectoral, or pectoral flaps.

Certain considerations must be taken into account when the question of myositis vs. soft part sarcoma arises. An adequate sample is one with proper markings that allow the pathologists to orient themselves to the periphery and central portion of the lesion. With myositis, the center may appear malignant while the periphery is seen to be benign. With most malignant soft part sarcomas, the central area may show necrosis or normalization while the more malignant areas can appear peripherally.

OPERATIVE DECISION

Biopsies obtained in the operating room should be interpreted along with clinical findings and accompanying x-ray films. Therapeutic approaches should never be based on the results of the biopsy alone. Grading of the tumor is important and at times may alter how extensive the approach should be, especially for older patients. One may choose to preserve an extremity with poor margins of tumor resection if the lesion proves to be desmoid or an equivalent low-grade neoplasm. Low-grade sarcomas tend to offer an opportunity for en-bloc resection without compromising the extremity. Grade III or anaplastic sarcomas frequently require amputation for cure. Regardless of the grade, however, resection too close to the tumor margin or to the pseudocapsule does not bode well for cure. There is some suggestion that implanting the periphery of the tumor bed or periphery of the resection with radioisotopes (brachytherapy) or the use of high-dose external radiation therapy to the bed may reduce the incidence of local recurrence. In our experience, too many recurrences have followed such therapy, especially if the tumor is high-grade. As such, we have opted to use these methods only in very selected instances.

There is little question, even when dealing with grade III tumors, that the disease may be perfectly curable, especially if one can define normal and wide margins around the tumor. Here, one must use judgment aided by information from the CT scan and arteriograms, as well as clinical knowledge of the patterns of local spread, to estimate the width of resection about the tumor in order to ensure removal of all microscopic disease. One should recognize that lesions such as epithelioid sarcoma, embryonal rhabdomyosarcoma, and recurrent or advanced synovial sarcoma may travel to regional node-bearing areas. The surgeon must know which structures can be sacrificed—e.g., nerve, artery, bone—so that plans for possible nerve graft or en-bloc bone resection can be designed into the operative procedure. To obtain adequate margins, it may be necessary to include periosteum with overlying muscle. If the tumor approximates deep structures and is high-grade, however, the incidence of recurrence is usually high and simultaneous metastasis may be noted.

Local resection should be performed only when adequate margins free of tumor and distant from the periosteum of bone can be obtained. Healthy muscle and adjacent fat should be removed en-bloc when attempting to remove a tumor cleanly. When tumor approximates bone, removal of the periosteum is inadequate; resection of underlying bone, such as removal of the scapula for tumors in the region of the infraspinatus muscle, is usually necessary.

Clavicle

When a tumor encroaches on the clavicle, resection of that bone and occasionally of the node-bearing tissue of the lower neck will achieve adequate margins. When the tumor approaches the medial clavicle, adequate margins cannot be obtained unless a portion of the sternum and rib cage are removed. The sternum should be split longitudinally from the manubrium to at least the second interspace; the medial half of the clavicle is sectioned to include the underlying ribs and the surrounding pectoralis and intercostal muscles. En-bloc resection of the required portion of the chest wall is then accomplished with adequate surrounding normal tissue about the tumor. Stability is achieved with the use of Marlex mesh. This is essential because of the anatomic position of the medial clavicle—i.e., sitting adjacent to the sternum and on the first rib. Halstead's ligament is a good landmark to identify; the clavicle can be divided several centimeters lateral to the sternum. This allows identification of the underlying neurovascular bundle (Fig. 3–5). One should not

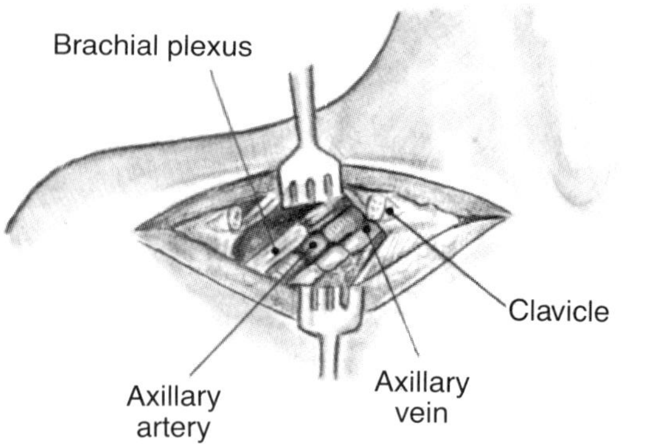

FIGURE 3–5. *Neurovascular bundle under site of resected clavicle.*

attempt to disarticulate the clavicle directly at the sternum, as the vessels arch up at this point and can be injured. Rather, the clavicle is divided somewhere just medial to its mid-third. The central portion of the clavicle is then elevated to expose the underlying vessels and now can be disarticulated from its sternal junction, carefully observing its proximity to vessels at all times. This technique is employed for high chest wall sternal resections, forequarter amputations, and the Tikhoff-Linberg reaction.[10]

Laterally placed tumors require that the acromion be resected along with clavicle. If one can save the central tendon of the deltoid to the outer clavicle, this will permit better shoulder function and radical clavicular surgery can still be performed. Once the clavicle has been removed, there is moderate functional impairment. We believe that if the adjacent musculature is brought together and the position of the shoulder is maintained without due stress on the sutures for a period of 3 months, then the shoulder will be remarkably strong, because the development of scar tissue required for adequate tensile strength necessitates that length of time to produce adequate function.

Hand-lifting or shoulder function that occurs too soon after repair of peripheral clavicular tissue will cause the tissue to stretch and pull out, resulting in shoulder function that may achieve only 50% of normal motion. If radiation therapy was previously employed and failed to control tumor growth, one can assume that healing will take longer and stress on the newly sutured tissue will be prolonged. Should fracture of the underlying clavicle occur, reduction can best be accomplished by using a Rush pin and drill holes placed medial and lateral to the lesion, so that cement can be poured over the pins. This will result in adequate stability with good shoulder function and relief from pain. The strength of the fracture treated by pinning and injection of methacrylate has been measured on cadaver bones and found to exceed twice the normal stress tolerance.

When soft tissue radiation has been initially employed, the underlying bone may develop osteoradionecrosis; bone fracture can then develop, resulting in penetration through the wound. This situation can be aggravated by the development of a "frozen" shoulder and further complications resulting from use of the arm on the affected side. Raising an object with rotation of the hand-elbow-humerus mechanism can cause further penetration of any fractured bone. A frozen shoulder under such circumstances will not resolve in the same manner as one that results from perforating fractured ends of the clavicle in resection of the head of the humerus. After this procedure, continuous narcotic therapy is required for relief of pain. Pain resulting from the rubbing ends of a fractured clavicle may also be handled by approaching the fracture above or below irradiated skin, then proceeding with excision (resection ends) of the fractured site. Attempts to do bone grafting at the site of resected irradiated bones will fail even with optimal fixation and mobilization. Should one be dealing with a pathologic fracture of the clavicle (Fig. 3–6*A*), one way to repair it is through a transverse incision along the clavicle after the biopsy. Holes are drilled into the bone proximally and distally, and a Rush pin is inserted (Fig. 3–6*B*). Cement is

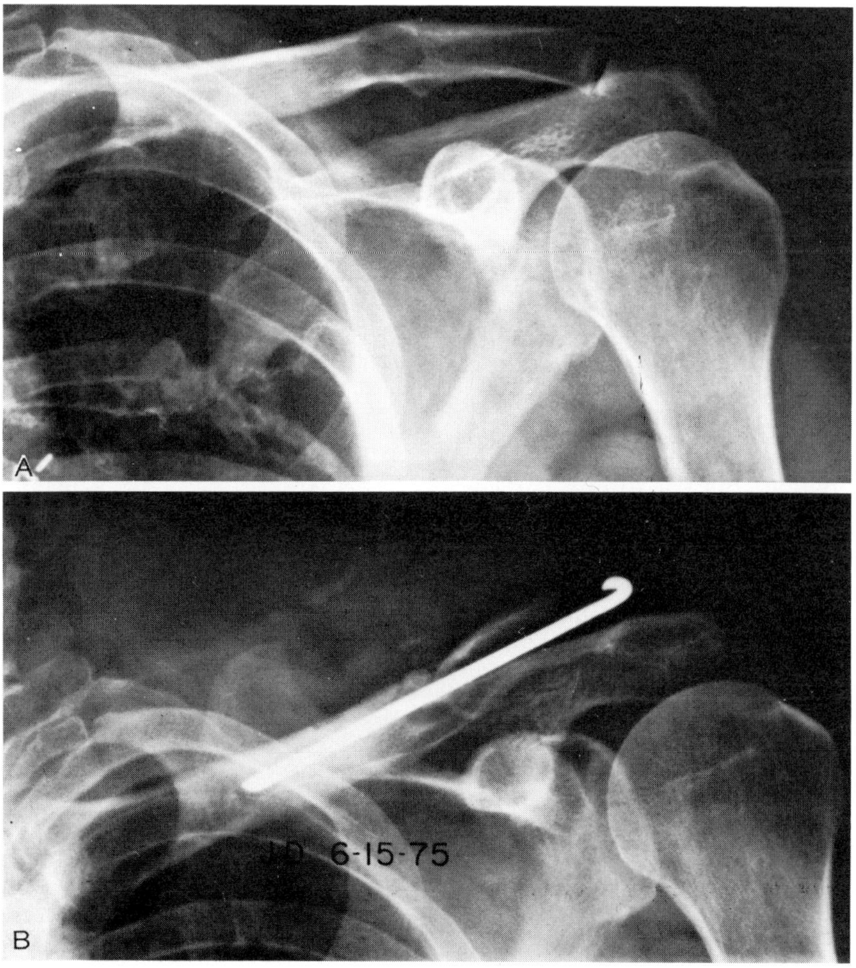

FIGURE 3–6. *A, Pathologic fracture of the left clavicle. B, Repair of fracture site with a Rush pin.*

then injected into the drill holes. No refractures have been found after this type of repair.

Scapulectomy

One should remember that occasionally primary soft tissue tumors are metastatic or inflammatory. Isolated soft tissue metastasis to the shoulder girdle can be seen with breast carcinoma (occult in the female patient), pulmonary lesions (metastatic squamous), renal cell carcinoma, and colon carcinoma. A 68-year-old man was first seen by us with a mass over the scapula. Biopsy proved the lesion to be a metastatic adenocarcinoma of the colon resulting from a bowel lesion that had been resected 2 years before and represented the only site for proven metastasis on work-up. A palliative scapulectomy was performed to control the pain.[15]

Scrofula of the axillary nodes may drain toward the clavicle with associated painful lesions; while not uncommon in the past, such lesions are now rare with the availability of anti-tuberculous therapy. Tumors sitting on the head of the humerus or at the glenohumeral joint are best treated by en-bloc resection of the entire glenohumeral joint and, if necessary, the adjacent clavicle. One should attempt as adequate a resection as necessary to encompass the tumor with normal surrounding tissue and, if necessary, underlying bone, with the goal of obtaining optimal function and reconstruction. If the area of the humeral head is infiltrated by high-grade neoplasm penetrating the subdeltoid coracoid bursa, one must envision extension throughout the entire bursa. Under this set of circumstances, the only effective way of managing the tumor is extensive en-bloc resection of the area to prevent unnecessary tumor spillage, which would result if limited glenohumeral resection were employed.

Tumors arise more frequently in the region of the supraspinatous and infraspinatous muscles than in any other sites about the shoulder girdle. Depending on the size of the tumor and its position, a portion of the scapula may be preserved by performing a muscle group dissection along with a partial scapulectomy. Here, good preservation of shoulder function is usually obtained since the glenoid cavity and rotator cuff remain intact. Most of the fully malignant sarcomas infiltrate the periosteum of the scapula and require total scapulectomy. Under such circumstances, the neurovascular bundle is preserved and forearm-hand function maintained, as with the (Marcove)-Tikhoff-Linberg resection.

Tikhoff-Linberg Resection

For tumors infiltrating the skin, the pectoralis or the deltopectoral myocutaneous flap can be used to close virtually any resulting cutaneous defect. A common error among many surgeons attempting resection is to be more concerned with retaining shoulder function than with assuring adequate margins of resection. Here the (Marcove)-Tikhoff-Linberg resection[11] allows the removal of the tumor with good margins and also preserves forearm function. With this procedure the neurovascular bundle is preserved, whereas it is sacrificed with a forequarter amputation.

It is important that adequate clearance of the neurovascular bundle be maintained. The end result of this procedure and others such as the scapulectomy is that postoperatively the patient can carry moderately heavy objects, use a fork and knife, and lace shoes and button shirts or blouses (Fig. 3–7). A description of the technique we employ can be found in the section on surgical amputative procedures.

Chest Wall Involvement

Tumors, on occasion, may arise from the chest wall or the ventral surface of the scapula. CT scanning can easily resolve the extent of invasion to the chest wall and the degree of scapular involvement. The procedure of choice under such circumstances is chest wall resection with scapulectomy; Marlex mesh is used to reconstruct the chest wall defect and maintain stability. Most patients require intubation and respiratory assistance for several days postoperatively. Eventually, moderate stability of the flail chest ensues. Huge areas of back musculature are easily sacrificed with minimal functional disability. Usually the patient notes some winging of the scapula, and it may be necessary to trim down the protuberant portion of the scapula. The limiting factor for resection in this area is the medial extension

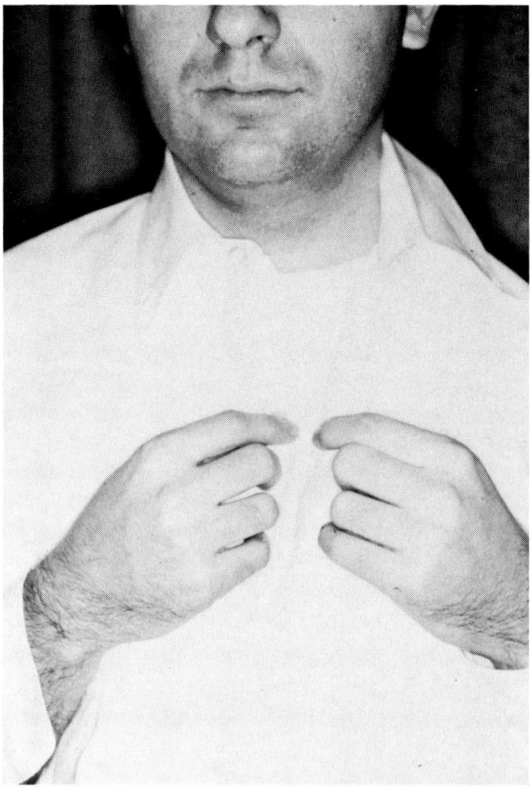

FIGURE 3–7. After scapulectomy, elbow function is retained, allowing patient to button his shirt.

of tumor to the region of the vertebral body and neural foramina. New techniques now allow the resection of portions of vertebral bodies. Marcove has developed a technique for repair of vertebral body defects by dowling into adjacent healthy bone and using fibular grafts for support, or by stabilizing the area with heavy Steinmann pins placed into healthy osseous structures. Methylmethacrylate can be injected along the spines to reinforce them.

Shoulder Function

In cases of resection of portions of the shoulder girdle that include the heads of the humerus, attempts have been made to insert a metal ball in place of the missing head. The only accomplishment here is an impressive x-ray film. No improvement in function is obtained, and the desired arm lengthening is not achieved. Ceramic devices have been used with no particular benefit. Figure 3–8 illustrates the placement of such a device at the time of a Tikhoff-Linberg resection of the upper end of the humerus. The authors now prefer to use a metallic prosthesis, such as a ground-down Neer shoulder prosthesis with a modified small head and flattened edges. Stabilization of the upper end of the humerus and prosthesis with surrounding muscle and fascia is worthwhile since it can improve flexion of the elbow. The results of various operative procedures we perform depend on the nature of the neoplasms that are resected—e.g., scapulectomy for most

FIGURE 3–8. Prosthetic replacement for the upper humerus during Tikhoff-Linberg resection.

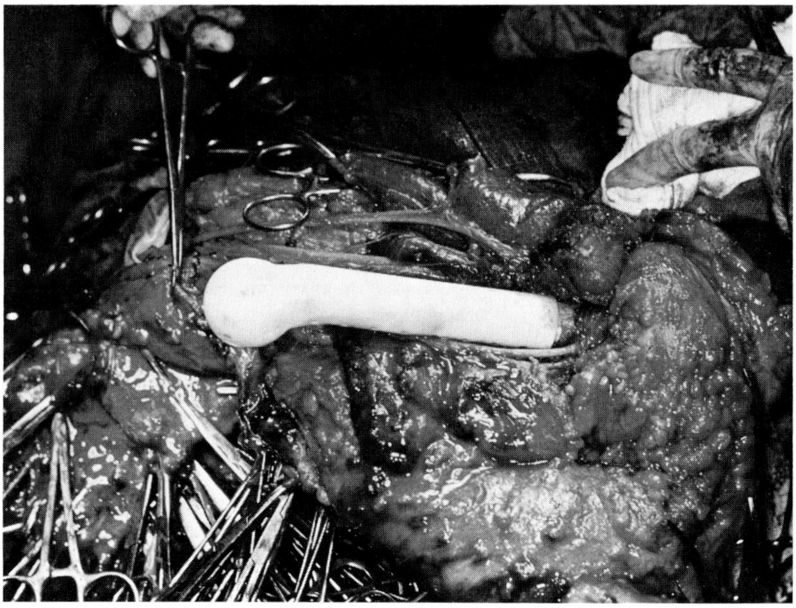

malignant synoviomas has been followed by rapid pulmonary dissemination. Other patients have survived after extensive resections for sarcoma, especially in cases of liposarcoma, well-localized adult rhabdomyosarcoma, and fibrosarcoma. In performing surgery in the region of the shoulder girdle, knowledge of the anatomy of the neurovascular bundle is essential since those tumors that approximate axillary structures or involve regional nodes in this area require en-bloc axillary node dissection. When chemotherapy and radiation therapy have been used preoperatively, the anatomy may be so distorted that the neurovascular structures can be compromised unless exceedingly careful, sharp dissection is used to enter the distorted anatomic planes. This problem is obviated with forequarter amputation since the vessels are ligated close to the chest wall and all node-bearing tissue is resected as part of the operative specimen. Several types of incisions have been employed for axillary dissection when axillary nodes are to be removed in a discontinuous procedure. When extensive nodal dissection is required, the procedure that Booher suggested was to employ an incision paralleling the axillary fold with a "T"-shaped extension coursing to the mid-clavicle to expose the pectoralis. We prefer a transverse axillary incision extending across the axillary folds from the pectoralis major to the latissimus dorsi (Fig. 3–9). Division of the pectoralis major to the clavicle can be accomplished when tumors in this region are bulky and require wider exposure. Dissection is performed sharply with a fine scalpel incision made into the adventitia over the axillary vessels. The tumor and nodes can then be swept inferiorly. Feeding vessels can be hemoclipped and further divided, thus freeing the tumor from the brachial plexus and axillary vessels. Long thoracic and subscapular nerves are preserved whenever possible. When the axillary vein is invaded or radiation necrosis has produced extensive edema in the face of viable tumor, amputation is probably in order. Further necrosis in this region secondary to progressive radiation effects usually results in a functionless arm or radiation arteritis with eventual vascular blowout. Forequarter amputation may be necessary to control vascular bleeding under such circumstances.

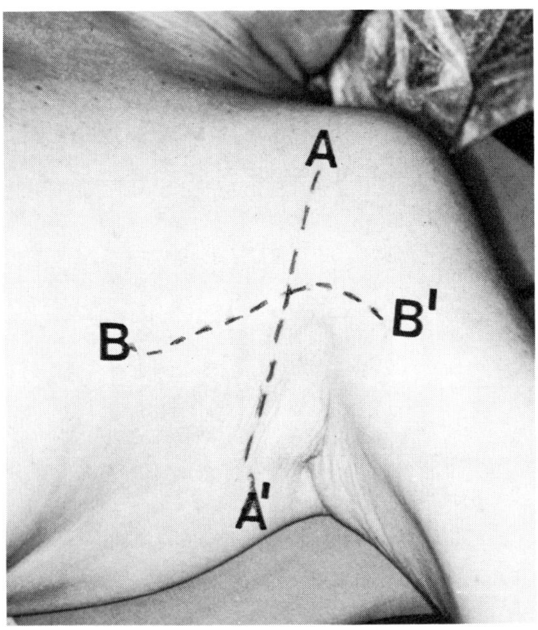

FIGURE 3–9. Approach to the axilla using the transverse axillary incision (A-A') in contrast to the classic incision paralleling the pectoralis fold (B-B').

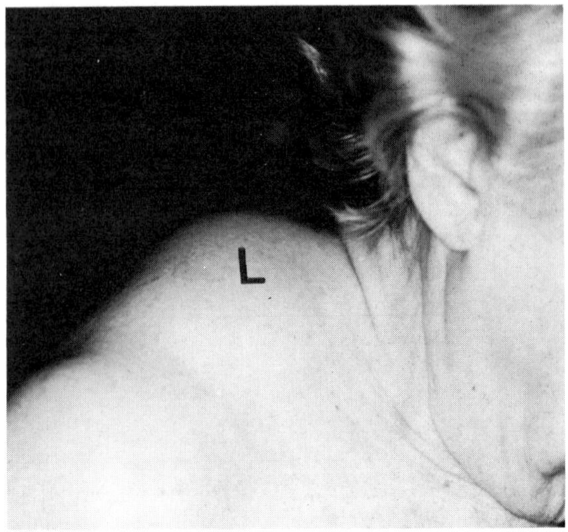

FIGURE 3–10. Lipoma (L) in the supraspinatus region.

PATTERNS OF TUMOR BEHAVIOR

The presence of an expanding firm tumor mass does not always signify that the lesion is sarcomatous. Frequently, benign fatty tumors arise in a closed subfascial space, which, when they expand, give the appearance of a firm tumor mass. This can occur in the area of the supraspinatus muscle (Fig. 3–10), or in the region of the intercostal

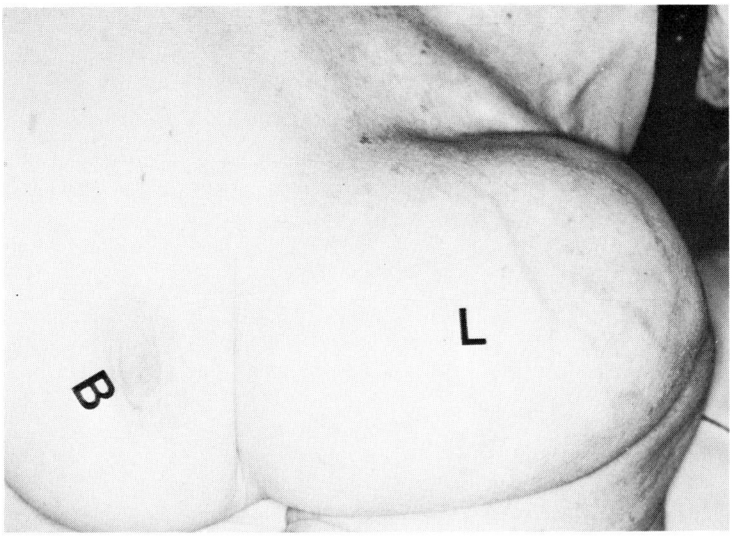

FIGURE 3–11. *Large lipomatous mass (L) arising in the region of the left anterior axillary fold above the breast (B).*

muscles under the female breast to suggest a deeply placed malignancy. As the tumor is approached and the fascia incised for biopsy purposes, the tumor pops out with its characteristic soft, yellowish appearance. Certain variants of the benign lipoma—especially the fibrolipoma, spindle cell lipoma, angiomyolipoma, and lipoblastoma—may clinically be confused with neoplasia. Lipoblastomas account for about 20% of the benign fatty tumors. Deep-seated lesions are the least common and tend to be larger than the cutaneous tumors. In the extremities they may arise from subperiosteal tissue or from juxta-articular margins. At times the lipomas of the chest wall–shoulder girdle may be enormous; Figure 3–11 shows a large benign lipomatous mass over the tail of the breast extending onto the shoulder girdle. Other large diffuse masses are seen with lymphomas of extranodal origin infiltrating soft tissue (Fig. 3–12) and giant cell tumors of osseous origin infiltrating the soft tissue of this region (Fig. 3–13).

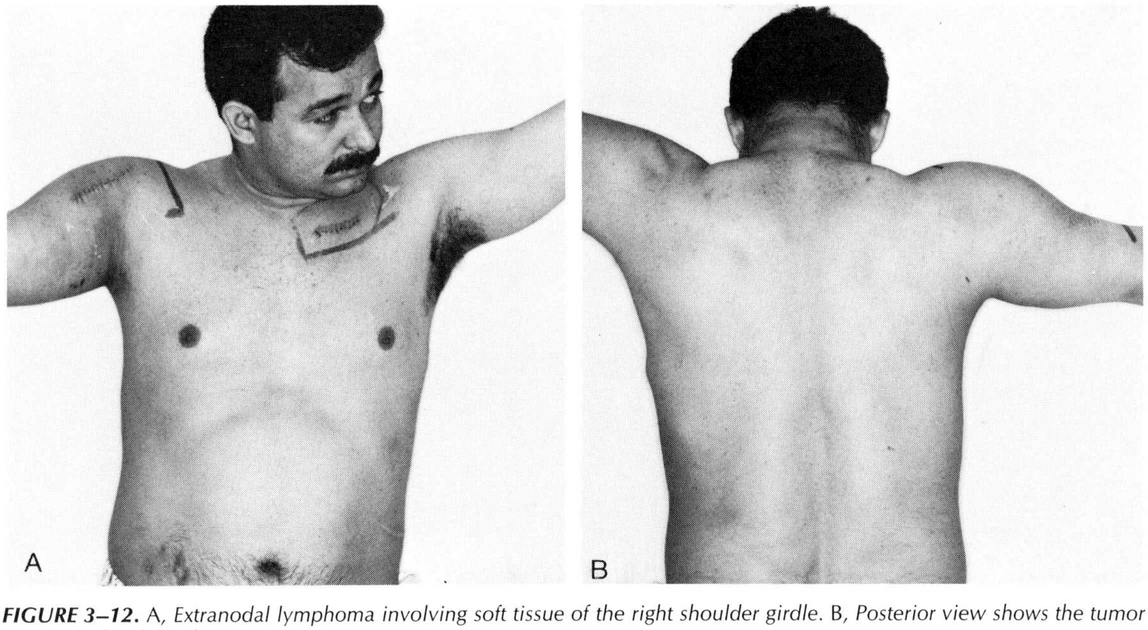

FIGURE 3–12. *A, Extranodal lymphoma involving soft tissue of the right shoulder girdle. B, Posterior view shows the tumor involving the deltoid region.*

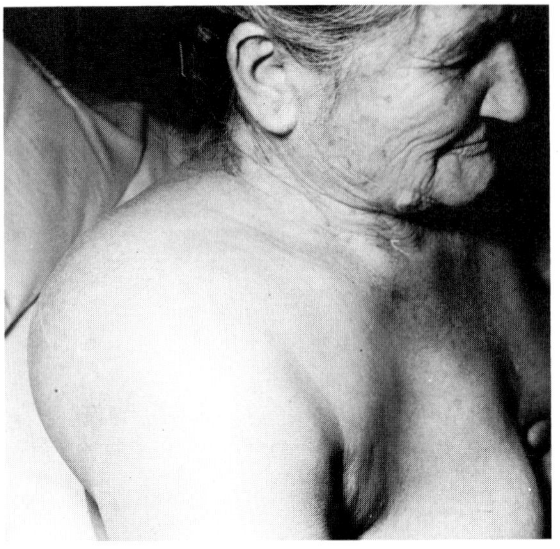

FIGURE 3–13. *Giant cell tumor of the right shoulder.*

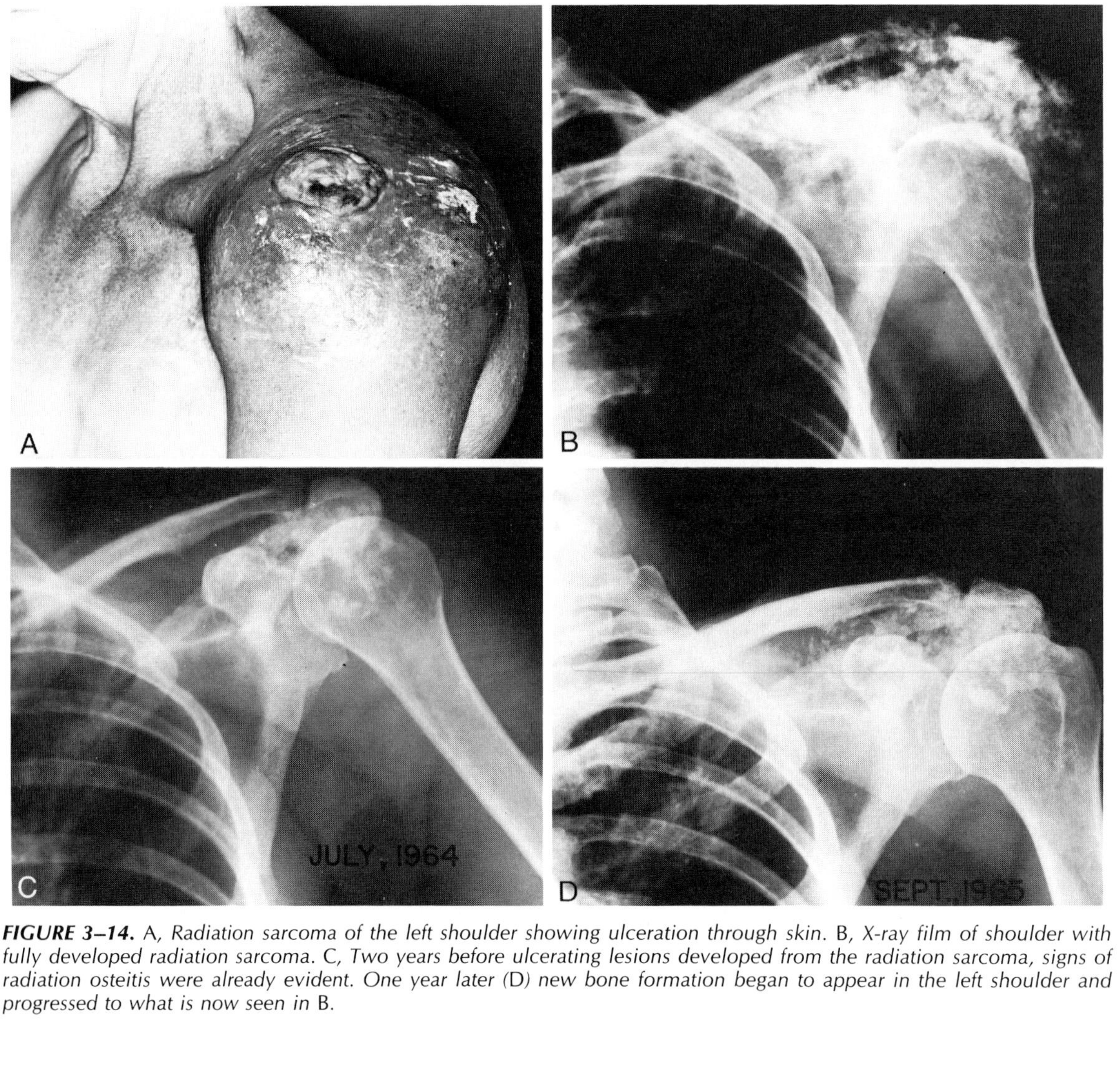

FIGURE 3–14. *A, Radiation sarcoma of the left shoulder showing ulceration through skin. B, X-ray film of shoulder with fully developed radiation sarcoma. C, Two years before ulcerating lesions developed from the radiation sarcoma, signs of radiation osteitis were already evident. One year later (D) new bone formation began to appear in the left shoulder and progressed to what is now seen in B.*

In certain instances a large soft tissue mass represents extension of soft tissue from a bone primary that may have resulted or been induced by prior radiation therapy. Figure 3–14*A* shows a large soft tissue mass with multiple cutaneous ulcerations secondary to breakdown of the overlying skin due to tumor and radiation necrosis. Radiography of the shoulder girdle (Fig. 3–14 *B* to *D*) shows the characteristic pattern of neoplastic new bone formation being laid down in the soft tissue component of the tumor. A review of previous x-ray films revealed that progression of disease from radiation osteitis to the present disease process had taken place over 3 years. Arlen et al.[1] evaluated radiation osteitis in 28 patients treated at Memorial Hospital between 1957 and 1970. Thirteen of these patients had soft part tumors as well as visceral lesions treated by radiation therapy. In 1957 Cruz and Coley[5] described 7 of 11 cases in which soft tissue primary tumors—including Hodgkin's disease, breast carcinoma, retinoblastoma, seminoma, hygroma, and squamous carcinoma of the head and neck—manifested malignant transformation of the underlying bone that was exposed to radiation therapy.

In the Memorial Hospital series[1] of radiation-induced tumors there were four cases of osteosarcoma arising as a result of radiation therapy for breast carcinoma: the clavicle was invaded in one patient, the scapula in another, and two patients eventually developed osteogenic sarcoma of the humerus. Osteogenic sarcoma eventually developed in the pubic bone of two patients with carcinoma of the cervix treated by radiation therapy. All of these patients had been cured of the primary lesion at the time of the appearance of the osteogenic sarcoma.

The histologic pattern that we see with these rare tumors is the same one that is seen with the conventional sarcomas. Profuse bone and tumor osteoid formation was always present. The pattern was intermixed with occasional areas of anaplastic spindle and giant cell sarcoma associated with exuberantly growing fibroblastic cells of aberrant shapes and forms.

Five patients underwent interscapulothoracic amputations: two had rib resections, one a laminectomy, and one a partial sacrectomy. The survival rate for patients who underwent surgery alone has been better than 30%.

When recurrence is noted following attempted ablation, the interval from primary treatment to recurrence is usually short and can be recognized within a 20-month period. The most common site for recurrence is at the amputation site or in the lung fields.

A possible sequence of events in radiation carcinogenesis was described by Cole,[5] who attempted to incorporate many complex interactions at the subcellular, cellular, and organic levels. The first step necessitates production of specific genetic alterations (possibly oncogene-derived) in one of a small number of irradiated cells. This effect may be produced directly by the action of radiation therapy on the genetic apparatus or indirectly by primary damage to extragenetic sites or activation of a latent virus. More recent studies have implicated factors such as dose rate and radiation quality.

SURGICAL PROCEDURES

Forequarter Amputation

Forequarter amputation has been the primary procedure for managing large sarcomas on and about the shoulder girdle. Among the more common malignant lesions that have required this form of surgery is the extra-abdominal desmoid.[6] A 48-year-old black woman was initially examined for a nodular tumor mass of the left shoulder. After wide resection, several nodules were noted in the region of biopsy excision site. The tumor proved to be an extra-abdominal desmoid. Numerous biopsies taken proximally and distally showed recurrent tumor spreading centripetally (Fig. 3–15*A*). Based on these findings, a forequarter amputation was performed. Any attempt at preserving her arm would have failed because of the diffuse spread of this low-grade fibrosarcoma into adjacent fascial planes. Such tumors have been seen to invade the mediastinum. Should the tumor have recurred only as a discrete nodular mass and other biopsies been negative, then a second wide resection, if not muscle group dissection, could have been employed. The postoperative appearance of the patient is shown in Figure 3–15*B* and *C*.

The term "desmoid tumor" was introduced by Mueller in 1838 to describe the tendon-like consistency of the tumor. In con-

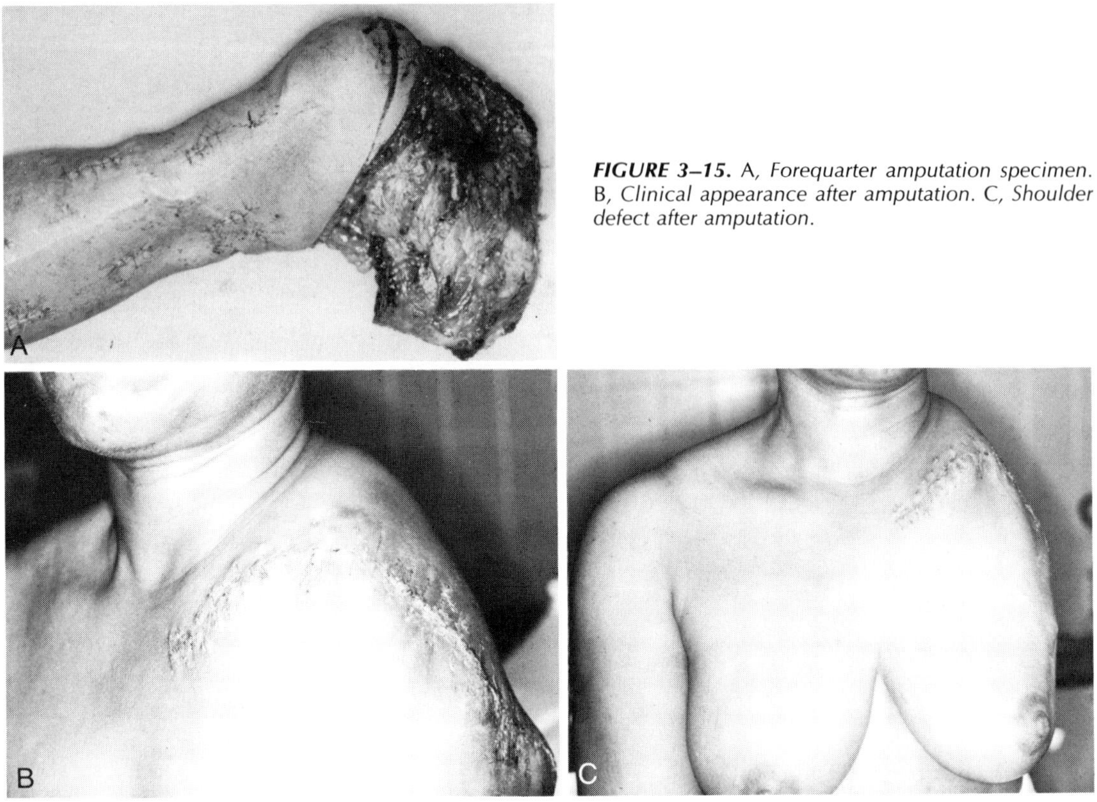

FIGURE 3–15. A, Forequarter amputation specimen. B, Clinical appearance after amputation. C, Shoulder defect after amputation.

trast to many of the fibrous tumors, these lesions are found to diffusely infiltrate the fascial and aponeurotic structures. They tend to be locally invasive with a high degree of recurrence when not completely removed. Giant cells are seen at the periphery of the zone of infiltration and are considered to represent muscle cell degeneration, with the remaining nuclei forming the giant cells (Fig. 3–16). The abdominal wall is the most common site, the frequency being three times that of extra-abdominal sites. Most extra-abdominal lesions occur around the shoulder girdle, but they can be found around the pectoralis major and buccinator muscles.

The proper management of extra-abdominal desmoid is critical when tumor approximates the major neurovascular structures. Otherwise, conservative wide resection can be employed so long as incisional biopsy suggests wide margins of removal have been achieved. Bone should be biopsied when it is suspected that the lesion infiltrates deeply. Resection of segments of long bones with prosthetic replacement may be necessary if it appears that the extremity can be saved. Vascular structures should be dissected free of tumor and nerves preserved by dissection within the perineurium. It is important that attempts be made to take biopsy specimens of the margins of resection at the time of surgery. While local recurrence of inadequately resected lesions is not uncommon, it takes many years for untreated recurrence to spread centripetally to involve central vital structures. In one case in which desmoid was dissected from the perineural sheath of the sciatic nerve and dissection was carried above the sciatic notch, the patient was free of disease 7 years after resection with no evidence of abdominal visceral involvement.

El-Domeri and Miller[7] reported results of the treatment of 105 patients undergoing forequarter (interscapulothoracic) amputation at Memorial Hospital. In 91 of the patients, surgery was performed for primary malignant tumors. Forty of the patients had soft part sarcomas in this series. In 79% of the patients, the tumor was located in the upper arm, axilla, or shoulder joint. The classic procedures were performed in 92 patients, for curative purposes in 85 and for palliation in 7. In 13 patients the operative procedure was extended to include adjacent regions, e.g., en-bloc radical mastectomy, ipsilateral neck dissection, and chest wall resection. The extension of the primary operation was performed to encompass all gross disease. When the tumor has extended over the superior or anterior aspect of the shoulder joint, the main approach to control of the neurovascular bundle will have been compromised. In this instance, Nadler and Phelan[13] have described a technique of entering the pleural cavity through the bed of the second rib to reach to the subclavian vessels and brachial plexus.

Holleb and Lucas[8] reported on six patients with breast carcinoma in whom failure to control disease in the axilla following radiation therapy led to a situation of necrosis and impending vascular necrosis. Forequarter amputation was employed for palliative purposes.

In 1737 Samuel Wood sustained a traumatic avulsion of the upper extremity and scapula when he was caught in the rope of his mill wheel; he was successfully treated at St. Thomas Hospital, London. Mosley described this case and illustrated this patient's appearance among 68 traumatic cases that occurred during the period from 1737 to 1956. The first surgical removal of an arm and shoulder girdle was performed for a gunshot wound by an English Naval surgeon in the 1820s. The first interscapulothoracic amputation for a malignant growth was performed by Crosby, an American surgeon in 1836. He removed an osteosarcoma that weighed 25 lb; the patient survived 28 months. Paul Berger's 1887 monograph detailed all aspects of the operation, so the operation is commonly attributed to him. Mosley considered Berger's work to be the basis for most writings since then. It covered the history, indications, and technique and stressed the preliminary ligation of the subclavian artery and vein, which had been described by Ollier in 1885. LeConte (1899, 1901, 1902) advised removal of the sternal end of the clavicle, in contrast to Berger's classic resection of the middle third of the clavicle and subperiosteal vascular ligation. Kocher (1895) advocated exposure of the subclavian vessels via an inferior approach through the costocoracoid membrane by prior resection of the pectoral muscles. Knoggs first described the Littlewood, or posterior, approach. Mosley considered the posterior approach capable of allowing faster execution of the procedure, except where en-bloc lymph node dissection of the base of the neck is required.[12] In the 1940 edition of Pack's encyclopedic volumes, there is a very lucid description of the procedure by Brunschwig. In 1961 Pack and McGraw[14] described the procedure for interscapulothoracic amputation and reviewed results of 109 cases. Byron et al.[3] reviewed seven patients who underwent surgery for soft part sarcoma. Adjuvant chemotherapy was ad-

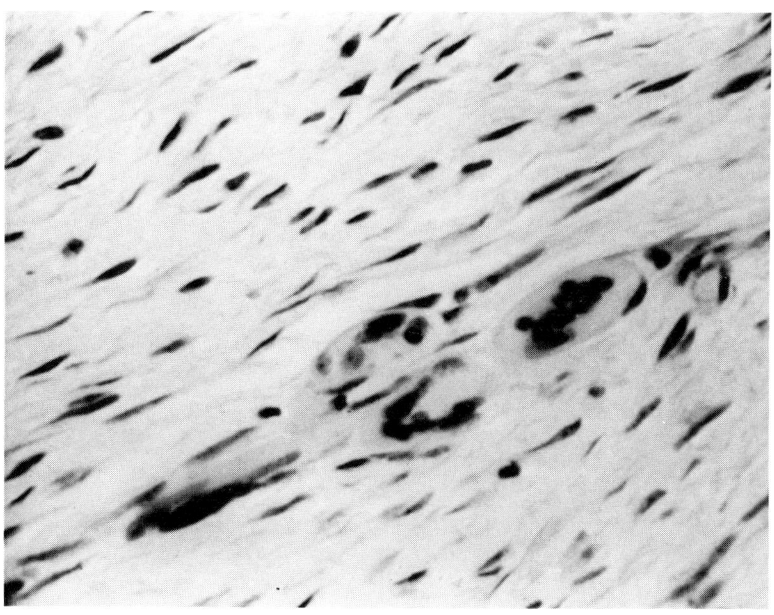

FIGURE 3–16. *Desmoid tumor infiltrating muscle at the periphery of the tumor.*

ministered intra-arterially, the axillary vessels having been exposed through an approach to the shoulder girdle. If the clavicle were involved by tumor, it would be taken at the junction with the sternum; otherwise it would be divided at the junction of the proximal and middle thirds.

The spread of tumor through the chest wall was considered to be a contraindication to performing forequarter amputation until Stafford and Williams[17] described the radical transthoracic forequarter amputation. A variation of this procedure was described by Wurlitzer[19] for recurrent sarcoma, where a major portion of the upper chest wall and upper sternum and the upper lobe of one lung were successfully removed en bloc with forequarter amputation.

When forequarter amputation is utilized for primary control of disease, approximately 30 to 40% of patients can be cured. En-bloc and Tikhoff-Linberg resections have been used whenever possible in an attempt to leave a functioning forearm and hand. Other procedures have also been employed with local disease that appears not to involve the neurovascular bundle. A 30-year-old man had been followed for a mass present over the scapula. The lesion had not increased in size for 1 year and had initially been considered to be a lipoma by his physician. When the tumor was finally biopsied (Fig. 3–17*A*), it proved to be a fully malignant fibrosarcoma, deeply infiltrating the muscles and extending through the periosteum of the scapula. A total scapulectomy was performed (Fig. 3–17*B*) with preservation of function in the forearm (Fig. 3–17*C* and *D*). The type of defect in the operative field with scapulectomy is seen in Figure

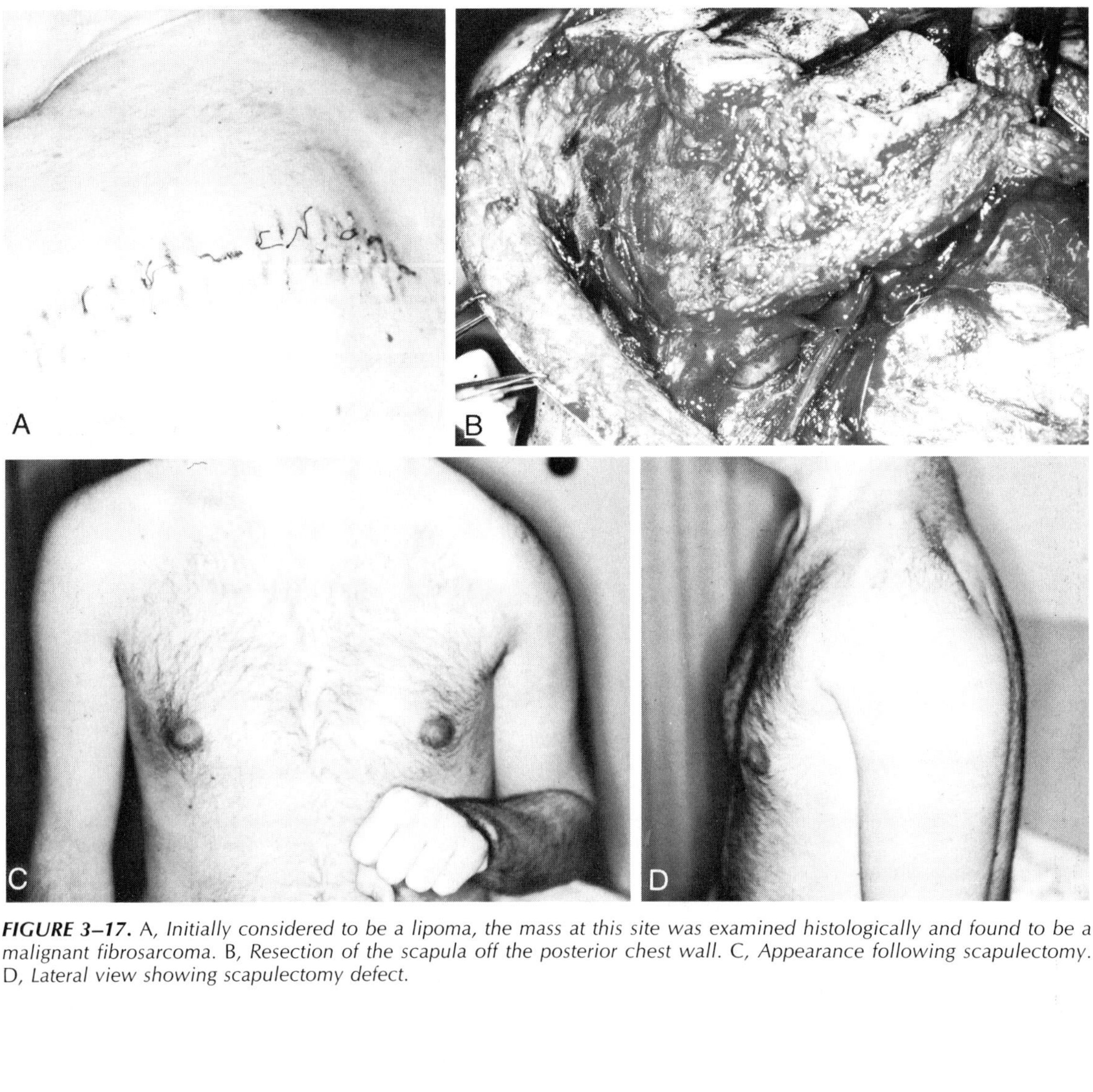

FIGURE 3–17. *A, Initially considered to be a lipoma, the mass at this site was examined histologically and found to be a malignant fibrosarcoma. B, Resection of the scapula off the posterior chest wall. C, Appearance following scapulectomy. D, Lateral view showing scapulectomy defect.*

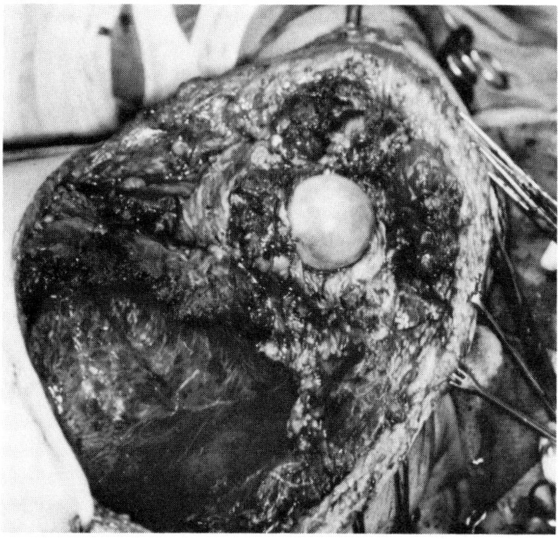

FIGURE 3–18. Operative defect showing the humeral head.

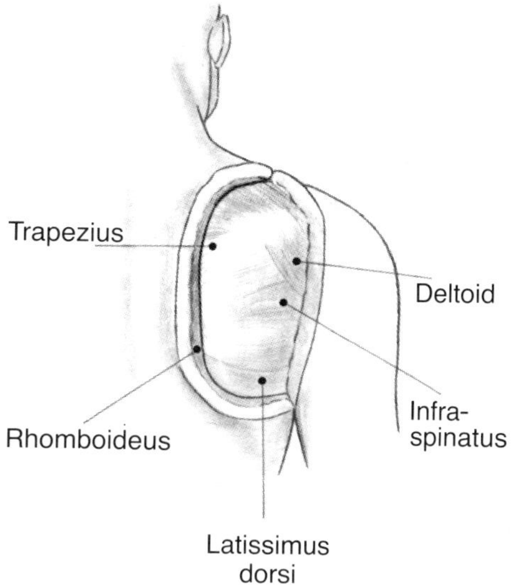

FIGURE 3–20. Muscles to be exposed and transected during scapulectomy, Tikhoff-Linberg resection, and forequarter amputation.

3–18. Here the posterior rib cage is clearly defined and head of the humerus identified prior to its fixation to the chest wall. The technique for suspension of the humerus has been described by Burnel.[2] Scapulectomy has been the ideal procedure when tumors such as the synovioma arise on the scapula. Samilson has described the array of neoplasms in this region.[16] Figure 3–19 shows the appearance of a transected specimen, exposing tumor as it infiltrates the muscles down to the periosteum of the scapula. Figure 3–20 illustrates the exposed muscles on the back that must be divided prior to scapulectomy, Tikhoff-Linberg resection, and forequarter amputation.

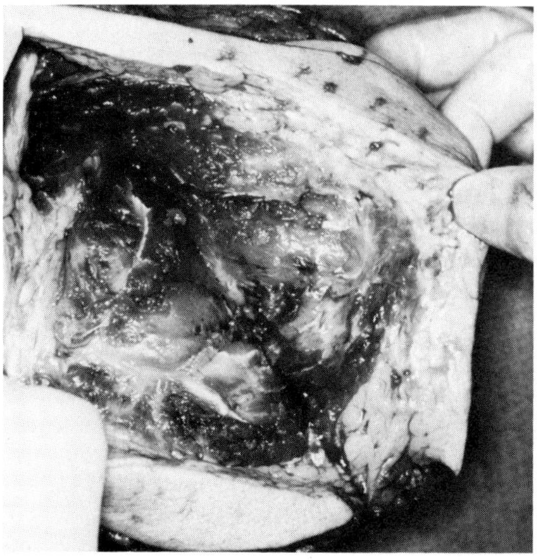

FIGURE 3–19. Scapulectomy specimen exposing synovioma invading the surface of the scapula.

Tikhoff-Linberg Resection

The Tikhoff-Linberg resection has gradually become the primary modification among shoulder resections to be considered when attempting to preserve arm function.[9] It supercedes scapulectomy when shoulder girdle neoplasms approximate the glenoid cavity or even involve the humeral head. Although such a resection results in loss of shoulder function, it does preserve axillary vessels and the branchial plexus so that the elbow can be fully flexed and full forearm and hand function remains.

A 36-year-old white man was admitted for evaluation and treatment of a large shoulder mass. There was a 7-year history of pain and swelling in the left shoulder and a working diagnosis of bursitis or tenosynovitis, or both. In the several months prior to admission the patient noted a rapid increase in the size of the swelling and increased pain in the area. Past medical history and review of systems were unremarkable. Physical examination revealed a well-developed, well-nourished patient in no acute distress; the left shoulder had limited motion. A very firm tender mass (11 by 7 cm) was palpable over and firmly attached to the left scapula, moving with that structure. Abduction in the left upper extremity was limited to 90° secondary to pain and muscle infiltration. There was no evidence of neurovascular compromise in the extremity.

Review of x-ray films taken over the past 7 years revealed the presence of a slowly enlarging lytic lesion of the left scapula with eventual appearance of an overlying soft tissue mass (Fig. 3–21*A*). The lytic lesion was smooth-walled and adjacent to the glenoid cavity, giving the appearance of a benign cyst. A left selective subclavian arteriogram revealed a highly vascular soft tissue mass of 10 to 15 cm, which was suggestive of a primary vascular tumor (Fig. 3–21*B* and *C*). Blood supply was derived by way of branches from the thyrocervical trunk, directly from the third portion of the subclavian artery, and from the axillary artery. The central portion of the tumor showed marked neovascularization with early draining veins. CT scan revealed a large homogeneous soft tissue mass arising from the left scapula. No calcification could be seen within the lesion. Enhancement with contrast material was diffuse and nonspecific. Biopsy (Fig. 3–21*D*) confirmed the highly vascular nature of the lesion. Exact histopathologic diagnosis could not be made from the biopsy, but the differential diagnosis was consistent with a malignant connective tissue neoplasm, possibly hemangiopericytoma.

The patient subsequently underwent primary resection of the tumor by Tikhoff-Linberg resection (Fig. 3–21*E*). Control of blood supply was obtained with preservation of the neurovascular bundle. The tumor was found to involve the scapula, specifically in the area of the glenohumeral joint, with extension into a major portion of the joint and surrounding muscle, and with fixation to the deltoid muscle and rotator cuff. En-bloc resection was accomplished by scapulectomy, muscle group dissection, and removal of upper humerus and glenoid (Tikhoff-Linberg). Preservation of the neurovascular bundle allowed for virtually complete function of the forearm and hand. Mobilization of the scapula off the chest wall is shown in Figure 3–21*F*. The opened specimen shows tumor in approximation to the head of the humerus (Fig. 3–21*G*). The postoperative course was uneventful.

This tumor, which is primarily a soft part sarcoma, is most commonly found in the lower extremity and retroperitoneum. Among the 106 cases seen at the Armed Forces Institute of Pathology, 37 were in the lower limb and 26 in the retroperitoneum. It was defined as a distinct entity by Stout and Murray[17a] in 1942. The increased vascularity of the tumor may be associated with pulsation and bruit, but this was not felt in this patient. Many of the tumors have a benign clinical course, even in the face of pulmonary metastasis, which can progress slowly over many years. The tumor, however, may be very aggressive. In one patient in whom a lesion of the rectus and abdominis had been removed, a solitary pulmonary metastasis was noted prior to discharge from the hospital and required resection. However, progressive disease occurred and the patient died within 1 year of the abdominal resection. Late metastasis with this tumor is not uncommon and can occur 5 years after the primary surgery. Radiation therapy is occasionally found to be of some benefit in controlling local recurrence.

The occurrence of this tumor in bone is relatively infrequent; six patients have been treated at Memorial Hospital, and pain was the most common complaint. Both the femur and humerus were affected in two cases. Three died of widely disseminated disease. As with the soft tissue lesion, morphology of the tumor in terms of cellular pleomorphism and mitotic activity can probably be correlated with clinical behavior. A 70-year-old man had originally presented with a malignant fibrous histiocytoma in the gastrocnemius muscle. The tumor had been locally resected, only to reappear in the right shoulder. Approximately 1 year after leg surgery he had symptoms of bursitis in the shoulder. A routine x-ray film revealed destruction of the humoral head, glenoid cavity, and scapula (Fig. 3–22*A*). An angiogram showed displacement of major vessels (Fig. 3–22*B*). Because this was a second lesion it was believed that amputation (forequarter) might be avoided. This patient presented us with our first opportunity to perform the Tikhoff-Linberg resection. The specimen is seen in Figure 3–22*C*, and the postoperative appearance of the patient in Figure 3–22*D*. Because the patient remained free of disease with no evidence of local recurrence, this operation initiated the series that was to be performed at Memorial Hospital.

Another patient was treated for a large sarcoma in the left upper arm. At surgery the radial nerve had to be resected with the tumor. This patient underwent forearm

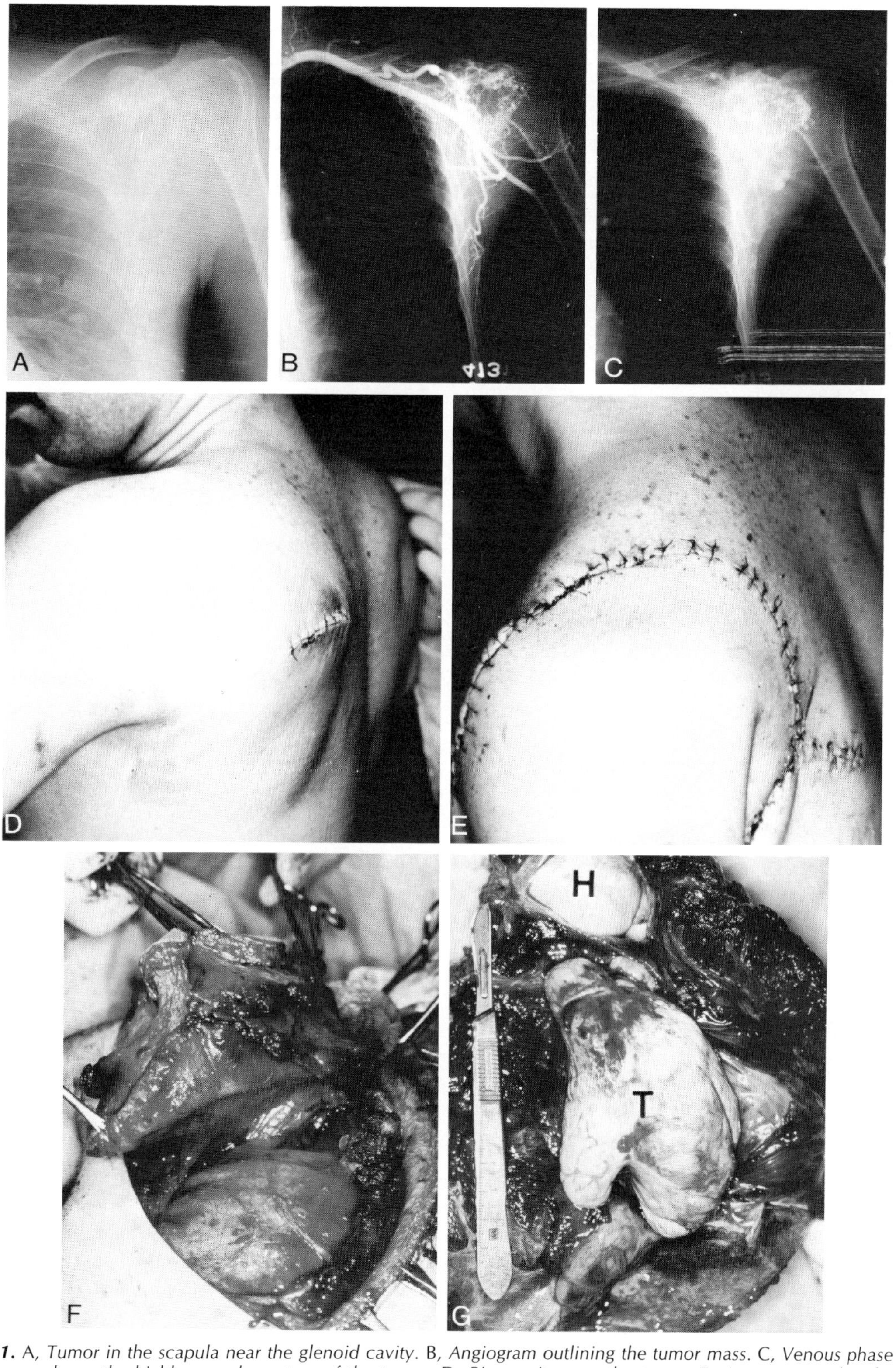

FIGURE 3–21. *A, Tumor in the scapula near the glenoid cavity. B, Angiogram outlining the tumor mass. C, Venous phase of the angiogram shows the highly vascular nature of the tumor. D, Biopsy site over the tumor. E, Appearance after the Tikhoff-Linberg resection. F, Mobilization of the scapula in the initial stage of the Tikhoff-Linberg resection. G, Specimen showing proximity of the tumor (T) to the humeral head (H).*

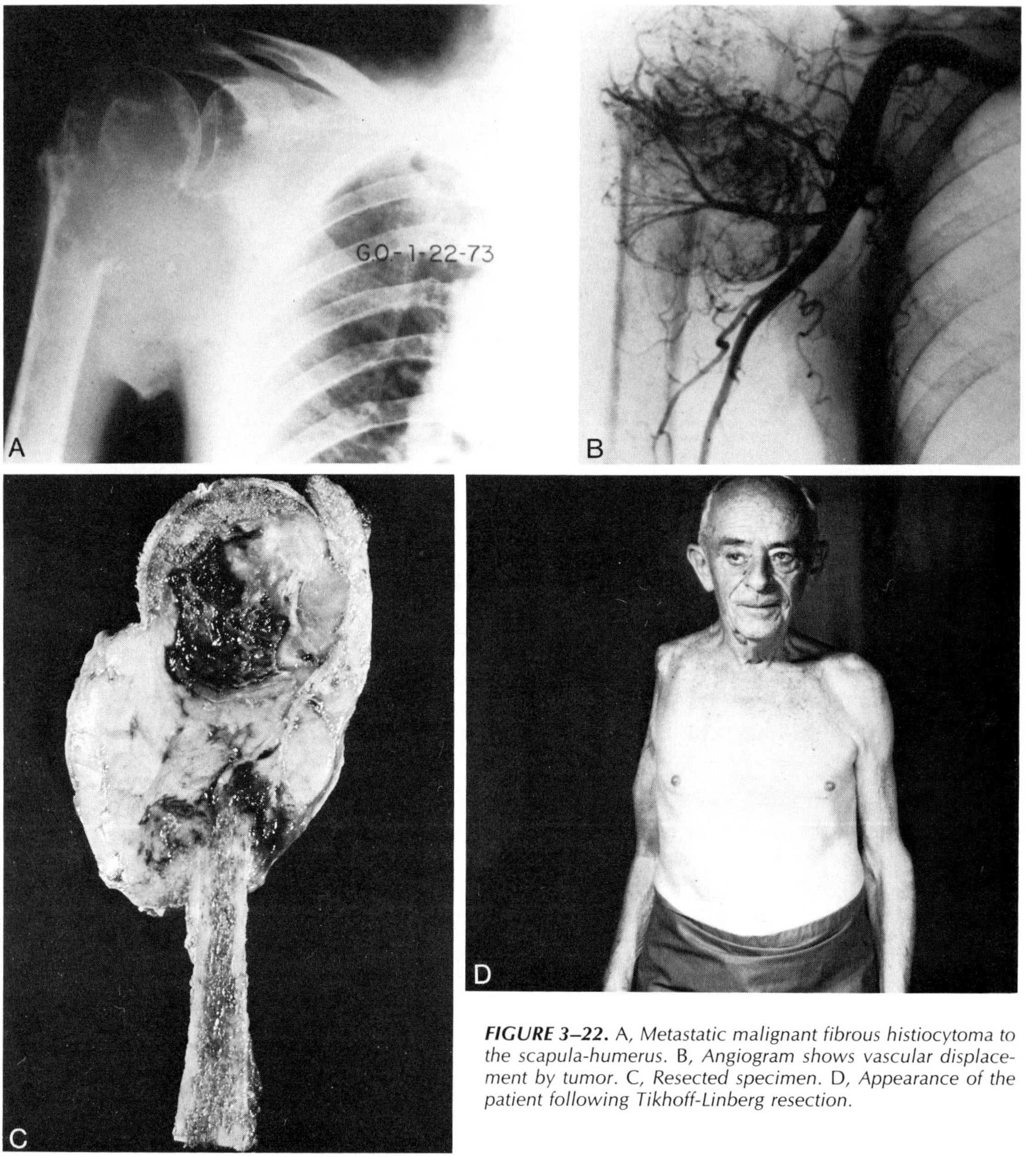

FIGURE 3–22. A, Metastatic malignant fibrous histiocytoma to the scapula-humerus. B, Angiogram shows vascular displacement by tumor. C, Resected specimen. D, Appearance of the patient following Tikhoff-Linberg resection.

flexor muscle transfer to prevent wrist drop (Fig. 3–23*A* and *B*), and this allowed him to discard his brace. Six years later a solitary intracardiac metastasis developed, and the patient died 2 years later. Because of the short residual humerus, elbow flexion was weak. Figure 3–23*C* shows the radiologic appearance of the residual resected end of the humerus after an extensive resection of a major portion of the humerus along with tumor. A Küntscher rod was placed into the remaining distal end. The upper end of the rod was fixed to the chest wall, allowing greater elbow strength on flexion, which is essential when this much humerus is removed. Whitehill et al. have described an improved technique for reconstruction after such surgery.[18]

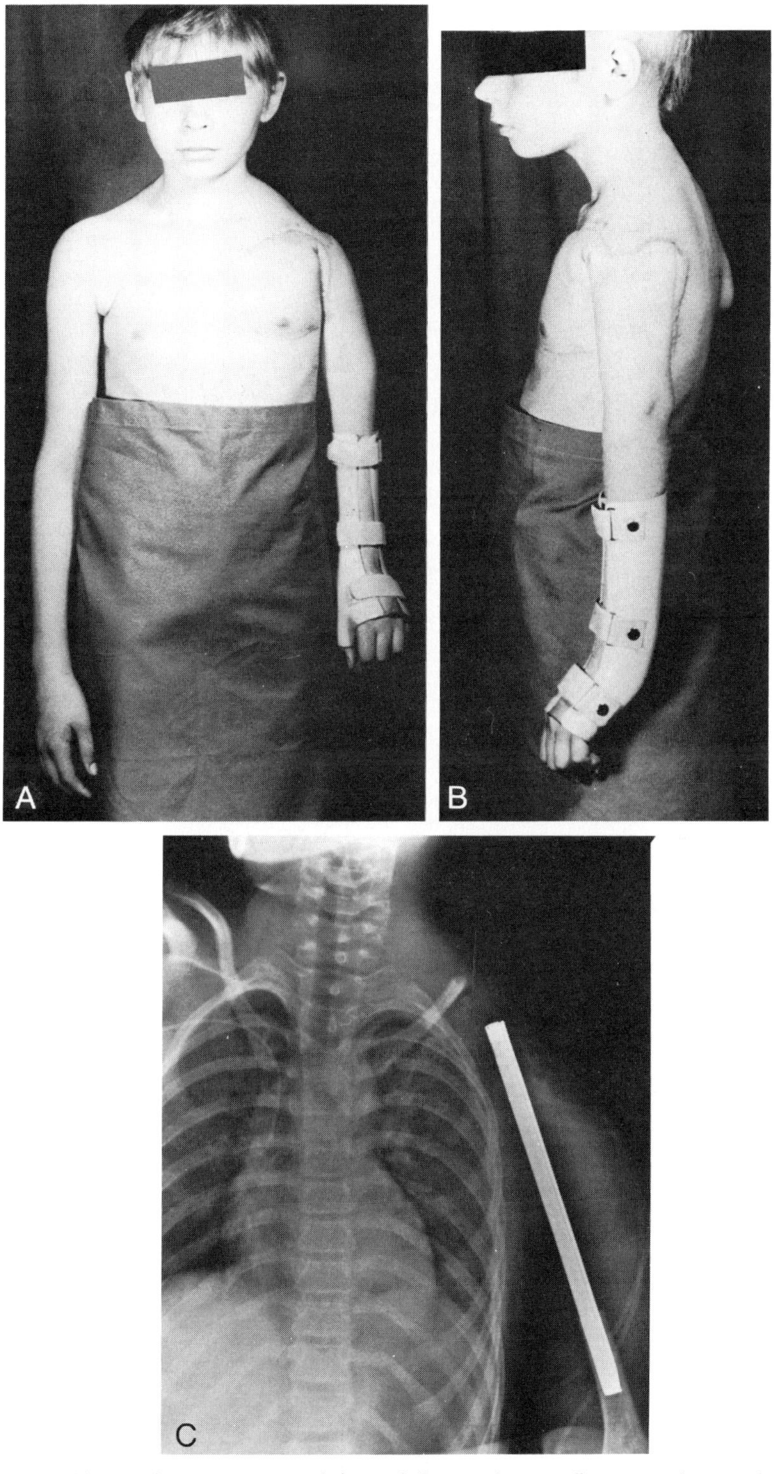

FIGURE 3–23. *A and B, Tikhoff-Linberg resection with brace following forearm flexor muscle transplant. C, Küntscher rod in remaining portion of the humerus to provide length.*

REFERENCES

1. Arlen M., Higinbotham N. L., Huvos A. G., et al.: Radiation-induced sarcoma of bone. Cancer 28:1087–1099, 1971
2. Burnel H. N.: Resection of the shoulder with humeral suspension for sarcoma involving the scapula. J. Bone Joint Surg. [Br] 47:300–303, 1965
3. Byron R. L., Cronemiller P. D., Bierman H. R., Yonomoto R. H.: Interscapulothoracic amputation and sacroiliac disarticulation with adjunctive arterial chemotherapy. Surg. Gynecol. Obstet. 111: 457–463, 1960
4. Cole L. T., Nowell P. C.: Radiation carcinogenesis: Sequence of events. Science 150:1782–1786, 1965
5. Cruz M., Coley B. L.: Post-irradiation bone sarcoma. Cancer 10:72–88, 1957
6. Das Gupta T. K., Brasfield R. D., Ohara J.: Extra-abdominal desmoids: A clinico-pathologic study. Ann. Surg. 170:109–121, 1969
7. El-Domeiri A. A., Miller T.: The role of interscapulothoracic amputation in the treatment of malignant tumors. Surg. Gynecol. Obstet. 129:1203–1206, 1969
8. Holleb A. I., Lucas J. C.: Palliative interscapulothoracic amputation in the management of breast cancer patients. Cancer 12:643, 1959
9. Linberg B. E.: Interscapulo-thoracic resection for malignant tumors of the shoulder joint region. J. Bone Joint Surg. 10:344–349, 1928
10. Marcove R. C.: Neoplasms of the shoulder girdle. Orthop. Clin. North Am. 6:541–551, 1975
11. Marcove R. C., Lewis M. M., Huvos A. C.: En-bloc upper humeral interscapulothoracic amputation: The Tikhoff-Linberg procedure. Clin. Orthop. 124:219–228, 1977
12. Mosley H. F.: The Forequarter Amputation. Edinburgh, E.S. Livingston Ltd., 1957
13. Nadler S. H., Phelan J. T.: A technique of interscapulothoracic amputation Surg. Gynecol. Obstet. 22:359–364, 1966
14. Pack G. T., McGraw T. A.: Interscapulothoracic amputation for malignant melanoma. Arch. Surg. 83:694–699, 1961
15. Ramirez J., Arlen M., Jordain L. M.: Total scapulectomy for soft part tumors of the shoulder girdle. Surgery 69:271–275, 1971
16. Samilson R. L., Morris J. M., Thompson R. W.: Tumors of the scapula. Clin. Orthop. 58:105–115, 1968
17. Stafford, E. S., Williams G. R.: Radical transthoracic forequarter amputation. Ann. Surg. 148:699, 1958

17a. Stout A.P., Murray M.R.: Hemangiopericytoma: A vascular tumor featuring Zimmerman's pericytes. Ann. Surg. 116:26, 1942.

18. Whitehill R., Wanebo H. J., Mabie K. N., et al.: Reconstruction after the Tikhoff-Linberg procedure. Arch. Surg. 117:1248–1249, 1982
19. Wurlitzer F. P.: Improved technique for radical transthoracic forequarter amputation. Ann. Surg. 177:467–471, 1973

CHAPTER

4

Tumors of the Upper Extremity

Sarcomas that involve the upper extremity are not as frequent as sarcomas of the lower extremity. Such lesions must be suspected in the differential diagnosis of any firm mass found in relationship to the neurovascular bundles or muscular groups of the arm and forearm. For the purpose of this discussion, those tumors that occur on or about the shoulder girdle will be treated as separate entities, since the surgical approaches that are required to manage them are separate and distinct. The tumors of the arm arise in two distinct areas: (1) the upper arm below the deltoid, to the region above the elbow, and (2) the forearm, from the elbow to the wrist bones. Few of the sarcomas that appear in the upper extremity are unique to this region—e.g., the epithelioid sarcomas, which are extremely rare, occur more frequently about the wrist than elsewhere. In general, however, the tumors that are usually encountered in upper extremity are those also found in the lower extremity: liposarcomas, fibrosarcomas, and malignant fibrous histiocytomas.

Clinically, most of the tumors present as nodular masses arising within muscle groups and occasionally crossing fascial planes to involve several muscle groups. They occasionally appear in fascia or fat, or arise from neurogenic structures of the arm and forearm. Few of the lesions grow to the enormous size that can be seen for tumors encompassing the thigh, or ulcerate to the degree seen with many extensive lower extremity sarcomas.

DIAGNOSTIC STUDIES

Plain x-ray films are frequently used to define whether there is an existing lipomatous lesion or fatty component to the tumor, whether calcification has occurred within the tumor, or whether bone erosion can be seen. Xeroradiography is often useful in giving sharper delineation to such findings. Angiography may be essential in determining the extent of the vascular supply to the tumor, as well as which principal feeding vessels are involved. The angiogram can also define the limits of the tumor should clinical extension not be clear. Tumor vessels may not be prominent; under such circumstance bowing of the vessels by a nonvascular lesion may help to define its dimensions.

We have routinely performed these studies as an additional aid for planning the extent of resection of the malignant lesion, especially when trying to define the extent of the muscle group resection in the planned dissection. The CT scan and other x-ray studies may be fairly accurate in portraying tumor limits. On occasion the scan may suggest that the tumor has infiltrated the periosteum of bone, but on exploration the lesion is found to be mobile with adequate normal tissue intervening between tumor and bone. Here, the presence of free periosteal planes may obviate amputation and allow en-bloc removal of tumor. This is especially true if the tumor is considered to be low-grade. The confusion in interpretation of CT scans may be the result of edema that frequently develops in tissue planes around the tumor. When there are questions of safety, in terms of the margins of resection, then intra-arterial chemotherapy and postoperative radiation therapy should be considered. If histologic study reveals that the margins of resection are considered too close, the treatment plan must be reevaluated; amputation, however, should not be performed unless it has been planned for preoperatively.

Neifeld[26] reported results of experience with CT scan studies of 16 extremity lesions. The scan was found to be useful in defining not only the limits of the primary lesion, but also extension of tumor that was not appreciated clinically, such as the presence of nodal involvement in the axilla and growth of the tumor under the pectoralis major to invade the chest wall. In such instances, appropriate procedures could be planned in advance of the surgery and one could decide whether axillary dissection and chest wall resection would be of value. Certain scans were misinterpreted, resulting in overestimation of tumor size with suggestion of neurovascular or even osseous involvement probably as a result of secondary edema of the surrounding structures.

The findings obtained from the CT scan and angiography should be used as a guideline and must, of necessity, be confirmed at the time of exploration. Although the presence of benign fatty tumors can be anticipated from radiographic analysis of a tumor, low-grade liposarcomas can be misinterpreted as being benign. As such, the potential for malignancy should be considered in any differential diagnosis of a fatty tumor. Neifeld has suggested that if the tumor appears to be clinically resectable with limb salvage surgery, then this should be attempted even if the scan suggests a greater extent of tumor involvement. Such a judgment, however, must be confirmed at the time of surgery. In numerous instances in which the scan has implied that the periosteum has been infiltrated, we have discovered at surgery that a more than adequate plane is present. If, on preliminary biopsy, the pathology report suggests a low-grade malignancy or a histologic type that is amenable to preoperative radiation therapy or infusion of Adriamycin, then the borderline case may be given the benefit of such preoperative therapy.

Histologic confirmation is essential in diagnosing and treating all lesions. Pitfalls, however, should be known and anticipated. Small lesions (less than 2 cm) that appear superficial may be biopsied by total excision in the office. Deeper lesions that are larger than 2 cm should probably be sampled in an ambulatory facility, which can offer intravenous sedation and general anesthesia, if necessary. Tumors larger than 5 cm may be sampled by incisional biopsy, bearing in mind the heterogeneous nature of many of these lesions. Bulky lesions arising in muscle and fascial planes should probably be radiographically imaged. Multiple incisional biopsies with frozen section are then performed to guarantee that areas of distinct malignancy have been obtained for further study. Frequently we remove an additional small sample for fixation in gluteraldehyde to be used for possible electron microscopic examination at a later time if needed. Aspiration biopsy can be of value, but only when an experienced cytopathologist is available to study the material. Major muscle group dissections and amputations should never be planned until all radiographic and histologic studies have been completed, and grade as well as tumor type assured. Figure 4–1 illustrates an aspiration biopsy performed for an infiltrating fibrous lesion of the forearm using a Martin aspiration syringe. This glass-barreled metal-plunger syringe allows the build-up of adequate negative pressure. The needle and trocar are delivered to the surface of the tumor; the trocar is removed and, with negative pressure applied to the syringe plunger, three stabs are made into the tumor. With one continuous motion the syringe and needle are pulled away, the cutting edge of the needle having transected portions of the tumor, which are aspirated into the syringe. We also employ TruCut Vim-Silverman biopsy needles for similar purposes.

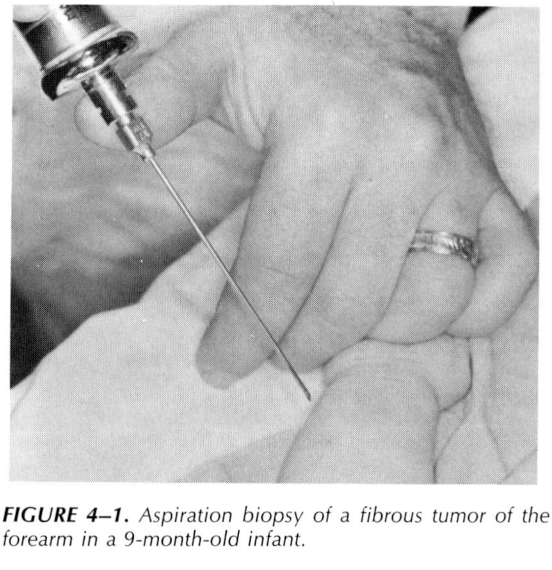

FIGURE 4–1. *Aspiration biopsy of a fibrous tumor of the forearm in a 9-month-old infant.*

SURGICAL APPROACHES

After a biopsy has been performed and we are now in the process of exploring the tumor for resection, we have often found that an outflanking technique may be helpful to guarantee that the tumor is adequately encompassed. In this approach to the tumor, the surgeon resects areas where margins are easiest to approach. By constantly palpating and displacing the tumor from the operative field, sharp dissection will achieve clean margins of resection. This approach allows better evaluation of the more difficult, deeper areas to be resected later.

When performing the deeper dissection, constantly palpating through the normal tissue surrounding the tumor mass, the surgeon may find that the lesion is suddenly more mobile but that nerves, vessels, and bone in the proximity do not have adequate margins of freedom from the tumor. In such cases, it may be necessary to include such tissues in the specimen. Indeed, the entire local procedure as planned may need to be discarded. If prior permission has been obtained, the surgeon may then choose to amputate, but only as a last resort. The exact distance one must be from a malignant tumor margin is actually unknown. In certain cases it may suffice to resect within millimeters of the tumor pseudocapsule, whereas in other cases recurrence will be rapid. So-called margins are measurements that have more validity for the pathologist than for what is actually found in the operating room. We have all seen instances in which a separate nodule has developed outside the original resection scar and where the pathology report has indicated an adequate margin of resection. In our opinion this recurrence is the result of one of three possibilities: (1) false margins of resection due to inadequate sampling from the tumor, which was considered to have been adequately resected; (2) a multifocal situation not under the control of the operating surgeon; or (3) skip metastasis, which the pathologist cannot define. In either case we have still relied on primary resection as the initial approach for cure and have found that in the presence of local recurrence, adequate en-bloc resection of this recurrence may allow an additional opportunity for salvage. Should one note a local recurrence rate in excess of 5% where the belief has been that adequate margins have been obtained at the time of resection, and this has been confirmed by the pathologist, then either the surgeon or the pathologist or both are in error. In approximately 60% of patients referred to us for re-resection of a tumor field that was supposed to have been widely resected initially, residual disease has been found in the secondarily removed en-bloc specimen. After wide local excision of any sarcoma, one must reevaluate previous surgery, pathologic specimens, size of tumor, and extent of margins before deciding on the need for re-excision.

In the arm, margins of resection are often less easily obtained than with tumors in the leg. One should contemplate the need to resect neurovascular structures, skin, and bone more frequently in order to cure upper extremity lesions. While it is true that upper arm lesions are easier to handle than ones arising in the forearm, the aforementioned rule that all malignant tumors below the elbow require amputation does not hold up, provided that the previously stated principles are followed. Certainly one can follow an en-bloc resection with amputation if necessary. The classic approach of en-bloc resection with surrounding normal muscle and fascial planes is to be utilized whenever possible. Figure 4–2*A* illustrates the incision used with a fully malignant sarcoma. The tissue planes that must be exposed and resected are shown in Figure 4–2*B*.

When soft tissue lesions of the mid or distal radius are resected, transposition of the hand to the ulna (one-bone forearm) yields a strong functional hand.

PATTERNS OF TUMOR PRESENTATION

Fibrous Tumors

One of the common types of malignant tumors of the arm is that of fibrous tissue origin. Such tumors can occur in patients of all ages. Occasionally, a very young child is found to have such a fibrous tissue tumor, one that appears to be clinically aggressive and suggestive of malignancy. Such young patients can present with a histologic pattern of benign fibromatosis infiltrating bone, giving the clinical impression of sarcoma. We examined a 1-year-old male infant with a bulging tumor mass in the forearm. Using a Martin aspiration syringe, aspiration biopsy of the lesion was performed in the interosseous membrane, where x-rays had shown

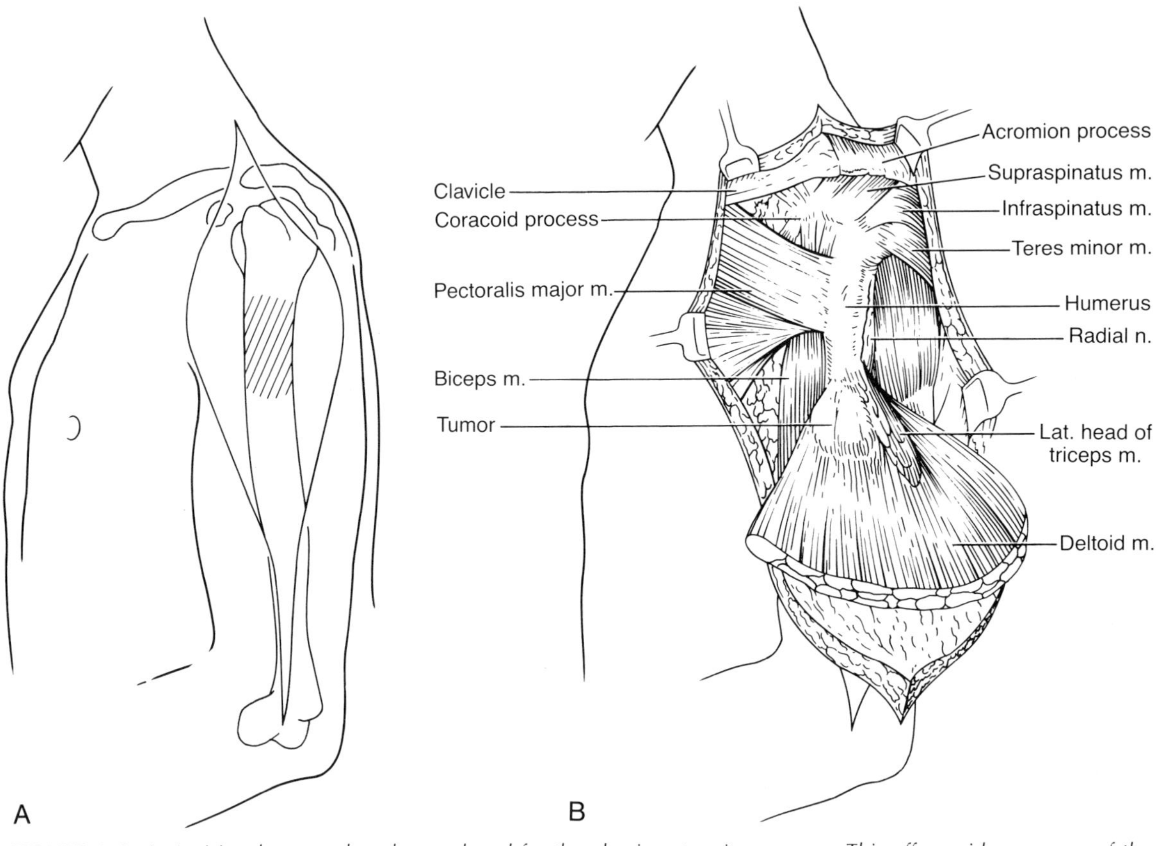

FIGURE 4–2. *A, Incisional approach to be employed for the classic extremity sarcoma. This offers wide exposure of the anatomic structures to be resected. B, Anatomic structures that have been exposed and are being resected as part of the procedure of muscle group dissection.*

the tumor to infiltrate the radius and ulna (Fig. 4–3*A* and *B*). Treatment consisted only of local excision of the lesion from the interosseous membrane and the ulna (Fig. 4–3*C*). Initially it was believed that the lesion resembled low-grade fibrosarcoma; however, the final diagnosis was juvenile fascial fibromatosis (Fig. 4–3*D*). Radiographs taken within the year showed healing of bone (Fig. 4–3*E*), which would be expected with fibro-

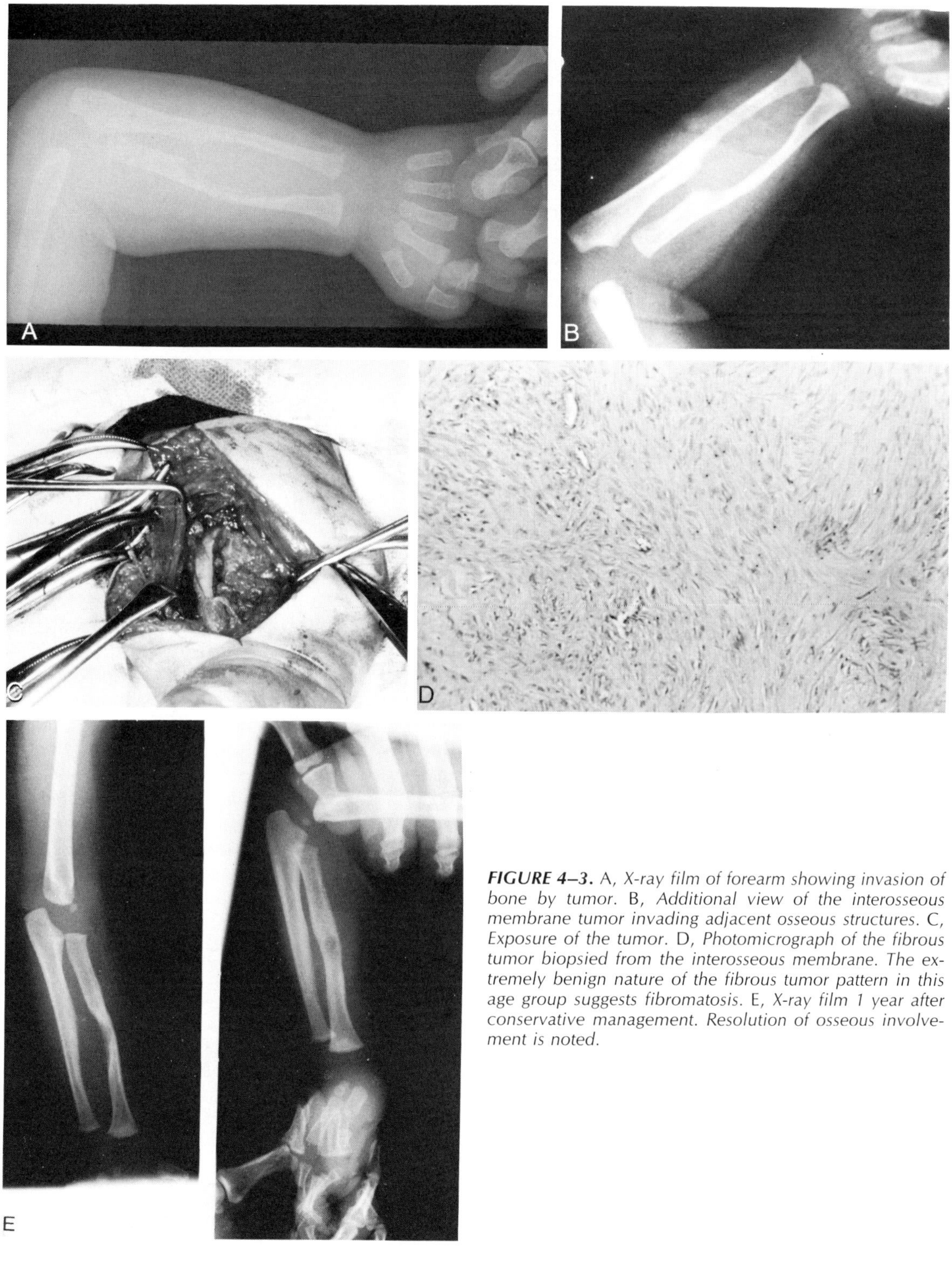

FIGURE 4–3. *A, X-ray film of forearm showing invasion of bone by tumor. B, Additional view of the interosseous membrane tumor invading adjacent osseous structures. C, Exposure of the tumor. D, Photomicrograph of the fibrous tumor biopsied from the interosseous membrane. The extremely benign nature of the fibrous tumor pattern in this age group suggests fibromatosis. E, X-ray film 1 year after conservative management. Resolution of osseous involvement is noted.*

matosis. Otherwise, progression of the disease would have occurred, necessitating amputation. Similar instances of the invasion of bone by fibrous neoplasia have been described in young children. Kindbloom and Angerval[23] described a case with invasion of bone similar to the one we had treated. After curettage, the bone lesion healed with no evidence of recurrence or dissemination. The tumor was composed of leiomyoma-like regions with areas of spindle-shaped cells and abundant collagen, similar to what was found in our patient. Ultrastructurally, the tumor cells resembled primitive fibroblasts suggestive of leiomyoblastic differentiation; however, such a case must be followed very closely to confirm the clinical and pathologic diagnosis. There have been reports of amputation for this tumor, similar to the procedure followed for the initial group of patients with benign plantar fibromatosis. If a nodule reappears after resection of such a lesion, then a more serious situation probably exists, unless the primary resection was inadequate. Clinical and pathologic confirmation of the nature of the primary tumor and of the recurrent lesion must be established and the entire clinical picture reviewed. Each discipline available for diagnosis and treatment must be utilized with the soft tissue tumors, as with osseous neoplasms.

In the spectrum of fibrous tissue tumors, fibromatosis especially in the juvenile period, can behave like and be mistaken for a malignant lesion. In the case illustrated, aspiration biopsy was performed and the lesion initially considered to be a fibrosarcoma. Because of the age of the patient, the possibility of aggressive fibromatosis was entertained. After analyzing the pathologic material and the clinical picture, we resected the lesion conservatively and followed the postoperative course closely. Our evaluation proved to be correct, since the lesion did appear to heal spontaneously through what was believed to be a process of maturation.[3]

This particular tumor is one of a wide array of fibroblastic tumors that can occur in the neonatal period. While such tumors are infrequent, they are the second most common form of tumor to be found in the early age group, exceeded in frequency only by lymphangiomatous lesions. There are other situations in which bowing of bone and failure to tubulate normally may indicate a great likelihood for the development of soft tissue tumors at other levels in the extremity. We have found that such tumors tend to be progressively more malignant with each recurrence.

In a review by Kaufman and Stout,[20] congenital mesenchymal tumors were categorized according to their appearance and behavior. There appears to be a wide spectrum of fibroblastic responses, progressing from the well-known keloid to Dupuytren's contracture, fascial fibroma, and desmoid tumor, to low-grade fibrosarcoma and dermatofibrosarcoma. Touraine and Ruel[33] suggested that such lesions should be linked together as a clinical entity and labeled them "hereditary polyfibromatosis."

Microscopically, the degree of cellular activity of these tumors may be misinterpreted—e.g., invasiveness may appear to be a strong possibility and yet may not occur; the reverse may also be seen. In a case reported by Prior and Sisson,[29] amputation was performed for a fibroma of the thumb; later the metacarpal bone stump was removed because of an unhealed wound at the site of amputation. A lung lesion subsequently appeared and was removed by pneumonectomy. The lung lesion proved to be a fibroma, believed to be metastatic and histologically identical to the one removed from the finger. Fibromatosis most often appears as discrete, usually circumscribed masses, but on occasion it may diffusely infiltrate the surrounding tissue and even occur at multiple sites. A generalized form involving the viscera has also been described.[12, 20]

In 10 of the cases reviewed by Stout,[32] there were three instances of diffuse involvement of extremities. In the first of these there was extensive involvement of the forearm at birth, yet at 4 years of age, without undergoing any therapy, the child was healthy and had no evidence of residual disease. In the second case there was extensive involvement of the hand, but no follow-up was obtained. Diffuse involvement of the leg was noted in the third case, and amputation was performed because of the bizarre histologic appearance of some areas of biopsy. Nine months after surgery, the patient was described as being free of disease. Infiltrative growth patterns of these and other juvenile lesions, such as lipomatosis and massive hemangiomatosis, may make surgical excision impossible and amputation, in many cases, the required procedure. The major consideration in treating patients with fascial fibromatosis is whether progression of disease will continue to the extent that amputation of the extremity must be performed. We have also seen a patient who had undergone cosmetic toe surgery and epiphyseal stapling of the knee on the same side with fibrosarcoma developing in both operative scars. This patient had abnormal tubulation of bones. After multiple local recurrences, hemipelvectomy was eventually performed, as each succeeding lesion had behaved more aggressively.

There is some indication that maturation of such a disease process may occur at least in early childhood. Noting that the diffuse form of juvenile aponeurotic fibroma occurs in young children and the circumscribed fibroma in an older age group, Keasby suggested that this difference represented a transitional growth pattern.[22] Booher and McPeak[6] reported a case of fibrous tumor of the wrist in a 7-day-old infant. The diagnosis was first thought to be lipofibrosarcoma, but was later changed by Stewart to fibrolipoma. Despite several attempts at excision, the tumor always recurred and eventually showed diffuse involvement at the wrist. This tumor continued to grow, extending around the tendons, median nerve, and carpal bones. Extensive biopsies over a period of time showed a histologic transition, the final specimen being considered a desmoid. At the age of 5, a discrete recurrence appeared with interstitial calcification within the mass. Histologically, this tumor was finally considered to be a compact fibroma. The arm was left otherwise intact.

Twelve cases of infantile fibromatosis presenting with an aggressive pattern was reported from the Armed Forces Institute of Pathology.[12] In all of these instances, the question of fibrosarcoma had arisen, but lack of metastasis in every instance, followed by reevaluation, led to their classification among the fibromatoses. The findings in one of these cases were similar to those in the case we described above, namely, osseous involvement of the radius and ulna by a spindle cell tumor of the forearm present since birth. Although the lesion was partially removed when the patient was 4 years old, roentgenograms of the forearm made at the age of 14 showed a normal ulna and radius. Conservative therapy in this patient was followed by eventual maturation of the lesion and preservation of the extremity with normal function.

True osseous involvement by fibromatosis seldom occurs. In the case of diffuse involvement of the lower extremity reported by Kaufman and Stout,[20] invasion of bone was noted. These authors also reported another case of osseous involvement, in an infant who had the generalized form of fascial fibromatosis with 31 recognized bone lesions and massive involvement of one kidney. The bone lesions regressed following nephrectomy and removal of a parietal mass from the skull. Condon and Allen[8] reported a case of generalized fibromatoses associated with lytic lesions in the long bones, ribs, vertebrae, and skull. The extent of this involvement made survival impossible and the patient died shortly after birth. Osseous lesions of this nature are rare in infancy, but when present, the differential diagnosis includes neurofibromatosis and reticuloendotheliosis. Should biopsy reveal only disorganized fibrous tissue with both osseous and soft tissue lesions, the diagnosis of fascial fibromatosis should be strongly entertained.

Another benign nodular lesion of the upper extremity is nodular fasciitis.[25] Also known as pseudosarcomatous fasciitis, this lesion can at times be found in other sites of the body, except for the viscera.[32] We have noted several lesions in the upper extremity that orginally were reported to be sarcomatous and the patients referred for either muscle group dissection or amputation. Review of submitted pathology material, however, proved these lesions to be totally benign. The most frequent error has been to misinterpret such tumors as fibrosarcoma or liposarcoma. The suspicion that the physician is dealing with a sarcoma is usually based on the fact that these lesions are rapidly growing and tender, often presenting on the volar surface of the arm and forearm. Rarely does the clinical history date back more than 3 months before the patient is referred for surgery. The tumor itself is typically small, with most no larger than 2 cm and few ever reaching 4 cm in diameter. Histologically, one finds reparative tissue composed of plump fibroblasts arranged in a random pattern; mitoses are present. Blood vessels infiltrate the lesion, which contains plump endothelial cells with variable inflammatory infiltrates, which probably account for the tenderness. Occasionally, the lesion blends in histologically with other lesions such as proliferative myositis, myositis ossificans, and granulation tissue.[19]

Four microscopic features are to be noted: (1) With nodular fasciitis the nuclei are never hyperchromatic, and when there is cellular atypia the cells are plump with abundant cytoplasm, large nuclei, small nucleoli, and a diffuse, lightly staining chromatin pattern. (2) The lesion has never been observed to extend to or through the skin. (3) Small collections of dense mononuclear cells are found in the periphery of the lesion, but within the central area there are fewer, but a variable amount of, mononuclear cells. (4) There is a limit to the number of mitoses, which are not tumor-related, i.e., one per high-power field. When a lesion originally diagnosed as nodular fasciitis is found to recur, one should consider that the original diagnosis may not have been correct. In a report of 114 patients with 116 lesions, no recurrence was noted among any of the patients.[5]

Among the more malignant fibrous tumors encountered, dermatofibrosarcoma should be considered in the differential diagnosis, although it occurs rarely. Of 119 cases of dermatofibrosarcoma treated at Memorial Hospital, 7 tumors arose in the region of the arms and legs. Essentially, this is a tumor of the trunk and shoulder girdle, but it must be considered when a firm fibrous tissue tumor is found in the upper extremity. The characteristic cartwheel pattern of fibroblasts was originally described by Hertzler.[18] At times, the lesion can be mimicked grossly by the fibroblastic phase of malignant melanoma. Complete resection of the tumor is essential, since this nonaggressive tumor has a high incidence of local recurrence and at times metastasizes. McPeak[24] and Penner[28] reviewed 402 cases, 23 of which had proven metastatic disease. At Memorial Hospital, 64 patients had recurrence of their tumor, mostly within the first year of surgery. Nine of the 10 patients with metastases died of pulmonary disease. Surgery must include not only wide resection of at least 2 to 4 cm about the tumor, depending on its size, but also the underlying fascia. In most instances, a full-thickness graft or pedicle flap is necessary for adequate closure.

The desmoid tumor, considered by many to be an essentially benign neoplastic process, is a variant in the spectrum of fibrous tissue tumors that should be considered to represent low-grade fibrosarcoma. This concept was held to be true by Ewing and is the prevailing philosophy at institutions with experience in managing this tumor. Among 162 cases at Memorial Hospital, 11 occurred in the upper extremity, including the shoulder. These "extra-abdominal desmoids" appear to be somewhat more aggressive than their "abdominal" counterpart. Because of the tendency for these cells to appear innocuous, especially at the periphery, where the lesions infiltrate into fascial planes, adequate resection may be difficult. A 50-year-old female patient with a previous history of extra-abdominal desmoid tumor of the upper arm was found to have recurrent lesions extending along the biceps and triceps, reaching centripetally toward the deltoid and clavicular regions. In order to obviate further spread, which has in the past been reported to extend well into the mediastinum, four-quarter amputation was performed. Multiple biopsies had indicated that recurrent tumor was present at all sites sampled. A four-quarter amputation was performed to minimize the possibility of further retrograde extension of tumor into the thoracic cage. We have seen desmoid tumors that extended up one arm into the mediastinum and cross into the other arm.

In 1865 Paget first described the existence of the extra-abdominal form of desmoid tumor. While common in the second to fourth decades, this lesion can also occur in childhood. Exelby et al.[14] reported 22 cases in children. In resecting such tumors it is essential that adequate margins of resection be achieved. This may be difficult owing to blending of the tumor cells into the surrounding fascial planes that envelop the muscles of the extremity. At those sites where tumor does infiltrate, destruction of muscle cells can occur with clumping of the nuclei to form pseudogiant cells. Samples from the periphery of the lesion should be submitted for frozen section, as it is important to decide whether wider margins of resection should be obtained at the time of the initial procedure. One should remember, however, that examination of frozen section can be difficult with this tumor, even in the hands of an experienced pathologist. Metastatic lesions are rare, in contrast to the somewhat higher incidence of metastases reported with dermatofibrosarcoma protuberans.[28]

Fully malignant fibrosarcomas are not too different from desmoid tumors in clinical appearance. They usually appear as firm, pseudoencapsulated nodular masses that may develop over a period of months to years. Skin ulceration may be noted late in the clinical course. The behavior of these tumors can generally be inferred from the histologic pattern. Quick and Cutler, in 1927, introduced a grading system for these sarcomas. In 1935, Geschicter and Lewis[15] reported their experience with classifying them into differentiated and undifferentiated forms. Follow-up studies using such a classification have shown that the 5-year survival is closely related to the histologic pattern of the tumor. We have found a counterpart in fibrosarcoma arising primarily within the medullary canal of bone (medullary fibrosarcoma of bone) and rupturing through the cortex into the soft tissues, presenting as a large soft-part sarcoma. Survival in these patients depends entirely on grading and not on size.[9] Cryosurgery may be one of the ways to manage such lesions, as it has been successfully employed in the management of low-grade fibrosarcomas of bone followed for 15 years with subsequent negative biopsies. The low-grade fibrosarcomas tend to be monomorphic with no mitoses and no giant cells; high-grade lesions are pleomorphic and have mitotic figures and isolated tumor giant cells. The fibrosarcomas are seen most frequently in the extremities, and twice as often in the lower extremity.

Neurogenic Tumors

Benign neural tumors such as the schwannoma are not uncommon in the arm. A 60-year-old man had a firm 3-cm mass in the cubital fossa of his right arm. The mass was firm, somewhat mobile, and nontender. The possibility of schwannoma was raised. There was no evidence of von Recklinghausen's disease. The tumor was explored, dissecting it from the brachial artery. It appeared to arise from a branch of the radial nerve (Fig. 4–4*A*). The cut section of this tumor is shown in Figure 4–4*B*. On dissecting tumors in the cubital fossa there is a profuse arterial anastomosis in this region derived from the brachial artery. The ulnar nerve lies superficially, behind the medial epicondyle and out of the operative field. The radial nerve runs adjacent to the artery under cover of the brachioradialis, and the median nerve runs on the medial side of the artery, exiting beneath the pronator teres. Neurogenic sarcomas associated with von Recklinghausen's disease do not usually appear in the upper extremity per se, but rather within the axilla, where branches of the brachial plexus may be involved by tumor. Approximately 16% of these tumors appear in the lower extremity. Those tumors not associated with von Recklinghausen's disease have an incidence of approximately 15% of developing in the region of the arm. To prevent recurrence, the treatment of choice for these sarcomas of the upper extremity is muscle group dissection, as for sarcomas in other areas of the body.[10, 16] These tumors are most difficult to manage in the forearm, especially in the region of the wrist. In this area are structures that cannot be sacrificed without producing

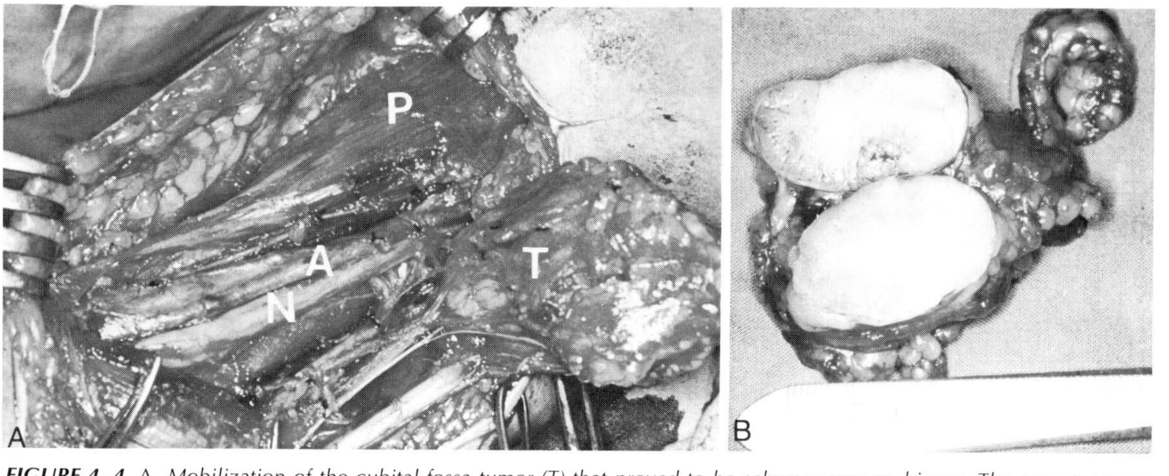

FIGURE 4–4. A, *Mobilization of the cubital fossa tumor (T) that proved to be schwannoma on biopsy. The pronator teres (P) is noted. The neurovascular bundle (A) consists of brachial artery and vein just above their division into radial and ulnar structures. The median nerve (N) and ulnar artery pass under the fibrous "sublimis arch" that connects the radial and humero-ulnar heads of the flexor digitorum sublimis.* B, *Appearance of the resected specimen.*

moderate to marked disability, and amputation frequently is required.

Tenosynovial Tumors

Synoviomas may appear in the upper extremity, usually as a nodular lesion or mass. Occasionally, symptoms suggest that a pathologic process may be present, but no discrete lesion is found at the time of examination. Rajpal et al.[30] reported on a patient who manifested signs of the carpal tunnel syndrome. On exploration of the wrist, suspicious tissue was found, which proved to be a synovial sarcoma on biopsy. Definitive surgery one month later consisted of resecting the biopsy site, dividing the palmaris longus with en-bloc resection of the palmar aponeurosis and the flexor retinaculum. Since microscopic examination revealed that tumor involved the margins of resection, 6000 rad was delivered to the site. The patient has remained free of disease 6 years after surgery.

Tumors of Adipose Tissue

Occasionally, benign tumors of fetal or embryonal adipose tissue are seen arising in the extremity, usually in infants and children. At times these lesions bear close resemblance to a myxoid or well-differentiated liposarcoma. In 1958 Vellois[34] coined the term "lipoblastomatosis." The Armed Forces Institute of Pathology has recorded 35 such cases, 88% occurring before 3 years of age and involving the soft tissues of the upper and lower extremities. The circumscribed form was more commonly seen and was superficially located and clinically comparable to a lipoma. Diffuse forms were deeply situated. Both forms showed an identical picture histologically: lobulated immature adipose tissue composed of lipoblasts, a plexiform capillary pattern, and a rich myxoid stroma. The clinical course was benign, with occasional recurrence probably the result of incomplete excision. Other fatty tumors such as liposarcoma must be included in the differential diagnosis of any nodular mass arising in the upper extremity. Figure 4–5 shows the appearance of a recurrent liposarcoma of the volar surface of the forearm just above the wrist. The patient, a 59-year-old woman, originally had under-

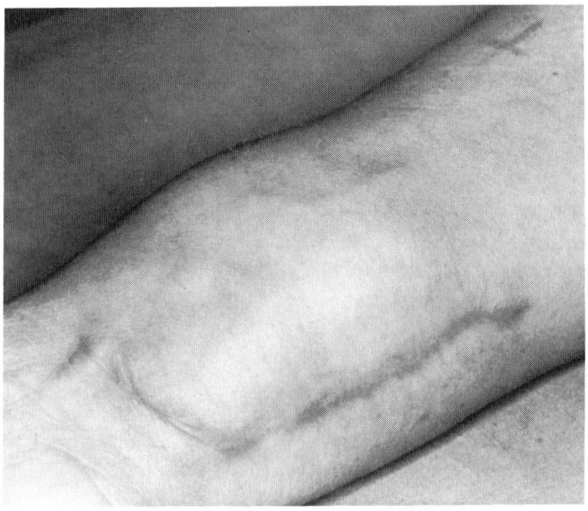

FIGURE 4–5. Recurrent liposarcoma of the forearm just above the wrist.

gone wide resection of a liposarcoma that recurred within 6 months after surgery. The bulge noted in the wrist area resulted from tumor expansion in proximity to the flexors of the hand. The recurrent tumor was resected widely, down to the region of a flexor pollicis longus. Postoperative radiation therapy (5000 R) was used one month after resection and skin graft. Within 3 months, recurrence was again noted and the limb was amputated through the mid-humerus. The patient has since remained clinically free of disease. With this particular lesion, survival depends on complete removal at the site of recurrence, and the tumor's histologic type, size, and histologic grade. Enzinger and Winslow[13] reported a survival rate of 85% for well-differentiated liposarcomas versus 21% for pleomorphic liposarcomas in a series of 103 patients. We have frequently found that radiation to the site of resection of pleomorphic liposarcoma has failed to control disease if good margins of resection were not achieved.

Muscle Sarcomas

Rhabdomyosarcoma is one of the more common malignant sarcomas of the arm. This tumor can occur as a single or lobulated lesion and at times may present with a multicentric pattern containing discrete nodular masses. Figure 4–6*A* shows the appearance of the solitary nodular form of rhabdomyosarcoma. Muscle group dissection was employed (Fig. 4–6*B* and *C*), with

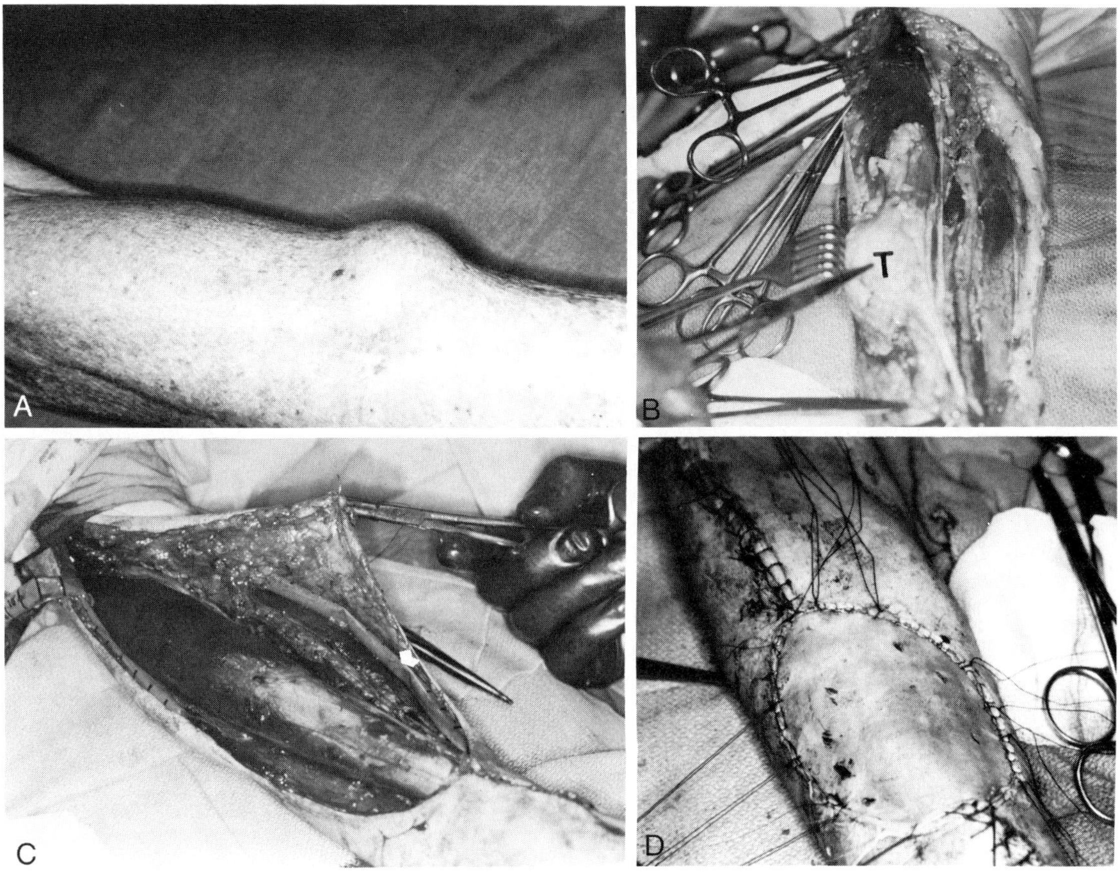

FIGURE 4–6. *A, Rhabdomyosarcoma of the forearm. B, Mobilization of tumor after skin flaps have been raised and margins of tumor (T) defined. C, Operative field after tumor removal. D, Skin grafting of defect.*

removal of a portion of the overlying skin, which then required skin grafting (Fig. 4–6*D*). Occasionally, a deeply placed mass may so diffusely infiltrate the surrounding tissue of the arm that it may be difficult to describe it as a discrete lesion. This pattern is more common in the leg than in the arm. While most of the lesions have a firm consistency, the variations and behavioral patterns at the capsular margin (tumor-tissue interface) are numerous and result in either a circumscribed or an infiltrative picture.[27] Hemorrhagic lesions are not uncommon with extensive areas of necrosis, so clinically the mass may resemble a large hematoma. Attempts at biopsy or even local resection can result in tumor spillage and the loss of large amounts of blood, which then serves to seed the wound. In some patients, anemia may be noted as a result of a large volume of intramural hematoma and suppression in red cell production by the tumor. When such lesions are defined, muscle group dissection usually does not satisfy the situation because of the rapid growth pattern. Tumor doubling appears to take place in days, so there is little time to attempt local control with techniques such as preoperative radiation therapy. For the occasional discrete solid nodular lesion that we do find, postoperative radiation therapy and chemotherapy can be offered to control the tumor bed and prevent possible vascular dissemination. Frequently, following biopsy of an extensive tumor whose operability is questionable, preoperative radiation therapy and chemotherapy will alter the status of the tumor, converting it to an operable lesion.

Various growth patterns have been defined for rhabdomyosarcoma that can be determined by history prior to initiation of therapy: (1) The neoplasm may remain small and quiescent for many months or even years and suddenly exhibit growth, either spontaneously or induced by trauma. (2) The tumor may grow in a fulminant manner. (3)

The tumor may grow slowly for weeks and appear to be dormant. It is only rapid recurrence occurs following a conservative surgical approach that the true nature of the tumor can be recognized.

Because of the high incidence of pulmonary metastasis, the status of the lung fields must be evaluated before any definitive procedure is employed. In the face of known metastases, amputation may still be necessary to control bulky, ulcerating, and hemorrhagic tumors. Chemotherapy can then be introduced in an attempt to manage the more distant lesions.

There are some instances in which these tumors prove to be multicentric. The need for muscle group dissection is therefore quite important, especially for lesions larger than 5 cm in the arm and 3 cm in the forearm.

Histopathologically, these tumors are classified as adult pleomorphic and embryonal; within each group there are subclassifications. Of the 100 cases reported by Pack,[27] 27 occurred on the arm, in contrast to 41 arising in the thigh. This is probably due to the greater muscle mass in the thigh region. There is an unexplained phenomenon of a higher incidence of cures for lesions of the upper extremity. Because of a high propensity for lymph node involvement, with forearm and arm lesions, axillary dissection should be considered. This should probably be carried out on a prophylactic basis for the larger lesion and especially when the tumor is embryonal in nature. While wide en-bloc resections may be important, an attempt to preserve arm and hand function must be made.[2]

It is of interest that for its weight and extent, skeletal muscle has fewer tumors than any other tissue in the body. The comparative rarity of rhabdomyosarcomas as a muscle tumor may be attributed to the fact that striated muscle cells are completely differentiated and do not undergo cellular division after birth as do most of the other cells in the body.

Malignant Fibrous Histiocytoma

Among the nodular lesions, malignant fibrous histiocytomas should be considered in the differential diagnosis. At the Mayo Clinic, Kearney[21] reviewed the records of 40 of 467 patients who presented with upper extremity lesions. Sixteen cases of malignant fibrous histiocytoma were found in the shoulder girdle region, 6 in the arm, 3 in the region of the elbow, 13 in the forearm, and in the hand. The treatment of choice is identical to that for malignant fibrosarcoma, liposarcoma, and rhabdomyosarcoma.

Extranodal Lymphoma

A rare soft tissue lesion is the extranodal component of lymphosarcoma, in which abnormal lymphocytes are deposited in the soft tissues to produce the classic appearance of a soft tissue sarcoma (Fig. 4–7). After biopsy or local excision, radiation therapy followed by chemotherapy can prevent the

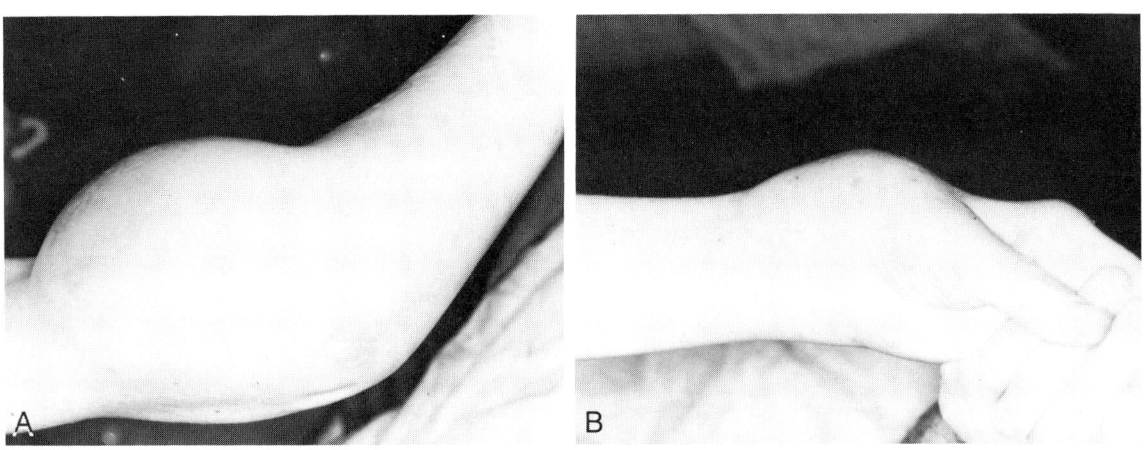

FIGURE 4–7. *A, Extranodal lymphoma of soft tissue of forearm. B, Extranodal lymphoma with additional involvement around wrist.*

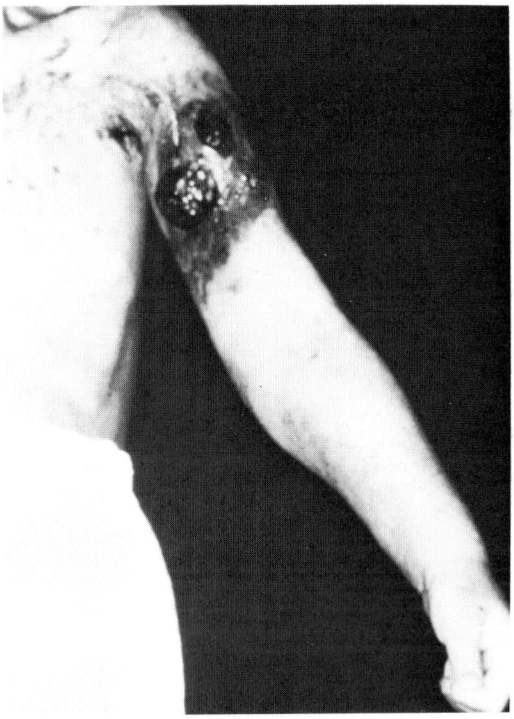

FIGURE 4–8. *Stewart-Treves syndrome showing tumor involvement of upper arm.*

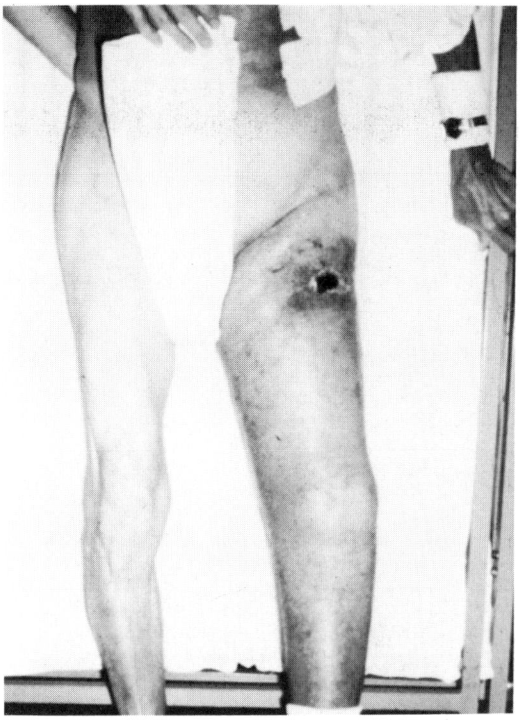

FIGURE 4–9. *Angiosarcoma of the lower extremity secondary to lymphedema.*

reappearance of such tumors. Berg et al.[4] described two cases of undifferentiated tumor arising in soft tissue and suggestive of sarcoma. Immunohistochemical staining revealed that the tumors did not react with antisera to actin, myosin, or myoglobin but were intensely positive with antisera to T-200 (a panleukocytic marker) and B1 (a pan-B-cell antibody). The studies allowed the proper combination chemotherapy to be instituted.

One of the complications of axillary surgery for carcinoma of the breast, especially following radiation therapy, is the development of lymphedema. In 1948 Stewart and Treves described a virulent form of lymphangiosarcoma arising in the engorged lymphatics of such extremities. Figure 4–8 shows the appearance of this form of lymphangiosarcoma in the lymphedematous arm of a patient who had undergone mastectomy. Characteristically lymphedema was present for 5 to 25 years after mastectomy, after which an ecchymotic purplish patch appeared in the skin. This led to progression in the form of multiple nodular, purple, ulcerating lesions followed by visceral and pulmonary metastases. Southwick and Slaughter[31] suggested the use of radiation therapy as the primary form of therapy, but surgical ablation, most frequently interscapulothoracic amputation[11] would seem to be more effective. Such lesions also appear in the lower extremity (Fig. 4–9) as a complication of lymphedema.

REFERENCES

1. Allen P. W.: The fibromatosis: A clinicopathologic classification based on 140 cases. Am. J. Surg. Pathol. 5: 255–270, 1977
2. Ariel I. M., Briceno M.: Rhabdomyosarcoma of the extremities and trunk: Analysis of 150 patients treated by surgical resection. J. Surg. Oncol. 7:269–287, 1975
3. Arlen M., Kouen L., Frieder M.: Juvenile fascial fibromatosis of the forearm with osseous involvement. J. Bone Joint Surg. 51-A: 591–595, 1969
4. Berg A. R., Linder J., Anderson R. W., et al.: The undifferentiated malignant neoplasm: Identification of lymphoma arising in skeletal muscle by immunohistochemical analysis. J.A.M.A. 254: 2625–2626, 1985
5. Berstein K. E., Lattes R.: Nodular (pseudosarcomatous) fasciitis: A non-recurrent lesion. Cancer 49:1668–1678, 1982
6. Booher R. J., McPeak C. J.: Juvenile aponeurotic fibromas. Surgery 46:924–931, 1959

7. Chung E. B., Enzinger F. M.: Benign lipoblastomatosis. Cancer 32:482–491, 1973
8. Condon V. R., Allen R. P.: Congenital generalized fibromatosis. Radiology 76:444–448, 1961
9. Cunningham M. P., Arlen M.: Medullary fibrosarcoma of bone. Cancer 21:31–37, 1968
10. Das Gupta T. K., Brasfield R. D.: Solitary malignant schwannoma. Ann. Surg. 171:419–429, 1970
11. Dembrow V. D., Adair F. E.: Lymphangiosarcoma in the postmastectomy lymphedematous arm. Cancer 14:210–212, 1961
12. Enzinger F. M.: Fibrous tumors in infancy. *In* Tumors of Bone and Soft Tissue. Chicago, Year Book, 1965
13. Enzinger F. M., Winslow D. L.: Liposarcoma. Virchows Arch. (Pathol. Anat.) 335:367–388, 1962
14. Exelby P. R., Knapper W. H., Huvos A. G., Beattie E.: Soft tissue fibrosarcoma in children. J. Pediatr. Surg. 8:415, 1973
15. Geschicter G. F., Lewis D.: Tumors of connective tissue. Am. J. Cancer 25:630, 1935
16. Gosh B. C., Ghosh L., Huvos A. G., Fortner J. G.: Malignant schwannoma. Cancer 31:184, 1973
17. Hachisuga T., Hashinoto H., Emjoji M.: Angioleiomyoma. Cancer 54:126–130, 1984
18. Hertzler A. E.: Fibrosarcomatous tumors of skin of the trunk characterized by attenuated dermal surfaces. Ann. Surg. 83:489, 1926
19. Hutter R. V. P., Stewart F. W., Foote F. W., Jr.: Fasciitis: A report of 70 cases with follow-up proving the benignity of the lesion. Cancer 15:992–1003, 1962
20. Kaufman S. L., Stout A. P.: Congenital mesenchymal tumors. Cancer 18:460, 1965
21. Kearney M. M., Soule E. H., Ivins J. C.: Malignant fibrous histiocytoma: A retrospective study of 167 cases. Cancer 29:961–976, 1972
22. Keasby L. E.: Juvenile aponeurotic fibroma (calcifying fibroma). Cancer 6:338–346, 1953
23. Kindbloom L. G., Angervall L.: Congenital solitary fibroma of the skeleton. Cancer 41:636–640, 1978
24. McPeak C. J., Cruz T., Nicastri A. D.: Dermatofibrosarcoma protuberans: An analysis of 86 cases, five with metastasis. Ann. Surg. 166:803, 1967
25. Mehregan A. H.: Nodular fasciitis. Arch. Dermatol. 93:204, 1966
26. Neifeld J. D., Walsh J. W., Lawrence W., Jr.: Computed tomography in the management of soft tissue tumors. Surg. Gynecol. Obstet. 155:535–540, 1982
27. Pack G. T., Eberhardt W. F.: Rhadomyosarcoma of skeletal muscle: Report of 100 cases. Surgery 32:1023–1064, 1952
28. Penner D. W.: Metastasizing dermatofibrosarcoma protuberans: Case report. Cancer: 1083–1086, 1951
29. Prior J. T., Sisson B. J.: Dermal and fascial fibromatosis. Ann. Surg. 139:453–467, 1954
30. Rajpal S., Moore R. H., Karakousis C. P.: Synovial sarcoma: A review of treatment and survival in 52 patients. N.Y. State J. Med. 84:17–19, 1984
31. Southwick H. W., Slaughter D. P.: Lymphangiosarcoma in postmastectomy lymphedema. Cancer 8:158, 1955
32. Stout A. P.: Juvenile fibromatosis. Cancer 7:953–978, 1954
33. Touraine A., Ruel H.: La Polyfibromatose Hereditaire. Ann. Dermatol. Syphilgraph. 5:1, 1945
34. Vellois F., Baez J. M., Schumacher H. B.: Lipoblastomatosis. Am. J. Pathol. 34:1149, 1958

CHAPTER

5

Tumors On and About the Pelvic Girdle

Tumors on and about the pelvic girdle most frequently represent soft part lesions arising from the gluteus muscles or the surrounding fibrofatty tissue of the buttock. Occasionally a tumor presents in a manner identical to that of a soft part tumor but actually is derived from osseous structures underlying the muscle of the buttock (Fig. 5–1). Such tumors are represented by the osteosarcomas, chondrosarcomas, fibrosarcomas and, at times, sacral chordomas.[4, 6, 8]

The soft tissue lesions present as a unique group of neoplasms that more often than not require imaginative approaches in their management. The majority of these tumors are seen as nonspecific swellings in the area of buttock (Fig. 5–2) if not in the entire buttock itself. Figure 5–3 shows the CT appearance of an extensive liposarcomatous mass that replaces essentially all of the buttock. At times, such soft part lesions may erode the sacrum, extending into the true pelvis to impinge on the pelvic viscera. Such lesions may be confused with sacral chordomas or giant cell tumors of the sacrum and must therefore be defined by biopsy. It is not unusual for a deeply placed rhabdomyosarcoma arising in gluteus to be forced by the overlying fascial planes to erode into the sacrum. In other instances, sarcomas of the gluteus may extend through the sciatic notch into the true pelvis (Fig. 5–4).

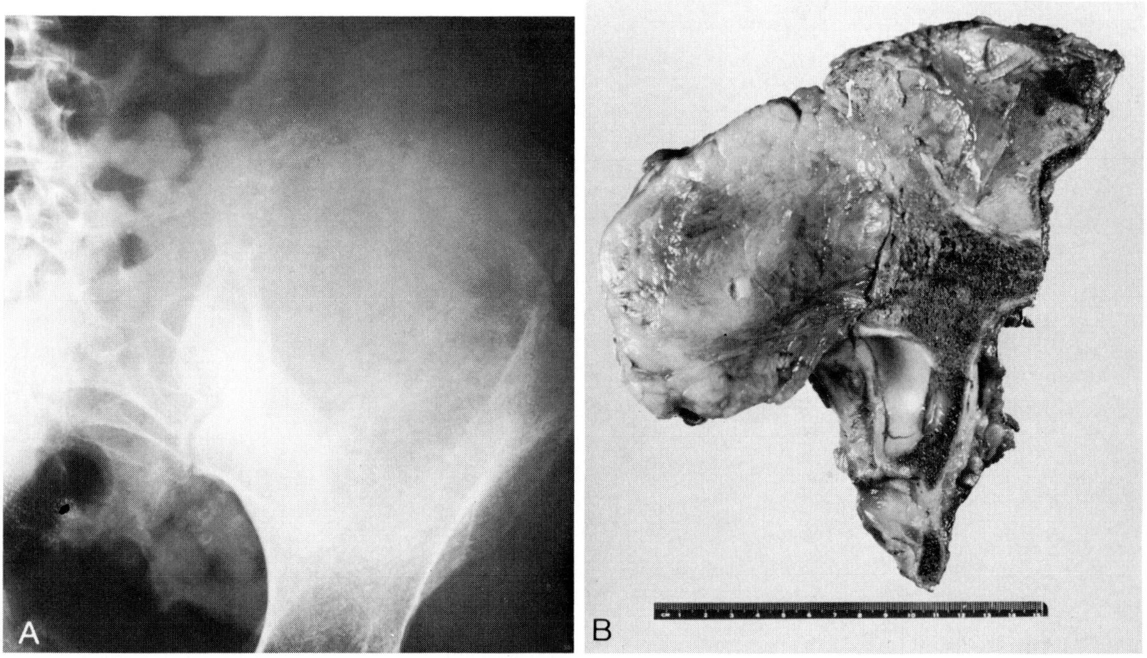

FIGURE 5–1. A, Medullary fibrosarcoma of bone arising from the ilium. B, Resected tumor with ilium.

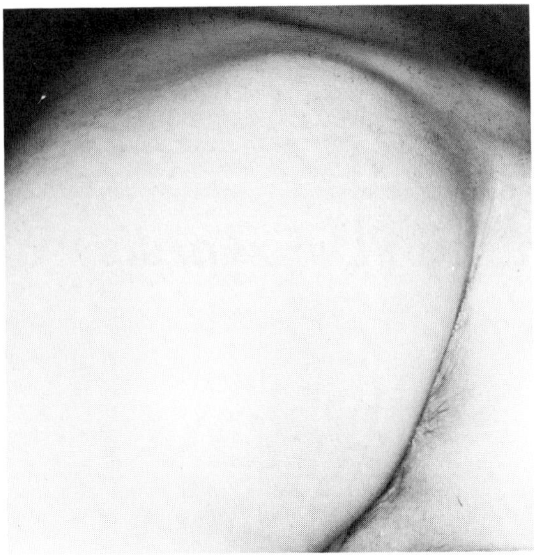

FIGURE 5–2. Sarcoma of the buttock.

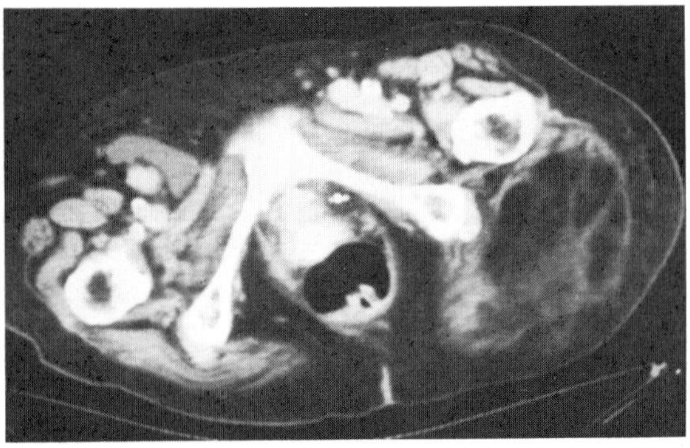

FIGURE 5–3. Liposarcoma of the left buttock seen on CT scan.

An 18-year-old female patient was referred for what was initially thought to be an inoperable embryonal rhabdomyosarcoma of the left buttock, which was confirmed on open biopsy. CT scan showed a large lesion arising in the deep gluteal muscles, entering the pelvis to impinge on and displace the viscera. Chemotherapy was started and resulted in prompt shrinkage of the tumor, as shown on CT scan (Fig. 5–5*A*). Based on these findings it was believed that surgical intervention was a possible means for effecting a cure; at the very least, palliation could be achieved with radiotherapy and chemotherapy. An abdominosacral laparotomy[9, 11] was performed for the following reasons: (1) The pelvic viscera could be separated from tumor that remained in the pelvis after shrinkage by chemotherapy. Then, when dissection was carried out from the buttock side in the second phase of the procedure, the deepest limit of dissection defined on entry into the pelvis could be clearly defined. (2) A pelvic iliac node dissection could be performed to assure that no metastasis had occurred. If nodes were found to extend to or above the iliac bifurcation, the limits for postoperative radiation therapy would be defined. (3) Hypogastric artery ligation could be performed to reduce the extent of bleeding that might occur at the time of the buttock resection.

On completion of the pelvic dissection in this patient, which essentially revealed minimal disease as a result of chemotherapy, the external iliac artery was dissected away from the psoas muscle. The obturator space was entered and the obturator nerve completely dissected. At this point, the sciatic nerve roots were defined just under the point where the obturator nerve exited from the sacrum into the lateral pelvic wall. The sciatic roots were dissected to the sciatic notch. Surgicel was placed under obturator

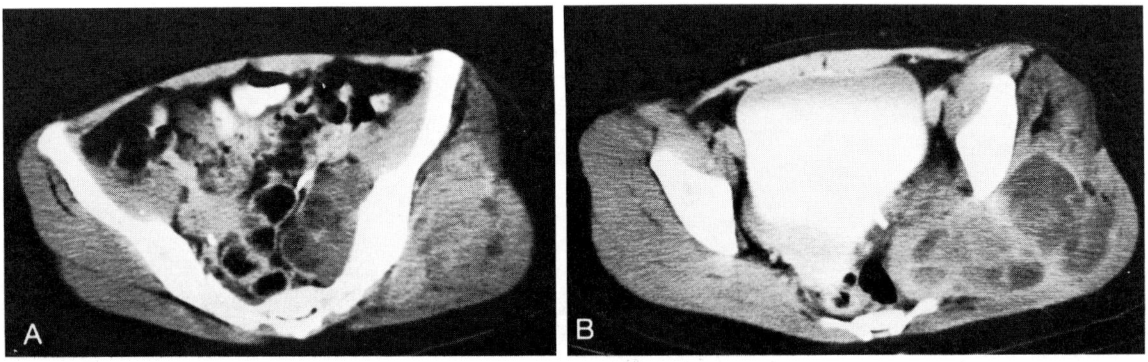

FIGURE 5–4. A, Rhabdomyosarcoma of the left buttock with a large pelvic component. B, Lower cut on scan shows pelvic extension through the region of the sciatic notch.

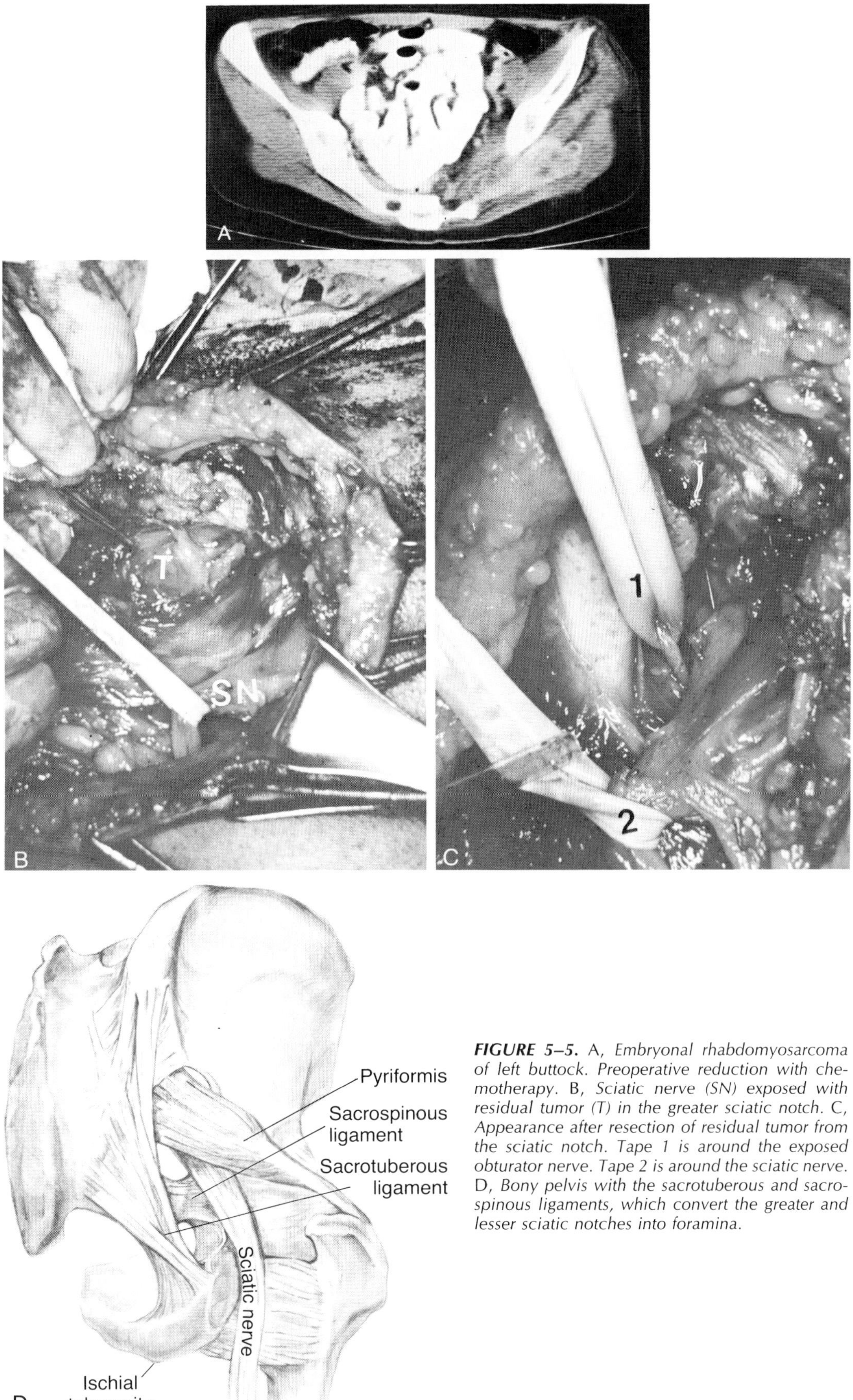

FIGURE 5–5. *A, Embryonal rhabdomyosarcoma of left buttock. Preoperative reduction with chemotherapy. B, Sciatic nerve (SN) exposed with residual tumor (T) in the greater sciatic notch. C, Appearance after resection of residual tumor from the sciatic notch. Tape 1 is around the exposed obturator nerve. Tape 2 is around the sciatic nerve. D, Bony pelvis with the sacrotuberous and sacrospinous ligaments, which convert the greater and lesser sciatic notches into foramina.*

nerve to serve as a marker for the deep phase of the buttock dissection; the abdomen was then closed.

The patient was turned in a lateral decubitus position, and an elliptical incision encompassing the original biopsy site was made. This incision extended from the posterior aspect of the greater trochanter to the mid-sacrum. Skin flaps were raised superiorly and inferiorly to expose the gluteus maximus. Because the tumor was palpable within gluteus maximus it was decided to define the sciatic nerve and trace it from the posterior upper thigh to the sciatic notch.

SCIATIC NERVE

The sciatic nerve normally emerges from the greater sciatic foramen, appearing as a large flattened band just under the lower border of the piriformis muscle, and comes to lie between the other external rotators anteriorly and the gluteus maximus posteriorly. The rotators and the nerve itself can be found situated in the groove between the ischial tuberosity medially and the greater trochanter laterally. The nerve descends at the lateral base of the ischial tuberosity and lies on the adductor magnus muscle, very close to the back of the femur. After resecting the gluteus with tumor, the main nerve trunk was identified and traced proximally toward the sciatic notch. A Penrose drain was placed around the nerve. The nerve was then traced under the piriformis muscle to the sciatic notch. At this point, a soft bulging tumor mass was felt impinging in the region of the nerve roots in the pelvis (Fig. 5–5*B*). The tumor was lifted off the nerve. The operative field at this time showed not only the sciatic nerve arising from the pelvic nerve roots, but also the intrapelvic obturator nerve. A Penrose drain was placed around the obturator nerve (Fig. 5–5*C*). The margins of resection were found to be clear, except at the sciatic notch, where the sciatic nerve had been compressed by tumor. Figure 5–5*D* shows the landmarks that are defined in relationship to the sciatic nerve and the course the nerve takes as it exits the pelvis. The patient had an uneventful postoperative course; approximately 3 weeks after discharge from the hospital, radiation therapy was initiated, with the center of the field being directed at the sciatic notch. After radiation therapy, chemotherapy was given. The patient remains free of disease.

SURGICAL APPROACH

The approach to most large buttock tumors was initially defined by Bowden and Booher.[2] Their surgical procedure has been described as a radical gluteal resection (buttectomy), wherein the entire gluteal system is resected to the sciatic nerve and sacrum.[16] The incision for this operation is created about the tumor, with skin flaps raised above and below the mass (Fig. 5–6*A*). Primary dissection is performed around the tumor down to the gluteal fascia. The origin of the gluteus maximus muscle from the lateral edge of the sacrum and coccyx and from the posterior portion of the iliac crest is exposed medially. The largely aponeurotic insertion into the gluteal (third) trochanter of the femur and to the iliotibial band is next exposed laterally. The gluteus maximus is transected off the trochanter and retracted upward in an everting fashion to expose the underlying piriformis muscle and, at this point, the sciatic nerve (Fig. 5–6*B*). Medial detachment is performed next. By palpation of the tumor mass within the gluteus, the extent to which a deeper resection is required can be defined. The operative field following resection of tumor and muscles is shown in Figure 5–6*C*. Figure 5–6*D* illustrates the postoperative appearance of a patient who underwent this procedure for rhabdomyosarcoma of the gluteus maximus 10 years before.

Wanebo et al.[18] reviewed the experience with sarcomas of the buttock treated at Memorial Hospital between 1934 and 1966. Seventy-one patients were examined, of whom 52 had resectable lesions by either buttectomy or, if the lesion was considered too extensive, hemipelvectomy. Nineteen tumors were considered unresectable owing to neoplastic extension beyond the proposed margins. Among those undergoing surgery, 21 had untreated primaries and 31 locally recurrent tumors. All had a mass as the primary sign, and 26 complained of associated pain. The selection for buttectomy was based on size, mobility of the tumor, clinical involvement of the sciatic nerve, and evidence of bony invasion. We use bony invasion as the primary factor in precluding the use of muscle group dissection. Buttectomy was performed in 36 patients. Preoperative radiation therapy was used to reduce tumor size in two patients, thereby making these tumors operable. We have found this effect to hold true for the rhabdomyosarcomas and

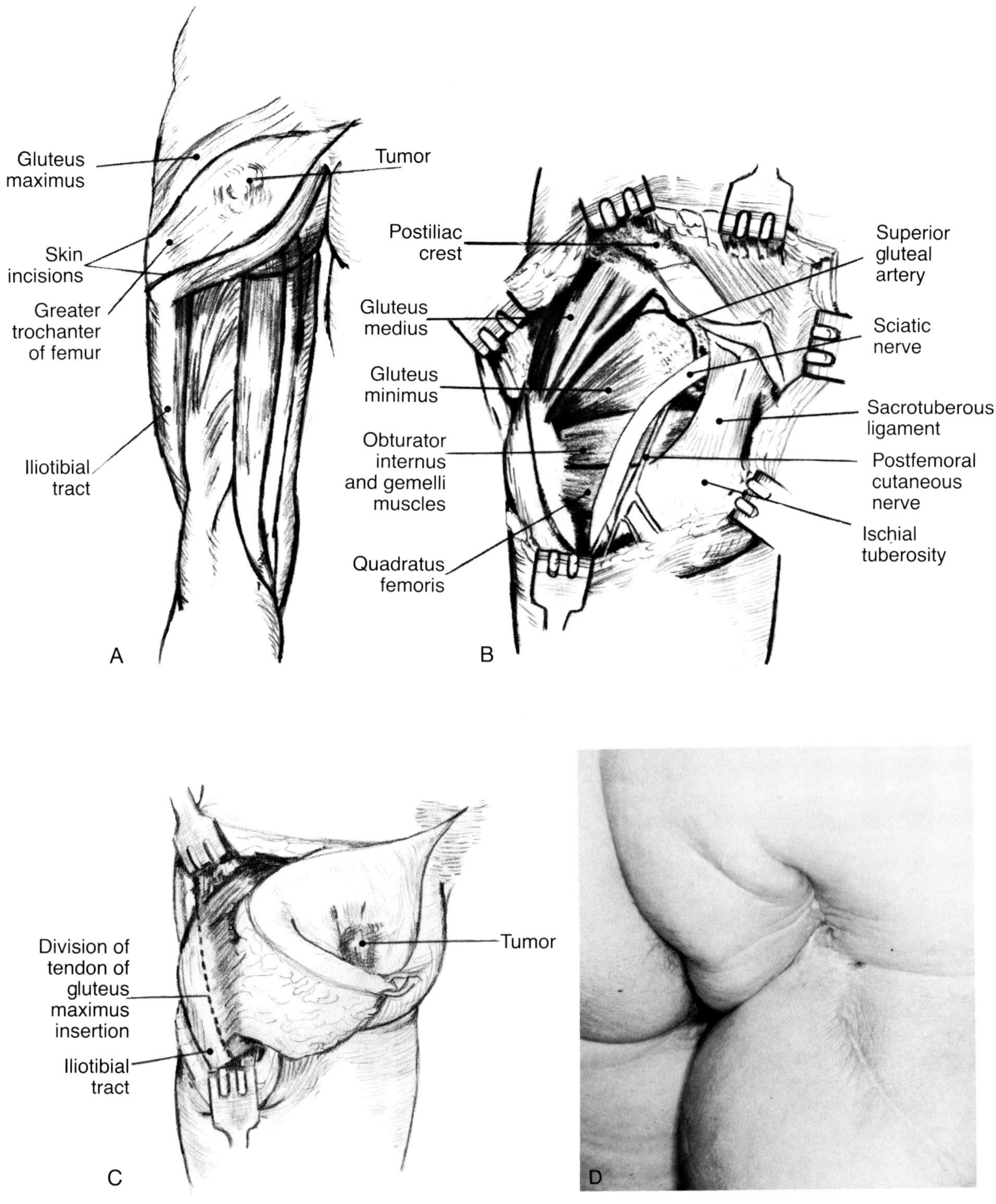

FIGURE 5–6. *A, Surgical approach to the buttock tumor. B, Mobilization of the tumor off the sacrum and posterior ilium. C, Operative field showing the sciatic nerve. D, Appearance after radical gluteal resection.*

liposarcomas. Five of the patients in the Memorial Hospital series had tumors that locally invaded either the ilium, sacrum, or ischial tuberosity. In this group of patients, a margin of bone was resected en-bloc with the primary tumor. All developed local recurrence, and four went on to have distant spread of tumor. Twenty-one of the 36 buttectomy patients survived for 5 years or more. The most frequently encountered sarcomas in this series were the fibrous tissue tumors (15 patients), rhabdomyosarcomas (8), and liposarcomas (7). In the buttectomy group the metastatic rate was doubled when the patients were operated on for recurrent disease. Cantin et al.[3] found that the incidence of metastasis increased from 27% in patients with local disease to 65% in those with recurrent disease.

TUMORS ARISING FROM THE BONY PELVIS

At times the tumor is found to arise off the posterior iliac wing or sacrum, necessitating osteotomy. Figure 5–7*A* shows the appearance of a chordoid chondrosarcoma presenting as a primary gluteal mass. The typical bubble cells (physaliphorous) of chordoma are not present in this lesion. This tumor was dissected off the sacrum by osteotomy, with the classic gluteal resection performed (Fig. 5–7*B*). Postoperative radiation therapy followed the resection. Deep margins were compromised by tumor. Because the patient was 81 years old, hemipelvectomy was not considered. The patient has remained clinically free of disease for more than 2 years.

A morphologic study of chordoid chondrosarcoma was done by Pardo-Minden et al.,[14] who compared this tumor with chondrosarcoma and chordoma. This tumor arises from soft tissue and bone and is relatively less aggressive than chondrosarcomas arising in this region. It bears a close morphologic resemblance to the chordoma, but its ultrastructural features are related to the chondrosarcoma. This tumor appears radiosensitive, in contrast to the chondrosarcoma, and long survivals can be anticipated following appropriate surgery or radiation therapy, or both. In one patient we treated, where chordoid chondrosarcoma arose from the interosseous membrane between the tibia and fibula, resection was followed by curettage of bone and cryosurgery to the tumor bed. Although amputation had been considered, this conservative limb-sparing procedure was chosen, and followed by radiation therapy. Three years later, the patient remains clinically free of disease. When cryosurgery is used for malignant disease, a follow-up biopsy is recommended, as local recurrence may be subtle and not recognizable until clinical mestastasis becomes evident.

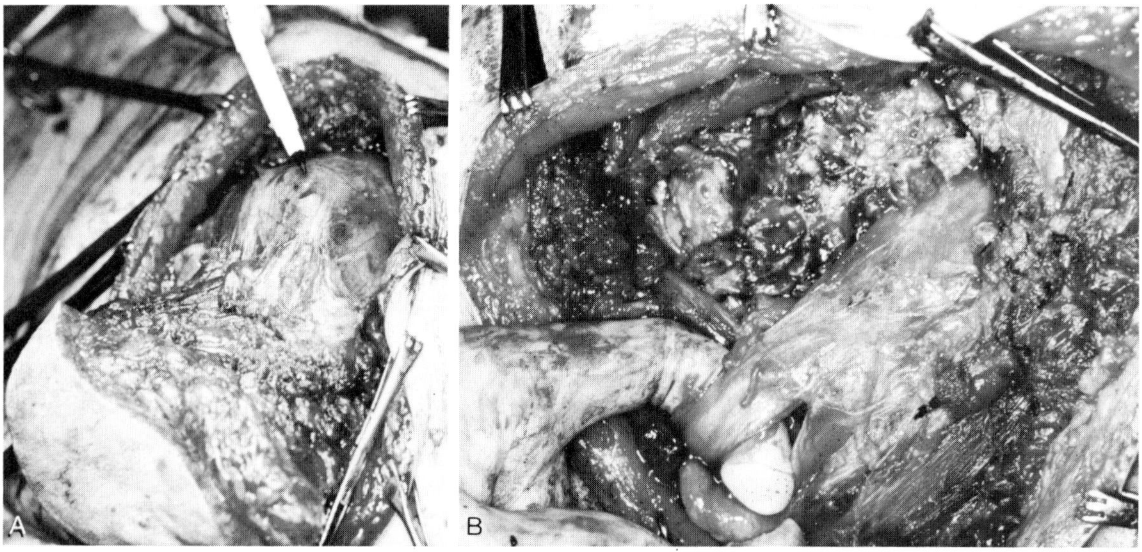

FIGURE 5–7. A, *Cautery tip pointing to sarcomatous mass.* B, *Sciatic nerve hooked by a finger as it passes into the greater sciatic notch.*

Chordomas that begin in the gluteal region usually present with dull or intermittent pain as invasion of nerve roots occur. Difficulty in walking can appear early, and patients can experience bladder and bowel incontinence as a result of nerve compression.[13] In the sacral region a large pelvic mass can form, infiltrating and displacing the rectum and pelvic viscera. Eventually a large mass in the buttock appears (Fig. 5–8*A*). An abdominosacral approach is required for resection, especially when barium enema reveals that the rectum is displaced and CT scan reveals a large pelvic component. The pelvis is entered to free viscera and ligate hypogastric vessels as the initial phase of the procedure. With the patient in a prone position, the procedure continues with sacral resection. The tumor has a characteristic bubbly, gelatinous appearance (Fig. 5–8*B*) and is almost impossible to remove completely. Partial resection has been found to be acceptable for palliation and is followed by intraoperative cryosurgery. Postoperative radiation therapy should then be offered. Figure 5–9 shows the appearance of recurrent sacral chordoma; tumor can be seen bulging from the upper midline incision of a previous resection. Repeat surgical decompression may be useful, especially if the tumor is following a chronic course and there is no evidence of distant metastasis. If radiation therapy has already been used and has failed, cryosurgery can always be repeated.[16]

MacCarty et al.[12] described 18 patients with sacrococcygeal chordomas. Tumors were identified during surgery and removed as completely as possible but preserving the nerves, especially the pudendal nerve. The coccyx and the lower three sacral segments were usually removed. Of the 18 patients one died in the immediate postoperative period, and four others died because of their disease at 4, 4.5, 6, and 7 years. Among the long-term survivors there were three patients surviving for 8, 9, and 12 years without evidence of recurrent tumor.

TUMORS OF SOFT TISSUE ORIGIN

Figure 5–10 shows the appearance of a large fibrosarcoma of the buttock. This lesion

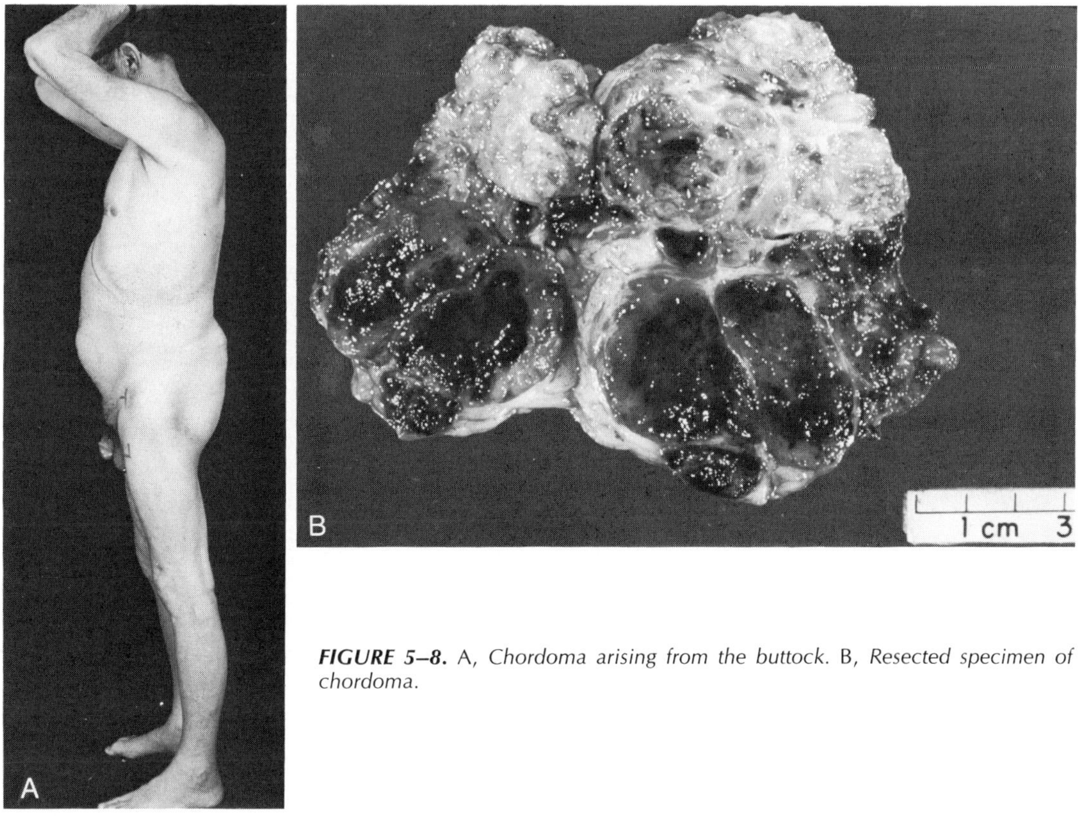

FIGURE 5–8. *A, Chordoma arising from the buttock. B, Resected specimen of chordoma.*

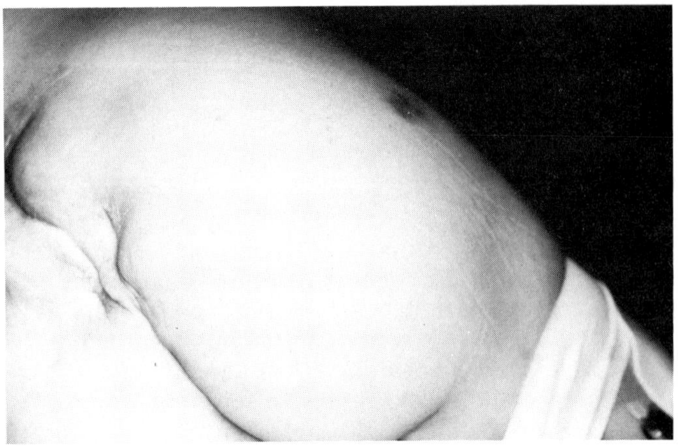

FIGURE 5–9. *Recurrent chordoma in upper incision.*

was fixed to and invaded the upper femur. Because of the patient's age, wide resection was performed without the necessary amputation needed for control of disease. Figure 5–3 illustrated the appearance of a liposarcoma arising in the gluteus maximus. The CT scan appears to be important in such instances because of its ability to define which groups of muscles are involved, the proximity to the sacrum and trochanter, and the possibility of sciatic nerve impingement. Most sarcomas can be dissected off the sciatic nerve at the time of transection of the trochaneric attachments. The one instance in which dissection is extremely difficult, if not impossible, is when the tumor has insinuated the nerve fibers, as occurs with sacral chordoma. Should nerve infiltration occur, the nerve should probably be resected as part of an en-bloc procedure, only if the surgeon believes this would be curative; otherwise, radiation therapy may be offered in managing the minimal disease left behind.

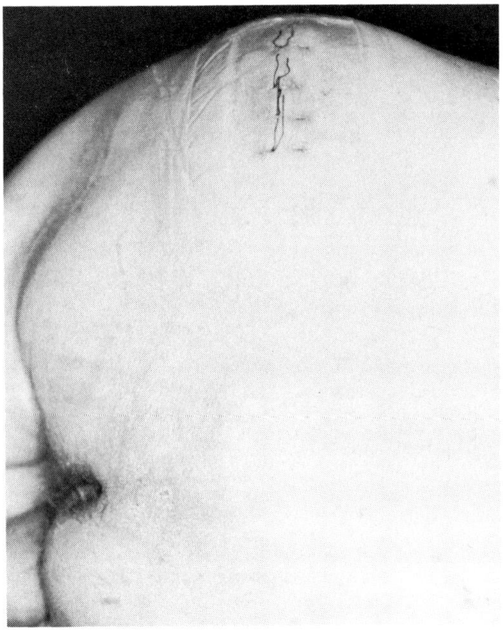

FIGURE 5–10. *Fibrosarcoma of the buttock.*

Other presentations for soft tissue sarcomas have been noted. In one instance, the entire gluteal region was replaced by necrotic rhabdomyosarcoma manifesting as a buttock abscess, and the patient was scheduled for hemipelvectomy. During drainage of the abscess, the tumorous condition was recognized. Because the tumor was too extensive for resection, amputation was considered, so the patient was referred to us for evaluation. On examination, we believed that even with amputation, cure would be highly improbable. Radiation therapy (4000 rad) was delivered to the buttock, and postradiation chemotherapy was used to prime the patient for a possible second-look radical gluteal dissection. The patient remains clinically free of disease 5 years following resection.

In most of the sarcomas arising from the buttock, there has been no evidence of necrosis through the skin. Recently, however, we examined a 40-year-old pregnant woman who had noted the appearance of a nodular mass in her right buttock. Her obstetrician thought the lesion was benign and failed to correlate it with the presence of café-au-lait spots on the trunk and extremities. There were no clinical signs of neurofibromatosis. Over the next few months the size of the lesion began to increase rapidly so that walking became difficult. The patient was now 5 months' pregnant and wished to carry the pregnancy to term or to the time when she could undergo a cesarean section. When we had the opportunity to see her the tumor appeared enormous (Fig. 5–11*A*). Extensive tumor was seen ulcerating through the skin of the buttock. CT scan suggested that the tumor was densely adherent to the sacrum (Fig. 5–11*B*). A radical gluteal resection was attempted without achieving the margins of resection. Tumor was found to invade sacral cortex. Histologic examination confirmed the presence of a triton tumor,[19] with a ratio of rhabdomyosarcoma to neurogenic sarcoma of approximately 3 to 2. It was believed that the only way to obtain a cure was to perform a hemipelvectomy. At this time pulmonary metastasis was found and further surgery was discounted.

Limb-sparing surgery can be considered with many of the larger tumors if it is preceded by brachytherapy, in which a concentrated dose of radiation is delivered to a suspicious area in which surgery cannot be thorough. Additional supplementary radiation therapy may bring the total tumoricidal dose to levels high-enough to be considered therapeutic. Again, later biopsy may be necessary to prove that all disease has been brought under control if supplemental diagnostic studies are inconclusive. We have not had exciting results with radiation therapy, even when higher doses can be delivered by afterloading. The exceptions, of course, are instances in which the tumor may be relatively radiosensitive, such as myxoliposarcoma or rhabdomyosarcoma. Radiation therapy should always be considered in situations in which it would make the difference between amputation and limb-sparing surgery.

Clinically, most tumors on and around the pelvic girdle and buttock region are benign. Biopsy is always necessary, even when the lesion appears innocuous. There is always the possibility that more radical surgery may be required. Therefore, potential margins of resection and flaps should be carefully planned. A 38-year-old man had a small 1-cm nodule under the buttock crease. Clinically the lesion was suspicious for a small lipoma or fibroma. There was no tenderness and the lesion was relatively mobile in the subcutaneous tissue. A CT scan had been ordered by the family physician and revealed a benign-appearing nodule (see Fig. 1–12*A*). Biopsy was performed under local anesthesia and revealed liposarcoma. The patient was taken to surgery for definitive wide resection, including the underlying fascia near the sciatic nerve.

The benign tumors are usually represented by large lipomas within the buttock region as well as angiomatous malformations. Wide resection here usually produces little deformity and no discomfort, and patients are usually able to function normally within 1 to 2 weeks following surgery.

On rare occasions, we may see unusual parosteal osseous tumors developing. Figure 5–12*A* represents the manifestation of a large sarcoma arising from the periosteum of the ilium. The extent of the tumor is seen in the angiogram (Fig. 5–12*B*). CT scan showed marked adherence to the periosteum; however, it was believed that local radical resection should be attempted prior to any am-

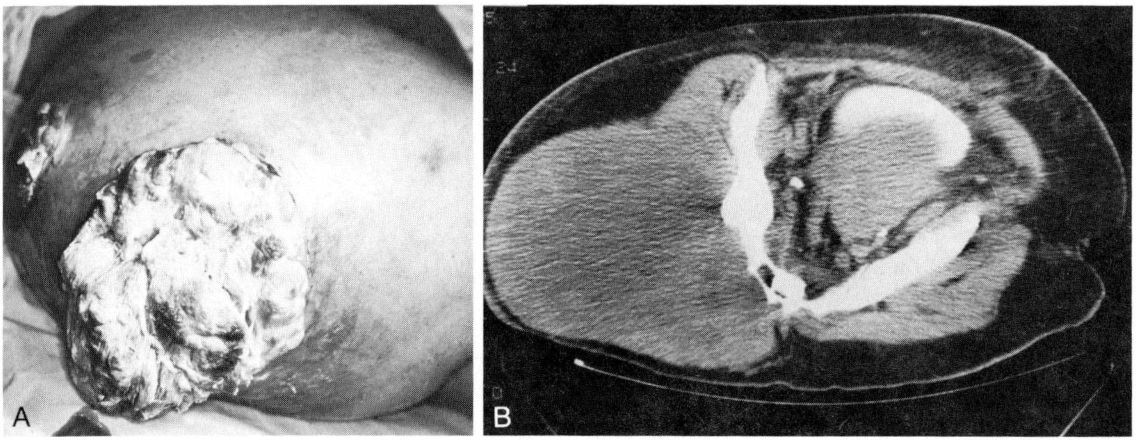

FIGURE 5–11. A, *Triton tumor of the buttock.* B, *CT scan of tumor.*

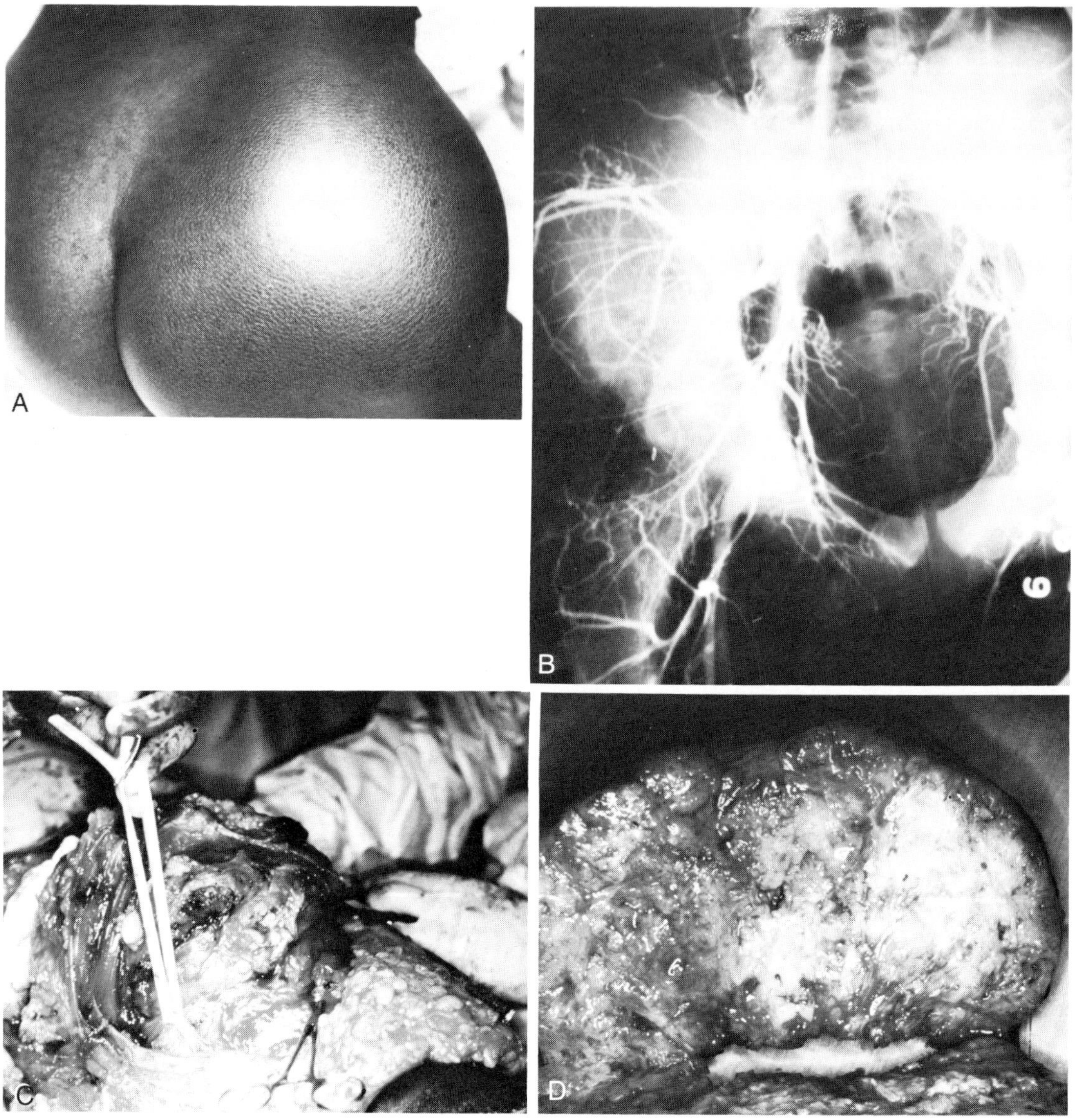

FIGURE 5–12. *A, Mesenchymal chondrosarcoma of the buttock. B, Angiogram of tumor. C, Exposure of tumor; tape is around the sciatic nerve. D, Resected specimen. Hand is behind tumor mass.*

putative resection. The grading of such a tumor is important. This patient had developed severe hip pain on walking, and this resulted in atrophy of the thigh over a period of several months. The pelvic region was explored first to define the major vessels feeding the tumor that had arisen from the hypogastic artery, as shown on angiography. The referring institution had performed an initial small biopsy, which showed malignant tumor that could not be defined histologically. Local resection was attempted (Fig. 5–12*C*). An elliptical incision was created over the tumor mass from S1 to the greater trochanter; this allowed raising of the skin flaps, detachment of the gluteus, and exposure of the tumor. After the sciatic nerve was defined, the tumor was separated off the sacrum with an osteotome. The tumor (Fig. 5–12*D*) was believed to be a mesenchymal chondrosarcoma.[10] Unlike other chondrosarcomas, mesenchymal chondrosarcomas are frequently responsive to chemotherapy. Such tumors are made up of a histologic array of chondroid tissue in various stages of differentiation mixed with cellular areas of small anaplastic cells that are frequently spindle-shaped or round. In this case, recurrence appeared within 1 month of surgery.

Thirty-five cases of mesenchymal chondrosarcoma arising in bones or soft tissue were seen at Memorial Hospital.[10] On histologic examination, the periphery of the chondroid nodules have been separated into small cell, undifferentiated, or even a predominant hemangiopericytoma-like pattern. Radical surgical treatment was used most often and included major amputation as well as muscle group resection for the soft tissue lesions. Thirty cases occurred in skeletal locations and five extraskeletally. Five cases occurred in the craniofacial bones. The humerus, ilium, and femur were the most common sites. The size of the lesions ranged from 4 to 30 cm. While some lesions appeared definitely cartilaginous, others were soft with large areas of necrosis and hemorrhage. On x-ray examination, the tumors exhibited a wide array of changes, characterized by osteolytic bone destruction, sclerosis, and intralesional amorphous calcification. Hematogenous and lymphatic metastasis complicated the clinical course either immediately or after a long delay. Pulmonary metastasis occurred in ten patients, and osseous metastasis in four. The median survival rate for this group was 7.9 months; the 5-year survival rate was 42%. Pain and swelling at the site of the tumor were more commonly noted by these patients than by those with the classic forms of chondrosarcoma. Among 28 extraskeletal lesions that have been reported, the brain and meninges have been involved in eight cases. The retroperitoneum and leg muscles were the primary sites in three cases each.

For many extensive tumors of the buttock and pelvic girdle, hemipelvectomy has been used to control the disease. Figure 5–13 is typical of the rapidly recurring rhabdomyosarcoma for which a hemipelvectomy with normal margins of resection was performed. The tumor recurred within several weeks of surgery and metastasized diffusely to the lungs.

Plain films of the buttock may reveal in many instances that the tumor being palpated is more deeply seated than thought and arises from or near the underlying osseous structures. CT scan is usually employed to define such margins, although MRI is beginning to offer additional information. If osseous structures are involved, en-bloc resection that includes a portion of the pelvic osseous structures must be considered. Hemipelvectomy may allow for more adequate removal of the tumor with better margins of resection. If a tumor is near a joint it may have already crossed that joint. Both hemipelvectomy and en-bloc resections should take this into consideration. One can perform segmental resection with removal of ilium, pubis, ischium, or sacrum.[5, 7, 15] Each site can be included as part of an en-bloc resection with preservation of limb function so long as one transects normal tissue away from the tumor pseudocapsule. To prevent subsequent limb telescoping and shortening, the gaps can be filled in with bone grafts either across the pubis or the sacroiliac resection. Even secondary scoliosis can be reduced. In the growing child these deformities may become quite severe. Subsequent limb lengthening procedures may be considered. If the sacrum is resected, the S2–S3 roots on one side must be preserved to avoid bowel and bladder dysfunction. When extensive neurovascular invasion has occurred, it may be impossible to attempt to preserve these structures and a hemipelvectomy or extended hemipelvectomy may be necessary.

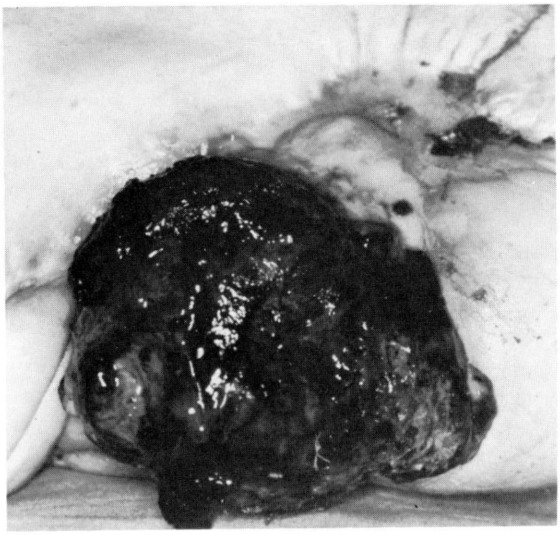

FIGURE 5–13. Recurrent rhabdomyosarcoma in hemipelvectomy stump.

Cutaneous sarcomas must be considered among the sarcomas that can involve the pelvic girdle. Figure 5–14 shows involvement of the scrotal and penile areas by Kaposi's sarcoma. At this stage of the disease treatment is extremely difficult since most of the lymphatics of the groin and pelvis are already involved by tumor and distant me-

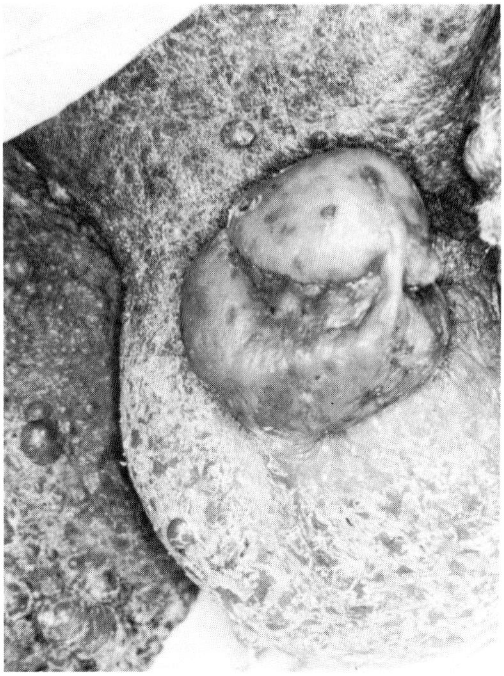

FIGURE 5–14. *Kaposi's sarcoma involving the scrotum.*

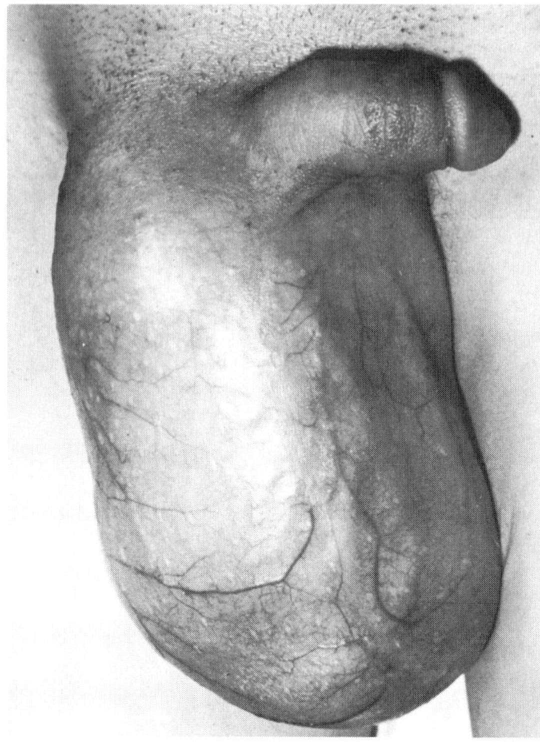

FIGURE 5–15. *Rhabdomyosarcoma of the spermatic cord.*

tastasis can be expected. Sarcomas are not only to be considered in the differential diagnosis of extremity and retroperitoneal lesions but should also be thought of in the differential diagnosis of intrascrotal masses of spermatic cord origin (Fig. 5–15). Here we see the intrascrotal presentation of embryonal rhabdomyosarcoma of the spermatic cord. Such lesions could easily be confused with hydrocele, yet must be considered neoplastic unless ruled out during the diagnostic work-up. Of the 13 cases of spermatic cord tumor reported from Memorial Hospital,[1] 11 were histologically malignant: embryonal rhabdomyosarcoma (5 patients), more mature sarcomatous lesions (5), and malignant mesothelioma (1). Among reported cases of spermatic cord neoplasms in the literature, rhabdomyosarcoma was the most frequent, followed by fibrosarcoma, leiomyosarcoma, and liposarcoma. Tumors were usually noted by patients 2 months prior to seeking medical attention. In one

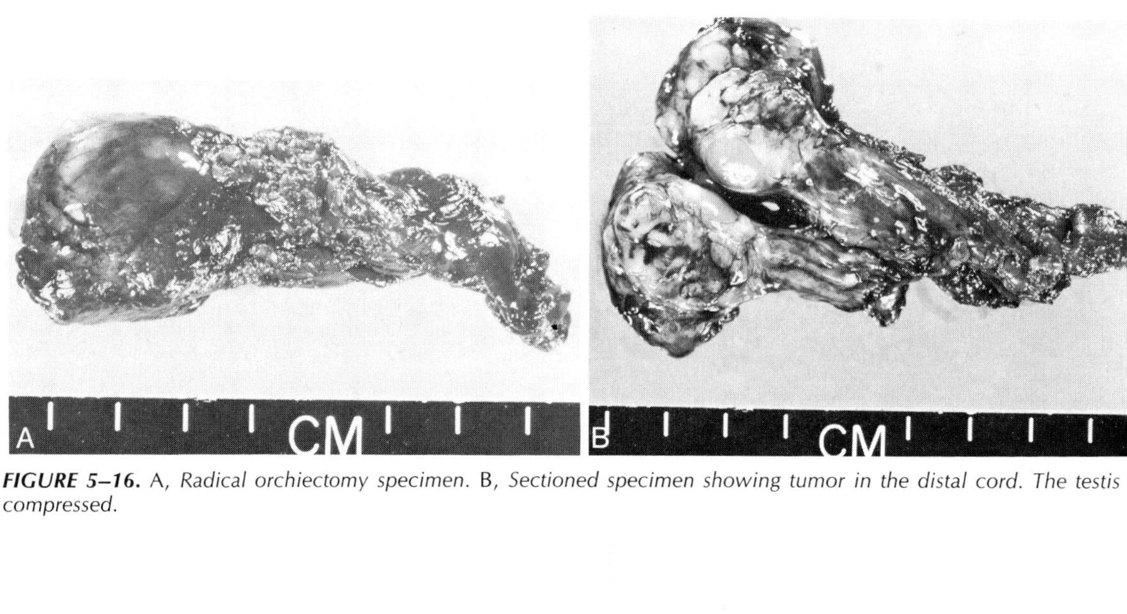

FIGURE 5–16. *A, Radical orchiectomy specimen. B, Sectioned specimen showing tumor in the distal cord. The testis is compressed.*

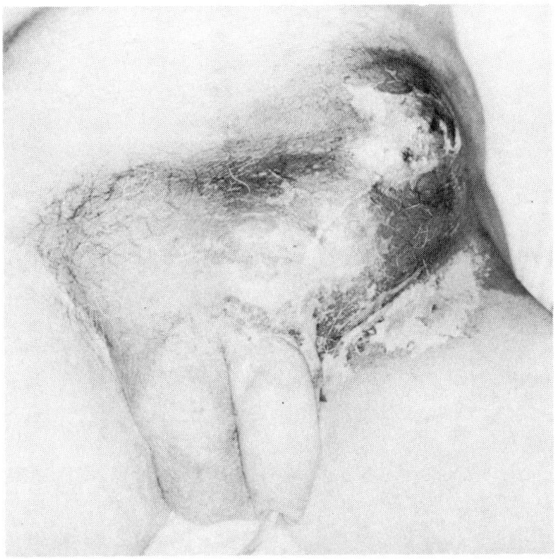

FIGURE 5–17. *Recurrent spermatic cord sarcoma involving the lower abdominal wall.*

instance, a painless scrotal mass had been present for 25 years before it was found to enlarge suddenly. The initial treatment for most cases has been orchiectomy plus high ligation of the cord at the internal ring (radical orchiectomy) (Fig. 5–16). When retroperitoneal node dissection was performed following initial resection of the primary tumor (1 to 2 weeks after orchiectomy), more than half of the patients were found to have positive retroperitoneal disease. In fact, the difference between survival and recurrence appeared to be related to node dissection and to defining whether nodal extension had occurred. Should extension of the disease be proved, certain lesions such as the embryonal rhabdomyosarcoma are best treated by radiation to the primary site and to the retroperitoneum, followed by maintenance chemotherapy. In several patients recurrence has been noted in the groin and lower abdominal wall (Fig. 5–17). No apparent relationship has been noted between this site of recurrence and the presence of prior retroperitoneal involvement.

REFERENCES

1. Arlen M., Grabstald H., Whitmore W. F. Jr.: Malignant tumors of the spermatic cord. Cancer 23:525–532, 1969
2. Bowden L., Booher R. J.: Surgical considerations in the treatment of sarcoma of the buttock. Cancer 6:89–99, 1953
3. Cantin J., McNeer G. P., Chu F. C., Booher R. J.: Problem of local recurrence after treatment of soft tissue sarcoma. Ann. Surg. 168:47–53, 1968
4. Cunningham M., Arlen M.: Medullary fibrosarcoma of bone. Cancer 21:31, 1969
5. Enneking W. F.: Local resection of malignant lesions of the hip and pelvis. J. Bone Joint Surg. 48-A:991–1007, 1966
6. Gray S. W., Singhabhandhu B., Smith R. A., Skandalakis J. E.: Sacrococcygeal chordoma. Surgery 78:573, 1975.
7. Gunterberg B.: Major resections of the sacrum. Acta Orthop. Scand. (Suppl. B):9–39, 1975
8. Halpern J., Kopolovic J., Catane R.: Malignant fibrous histiocytoma developing in irradiated sacral chordoma. Cancer 53:2661–2662, 1984
9. Huth, J. F., Dawson E. G., Eilber F. R.: Abdominosacral resection for malignant tumors of the sacrum. Am. J. Surg. 148:157–161, 1984
10. Huvos A. G., Rosen G., Dabska M., Marcove R. C.: Mesenchymal chondrosarcoma. Cancer 51:1230–1237, 1983
11. Localio S. A., Eng K., Ramson J. H.: Abdominosacral approach for retrorectal tumors. Ann. Surg. 191:555–560, 1980
12. MacCarty C. S., Waugh J. M., Coventry M. B., O'Sullivan D. C.: Sacrococcygeal chordomas. Surg. Gynecol. Obstet. 113:551, 1961
13. Mindell E. R.: Current concepts review: Chordoma. J. Bone Joint Surg. 63:501–505, 1981
14. Pardo-Mindan F. J., Guillen F. J., Villas C., Vazquez J. J.: A comparative ultrastructural study of chondrosarcoma, chordoid sarcoma, and chordoma. Cancer 47:2611–2619, 1981
15. Stener B., Guterberg B.: High amputation of the sacrum for extirpation of tumors: Principles and techniques. Spine 3: 351–366, 1978
16. Sugarbaker P. A., Chretien P. A.: A surgical technique for buttockectomy. Surgery 91:104–107, 1982.
17. Wanebo H. J., Marcove R. C.: Abdominal sacral resection of locally recurrent rectal cancer. Ann. Surg. 194:458–471, 1981
18. Wanebo H. J., Shan J., Knapper Hajdu S., Booher R.: Reappraisal of surgical management of sarcoma of the buttock. Cancer 31:97–104, 1973
19. Woodruff J. M., Chernik N. L., Smith M. C., et al.: Peripheral nerve tumors with rhabdomyosarcomatous differentiation (malignant "triton" tumors). Cancer 32:426–437, 1973

CHAPTER 6

Tumors of the Lower Extremity

PRINCIPLES OF MANAGEMENT

The management of soft part sarcomas of the lower extremity can be considered to represent the standard by which we plan for the management of most of the sarcomas arising elsewhere in the body. Not only are the soft part sarcomas found more frequently in the lower extremity, but in terms of management the techniques employed here can and frequently are adapted for use on other body sites. Muscle group dissection (Fig. 6–1), which is used to surgically encompass most of the lesions encountered, and vessel dissection, especially in the region of the groin (see Chapter 13), can be used for tumors in the arm-axillary region and extended for use on the muscles and vessels of the head and neck. Familiarity with the natural history of and mastery of the surgical techniques for controlling sarcomas arising in the lower extremity offers a broad base for the understanding and management of most sarcomas found at other sites.

Patterns of Presentation

The soft part sarcomas that arise within the lower extremity present an array of patterns that offer clues as to the tumor type and whether the lesion is benign or malignant. In general, these tumors arise as: (1) superficial cutaneous lesions, (2) nodular cutaneous masses, (3) ulcerating lesions, (4) expansile masses arising deep within the extremity, and (5) limb-girdling tumors that produce a generalized swelling within the leg. Within each tumor group, the differential diagnosis can usually be narrowed by analyzing information obtained from the patient's history, the duration of symptoms, clinical appearance of the lesion, and consistency of the tumor on physical examination. The site of origin, fixation of the lesion to surrounding structures, and invasion into the adjacent structures are important in the evaluation of the growth pattern of the tumor. For tumors that are categorized as expansile or limb-girdling, recognition of the nature of the disease is usually not established until late in the clinical course of development, as these tumors are usually painless and arise deep to the superficial muscle groups so that they are obscured from clinical detection.

The common sarcomas that one usually finds may involve cutaneous structures (as in Kaposi's sarcoma and angiosarcoma) or subcutaneous tissue (malignant fibrous histiocytoma, dermatofibrosarcoma protuberans, and leiomyosarcoma), or may arise from fascial planes of the extremity (fibrosarcoma and desmoid tumor). Fatty tumors can arise within the superficial structures and either appear as discrete nodular masses or may infiltrate these regions. They may also be found to insinuate deeply between muscle groups. They can also develop within the intramuscular structures as well as the subfascial regions of the extremity. This holds true for both the benign and malignant variations of the lipomatous tumors. As such, as easy as it is to make a clinical diagnosis of a superficial lipoma, many deeply seated subfascial lipomas frequently are clinically confused with infiltrating sarcomas. Other benign lesions may, on the basis of their presentation, be incorrectly labeled as malignant. In contrast to these

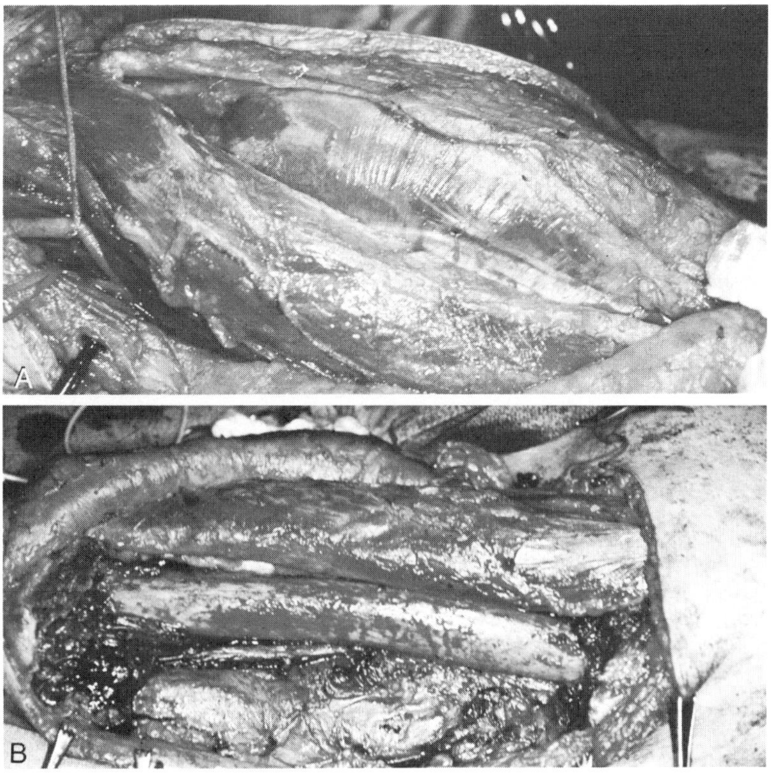

FIGURE 6–1. *A, Field of exposure for muscle group dissection of an extensive sarcomatous lesion situated deep to the vastus lateralis. The tape is around the sciatic nerve. B, Exposed femur after resection of the vastus lateralis and intermedius with tumor that proved to be a malignant fibrous histiocytoma.*

findings, the classic appearance of multiple subcutaneous lipomas may be mimicked as a result of disseminated subcutaneous metastasis arising from such lesions as carcinoma of the lung and kidney.

It is generally accepted that most malignant tumors arise in and around muscle groups and tend to infiltrate locally into surrounding fascial planes of the extremity, and as such set the stage by which we approach them surgically. Many have poorly defined margins at the time of resection so that it is difficult to ascertain adequate removal on the basis of gross examination of the operative specimen alone. This is typical for tumors such as the epithelioid sarcoma, which infiltrate surrounding tissue far beyond what can be predicted and probably can never be cured by wide resection.

In many cases that have been referred to us following wide local resection, further removal of surrounding tissue and of regional nodes, when indicated, has revealed the presence of residual microscopic disease. If the tumor has not been removed completely, then the result of such an inadequate resection will usually be followed by tumor spreading centripetally along the fascial planes of the extremity, but not necessarily within a given muscle group. If the primary tumor occurred in the upper thigh, it is probable that retroperitoneal structures will eventually be invaded as a result of invasion through the psoas region or the obturator membrane. Other sarcomatous lesions may extend deeply around muscle bundles or above the pubis, eventually reaching down to the periosteum of bone. Figure 6–2 shows the dissected leg after removal of a deep liposarcoma of the thigh. Resection has resulted in exposure of the femur. Some sarcomas, as they spread within the extremity, can occasionally involve lymphatic channels and invade the regional lymph nodes; most others must be considered in terms of their potential for vascular and neural invasion, spreading to distant sites along these pathways.

Factors Controlling Therapeutic Decisions

In any discussion of the management of such an array of neoplasms, optimal therapeutic decisions must be based on judgment and experience. It is difficult to assess the results of many of the reported small series,

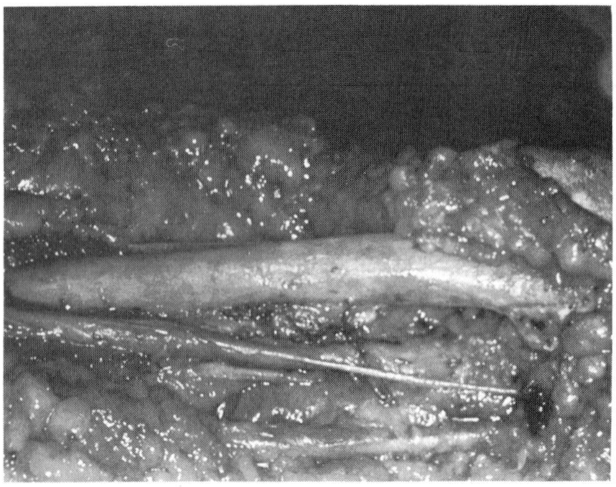

FIGURE 6–2. Femur visualized after en-bloc resection of an extensive liposarcoma involving the quadriceps femoris (rectus femoris and the three vastus muscles.)

especially since numerous factors control the patterns of behavior, including histologic type, size of the lesion, tumor grade, and site in the extremity (proximity to groin, knee joint, periosteum of bone, or neurovascular bundles). One must learn, through personal experience and analysis of existing case material, (1) the indications for the need for wide superficial resections in contrast to the use of muscle group dissection, (2) the methods for encompassing large aggressive lesions in proximity to bone, joint, and neurovascular pedicle, (3) the necessity for removing large areas of skin with tumor when so indicated, and (4) the methods for covering defects produced by resection of the tumors, using skin graft or myocutaneous pedicle flaps. The surgeon must be familiar with the techniques for vascular reconstruction and bone replacement when indicated.[10, 34, 43, 54] Furthermore, one must understand the indications for amputation when all other approaches have been ruled out.[18] We have attempted limb-sparing surgery whenever possible and have found that amputation may be avoided even with extensive tumor masses (Fig. 6–3), since good functional results can be achieved even when major muscle groups are resected. Indications for limb preservation can even be extended to those situations in which long bones such as the femur are involved by tumor. This has become feasible since the development of total femoral prostheses (Figs. 6–4 and 6–5).

The therapeutic benefits of limb infusion and perfusion with chemotherapeutic agents (before and after surgery)[60], hyperthermia, and radiation therapy or cryosurgery before and after surgery must be considered in their proper perspective as part of the overall management of the patient with extremity sarcomas.[13, 26, 47, 50, 72, 81, 88, 89] Management of recurrences in the operative wound, as well as recurrences in the amputation site, requires an understanding of possible neural and vascular invasion that may have compromised the initial operative procedure.

SUPERFICIAL LESIONS

For the most part, the majority of soft part lesions arising within the lower extremity fall within a spectrum of superficial benign lesions that are easily managed by the primary care physician. Most represent cutaneous or subcutaneous benign neoplastic processes, such as sclerosing angiomas, benign fibromas, lipomas, neurilemomas, and leiomyomas. It is important to be able to offer relatively accurate clinical diagnoses, followed by proper biopsy and histologic

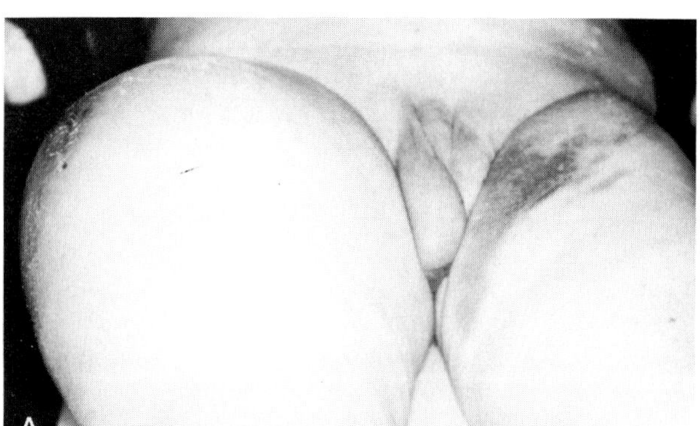

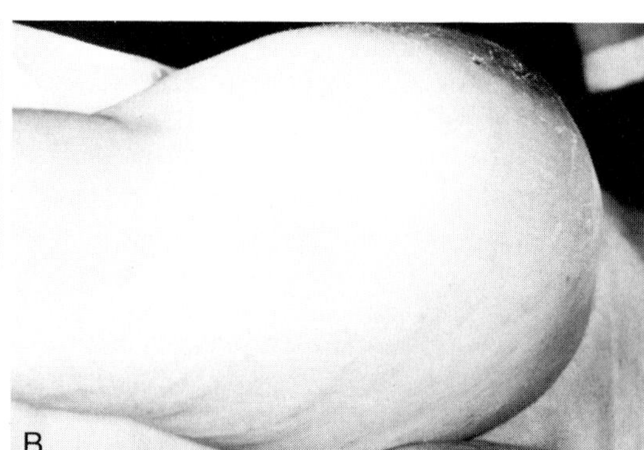

FIGURE 6–3. A, Large liposarcoma of the right anterior thigh. B, Medial view of the large tumor mass.

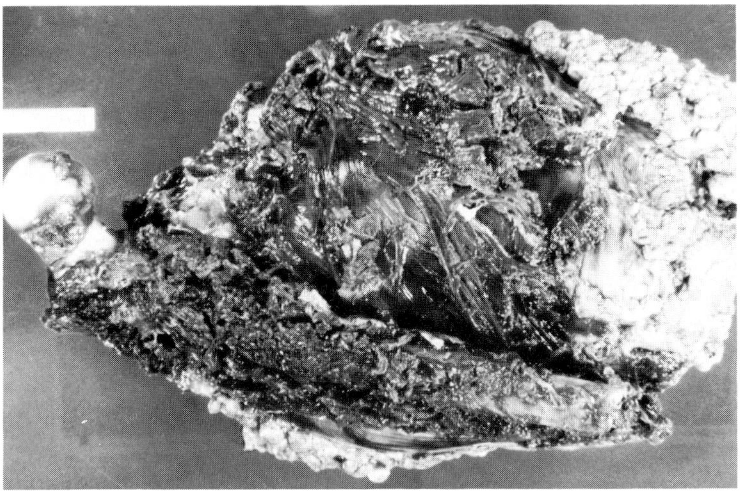

FIGURE 6–4. *Resected rhabdomyosarcoma of the anterior thigh with en-bloc resection of the upper half of the femur.*

examination. Innocuous lesions, such as ganglia, subcutaneous lipomas, benign fibrous histiocytomas, and neurofibromas, can easily be dismissed following adequate excisional biopsy and histologic review. Some of the benign presenting lesions may be worrisome in that pain is a primary complaint. Pain is known to be a factor accompanying malignant degeneration of certain lesions, but many subcutaneous tumors with such symptoms prove to be either painful lipomas or angiolipomas. Hachisuga et al.[37] reviewed 562 cases of angiolipomas, classifying them into capillary (374 tumors), cavernous (61), and venous (127). In 16 cases mature fat cells were found, suggesting a hamartomatous nature. Pain was though to be due to contraction of the vessels, giving rise to local ischemia.

In some instances, incorrect reassurances have been given when the patient has undergone resection of a small, somewhat benign-appearing lesion, such as Kaposi's sarcoma, Merkel's (neuroendocrine) tumor, or low-grade neurosarcomas.

DEEP LESIONS

While proper histologic classification remains of primary concern, equally important is the correct assessment of deeply placed lesions. In many instances, frank malignancies have been clinically assessed as lipomas

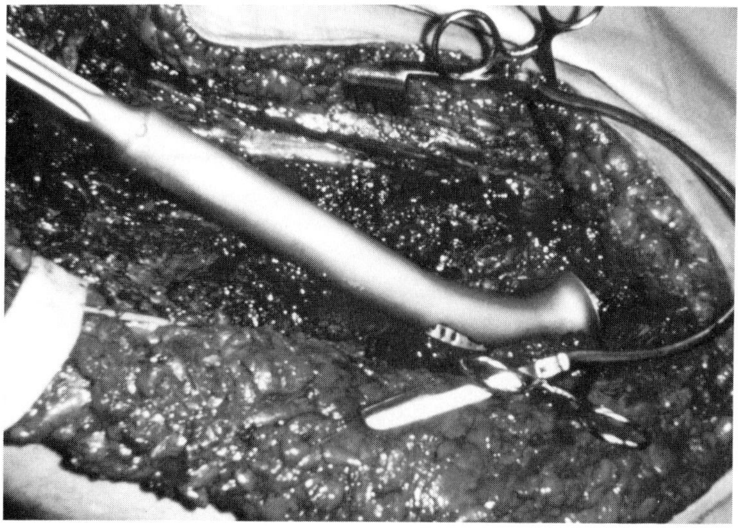

FIGURE 6–5. *Insertion of a femoral prosthesis after en-bloc muscle group dissection. (See also Color Plate I–2.)*

and dismissed as unimportant, when they actually were either malignant synovioma, liposarcoma, rhabdomyosarcoma, or fully malignant fibrous histiocytoma. Other tumors have been missed during initial examination or misinterpreted as a manifestation of phlebitis when they were found to arise deep to the superficial muscular structures or adjacent to periosteum of bone. In the latter instance, such lesions may be difficult to define even for experienced clinicians. Eventually, however, they will produce a diffuse swelling that was not easily appreciated in the early stages of the disease (Fig. 6–6). Clinical identification is usually defined only after the lesion has become quite sizable. The recent onset of asymmetry in an extremity should be considered as potentially serious and does require investigation to rule out such disorders as venous stasis, lipomatosis, lymphangiomatosis, and unusual hyperplastic muscle changes. Once these phenomena have been excluded, the examining physician must rule in or out the presence of a sarcomatous lesion. The presence of a lesion existing for several years (more than 5) does not eliminate malignancy. Recently we examined an 80-year-old man with an extensive mass occupying a major portion of the medial thigh (Fig. 6–7*A*). The lesion had been present for more than 14 years and only recently had begun to ulcerate at one point through the skin. He had been seen by numerous physicians over the past few years, each dismissing the lesion as of no concern because of the age of the patient and its potential for being benign or a slow-growing, low-grade tumor. The clinical and roentgenographic appearance of the mass was lipomatous. Our impression was that this tumor had the characteristics of lipogenic sarcoma. We chose to resect the tumor because of its size, the good medical condition of the patient, and the impending ulceration. A plain film of the leg had shown calcification near the ulcerating portion of tumor (Fig. 6–7*B*), which we erroneously presumed to be metastatic calcification. Pathologic examination showed that the tumor was a fully malignant mesenchymal sarcoma with malignant osteoid formation.

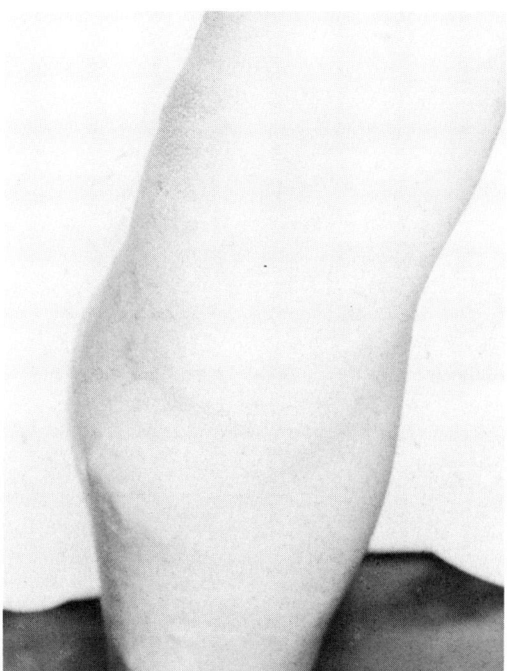

FIGURE 6–6. *Tumor arising in the tibialis anterior.*

We have frequently seen malignant sarcomas deeply placed in the leg so that their margins are adjacent to the periosteum of the femur, tibia, or sacrum; here the major mass of the tumor will be found to lie under such structures as the gluteus, quadriceps, or soleus. In rare instances, we have also noted such lesions in the region of the interosseous membrane between the radius and ulna or the tibia and fibula. It is improbable that such tumors could have been easily identified early in their clinical course, since most were asymptomatic during their initial growth phases. By careful questioning, however, the clinician can discern that symptoms in many of the patients actually were present for more than one year prior to recognition and biopsy. Sudden swelling of a limb may be a clue to vascular infiltration and blockage, especially with epithelioid sarcoma. Venograms with and without CT scan or arteriograms performed at this time could have proved helpful in some instances.

METASTATIC WORK-UP

In many of our patients who present with a tumor mass that has been diagnosed late in the clinical course of disease, there is a high likelihood that vascular dissemination has already occurred. This potential problem must be investigated as part of any work-up. Evaluation of lung fields by posteroanterior

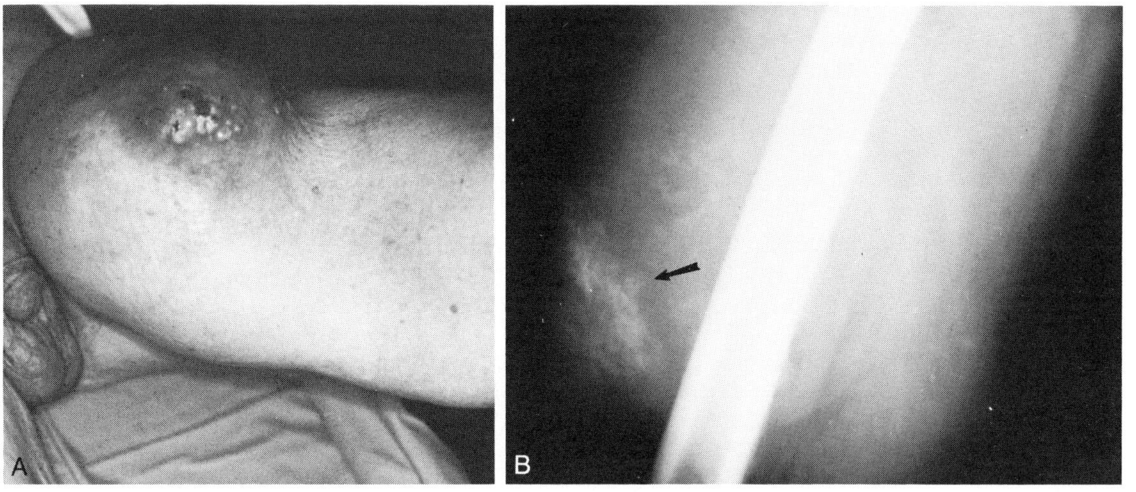

FIGURE 6–7. *A, Long-standing mass in the anterior medial thigh simulating liposarcoma with recent central ulceration. B, Plain film of the tumor shows calcification (arrow), which proved to be related to new bone formation in an area of malignant osteoid.*

and lateral chest films, as well as tomography or CT scanning of the chest, is indicated when one suspects a fully malignant sarcoma. This is especially true when the primary extremity lesion is greater than 5 cm in diameter and of high-grade malignancy. It is important to realize that no one test is absolute and that any one examination may reveal a lesion not detected by another method. Liver and bone scan may be indicated in appropriate cases. CT scan of the retroperitoneum, including the pelvis and abdomen, should be performed when any tumor is situated high in the muscle groups of the thigh and has the possibility of invading retroperitoneal structures by retrograde spread. There is little question that a delay in diagnosis is not in the patient's best interest. When a tumor is detected relatively early, biopsy and definitive resection usually offer the greatest possibility for cure. We have found that in some cases an exploratory laparotomy is indicated to help define the extent and nature of the lesion and to aid in planning treatment.

BIOPSY

The diagnosis obtained by biopsy is one of the major factors in deciding on the type of surgery to be employed. Which biopsy technique should be employed and which procedure should be utilized for definitive resection are of the utmost importance. Cutaneous lesions should be sampled by means of an adequate incision that should include not only the tumor but also a portion of the surrounding tissue. In case resection should be necessary, the biopsy incision should be placed in the region where the suture line will not interfere with any further attempt at surgery. Such primary biopsies may be repaired by simple suture ligatures. If the lesion is highly vascular the sutures should include the underlying base of the tumor bed in an attempt to control hemostasis. In such instances, a three-point suture should be used with the distal skin edge, base of tumor bed, and proximal skin edge as the foci. Nodular or deeper lesions can be biopsied by means of needle aspiration, incisional, or excisional biopsy. Because of the pitfalls of needle aspiration (false positives and false negatives) we generally prefer open biopsy. When performing any biopsy, consideration must be given to the malignant potential of the lesion and future surgery that may be necessary. If the tumor is malignant, the new incision line for resection must ellipse the previous incision site, which may have been seeded by tumor cells. It is important to plan the direction of the incision so that it will not only encompass the biopsy site, but also include those underlying structures that must be removed. The direction of the incision should also be aimed along the most common pathway for metastasis, so that the optimal degree of resection can be performed to include fascial planes that may have been involved.

In this chapter, we will evaluate the relative frequency with which various lesions arise in the lower extremity, those characteristics that might indicate the presence of a sarcomatous lesion, and the diagnostic procedures useful for defining the extent of involvement of the extremity tumors (dissemination into muscular planes, proximity to joints, vascular invasion, and bone involvement). In many instances, primary and secondary tumors must be distinguished. Biopsy techniques are important since inadequate sampling can lead to misdiagnosis.

TUMOR IMAGING

Angiography and CT scan imaging are important in the work-up of patients with extremity sarcomas that have been confirmed by biopsy.[33] The angiogram may reveal a pattern of extension not appreciated on clinical examination as well as the possibility of blood vessel involvement (encasement) or displacement. Figure 6–8 shows displacement of the profunda femoris artery in a medially bowed direction. This vessel usually arises from the lateral side of the femoral artery, about 1½ inches below the inguinal ligament. At the apex of the femoral triangle it lies behind the femoral vessels. It passes through the gap between the insertions of the pectineus and the adductor longus muscles, where tumor in this region has caused the displacement. Eventually it descends between the adductor longus and adductor magnus to end as the fourth perforating artery. Prior to definitive resection it may be necessary to ligate major vascular feeders to the tumor. Vascular displacement and infiltration by tumor can be noted, suggesting that possible vascular grafting may be required; this can be anticipated prior to the initiation of surgery. In those instances in which superficial infiltration of the adventitia of adjacent vessels may have occurred as a result of low-grade tumors, the tumor can still be resected with careful dissection of the blood vessels. Chemotherapy and radiation therapy would then be offered postoperatively to minimize the possibility of recurrence. Eilber has recommended the use of preoperative intra-arterial Adriamycin to diminish the incidence of local recurrence and to enhance survival.[26] The success of such treatment depends, to a great extent, on the vascular pattern defined by angiography. A vascularized lesion has a better chance of responding than one that has minimal vascularity.

The angiographic diagnosis of malignancy is fairly dependable and is based on findings such as (1) abrupt and irregular change in the caliber of the vessels, which is usually characteristic of invasion of the vessels by malignant tumor, and (2) perivascular leaking of contrast material outside the vessel wall, which probably represents vascularity within the neoplasm. Other findings seen in association with neoplastic growth but which also may be seen with occlusive vascular disease, inflammatory necrosis, and benign neoplasms include: distortion, dis-

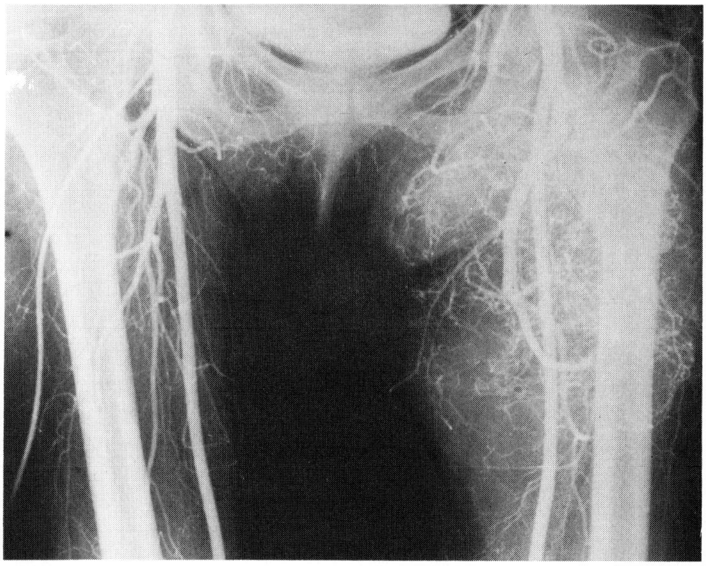

FIGURE 6–8. Angiogram of the left thigh shows pattern of tumor vascularity.

placement, and occlusion of normal vessels; hypervascularity; tumor stain; and arteriovenous shunting. In a review of the use of angiography in the management of musculoskeletal tumors, Hudson et al.[41] described 56 lesions, which included 19 fibrosarcomas, 13 liposarcomas, and 5 synoviomas. No correlation between the appearance on angiography and histologic type could be derived. Rather, the angiogram described the vascular pattern and origin of the blood vessels, and confirmed the feasibility of local resection over amputation in 14 of the patients. In our experience, vascularity may suggest histologic grading. Because one angiographic view can be misleading, it is best to take both the anteroposterior and the lateral views. A malignant vascular pattern may be found even after heavy radiation therapy, indicating the failure of that therapeutic modality. It also should be noted that fully malignant tumors may have no abnormal vascularity. At other times one may find that a biopsy-proven lesion may have no malignant vascularity but a short time later show a fully malignant vascular pattern. Weinberger and Lewinsohn[91] have shown that angiography has added substantially to a more precise preoperative histologic diagnosis and anatomic localization of sarcomatous tumors of the thigh. In the extremity, arterial infusion offers the ideal way of delivering drugs to the tumor. Denton et al.[19] have evaluated preoperative chemotherapy and rapid-fraction irradiation in 30 patients involved in a prospective randomized trial. Almost all had large, grade III tumors. Prior to excision of the mass all patients received a 3-day course of intra-arterial infusion with Adriamycin (total dose, 100 mg) followed within 2 days by rapid-fraction irradiation (3,000 R) over a 2-week period. After a mean follow-up period of 22 months, 90% of the patients had a useful extremity. The 3-year survival rate was 68% compared with an expected survival rate of 38% for patients with similar lesions who underwent excision alone.

Because it is important to completely extirpate the sarcomatous lesion within the normal tissues that surround it, more precise definition over that provided by standard x-ray films is required. In this regard, CT scanning has been formed to allow visualization of the exact muscle groups that encompass the tumor. Berger and Kuhn have described the value of CT in children.[6] DeSantos et al.[20, 22] have further defined the use of CT scanning to evaluate musculoskeletal neoplasms. A number of authors have confirmed the value of CT in defining the extent and pattern of tissue invasion by the soft part sarcoma.[24, 40, 51, 62, 91] When the vascular studies of the tumor show that vascularity is poor, a low-grade type of tumor can be assumed, but this does not always hold true. When the lesion is extremely vascular, one must consider angiosarcoma, hemangiopericytoma, and even metastatic renal or thyroid carcinoma. One patient we examined presented with an extensive destructive mass in the sacrum. Work-up, which included an intravenous pyelogram, was negative. Because needle biopsy was inconclusive, open biopsy through the buttock was performed. The lesion proved to be not only vascular but also pulsatile. A thyroid scan found a small nonpalpable lesion consistent with the metastatic sacral lesion, and proper therapy was initiated. On occasion, the marked vascularity of a tumor may signal the presence of rhabdomyosarcoma. Many of these tumors are not only extremely vascular but rapidly outgrow their blood supply, causing massive vascular breakdown within the tumor and erroneously suggesting the lesion is a benign hematoma. Biopsy of these lesions can produce extensive bleeding, and the physician may elect to refrain from further attempts at resection. Angiographic evaluation at this time usually reveals the underlying neoplastic process. Many of these tumors do call for amputation of the limb, as they approach regions such as the inguinal ligament or the upper shoulder joint.

PATTERNS OF BEHAVIOR

A number of benign lesions can easily cause concern at the time of presentation. Figure 6–9 shows the characteristic appearance of large nodular lesions in the region of the patella. The large giant cell tumor of tendon (villonodular tenosynovitis; Fig. 6–9*A*) is more commonly found in the hands and probably represents the second most common tumor to be found in that region. Figure 6–9*B* shows a large hemangioma of the suprapatellar region totally covering the patella. After the benign nature of this tumor

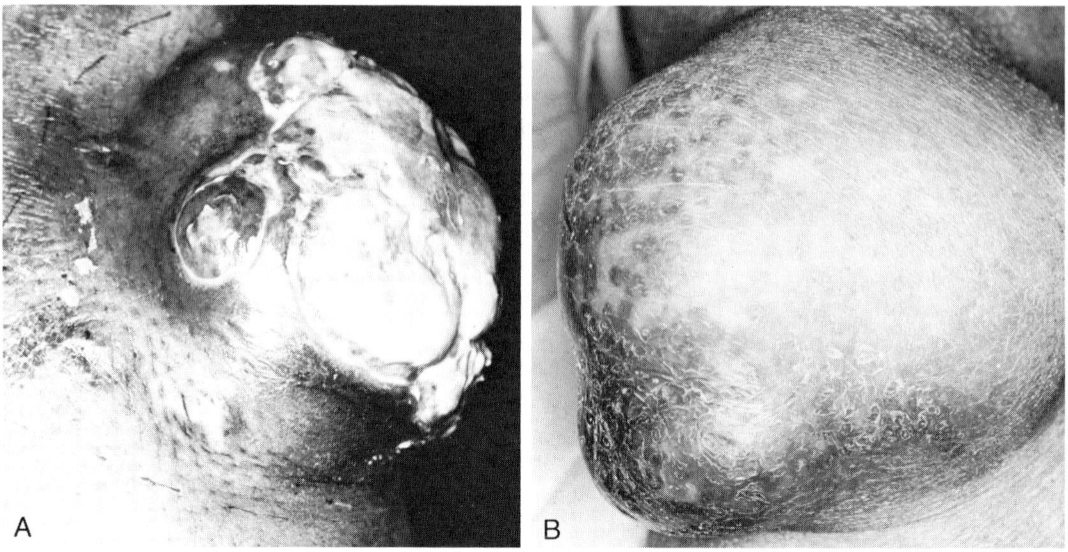

FIGURE 6–9. *A, Giant cell tumor of tendon in region of the patella. B, Suprapatellar hemangioma.*

was defined by biopsy, conservative wide resection and reconstruction was performed.

Pseudomuscular Hypertrophy

The appearance of a swelling in an extremity is usually presumptive evidence of a tumor mass. The use of imaging techniques and biopsy are considered essential in determining the extent and nature of these neoplasms. One of our patients at North Shore Hospital presented with an apparent lesion in the region of the gastrocnemius muscle, suggestive of a sarcomatous tumor. Biopsy showed hypertrophic muscle and fatty infiltration. Masdeu et al.[59] reported a similar case with pseudohypertrophy and fatty infiltration, findings that usually accompany muscular dystrophy. Other causes of such hypertrophy have been attributed to endocrine disorders, infection, and what now appears to be trauma to the lower leg. Benign tumors not only may appear to be clinically malignant, but also may have a histologic appearance that initially can be very worrisome. One of our patients presented with a nodular mass just above the medial malleolus. At the time of biopsy a mass that appeared to be sarcomatous was resected, with plans made for further surgery. Microscopically the cells appeared pleomorphic and sarcomatous, with multiple giant cells present. No signs of mitosis, however, could be identified. Such a tumor is characteristic of proliferative myositis.

Lipomatous Tumors

In contrast to lipomas, which are the most frequent primary masses of the lower extremity, the infiltrating lipomas and angiolipomas[4] are uncommon and are found within the musculature of the upper and lower extremities. Because of extension within the muscular planes, they are difficult to excise totally and are therefore prone to recurrence. Rarely, infiltration becomes so extensive that muscle dysfunction results or sensory changes appear as a result of pressure on nerve trunks. The vascular component of these tumors is inconspicuous and consists mostly of capillaries. The absence of large hyperchromatic nuclei and abnormal mitosis rules out the diagnosis of liposarcoma. Similar lesions to be excluded from the diagnosis of infiltrating lipoma include intermuscular lipoma, benign lipoblastomatosis, hibernoma, intramuscular lipoma, and spindle cell lipoma.[12, 62] Hibernomas are predominantly composed of multivacuolated fat cells and occur more commonly in the subcutaneous tissue of the back. The infiltrating angiolipomas appear firm and fixed and are frequently associated with pain and swelling. Histogically, a prominent vascular pattern can be found and may be reflected by severe bleeding at the time of resection.[4]

Angiomatous Tumors

In children, especially newborn infants, large vascular tumors may appear on the extremities. Such hemangiomas are the most common tumor occurring during infancy and childhood and about 75% of them are present at birth. These hemangiomas occur twice as frequently in female children, and occur singly in 80% of all patients. These tumors can grow to be fairly extensive, though they remain localized within the extremity. An entire extremity may be completely involved, and there may be evidence of extension to the viscera. They can also involve the retrobulbar space, breast, scrotum, tongue, liver, brain, and joints. Spontaneous ulceration frequently appears as a result of vascular thrombosis or trauma. These tumors are frequently associated with thrombocytopenia due to platelet entrapment (Kasabach-Merritt syndrome) within the cavernous portion of the hemangioma. Intratumor hemorrhage and thrombosis with involution can result. Various neurocutaneous syndromes can be associated with this form of angiomatosis: (1) von Recklinghausen's neurofibromatosis with hemangiomas of the skin; (2) Bourneville's disease (tuberous sclerosis) and Pringle's disease, in which angiofibromas are scattered in a butterfly pattern over the face and are associated with regional hemangiomas; (3) Sturge-Weber's disease and encephalofacial hemangiomatosis; and (4) Lindau-von Hippel's disease and hemangiomatosis of the retina and cerebellum. Cryosurgery, sclerosing therapy, and radiation therapy have all been used in the past to attempt to control such diseases. The possibility of neoplastic transformation many years later has led to a marked reduction in the use of radiation therapy. Occasionally, thrombosis of feeding vessels may be accomplished angiographically. Heavy sutures taken through the skin can be tied over the tumor and used for thrombosis of intratumor vessels. Angiomatous lesions occasionally can present in the subcutaneous regions of the leg as a nodular mass. Figure 6–10 illustrates the CT appearance of a nodular density in the posterior thigh of a 5-year-old child. On excision it proved to be a vascular malformation.

In adults, intramuscular hemangiomas

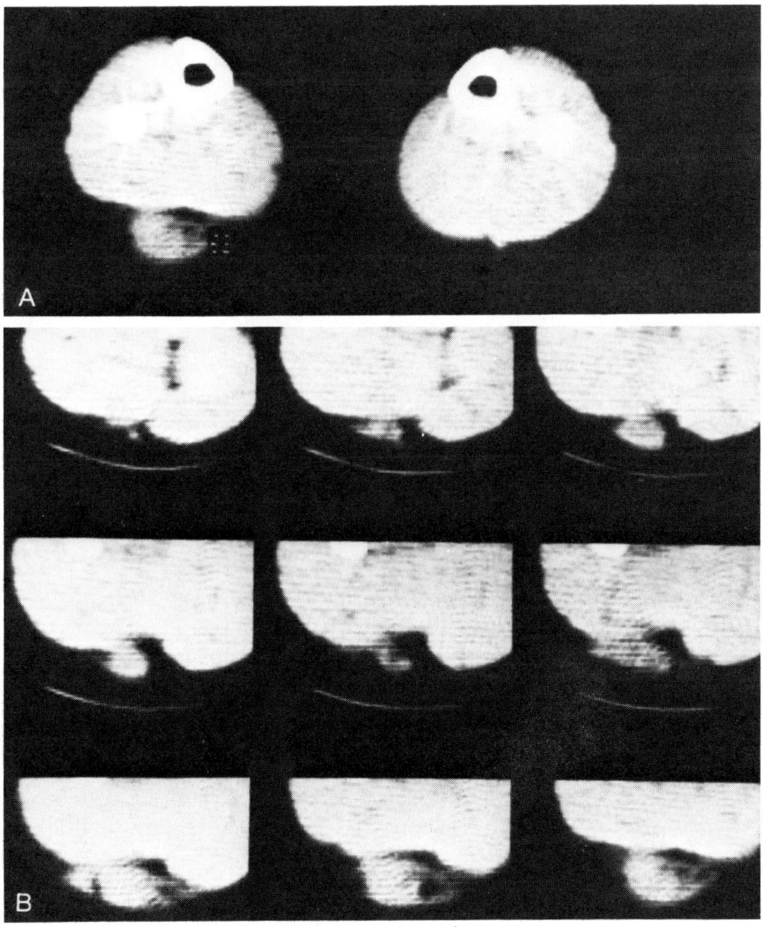

FIGURE 6–10. *A, Angiomatous lesion of posterior thigh seen on CT scan. B, Serial CT scan views.*

have been seen as primary extremity neoplasms.[2] Many of these have been biopsied and noted to be highly vascular neoplasms that deeply penetrated the muscular planes and were not clearly defined by limited biopsy. Most frequently they involve large anatomic segments of the body and are classified as angiomatosis. In the entire spectrum of vascular tumors these large lesions of the muscle represent 1% or less of the lesions encountered. Though any muscle mass can be involved, we have particularly noted that such tumors affect the neck, buttock, and arm, and most often the muscles of the thigh. Plain films of the extremity may reveal phleboliths. Angiography demonstrates the extensive vascular pattern that is usually encountered when attempting resection. In the presence of arteriovenous fistulas, some abnormal pattern of growth, particularly of an extremity. Statistically, the benign lesion is the most common type encountered. When resected, the vascular supply must be carefully traced and brought under control with fine vascular clips or ligatures. Figure 6–11*A* shows a large mass in the anterior medial thigh of a 30-year-old man that had been present and enlarging over a 20-year period. We carefully dissected the femoral vessels from the tumor, attempting to control all feeding vessels that could be identified. The defect where the lesion was present can be seen in Figure 6–11*B*. Marked displacement of the vessels is evident. The ill-defined lesion with numerous vascular clefts in a sclerotic stroma is apparent in Figure 6–11*C*. This lesion, known to be present for many years, had caused abnormal enlargement of the thigh, probably as a result of arteriovenous fistulization. It was necessary to identify the femoral artery in the region of the femoral canal and closely hug the vessel as the fine tributaries to the tumor mass were carefully brought under control. Failure to completely excise such lesions may lead to their recurrence. Cohen et al.[16] described two cases of intramuscular hemangiomas of the paraspinous muscles, in which arteriographic embolization was followed by immediate local excision. This technique was found to create a hypovascular surgical field that facilitated dissection. This type of recurrence was studied by Allen and Enzinger,[2] who reviewed 89 cases, in which recurrence had occurred in 18% and multiple recurrence in 7%. These recurrences were attributed to incomplete resection, which can be avoided in many instances by ensuring total control of the vascular supply during resection. Since these tumors rapidly revascularize following embolization, conservative management cannot be considered to be adequate; tumor resection is essential. The resected specimen seen in Figure 6–11*C* typifies the classic sclerotic lesion with numerous vascular spaces defined within it.

Kaposi's Sarcoma

Cutaneous vascular lesions are not uncommon and usually present as small, superficial, nodular, easily palpable masses. Occasionally, when present for long periods, these lesions are usually larger than normal but tend to remain in one discrete area. Frequently, one must rule out the presence of a vascular or hemangioendotheliomatous tumor such as Kaposi's sarcoma, which, while multifocal, can and often does arise as small nodular areas, often mimicking sclerosing angiomas in its initial stages of development. Such tumors may easily be managed by excision alone or in conjunction with the use of radiotherapy. Figure 6–12 illustrates the microscopic findings of such a lesion, composed of the typical admixture of plump endothelial cells, slit-like vascular channels with extravasated erythrocytes, and a polymorphic inflammatory infiltrated. If the lesions are known to be associated with diffuse areas of involvement, radiation therapy may be useful in bringing the problem under control during the early stages of disease. The tumors may reach a stage of local dissemination, with complications related to lymphatic and nodal involvement. Elephantiasis and severe cornification of the skin usually develops, resulting in the virtually complete incapacitation of the patient. Prior to such an event, radiotherapy coupled with hyperthermia or even chemotherapy delivered by arterial infusion can be employed in an attempt to achieve a better response. For this variant of lymphangioendothelial sarcoma, amputations have not been useful. Multifocal lesions above the amputation site can usually be expected, and these tend to spread to retroperitoneal lymphatics and eventually to the viscera. Bone metastasis can eventually appear in many patients as part of the end stage of disease. We have seen instances in which skull films

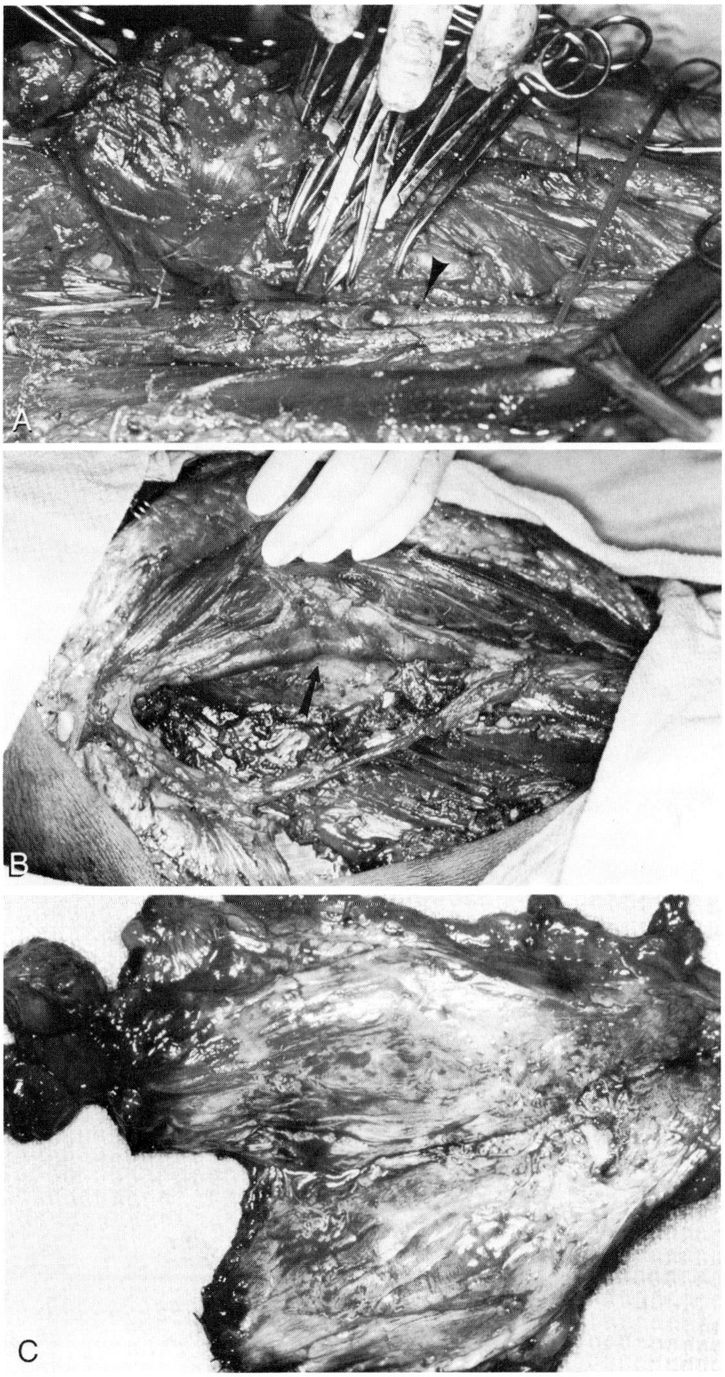

FIGURE 6–11. *A, Angiomatous tumor being resected from the anterior thigh. The tumor was found to be densely adherent to the femoral vessels. Arrow points to the femoral artery. B, Defect at the time of completion of tumor resection. Arrow points to displaced femoral vessels. C, Resected specimen.*

revealed disease that was so extensive that the lesions were interpreted as secondary to multiple myeloma. It has become apparent that many vascular sarcomas can and do metastasize to bone.

Lymphangiosarcoma

Lymphangiosarcomas, which occur secondarily in the lymphedematous extremity, can occasionally be identified and should be

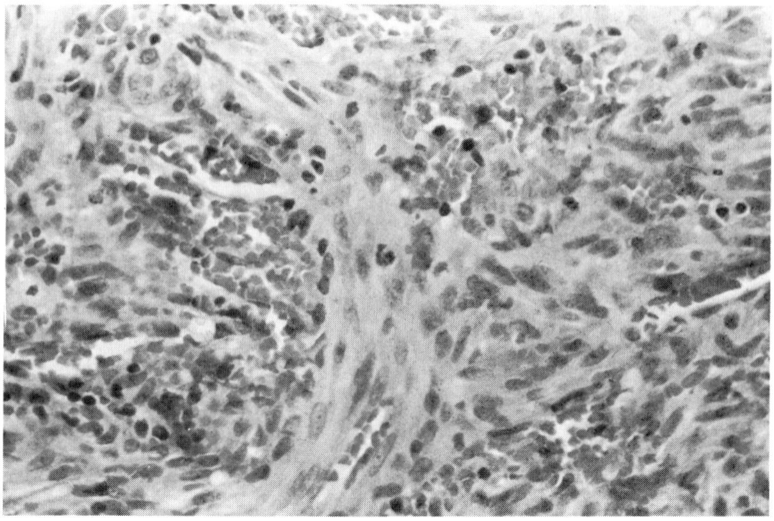

FIGURE 6–12. Microscopic appearance of Kaposi's sarcoma (× 100).

expected in any area of chronic lymphedema where discoloration and a cutaneous lesion develop. These tumors were first recognized by Stewart and Treves[84] in patients who underwent radical mastectomy. Clinically one notes the appearance of a macular, usually purplish, skin lesion that develops areas of nodularity. The tumors usually arise in the lymphedematous extremities, secondary to lymphatic obstruction from surgery and/or radiotherapy. Both the upper and the lower extremities have been involved by this type of lesion. One of our patients, a 65-year-old man, had originally undergone prophylactic groin dissection for a malignant melanoma. Moderate lymphedema of the right leg developed within 1 year of surgery. Despite attempts to reduce the swelling through elevation and use of elastic stockings, edema persisted. Seven years after groin surgery and the presence of marked lymphedema, he noted an excoriated cutaneous area over the pretibial region, with areas of purple discoloration. Within 2 months, the tumor had spread over a large area of the leg and nodular masses developed cutaneously (Fig. 6–13). Biopsy confirmed lymphangiosarcoma arising in the lymphedematous leg. An above-the-knee amputation was performed immediately. Amputation may effectively control this disease, whereas the efficacy of such ablative surgery for classic Kaposi's sarcoma is to be questioned. Although histologically similar, both lesions have differ-

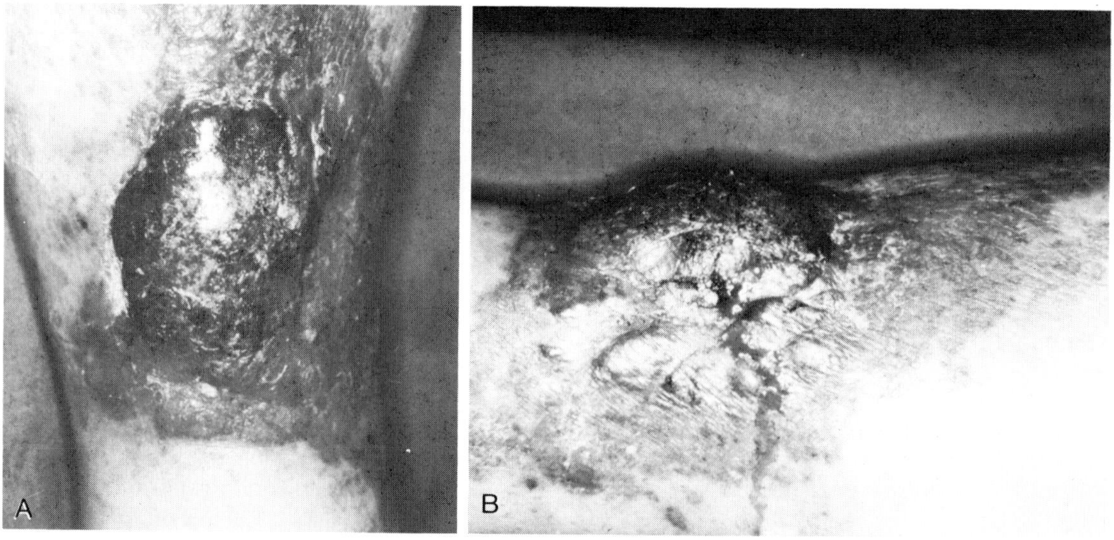

FIGURE 6–13. A, Lymphangiosarcoma of the pretibial area. B, Lateral view.

ent behavioral patterns in terms of how rapidly they spread and how widely they disseminate. Both lesions may be induced by an infective agent. Kaposi's sarcoma has been known to occur in homosexuals, where it is associated with acquired immunodeficiency disease (AIDS). In these patients, immunologic evaluation has shown a decrease in helper T-cell function and the possible association of an HTLV virus. The edematous extremity may provide a milieu for viral replication and irritation of underlying cells, allowing development of a similar type of tumor. Since the report by Stewart and Treves (1948), approximately 200 cases of this variant of angiosarcoma have been reported in the literature. It has been suggested that some of these tumors could represent metastases from antecedent carcinomas, but Salm has described cases without the association of preexisting disease.[75] In a review of the results of approximately 160 cases of angiosarcoma associated with a lymphedematous extremity, Woodward et al.[94] indicated that 50% of the patients were dead within 19 months of treatment and only 6% survived for 5 years. Centripetal spread and vascular dissemination to lungs and abdominal viscera are usually noted.

Cutaneous Leiomyosarcoma

Other sarcomas arising in the skin of the lower extremity are less common. Fields and Helwig[31] reported on a group of primary cutaneous and superficial subcutaneous leiomyosarcomas, most of which appeared in the extremities. The 65 cutaneous and 15 subcutaneous lesions that were described were believed to clinically represent an array of lesions that include skin carcinoma, malignant fibrous histiocytoma, fibroma, lipoma, granuloma, and neurogenic tumor. All developed as painful or tender intracutaneous nodules. Only after biopsy was performed did the diagnosis of leiomyosarcoma become established. Stout and Hill[87] initially reviewed cutaneous and subcutaneous leiomyomas of the skin, a group of smooth muscle superficial tumors, selecting only those cases that were considered to be malignant. In updating their analysis they found 36 malignant lesions, which microscopically were seen to consist of a poorly differentiated proliferation of spindle-shaped atypical myxomatous cells arranged in interlacing fascicles emerging into a collagenous stroma. At times, the benign lesions grew large and became calcified. Fields noted that local recurrence of such lesions was high among his group of patients. There was a 40% distribution of cutaneous lesions and a 50% incidence for subcutaneous tumors. In the latter group, one third eventually manifested metastasis or tumor-related death. Stout found a 61% incidence of local recurrence and a 56% incidence of metastasis in the deeper lesions. All of those that disseminated (19 tumors), involved metastasis to the lung, and an additional four patients showed signs of spread to the regional lymph nodes.

The median size of the resected cutaneous smooth muscle lesions was 1.8 cm, with a somewhat larger size (4 cm) for the subcutaneous tumors. Both groups are usually found to be slow-growing, with the interval from onset to diagnosis being 1 to 2 years. Cutaneous lesions develop either as a circumscribed nodular, lobular, or pedunculated tumor mass, or as a poorly defined induration of the skin. The subcutaneous variant is noted to be round oval, or lobulated with a rubbery hard texture, and white to yellow in color. Because of the high likelihood of recurrence, wide local excision of the cutaneous lesions will probably result in cure. Skin grafting may, however, be necessary when one utilizes a sufficiently wide resection to minimize the possibility of local recurrence. Deeper lesions may require more aggressive resection to the underlying fascia. It is essential that wide margins be histologically free of tumor. Occasionally, the benign form of leiomyoma may present as a large tumor mass. Ross et al.[74] reported a case involving a 6½-year-old boy with pain and swelling behind his left knee. A hard, slightly tender mass was palpated posterior to the tibia, just below the popliteal fossa. X-ray films showed a large cluster of calcified deposits in a mulberry configuration, surrounded by a thick band of calcification suggesting a capsule. The mass was adjacent to but separated from the tibia. On angiography, the mass was believed to be vascular. Radionuclide scanning demonstrated considerable uptake in the region corresponding to the calcified mass. It was necessary to mobilize the proximal origin of the medial gastrocnemius belly to gain exposure. After the neurovascular bundle in the distal popliteal space was totally retracted, the lesion

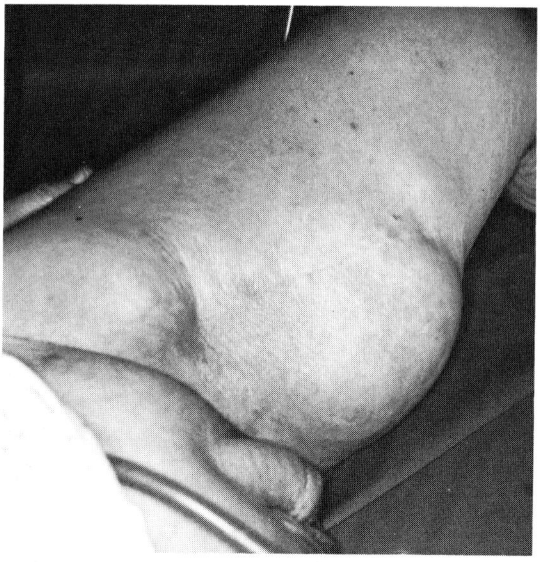

FIGURE 6–14. Large lipogenic sarcoma of the left thigh.

was separated by blunt dissection from the adjacent soft tissues and was completely excised. Fortunately, the tumor, which measured approximately 7 cm in diameter, was benign. Its pattern of spindle-shaped tumor cells arranged in fascicles was consistent with that of a benign leiomyoma with multiple areas of calcification.

Liposarcoma

Those tumors arising in the deep subcutaneous structures, such as dermatofibrosarcoma, are less common in the lower extremity than on the trunk and upper extremity. The most frequently encountered subcutaneous nodular masses are the lipomas. A lipogenic sarcoma can have many of the characteristic gross features of a benign fatty tumor. The pathologist should be able to identify such lesions by their greater degree of cellularity and sometimes the presence of multinucleated cells. The tumor may be completely enucleated and still have no suggestion of the firmness needed to consider it sarcomatous. Such lesions may be confused with benign lipomas even at the time of surgery. Figure 6–14 shows the clinical appearance of a large tumor of the medial aspect of the thigh that had been primarily resected 13 years before. Seven years ago, the lesion recurred and at that time it became apparent that the original tumor was a lipogenic sarcoma. CT scan on recent admission showed marked muscle involvement (Fig. 6–15) by a tumor with a high fat content totally surrounding the major vascular structures of the thigh. Considering the advanced age of the patient, debulking was believed to be the treatment of choice. In a younger patient, one might consider amputation or debulking with the knowledge that amputation might later be indicated. Because of the low-grade nature of the tumor, local recurrence would be more likely than distant spread.

Occasionally, atrophy and myxoid changes occur in a lipoma to mimic a low-grade myxoid liposarcoma. Fat necrosis may also simulate a well-differentiated liposarcoma. The above-mentioned patient was taken to surgery, and Figure 6–16 shows the clinical appearance of the large recurrent lipogenic sarcoma of the thigh as it was resected and the appearance of the tumor as it was being dissected away from the femoral vessels in the groin. Low-grade tumors like this would probably recur locally before metastasizing; therefore, one may attempt limb-sparing surgery before amputation.

If the tumor that has been resected represents a fully malignant liposarcoma, the incidence of recurrence and even possible me-

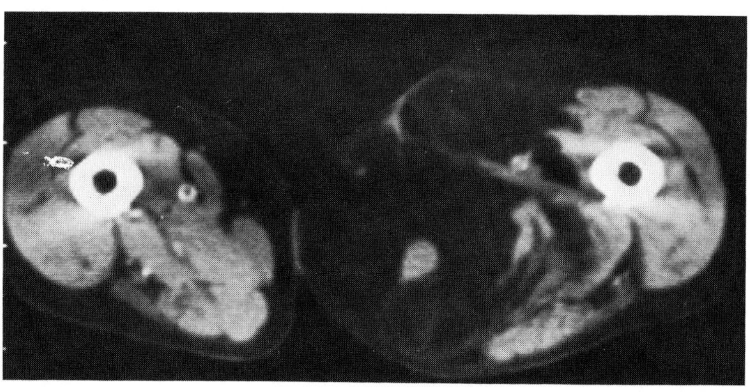

FIGURE 6–15. CT scan of the lipogenic sarcoma shown in Figure 6–14, showing extensive muscle involvement.

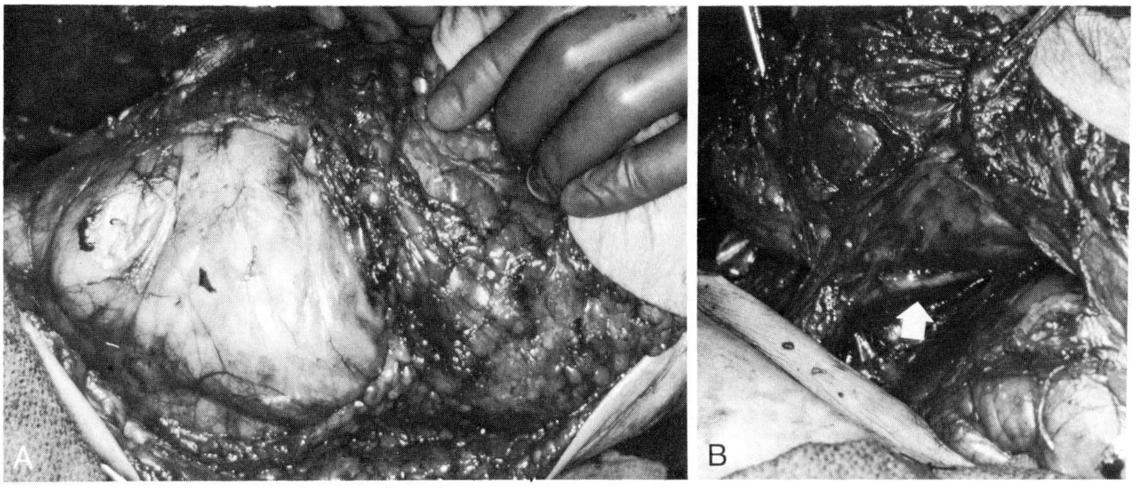

FIGURE 6–16. A, *Tumor being mobilized from the medial thigh.* B, *Dissection of tumor off the femoral vessels (arrow).*

tastasis can be fairly high.[20, 22, 30, 44, 49] As a small fatty tumor enlarges, especially if it has been observed for a long time, the possibility that it is malignant increases. When confronted with any fatty tumor larger than 5 cm in diameter, where enlargement appears to be continuing, one must take a biopsy to prove its actual histologic composition. For many fatty tumors, areas of malignant transformation are not usually uniform, so that random biopsy may not show the true nature of the lesion. Only adequate sampling or complete removal of the lesion will ascertain malignancy or benignity. When enucleation for biopsy purposes has been performed, the normal dimensions of the original lesion are obscured and a definitive local radical procedure may be more difficult to accomplish. This must be taken into account when planning the biopsy and the operation.

In several instances, we have seen lesions reported to be classic liposarcoma. Later, distant metastatic deposits were identified and resected. In such instances, careful review of the primary tumor and the metastatic foci suggested that the tumor was actually a mesenchymal sarcoma. Only after the initial primary tumor can be reevaluated and compared with the metastatic focus can one arrive at a more accurate diagnosis. For the most part, however, large fatty tumors of the thigh do represent malignant sarcomas, i.e., the liposarcoma. The liposarcomas themselves appear as discrete masses in the extremity, usually displacing surrounding muscles rather than extending into them as many of the fibrous tissue tumors do. Figure 6–17 shows a bulky discrete lesion in the posterior aspect of the thigh. In many instances such lesions may have a well-defined pseudocapsule (compressed tumor cells), which can be misinterpreted by the surgeon as a good plane for tumor dissection. Resection of the tumor proved that it was a liposarcoma. The CT scan in Figure 6–18 shows the appearance of a similar well-defined lesion in the posterior thigh. The tumor is seen sitting deep to the medially placed semimembranosus and semitendinosus muscles, with the biceps femoris completing the hamstring group of muscles. In actuality, this and other types of lesions require wide resection of surrounding tissue to ensure adequate margins (muscle group dissection). In this type of case, total muscle group dissection may not be necessary. Rather, taking a generous margin of normal surrounding muscles, including adjacent muscle not of a particular muscle group, can be employed to achieve adequate resection (Fig. 6–19). Intramuscular septa alone are not adequate margins for resection. As the tumor enlarges in size, it can present as a sizable mass. In rare instances, these tumors can reach enormous proportions before the patient seeks assistance (Fig. 6–20*A* and *B*). To ensure adequate resection with surrounding tissue, muscle group dissection must include all normal surrounding muscle planes, even extending to the femur if necessary. Figure 6–20C illustrates a problem

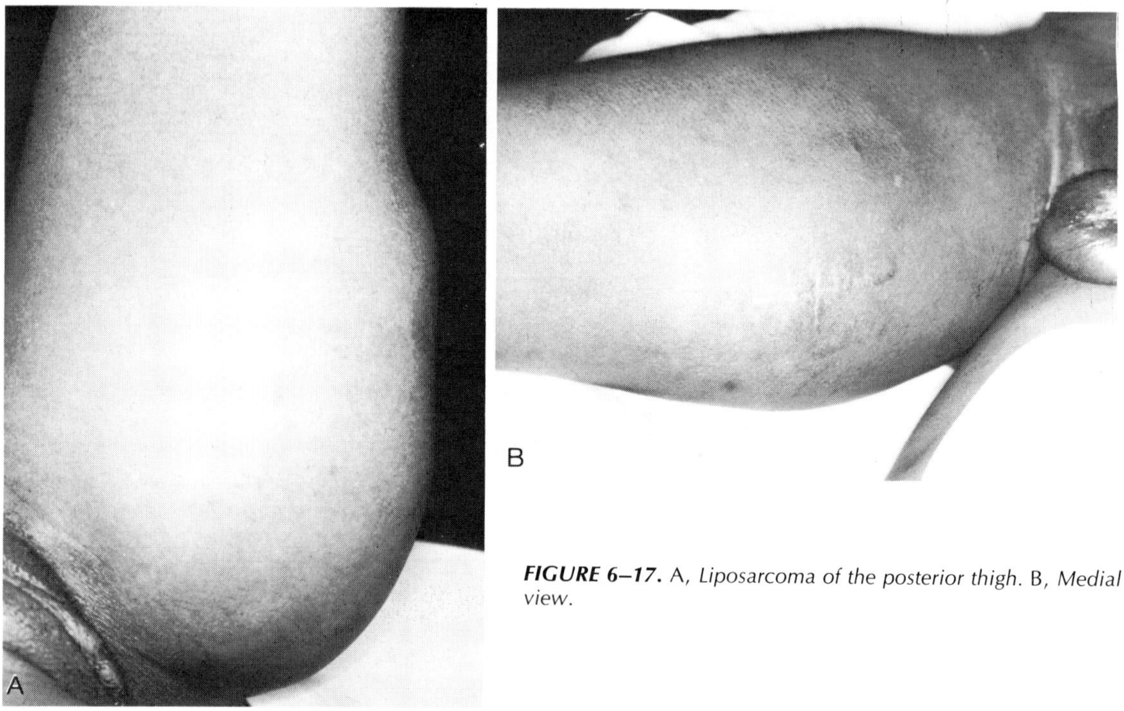

FIGURE 6–17. *A, Liposarcoma of the posterior thigh. B, Medial view.*

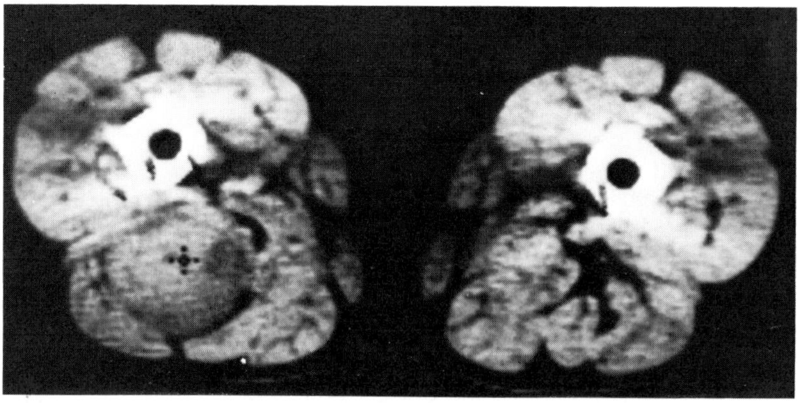

FIGURE 6–18. *CT scan showing sarcoma deep to the hamstrings.*

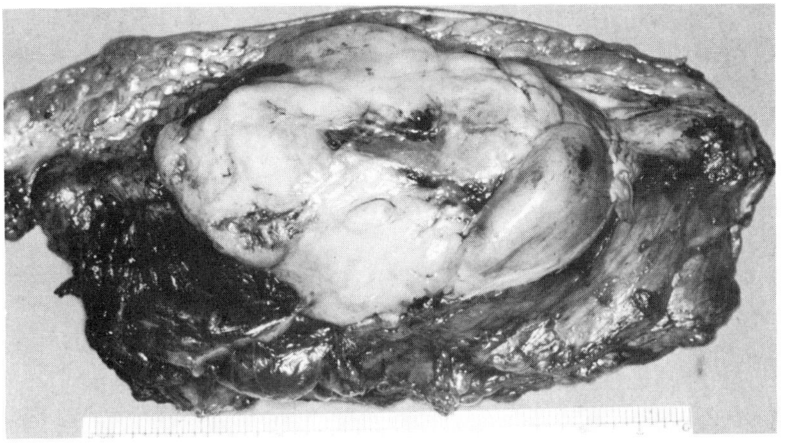

FIGURE 6–19. *Liposarcoma from the thigh with muscles (portion of quadriceps) removed to achieve margins of resection. Tumor is seen extending into subcutaneous fat.*

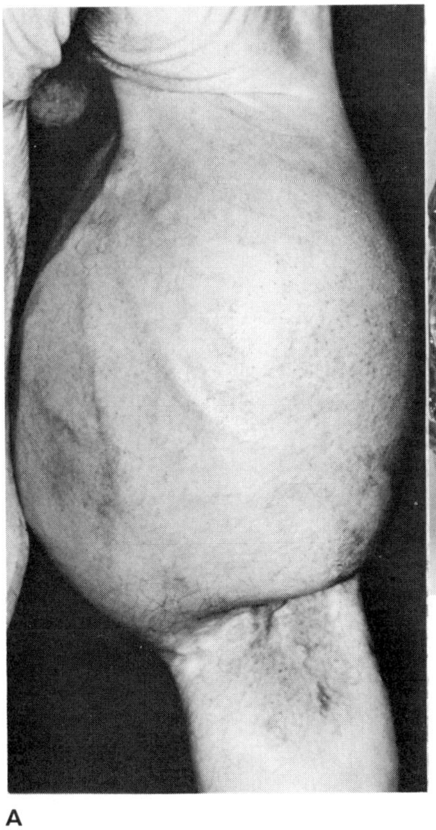

A

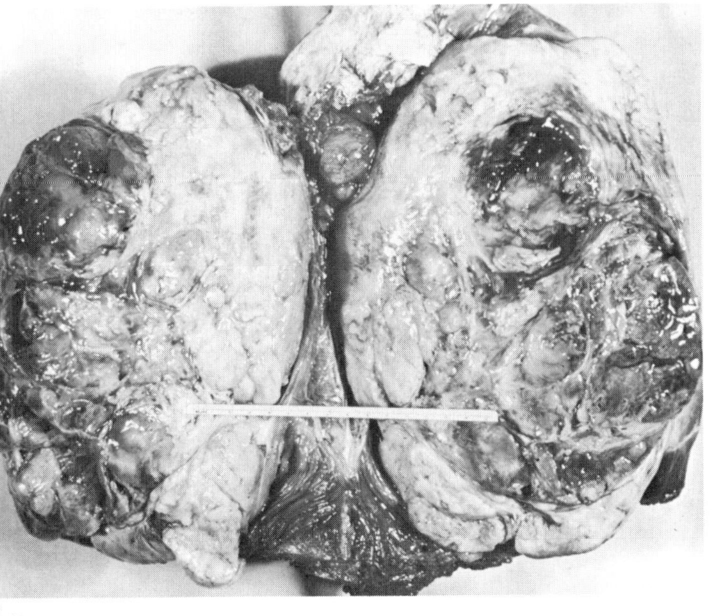

B

FIGURE 6–20. *A, Bulky liposarcoma of the posterior thigh. B, Resected specimen.*

that is not uncommonly encountered: a patient who has recently undergone resection of a liposarcoma of the medial thigh. A review of the specimen indicated that adequate normal muscle planes had not been removed with the tumor, which arose within the adductor group. We expected to find residual tumor at the time of reexploration. At surgery gross residual tumor was seen within the distal adductor muscle groups, adjacent to femur. Femoral vessels had been dissected to the popliteal space, separating them from the operative field; following this, completion of the dissection was carried out. If there is evidence of extension to the periosteum, one could, in the case of a low-grade sarcoma, dissect to and remove the periosteum (see Fig. 6–2) and follow through with cryosurgery to the bone. In the presence of a fully malignant sarcoma, however, one should consider removing underlying bone with the lesion. Preoperative chemotherapy followed by postoperative radiation is another option.[25, 35, 73] Should resection of bone be indicated because of the size of the tumor and invasion into cortical surfaces, replacement of the femur should be attempted before amputation.[54]

In the pretibial region, sarcomas are in close approximation to bone since the muscle mass is smaller here than in the thigh. Figure 6–21 is a cross-sectional view of this area showing the problems that can arise anatomically in the handling of tumors in this region. A CT scan in this instance appeared to show periosteal infiltration (Fig. 6–22*A*), but at the time of exploration the leg tumor could be removed with what appeared to be adequate margins (Fig. 6–22*B*). It was necessary to define the anterior tibial artery and vein, which were in proximity to the tumor and were removed with it. This artery, which arises from the popliteal artery, can be found to pass through the interosseous membrane into the anterior compartment, where the tumor was defined. After the vessels pass close to the neck of the fibula, they cross medially, descending against the anterior shaft of the tibia in the lower leg. Proximally the artery can be defined between the tibialis anterior and the extensor digitorum longus muscles. In the mid-leg the artery can be located between the tibialis anterior and the extensor hallucis longus muscles, which were resected with the specimen (Fig. 6–22C). When it approximates ankle the artery is crossed by the tendon of the extensor hallucis longus, and just above the transverse ligament it becomes superficial. It was also found necessary to sacrifice the anterior tibial nerve (deep peroneal nerve), which accompanied the artery along its lateral path in the leg. This nerve is one of three branches derived from the common peroneal nerve: superficial peroneal (musculocutaneous) nerve, passing forward between the fibula and the peroneus longus muscle; the anterior tibial recurrent nerve; and the anterior tibial (deep peroneal) nerve. The deep peroneal nerve can be lo-

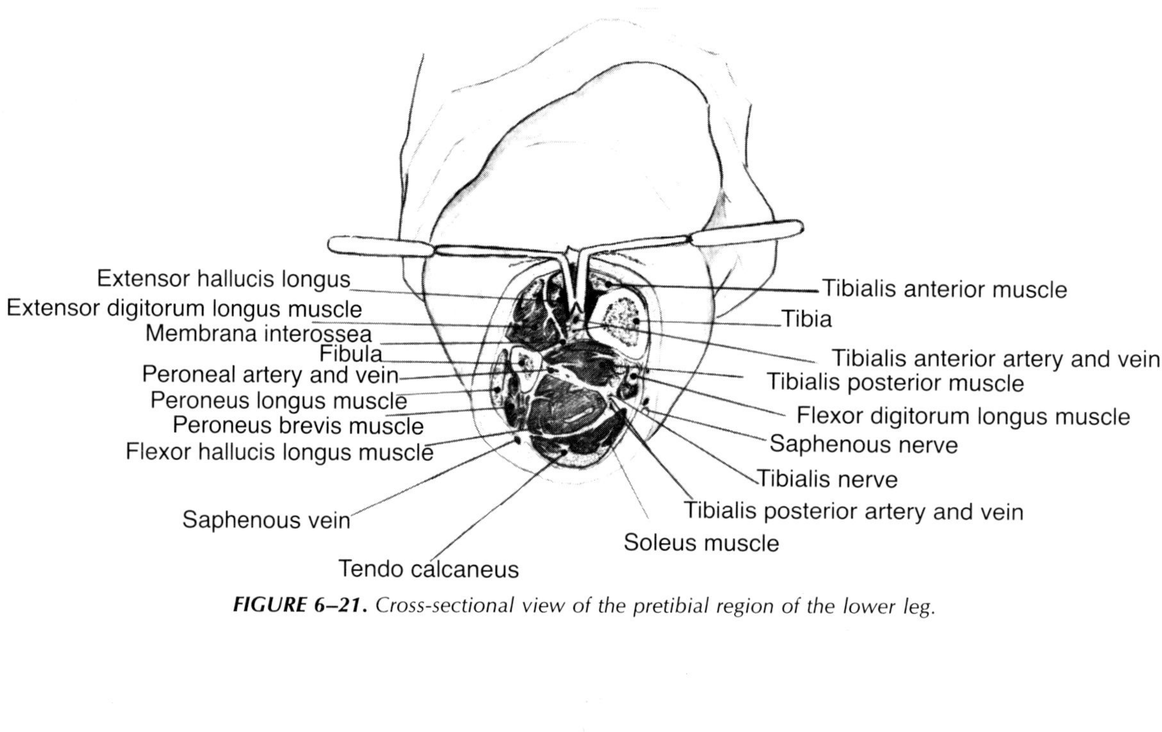

FIGURE 6–21. *Cross-sectional view of the pretibial region of the lower leg.*

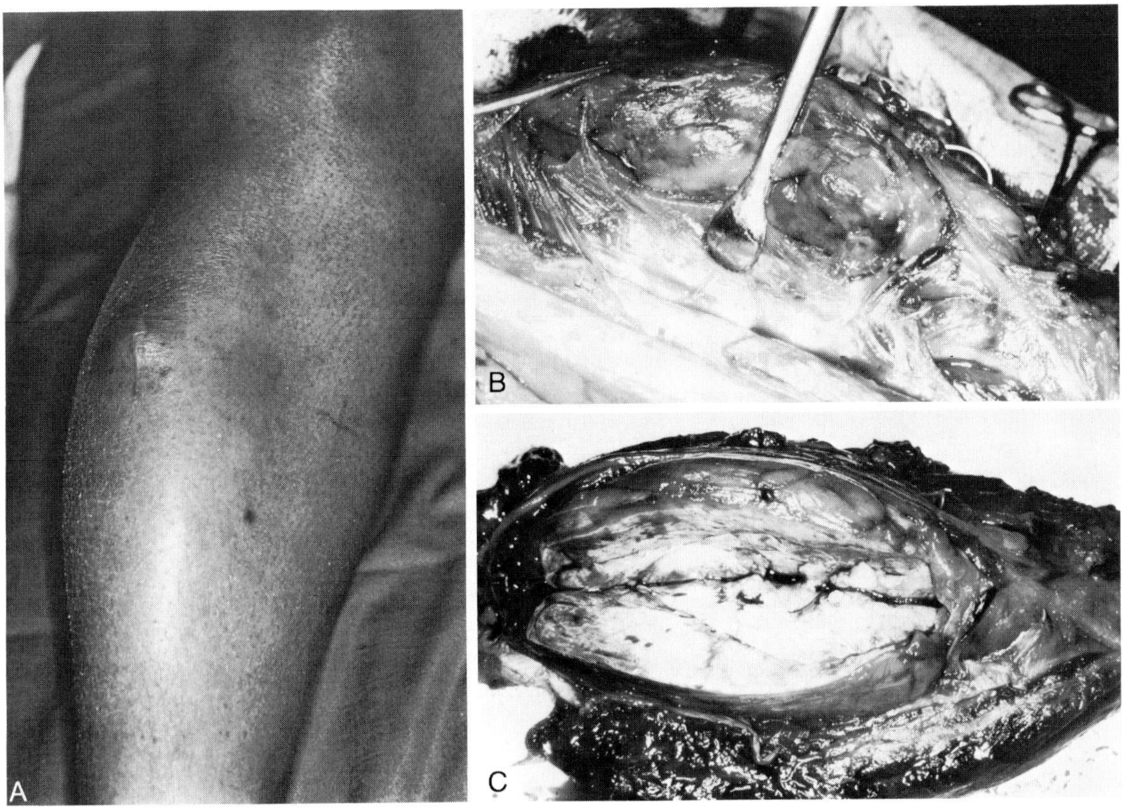

FIGURE 6–22. A, *Liposarcoma in the pretibial region.* B, *Resection of tumor from the tibia.* C, *Resected specimen.*

cated in the lateral aspect of the fibular neck, descending through the anterior compartment in proximity to the anterior tibial artery.

The fatty tumor masses that we encounter in the lower extremity are often heterogeneous, containing areas of benign-appearing lipomatous tissue, fully malignant sarcoma, and areas of myxoid composition. It is essential that adequate biopsy samples be taken, so that there is no confusion about the type of tumor involved and the margins of resection to be planned. Needle aspiration biopsy has not been adequate in these regards and, therefore, may be dangerous. In certain instances with aspiration biopsy, only a positive diagnosis is valid and the reviewer must be well versed in the cytology of sarcomas.

At Memorial Hospital, approximately 20% of soft part sarcomas of the lower extremity are represented by liposarcomas.[76] They are commonly found in the inner thigh and the region of the popliteal space. The liposarcomas are usually painless masses originating in the deep soft tissues, and they frequently attain significant size without ulcerating the skin. Grossly these tumors, especially the lipoblastic tumors, may resemble fatty tissue. When cut into, if the tumor exudes yellow oily fluid, liposarcoma should be diagnosed. Angiographically, these tumors show vascular patterns related to the degree of differentiation: low-grade, well-differentiated tumors are usually more vascular than the more pleomorphic lesions.

As mentioned, liposarcomas may achieve enormous proportions. A 60-year-old man noted a moderate-sized swelling of the thigh 1 year prior to definitive surgery. He was told that surgery could not be performed because of the size of the tumor. Thus there was another period of delay before symptoms of pain and difficulty in walking became pronounced; he was then referred for a hemipelvectomy (Fig. 6–23A). In order to plan our surgical approach, we needed a better biopsy. We reviewed the angiograms, which showed that the femoral vessels were displaced but not invaded. At biopsy, because the femoral vessels were easily mobilized, the entire mass was debulked by muscle group dissection (Fig. 6–23*B*). Histologically the tumor was found to be

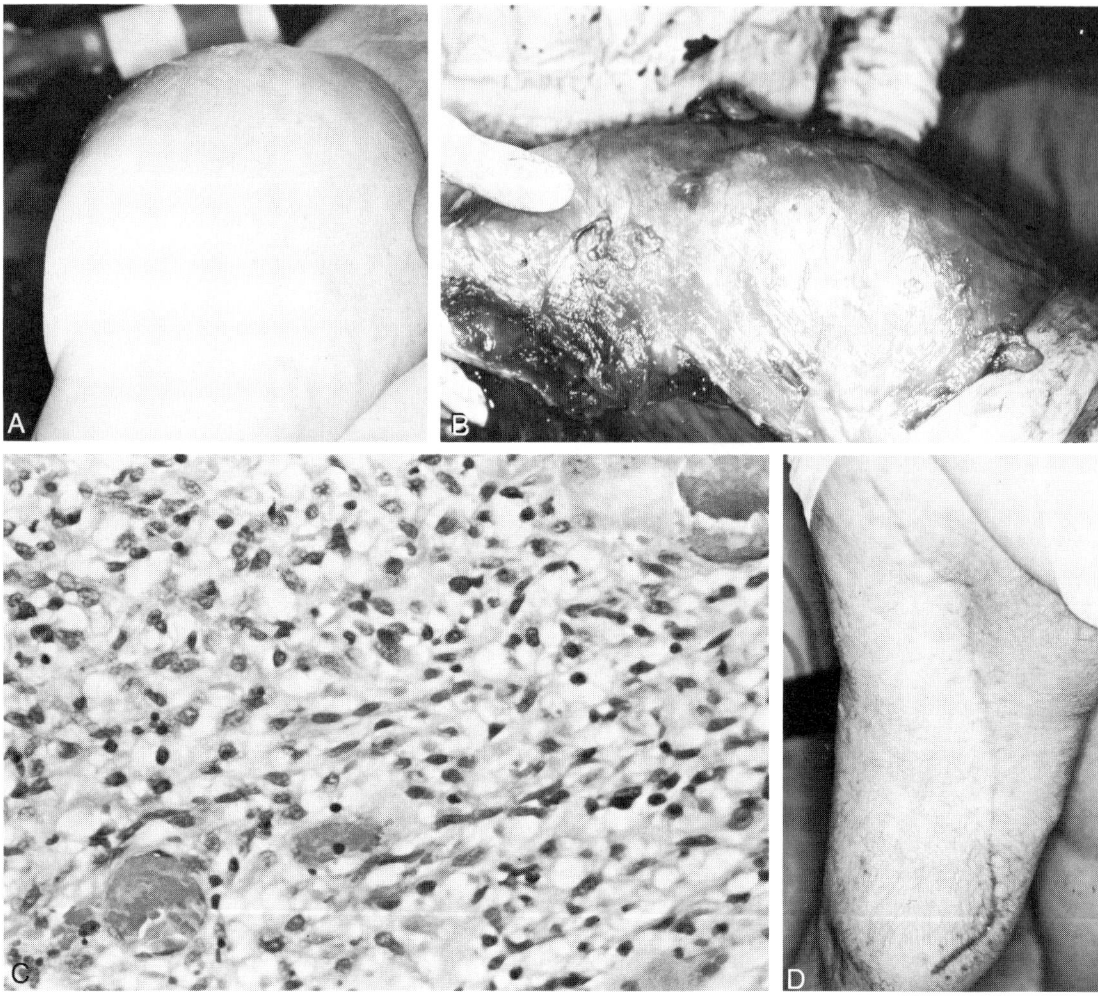

FIGURE 6–23. A, *Large myxoliposarcoma of the anterior thigh.* B, *Mobilization of the tumor mass.* C, *Microscopic appearance of the resected tumor (× 100).* D, *Appearance of the thigh after tumor resection.*

myxoliposarcoma (Fig. 6–23*C*) and contained abundant plexiform capillary vasculature, proliferating lipoblasts at varying stages of differentiation, and a supporting myxoid matrix. Despite extensive resection of the quadriceps and a portion of the adductors mucles, the patient was able to walk and returned to work without a leg brace (Fig. 6–23*D*). Radiation therapy was delivered to the operative field 1 month postoperatively. No recurrence developed in the extremity, in spite of the high incidence for these tumors to recur locally.

The report by Enzinger and Winslow[30] cited a survival rate of 53 to 85%, depending on the histologic type of the liposarcoma. In most reports the histologic patterns of recurrent tumor are usually similar to those of the primary tumor. In a few instances, higher grades of neoplastic recurrence may be seen, that is, the recurrence is more anaplastic than the primary from which it was derived. At Memorial Hospital, about 25% of the recurrent tumors were reported to develop less differentiated forms with each recurrence. In spite of the presence of a bulky tumor and the extensive infiltration seen with many lesions, infiltration of major structures such as skin, blood vessels, nerves, and bone is not common initially for the primary tumors. Many of the thigh tumors tend to be expansile and not infiltrative. This leads to an initial displacement rather than invasion of surrounding structures—one of the reasons why en-bloc muscle group dissection can be curative. In some instances the tumor may have represented a second primary tumor. Reszel et al.[70] reported five cases in which a second liposarcoma occurred in the opposite limb, one after 7 years and two after 10 years.

Myxoid liposarcomas are the most common form of malignant fatty tumor, accounting for 40 to 50% of the lesions. Regardless of the histologic type, however, recurrence is common when radical en-bloc resection is not performed. Failures are most frequent in the retroperitoneum because of the inability to completely encompass the tumors here. Failure also occurs when tumors of upper thigh approximate the region of the groin. More commonly, recurrences of the tumors are noted at 6 months to 1 year from the time of surgery. Occasionally, reappearance can be delayed for 5 to 10 years for the more differentiated tumors, giving a false sense of security to both patient and examining physician. Careful follow-up after 5 years is mandatory. The findings of a tumor mass more than 10 years after surgery must be considered a recurrence unless a new histologic diagnosis is established. Failure rates of 50 to 70% are described in most reported series of extremity liposarcoma. In many patients with liposarcoma, the tumor is deeply placed and has probably been present for many years prior to the patient's awareness of it. A good rule to remember is that the more deeply placed a lesion is, the more difficult it becomes to define by palpation, owing to stretching of the overlying structures in relation to the tumor. Thus we are confronted with an ill-defined swelling rather than an actual tumor mass. Such long-standing tumors have had a greater opportunity to infiltrate muscle and fascial planes widely, leading to a greater incidence for recurrence.

The reappearance of these tumors is related not only to histologic type but probably to the extent of local resection. In one of the cases of recurrent liposarcoma of the thigh that had been referred to us, the patient had undergone four previous resections with what was said to be adequate margins about the tumor. The patient, a 68-year-old woman, was referred for amputation because of the presence of a new bulky recurrence at the site of previous surgery. A fifth resection involved the removal of a large part of the quadriceps muscle, which was still intact, the vastus medialis muscle, and a portion of the adductor group. The skin was brought together by making multiple relaxing incisions on both sides of the resection site and undermining the skin completely around the entire thigh throughout its circumference. After adequate physiotherapy the patient was eventually able to walk. She has remained free of disease for more than 10 years.

Radiation therapy is indicated in those cases in which wide margins of resection cannot be adequately accomplished. Ewing and Stewart both reported on the radiosensitivity of these tumors. Spitle et al[82] noted that with postoperative radiation therapy the local recurrence rate could be reduced to 20%, in contrast to 74% without radiation therapy.

When a tumor is not widely resected, recurrences have been known to appear as long as 5 to 20 years later without signs of distant metastasis. Ewing described a liposarcoma that recurred 10 times in a 20-year period.

Lymph node metastases are rare but do occur with liposarcoma. Malignant lipomatous tumors tend to spread to the lung, frequently presenting with peppering of the pleural surface of the lung and diaphragm, rather than as discrete "cannonball" lesions. Enzinger[30] described the case of a 32-year-old woman with myxoid liposarcoma of the right thigh. Although it has been widely exised, the tumor reappeared locally five times over the next 26 years. Finally after the last recurrence and hemipelvectomy, metastases were found in the vertebrae and posterior mediastinum. The patient was 65 years old when the final metastasis was diagnosed.

Many liposarcomas of the thigh have been reported to be associated with a second lesion in the retroperitoneum. Enzinger quotes an incidence of 10% for the appearance of such tumors, either primary or metastatic.[30] We have noted that this situation may occur when adequate margins of resection have not been achieved in the upper aspect of the tumor dissection, in which case the tumor recurs above the inguinal ligament. Many of these recurrences probably result from extension of tumor along the muscle planes of the retroperitoneum.

While liposarcoma is one of the more frequent soft tissue tumors in adults, especially in elderly patients, these lesions have been described in children. Shmookler[79] reported 17 such cases. Sixty-five percent of these were in girls, primarily in the lower extremity (41%), particularly the thigh. The neck, back, and axilla were other sites for tumor growth. Only one case has been reported in the retroperitoneum. In children under 3 years of age lipoblastomatosis must be ruled out, as its characteristic lobules of embryonic-like adipose tissue may be confused with the malignant form of disease and misinterpreted by the pathologist.[62]

Myxosarcoma

The liposarcomas, especially the myxoid liposarcomas, are known to be radiosensitive.[35] In rare instances, pure myxosarcomas have been described; these must be differentiated from the predominantly myxomatous form of malignant fibrous histiocytoma.

Primary myxosarcomas of the extremity are extremely rare.[66] This tumor is of interest in its overall relationship to myxomatous tumors in general, and its natural history within the spectrum of soft tissue sarcomas. In Fig. 6–24*A* and *B*, a tumor mass situated on the outer aspect of the right calf is noted. The lesion, which developed in a 70-year-old man, was approximately 12.5 cm long.

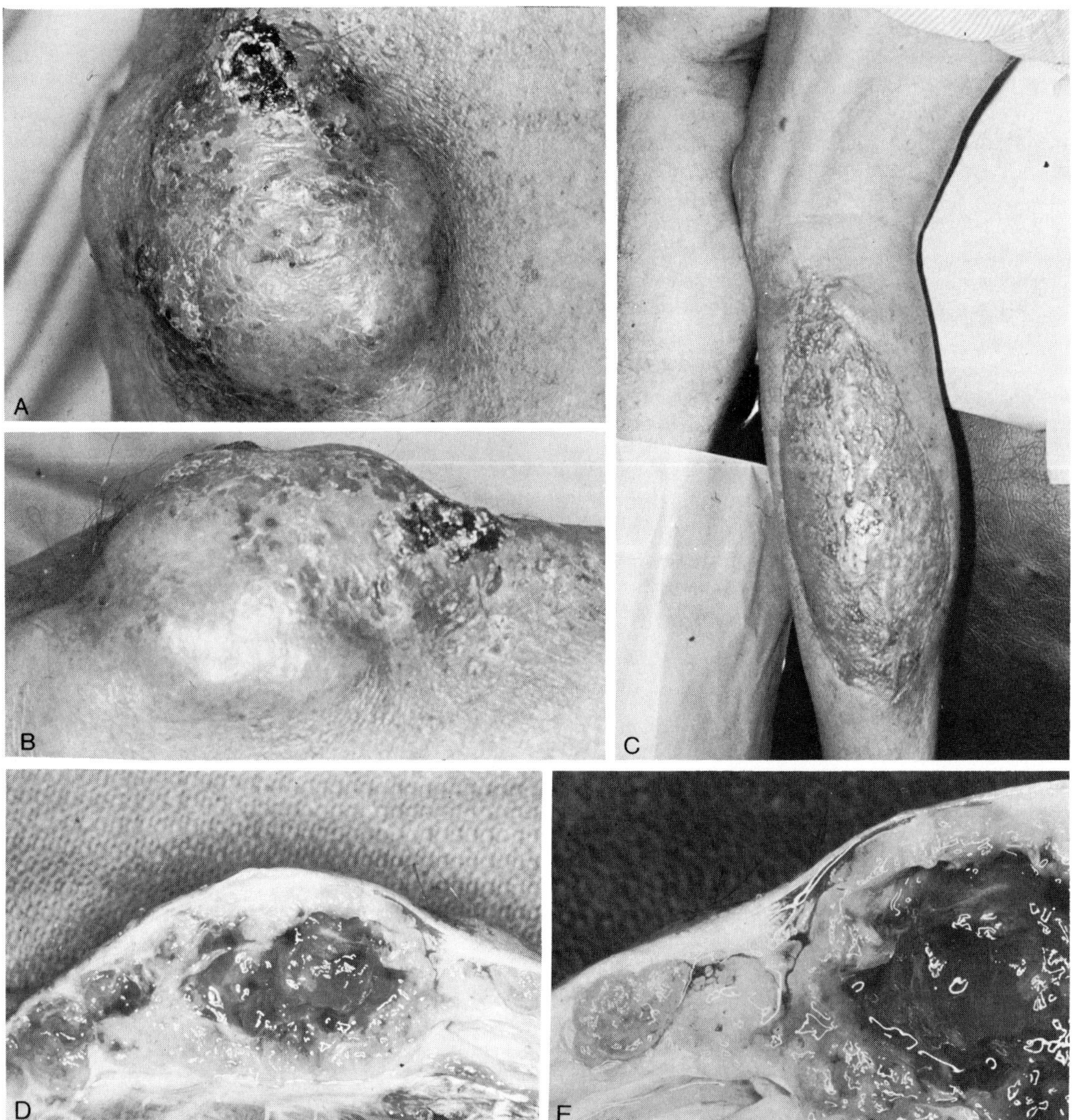

FIGURE 6–24. *A, Nodular tumor mass of right fibular region. B, Anterior view of lesion. C, Site of tumor resection with split-thickness skin graft. D, Section through lesion. E, Close-up view of sectioned tumor shows nodular spread of tumor through the subcutaneous plane.*

The skin in this case was raised in multiple nodules, with the more central primary lesion measuring approximately 5 cm in diameter. A nodular extension of the tumor continued inferiorly along the leg and at first was thought to represent venous infiltration by the tumor. The lesion was noted to be nontender, questionably fluctuant, and firmly attached to the superficial fascia overlying the lateral head of the gastrocnemius muscle. The initial impression was that this lesion was a sarcoma, requiring wide resection with underlying muscle and skin graft. Tumor was removed with the underlying lateral head of gastrocnemius muscle and part of the soleus muscle. A split-thickness skin graft was applied to the operative site for coverage (Fig. 6–24C).

Various methods of closing such defects have been tried. Pedicle closure has been attempted, but below-the-knee, split-thickness skin grafts function best. Rotation pedicle flaps raised from lower abdomen are of value, but only in closing defects in the upper thigh resulting from skin loss in association with removal of large ulcerating tumors.

The pathology report in this case showed that the tumor was essentially a myxosarcoma and that the margins of resection were free of disease. Grossly, the lesion consisted of a large gelatinous mass adherent to the underlying fascia but without muscle invasion (Fig. 6–24*D* and *E*). Microscopically, loose textured stellate cells in a myxoid stroma were noted; the stain for fat was negative. Close examination of the gross lesion revealed nodular extension of the tumor along the subcutaneous fascial planes. The patient had an uneventual postoperative course and has remained clinically free of disease for more than 5 years. Reports of such sarcomas are extremely infrequent. Some authors believe this tumor to be benign and only locally recurrent. All of the lesions reported were considered to have been derived from primitive mesenchyme growing in a pattern of loosely textured stellate cells set in a stroma of loose mucoid material. Approximately half of the tumors were reported to have occurred in the skin and subcutaneous regions of the extremity. Several cases have been reported in the retroperitoneum, intestine, muscle, breast, and pelvic viscera.[45] This particular lesion must be removed by wide resection, as with the majority of extremity soft part sarcomas. Local recurrence can be expected if excision is inadequate. Small subcutaneous nodules can be found extending for several centimeters distal to the central lesion in a pattern seen with the fibrous sarcomas.

Because discrete, seemingly innocuous nodular subcutaneous masses may, in reality, be fully malignant tumors, sound clinical judgment is necessary if biopsy is to be postponed. In many instances, the patient has been told by the physician, without benefit of such a biopsy, that there is no immediate need for surgical removal. A 58-year-old woman was referred for evaluation of a 4-cm lesion and was initially told that the tumor appeared entirely benign. This lesion has been present for more than 1 year prior to the eventual biopsy. Excision of the tumor and histologic examination revealed a fully malignant fibrous histiocytoma. Grossly, the lesion was resected at the time of excisional biopsy and a pathology report suggested that normal tissue margins were present about the tumor. Examination now showed a well-healed 4-cm scar over the site of resection, with no nodularity or thickening in the surrounding tissue (Fig. 6–25). A CT scan (Fig. 6–26*A*) showed that the tumor was located in the hamstrings, and angiography (Fig. 6–26*B*) showed that it was relatively avascular. Because of the highly malignant pattern seen on review of slides (Fig. 6–27*A*), a muscle group dissection was performed. The biopsy site was widely resected, with the incision extending to the groin because the question of clinically palpable nodes had been raised. Figure 6–27*B* shows

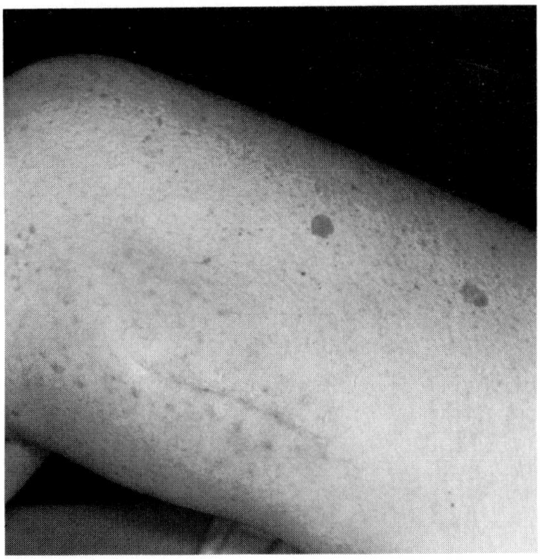

FIGURE 6–25. *Site of excisional biopsy.*

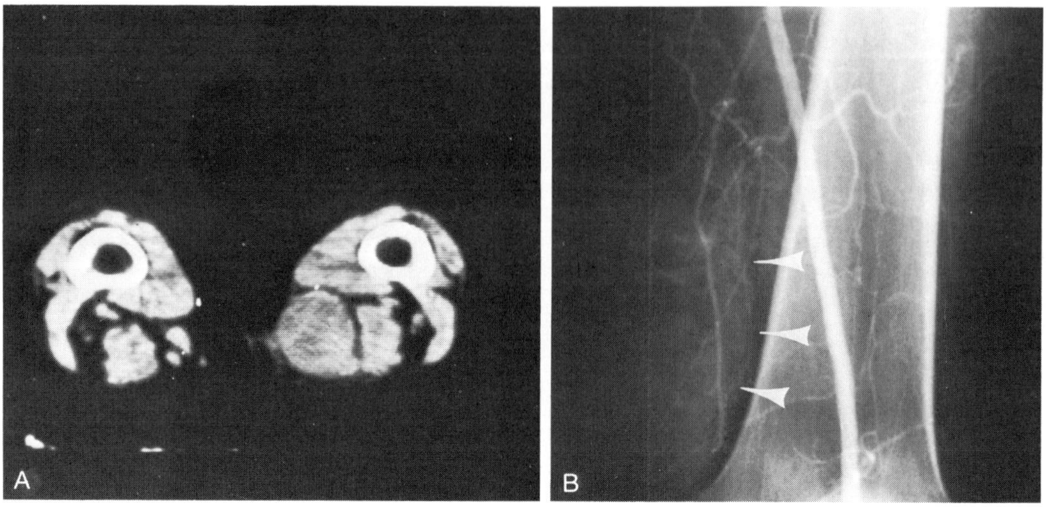

FIGURE 6–26. A, CT scan of the right thigh. A well-defined tumor mass is seen in the semimembranosus muscle. B, Angiogram shows a hypovascular lesion; arrows point to the medial margin of the mass.

exploration of the femoral triangle in anticipation of resection of nodes off the femoral vessel. Figure 6–27C shows division of the semimembranosus muscle above the tumor mass. Sections from the surrounding muscle following resection showed that residual tumor was present and that recurrence and dissemination would have resulted if further

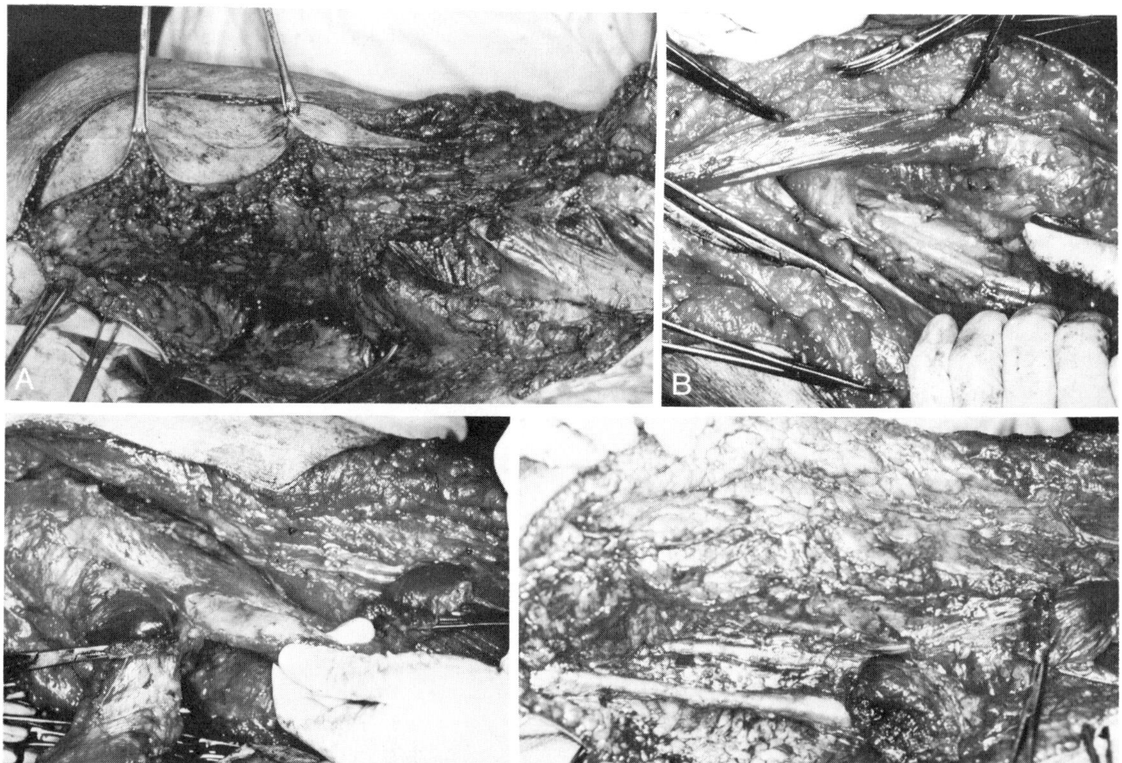

FIGURE 6–27. A, Field of dissection. An elliptical incision encompasses the biopsy site and extends to the groin, where nodes were taken in continuity with the muscles surrounding the tumor. B, Exploration of the superficial groin at the upper end of the operative field. The sartorius muscle is seen crossing the field. C, The semimembranosus muscle is divided above the tumor mass. D, Completed field of dissection. The semitendinosus tendon is seen. (See also Color Plate II–3.)

therapy had not been prescribed. We believe that total resection of surrounding normal tissue about a malignant tumor site is essential, especially in the face of a fully malignant sarcoma. Radiation therapy in such instances does not appear to be indicated as a primary form of treatment and, when possible, should never be used as the initial primary form of therapy. Rather, we rely on radiation therapy to shrink large bulky masses that may not be readily resectable but that may be radiotherapeutically sensitive. No attempt should be made to minimize the margins of resection. Radiation therapy should not be used as a definitive procedure in conjuction with enucleation for the treatment of fully malignant sarcomas. Postoperative radiation therapy should be delivered to the bed of a resection site where tumors are greater than 5 cm in diameter and where there is the possibility of microscopic spread. We feel that any modality offered to minimize the possibility of local recurrence and distant metastasis should be offered to the patient. For most sarcomas this should entail adequate surgical resection combined with significant adjuvant therapy.

SURGICAL PLANNING

In planning for the surgery of any of the deeply seated sarcomas, one should consider the amount of skin and extent of muscle and subcutaneous tissue to be resected. The biopsy site must be considered in planning for the incision. After creating an elliptical incision around the site of biopsy, to assure that the biopsy tract is included in the resection, relatively thick skin flaps should be raised as long as the tumor does not appear to infiltrate the subcutaneous tissues (Fig. 6–27A). Under these circumstances, 2 to 4 cm of normal skin can be removed with the biopsy site and the underlying subcutaneous tissue. As the deeper structures are transected, one must constantly palpate the lesion without actually visualizing it. The tumor mass may be found to extend into planes not appreciated by superficial palpation. The extent of the deeper structures to be included can then be evaluated so that additional surrounding normal tissue can be included around the tumor. Normal muscles should surround the lesion and, when the tumor mass is greater than 5 cm in diameter, the muscle groups should be traced to their origin and insertion and divided. If bone is near the pseudocapsule of the tumor it, too, can be resected. A complete set of Marcove-modified Guepar knee or hip resection prostheses makes bone and joint substitution easier and can be utilized immediately as required during resection. The prostheses are usually prepared prior to surgery, on completion of imaging studies.

Hemostasis is essential during such surgery by isolating perforating tumor vessels at their origin and controlling them with hemoclips or silk ligatures. When dissecting a lesion of the mid-thigh, it may be necessary to identify the femoral artery by extending the incision superiorly to the groin. Once defined, the artery can be dissected toward the tumor mass to insure that the lesion can be freed properly from the primary blood supply to the leg; blind dissection in such a situation could result in vascular injury. In most instances, if the angiogram and CT scan suggest that the vessel is free of tumor, adequate dissection to retract major vessels from the tumor site can usually be accomplished. If there is evidence of tumor invasion of vessels, then adequate dissection is not possible and resection of the main arterial supply may be performed with insertion of a vascular graft. In instances of extensive disease about the neurovascular pedicle, amputation must be planned.

Malignant Fibrous Histiocytoma

In the aforementioned case of malignant fibrous histiocytoma, complete vascular dissection beginning in the region of the groin had been performed, extending deep into the thigh with separation of muscle and tumor off the blood vessels. All nodes were removed in the dissection and found to be hyperplastic, probably as a result of an inflammatory response secondary to the initial biopsy. Malignant fibrous histiocytoma is one of the more common tumors of the extremity.[92] Previously, this lesion was known or described as pleomorphic liposarcoma or pleomorphic rhabdomyosarcoma. The major sign with this type of tumor, and with most tumors occurring in the thigh, is the presence of a discrete mass. Approximately 10% of the patients described have poorly localized pain. Thirty percent of the patients have also had osseous changes on radiography: lytic areas of the cortex and the periosteal region. Kearney[46] reported the results of 167 cases of this tumor treated at the Mayo Clinic between 1947 and 1976. Eighty-five occurred in the lower leg: 60 in the thigh, 15 in the leg, 8 about the knee, and 2 on the feet. Superficial tumors were those found entirely in the subcutaneous tissue; deep lesions arose in or involved the muscle groups. Of the 60 tumors in the thigh, 41 were classified as deep. Most of the tumors below the knee were classified as superficial. The fibrous variants were most commonly seen with the giant cell activity present; myxoid and inflammatory components were found to be lesser degree. Wide resection was the obvious treatment of choice. Of 36 patients referred with a history of complete excision and in whom en-bloc resection was later performed, 15 showed microscopic evidence of residual tumor. Among patients with superficial tumors, the local recurrence rate after complete excision was 71%; for those with deeper tumors it was 41%. One would suspect that complete excision of the superficial group was inadequate when compared with the surgery that was employed for more deeply placed tumors. In both groups we would have to assume that the en-bloc operation probably could have more comprehensively removed the tumor should proper neurovascular dissection have been performed. Patients with more proximal lesions situated above the knee appear to have worse long-term results than those patients with tumors that are distally placed. The proximal tumors were more likely associated with metastasis to lungs, regional nodes, and retroperitoneum. Ekfors et al.[27] reported 38 cases of malignant fibrous histiocytoma of the extremity among 246 sarcomas. The thigh was again the most frequent site. The predominant form of treatment was excision with postoperative radiation therapy. There were one or more recurrences in 17 patients and evidence of metastatic spread in 21. Eleven patients survived for more than 5 years. The number of recurrences suggested that the primary operation was usually not adequate. On reevaluation, radiation therapy appeared to offer no dramatic improvement in any of these patients.

The occurrence of malignant fibrous histiocytoma arising in previous surgical sites as well as their induction by other factors has been reviewed by Inoshita and Youngberg.[44] Radiation has been described as a possible causative factor; there are also several reports associating the tumor with bone infarct, woven dacron aortic graft, and trauma at the site of previous fracture. One case occurred in an amputation stump and another in a herniorrhaphy scar.

Calcification Within Soft Tissue Tumors

Many sarcomas tend to outgrow their blood supply, eventually resulting in necrosis of portions of the tumor. In certain instances calcification may develop. The presence or absence of ossification in normal soft tissue structures or in the lesion itself can therefore be important. If ossification is evident on a plain x-ray film, one must consider the possibility of benign traumatic calcification. Nonneoplastic heterotropic bone formation may be an important consideration in the differential diagnosis of a neoplasm, especially when the patient is young. Minor repeated episodes of trauma to the extremity are common among adolescents and may be a causative factor in the development of myositis, though a single major traumatic episode is more frequently associated with such a situation. When a localized area of myositis ossificans (circumscripta) is found without antecedent injury, this has been referred to as a pseudomalignant osseous tumor of soft tissue (Angerval). Patients may present clinically with a tender soft tissue mass, and a biopsy here may be mistakenly interpreted as showing malignant transformation if the central and peripheral margins are not adequately described to the pathologist.

Approximately 60 to 70% of patients with myositis ossificans circumscripta have a history of traumatic origin. The remaining have associated conditions such as paraplegia, poliomyelitis, burns, tetanus, or a spontaneous lesion of undefined origin. In a review of 16 cases with ossifying tumors occurring in soft tissue, it was found that four had benign histologic patterns; in twelve instances the ossification represented the presence of extraskeletal osteogenic sarcoma.[36] On the basis of histologic evaluation, the benign lesions are considered pseudomalignant osseous tumors of soft tissue. Ackerman[1] reported five cases of heterotopic bone formation, most in large muscle groups of the thigh and arms in close proximity to the periosteum of underlying bone. Pain may be an accompanying feature of heterotopic bone formation and is most severe in the early stage of the disease but diminishes over the clinical course; this is in contrast to the situation with malignant lesions.

The differential diagnosis that has to be considered in these cases includes periosteal osteogenic sarcoma, extraosseous (extraskeletal) osteogenic sarcoma, and synovioma. Synovioma is important not only in terms of its frequency as an extremity lesion but also because it represents a tumor that arises in the young with areas of benign calcification that frequently can be confused with myositis. These tumors do not always arise close to the joint but can appear in fascial planes close to the bone and at some distance from the joint spaces with which they are usually associated. At Memorial Hospital, patients with synovial sarcoma have been fairly young, with the ages ranging from 10 to 40 years (mean, 34 years for males and 31 years for females). In contrast, most patients seen with extraosseous osteogenic sarcoma are usually in their fifth or sixth decade of life.

Once heterotopic osteoblasts begin to form a matrix, the myositis lesion develops a fibrous capsule. Microscopically, three discrete histologic zones have been defined in such growths: (1) a central portion of the lesion containing rapidly proliferating fibroblasts with areas of hemorrhage and necrotic muscle, (2) a middle zone containing osteoblasts with islands of immature bone, and (3) a peripheral area composed of mature trabeculae clearly separated from the surrounding connective tissue. If a biopsy is taken from the central and middle zones, the pathologist may misdiagnose the lesion as malignant. In the benign lesions, maturation occurs in a centrifugal fashion, with the central area being the last to ossify. When the diagnostic work-up has been completed, plain x-ray films should be taken to aid in identifying calcification, soft tissue radiolucency, or osseous invasion. Angiographic studies also should be completed and CT scans of the extremity taken to define patterns of invasion into the surrounding tissue planes.

Synovial Sarcoma

Among other tumors of the lower extremity that should be considered in the differential diagnosis are synovioma, leiomyosarcoma, neurogenic sarcoma, and lesions such as alveolar soft part sarcoma. In those patients in whom synovioma has been confirmed, most of the lesions have appeared in the region of the thigh or about the knee (60 to 70%)[3, 11, 17, 38, 52, 77] Many of the recurring and metastatic tumors are less differentiated than the primary growths from which they arose. This is characteristic for many of the tumors, both epithelial and sarcomatous, that one encounters. The biphasic epithelioid cell features that one frequently finds in synovioma can be lost and the lesion will present as a monophasic spindle cell tumor at the time that it has been found to disseminate. In the young patient who presents with a history of trauma to the extremity and the presence of a mass with diffuse calcification, one should consider the possibility that the lesion is a synovioma. The trauma, of course, is unrelated to causative factors but seems to call the patient's attention to the existence of the lesion. Biopsy is essential for ruling out the presence of a benign traumatic mass. Once the diagnosis of synovioma has been established, wide resection with removal of surrounding muscle groups is employed. Approximately 5 to 10% of these lesions may spread to regional nodes; for this group of patients en-bloc regional node dissection should be employed, especially when a large lesion approximates the groin or there is a suggestion of nodal involvement.

The incidence of lymph node metastasis may be lower if one eliminates neglected cases of epitheloid sarcomas that have been confused with malignant synovioma. Figure 6–28 shows the appearance of an ulcerating synovial sarcoma of the thigh. Unfortunately

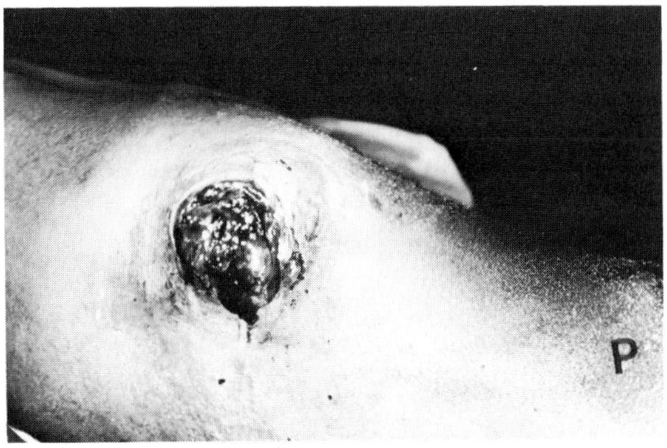

FIGURE 6–28. *Ulcerating synovioma presenting as a bulging mass above the patella (P).*

many of these tumors, in spite of adequate resection, do metastasize to the lungs. Radiation therapy has not proved to be effective, and chemotherapy does not appear to have had any major impact on the rate of either local recurrence or the growth pattern of the metastatic lesion.

Rajpal et al.[68] have reviewed with 52 patients treated at Roswell Park between 1967 and 1977. The ages ranged from 11 to 80 years (mean, 33.6 years). The lower extremity was most commonly involved (67.3%). Tumors tended to be relatively large, with 70.5% larger than 5 cm in diameter. Treatment consisted of simple excision in 15, wide resection in 12, and amputation in 14. Others received combination therapy with radiation and chemotherapy. The 5-year survival for all sites when the lesion was smaller than 5 cm (in 13 patients) was 72.7%, and when the lesion was larger than 5 cm (21 patients), 33.1%.

Leiomyosarcoma

Smooth muscle tumors such as leiomyosarcoma can on occasion appear in the extremities and usually are of venous origin.[63, 65] Fisher et al.[32] described the case of a 55-year-old woman who noted enlargement of an asymptomatic mass (1.5 by 2.0 cm) in the left groin. Excisional biopsy revealed what was thought to be metastatic leiomyosarcoma replacing lymph node. A diagnosis of an unknown primary tumor was considered. The patient underwent hysterectomy and pelvic node dissection for the possibility that an occult primary existed in the uterus. A groin dissection was performed to remove residual tumor that may have been left in the groin. During the radical groin dissection, the primary lesion was found in the region of the greater saphenous vein. Tumor protruded like a finger into the femoral vein, at the saphenofemoral junction. In such cases the interpretation of initial pathology specimens is significant. We have advocated that tumor masses in this area be removed by an en-bloc approach that includes the nodes in the saphenofemoral junction, thereby obviating any problem that would necessitate further reexploration of this region. This would hold true even if the tumor proved to be a lymphoma. In many of the tumors, removal of the superficial nodes above the saphenofemoral junction may reveal only hyperplastic changes. In actuality, the true pathologic change may have evolved deeper to the superficial site. Should an extensive mass of nodes be present, removal of the complete cluster of nodes sitting on the femoral vein may define the actual nature of the pathologic process. In this patient, a tumor of the saphenofemoral junction was resected by excision of the greater saphenous vein and tangential excision of the wall of the femoral vein with reconstruction. In a case referred to us from another institution a leiomyosarcoma had been incompletely excised in the region of the greater trochanter. More radical surgery was advised; however, the patient elected to have intensive local radiotherapy. This resulted in an area of brawny irradiated skin 12 inches in diameter. The tumor fungated through the skin several months after completion of the radiation therapy. The tumor was successfully excised by removing all irradiated skin, the outer wing of the ilium (which was adjacent to residual tumor), the upper femur, and the overlying muscles. A suitable prosthesis was set into the residual acetabulum and sutured into place by 3-mm dacron sutures. Because there was no remaining superficial tissue, a rubber dam was sewn watertight over two large drains placed for antibiotic circulation. Early granulation tissue formed beneath this dam; grafting was planned for a later date. Pathologic study of the specimen (Fig. 6–29) showed clear margins.

Neurogenic Tumors

Among the lesions to be considered in the lower extremity, those arising from nerve structures also have an important role in the clinical spectrum of neoplastic disease.[5, 9, 18, 71] Storm et al.[85] evaluated 20 patients with neurofibrosarcoma, 14 of whom had associated neurofibromatosis. This tumor represents approximately 5% of all soft part sarcomas. Analysis suggests that there is an excellent correlation between survival and tumor size, cellular pleomorphism, and mitotic activity. In this series, four lesions occurred in the proximal and five in the distal leg; local excision alone resulted in failure in two of three patients. The addition of radiation therapy and chemotherapy increased local control. Several years before this, Clark had noted that wide en-bloc re-

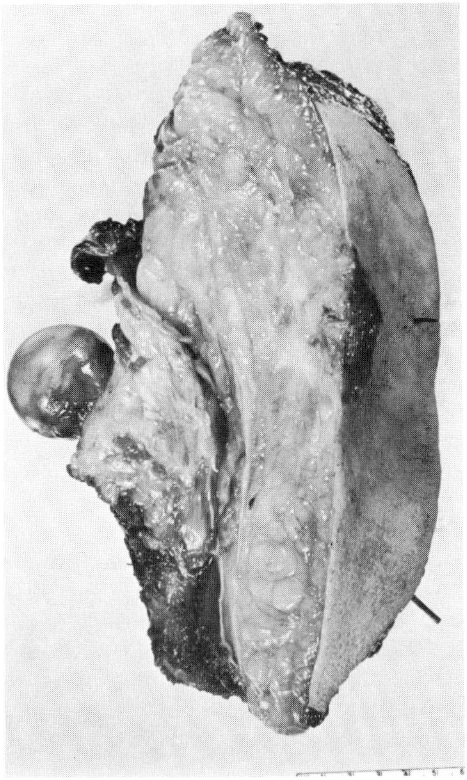

FIGURE 6–29. Resected specimen of a recurrent leiomyosarcoma involving the upper femur.

section of sarcomas could control local recurrence, decreasing the rate of their reappearance from 61 to 10%. We have advocated this type of surgical approach as the treatment of choice for most of these sarcomas. In Storm's group of patients, radical surgery combined with radiation therapy and chemotherapy helped control disease in more than 80% of patients. One of our patients, a 40-year-old man with von Recklinghausen's disease, presented with pain of sciatic nerve distribution. The patient had been seen at another institution, where laminectomy had been performed and a disc removed; amelioration of symptoms did not result. Our examination suggested a lesion of the right sciatic nerve. Biopsy of this area revealed a mass consistent with neurogenic sarcoma. He was scheduled for a more definitive resection of the large tumor mass, which replaced the entire sciatic nerve from its entry into the posterior thigh to its distal branches at the ankle. A radical muscle group dissection, including hamstrings and the entire sciatic nerve with tumor, was carried out. The leg was exposed with the patient in a prone position. Figure 6–30*A* shows the sciatic nerve tumor with a Penrose tape around it. Initially we thought that is patient would have a better prognosis with a hemipelvectomy; on reconsidering the extent of the tumor, the highly malignant nature of such lesions, and its propensity for proximal metastasis. We opted instead for limb-sparing surgery. The tumor was removed for palliative purposes by isolating it from the hamstrings, ensuring that the vascular pedicle was intact. The entire tumor appeared to have been completely resected. The complete nerve bundle appeared to have been totally replaced by tumor, with only very narrow margins of resection obtained in the region of the hip and ankle. A foot brace was used for the resulting foot drop. The patient did well for approximately 5 years, at which time he was noted to have become jaundiced. Work-up revealed a mass

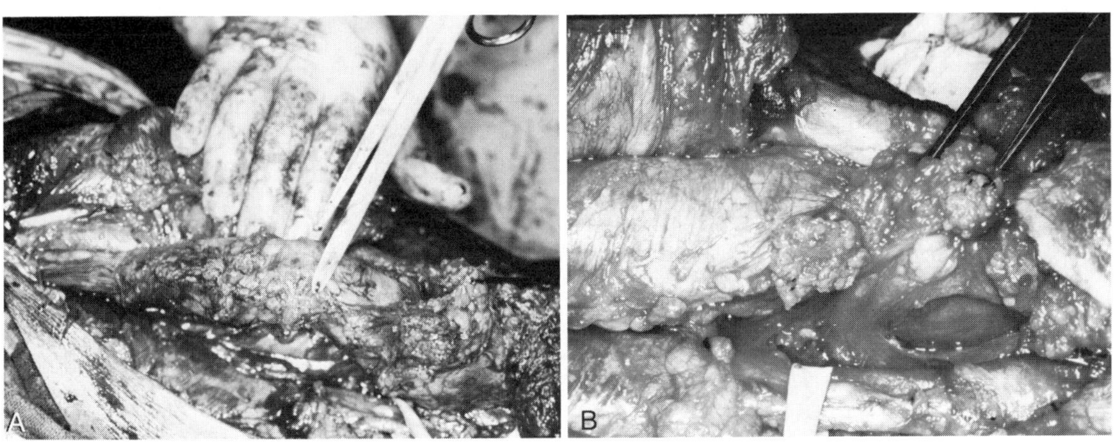

FIGURE 6–30. A, Exposure of a sciatic nerve sarcoma. Tape is around tumor mass. Patient is in prone position. B, Close-up view of neurogenic sarcoma. The Penrose tape in the lower field is around the vascular pedicle.

in the head of the pancreas. We considered the possibility that metastasis to the region of the porta hepatis had taken place. Exploratory laparotomy revealed a primary lesion in the head of the pancreas. A Whipple resection was performed, removing the entire head of the pancreas, the distal common duct, and the surrounding nodes. The tumor in the head of the pancreas proved to be a primary carcinoid tumor of pancreas with regional nodal metastasis. Four years following surgery, the patient remains free of disease.

The ability to define neurogenic malignancies in general, and the malignant schwannoma in particular, may be difficult. Histologically, the characteristic Antoni AB patterns of the benign tumor are absent. Morphologically, the tumors must be defined on clinical grounds as arising in nerve sheath. The pathologist's judgment is based on peculiarities in nuclear shape and hyperchromatism (now defined by DNA content during cell sorting), pallisading, and perivascular changes. The incidence of association with von Recklinghausen's disease is generally under 50% but may in some series reach 66%. Pain and the appearance of a possible nerve mass, especially when associated with von Recklinghausen's disease, should alert one to the possibility of malignant transformation in a preexisting nerve tumor. Most of the malignant schwannomas arise from major nerve trunks, such as the brachial plexus, sciatic nerve, and sacral plexus. They may be confused histologically with fibrosarcoma, monophasic synovioma, and leiomyosarcoma, so close association with nerve trunks or plexus should be clearly defined when considering neurogenic sarcoma.

When a neurogenic sarcoma develops in a patient with von Recklinghausen's disease, the prognosis is poor (39%). Survival of patients with neurogenic sarcoma is better (70%) when there is no von Recklinghausen's disease. Approximately 65% of patients with von Recklinghausen's disease and neurogenic sarcoma develop distant metastasis. While amputation has been advocated for tumors arising in most major nerve trunks, wide resection with en-bloc muscle group dissection can be performed and may be curative. Figure 6–31 shows a 1-year-old child who underwent resection of a posterior thigh lesion, which proved to be a neurogenic sarcoma arising from one of the branches of sciatic nerve. The original examining physician had scheduled a hemipelvectomy. Further work-up, including CT scan and angiography, revealed that the tumor was relatively well delineated, distant from the sciatic nerve, and well surrounded by hamstring muscles. We believed that this tumor could be easily removed without amputation. Characteristic café au lait spots were easily recognizable over the trunk of this patient. Wide resection was performed, and the patient remains free of disease more than 5 years later.

Peripheral nerve tumors can be found to contain heterogeneous components: osteoid, bone, benign striated muscle, cartilage, nevus cells, malignant melanoma, embryonic rosette-forming and glandular malignant neuroepithelial cells, liposarcoma, angiosarcoma, and embryonal and pleomorphic rhabdomyosarcoma. The compound nerve tumor in which rhabdomyosarcoma develops is referred to as the triton tumor. The muscle components of these peripheral nerve tumors are considered to be derived from Schwann cells of the neurolemmal sheath. In 1973 Woodruff et al.[93] described

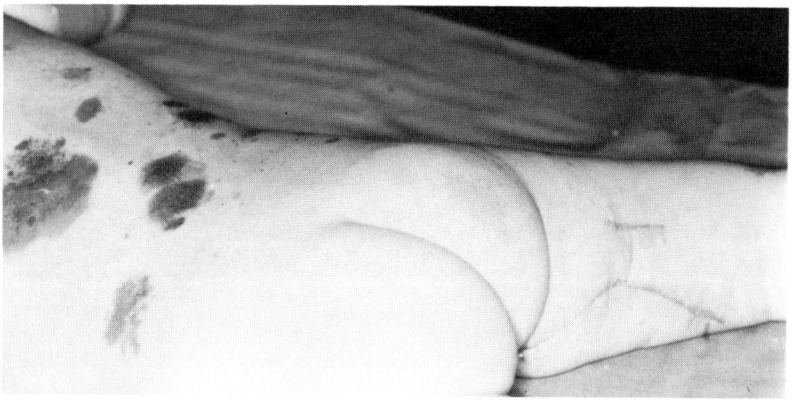

FIGURE 6–31. *Diffuse nevi of the trunk associated with neurogenic sarcoma of the right posterior thigh.*

three cases of peripheral nerve tumors with the rhabdomyosarcomatous components. All patients showed signs of von Recklinghausen's disease. Of nine patients reviewed by Woodruff, 7 were dead within 3 to 20 months. Markel and Enzinger[55] described the benign variation of the triton tumor, a neuromuscular hamartoma composed of mature neural and striated muscle elements.

Rhabdomyosarcoma

Fibrosarcomas and rhabdomyosarcomas are two other major lesions that produce extensive masses in the thigh and lower leg. Rhabdomyosarcomas can range in size from the extensive thigh mass shown in Figure 1–8, where circumferential swelling occupies most of the upper leg, to a small nodular mass presenting as a subcutaneous swelling on the thigh (Fig. 6–32*A*). The small nodular recurrence is one of the patterns exhibited after a small tumor mass has been locally resected in an incomplete fashion. Even with such a relatively minor presentation it becomes necessary to guarantee that adequate margins be obtained; therefore, underlying muscle must be resected, even if only to a limited degree. To assure that no damage to underlying vessels would occur here, femoral vessels were isolated in the groin and traced inferiorly as they coursed just under the site of resection. The specimen with underlying sartorius muscle is seen in Figure 6–32*B*. The patterns of growth with rhabdomyosarcoma may also vary: one lesion may enlarge over several months, while another may outgrow its blood supply almost overnight. In the latter case, there is marked necrosis and breakdown through the skin as illustrated by Figure 6–33*A*; this lesion of the mid-calf required amputation to achieve complete control of the disease. Because of rapidity of growth, these tumors can hemorrhage into themselves and even rupture through the skin surface as a large necrotic hemorrhagic mass, suggestive of a traumatic aneurysm or an extensive infected hematoma.

In many instances, the first clinical sign of rhabdomyosarcoma of the lower extremity is the appearance of an ill-defined swelling. This can also be seen in cases of liposarcomas that involve deep muscle groups. CT scanning followed by angiography when indicated, usually aids in deciding on the type of biopsy necessary to establish the proper diagnosis. If there is any question to the resectability of the lesion when it is exceedingly large, then preoperative radiation therapy with adjuvant preoperative chemotherapy can be delivered. This technique has produced excellent results in several of our patients. Such preoperative therapy has allowed preservation of the extremity.[80] Although these tumors in adults may be relatively radiosensitive, they do not respond to the same degree as the embryonal tumors.[81] In many instances, the embryonal sarcoma can virtually be cured with little more than wide resection of the primary tumor followed by radiation therapy and maintenance chemotherapy. The adult tumors must be widely resected to minimize the possibility of local recurrence and distant metastasis.

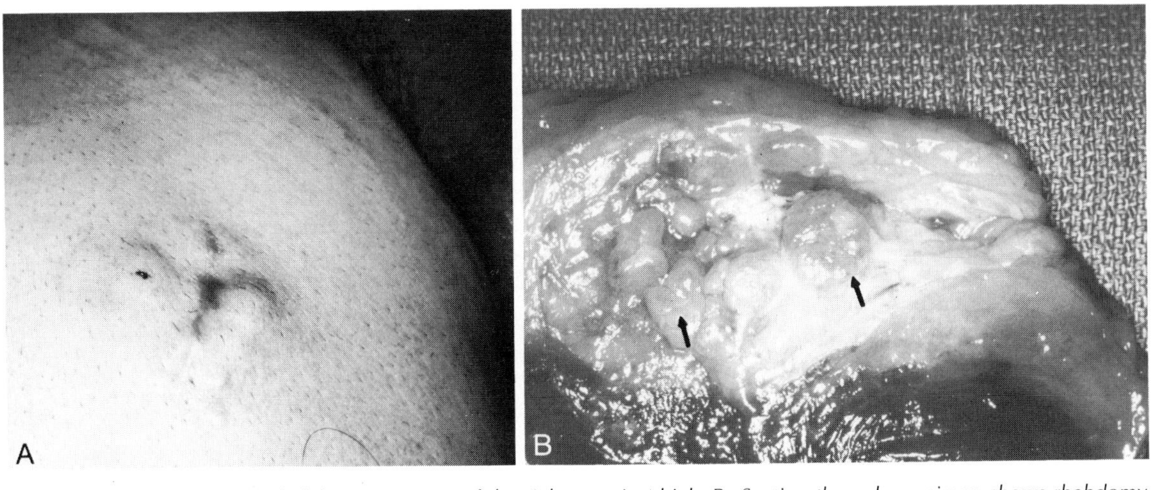

FIGURE 6–32. *A, Nodular rhabdomyosarcoma of the right anterior thigh. B, Section through specimen shows rhabdomyosarcoma (arrows) sitting above the sartorius muscle.*

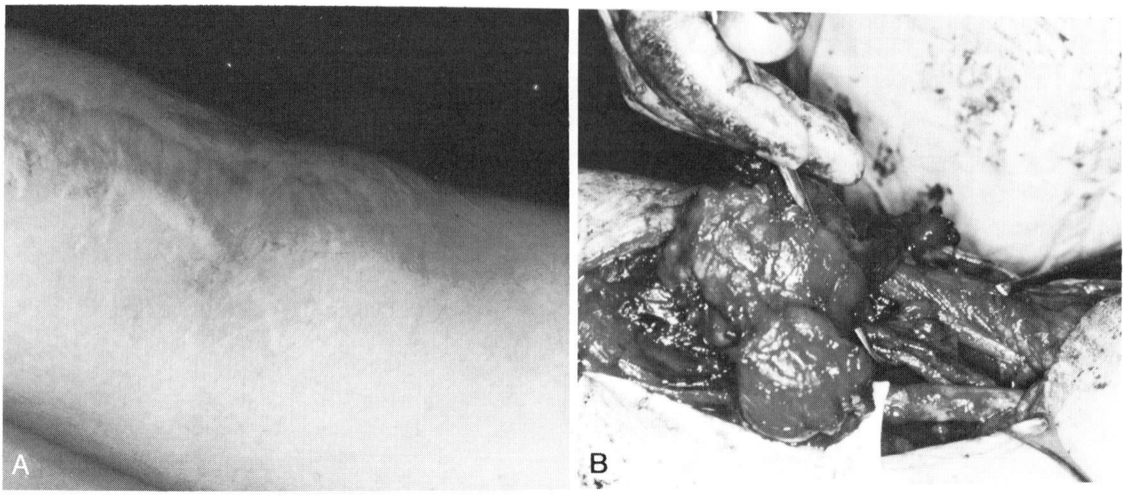

FIGURE 6–33. *A, Fibrosarcoma (desmoid) in the popliteal space. B, Dissection of tumor from the popliteal space. The Penrose drain is around the sciatic nerve.*

Postoperative radiation therapy to the tumor bed and maintenance chemotherapy should, however, be employed for all high-risk tumors when recurrence is expected to result following resection. The value of brachytherapy is still under study,[78] and it is not established as a well-defined form of therapy for the sarcomas. We believe that this form of implantation therapy should not be used to replace well-established radical surgery. Rather, it appears that brachytherapy is of some value when margins of resection are not available, e.g., adjacent to neural foramina. Better control can be achieved with implantation over external beam therapy in such select sites. We have however, seen many cases of recurrence in patients who underwent inadequate resection that was followed by brachytherapy.

When all potential sites for the development of rhabdomyosarcomas are considered, it is apparent that the extremities are not so frequently involved as one would anticipate, considering the relative distribution of muscle mass. At the Armed Forces Institute of Pathology, 558 cases were reviewed between 1970 and 1979, and alveolar rhabdomyosarcoma of the extremity was found to outnumber embryonal rhabdomyosarcoma by a ratio of 4 to 3. A few cases of pleomorphic rhabdomyosarcoma in adults were also seen. Pleomorphic lesions occurred predominantly in adults and were usually asymptomatic. Grossly, the lesions appear reddish-brown and are influenced by vascularity and the extent of necrosis. Much of this information can be obtained preoperatively by angiography. Cells with cross striations are extremely rare in the adult type of tumor, making exact diagnosis difficult at times. Special staining techniques, including fluorescein-labeled antimyosin serum and the immunoperoxidase technique for detection of myoglobin, have been described. In a report of the Intergroup Rhabdomyosarcoma Study, Hays et al.[39] noted that among the frequent sites for development of embryonal rhabdomyosarcoma, the extremities were associated with the highest relapse and lowest survival rates. An analysis of their data showed that five of six amputated patients had recurrence. Lymph node involvement in this group was approximately 20%. Seven of 21 group I patients and 9 of 27 group II patients had relapses despite adequate resection and follow-up therapy. Local radiation to the tumor site did not increase the disease-free interval or survival for group I patients; for group II patients administration of ACT-D and vincristine for 1 year appeared to be effective. In spite of the relatively favorable response to treatment that has been achieved with combination therapy for the embryonal group, about 20% still fail treatment and require additional modalities of therapy should they be applicable. Rancey et al.[69] evaluated the prognosis of children who had relapsed after having achieved complete response to initial therapy.

Fibrosarcoma

Fibrous tissue tumors are also among the more common lesions.[14, 67, 86] Among the 64 patients with fibrosarcoma followed between 1937 and 1969, Bizer[7] noted 11 tumors distributed to the upper extremity, 15 in the lower extremity, and 15 on the trunk. Seven of the patients (11%) had microscopic evidence of regional metastasis. Fifty patients underwent surgical resection, 20 having been treated by local resection. Local recurrence developed in 74% of these patients. Twenty were initially treated by radical resection, with a 30% incidence of local recurrence. In several patients, radical tumor extirpation necessitated amputation because of the size and position of the fibrosarcoma. The absolute 5-year survival rate for all cases was 44% with a marked difference in survival noted in relationship to effectiveness of the treatment. Figure 6–33 shows a recurrent desmoid tumor (low-grade fibrosarcoma) of the popliteal space presenting as a bulging mass, similar to a Baker cyst. The tumor, because of its low-grade nature, was sharply dissected off the sciatic nerve. This tumor has not recurred during 5 years of follow-up. Fibrosarcoma may at times be mimicked by spindle cell melanoma (Fig. 6–34). The patient, a 67-year-old man, had an enlarging mass developing over the upper lateral aspect of his right thigh. Clinically the mass was thought to be fibrosarcoma or malignant fibrous histiocytoma. On examination we noted a scar near the central area of the tumor mass. The scar represented the biopsy site of a pigmented lesion that had been removed 14 years before. We predicted that the tumor mass would prove to be melanoma. The tumor was resected with enbloc groin dissection. The final pathology

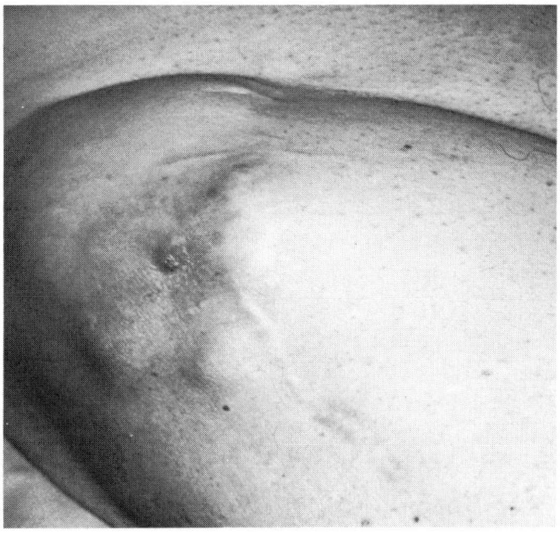

FIGURE 6–34. *Spindle cell melanoma of the right lateral thigh presenting as fibrosarcoma.*

report confirmed our speculation. DiMaio et al. evaluated such tumors ultrastructurally.[23] The feature found in common with the six desmoplastic melanomas studied (neurosarcomatous transformation occurring in malignant melanoma) was interpreted as evidence for Schwann cell differentiation. The ultrastructural findings provided further support for the concept that melanocytic lesions may simulate tumors of Schwann cell origin, presumably reflecting the common embryologic origin of the two cell types from the neural crest.

Alveolar Soft Part Sarcoma

In 1966 Leiberman et al. reviewed an unusual group of tumors that had arisen primarily in the extremities (see Chapter 1). These 53 cases presented a classic picture showing a pseudoalveolar pattern with glomerular structures present. An ultrastructural analysis by electron microscopy further revealed that within the lesions a protein carbohydrate crystal was present. Such crystals were found to be characteristic for this lesion and could be defined by specially stained preparations. The lesion was designated by the term "alveolar soft part sarcoma." Thirty of the 53 cases occurred in the lower extremity, and the right side appeared to be favored. Though the lesions were indolent, they almost always were found to be fatal, with metastasis to lung, bone, and brain common. The mean survival with local excision was 70 months. This could be extended to approximately 91 months by employing excision and radiation therapy. Extensive surgery did not appear to offer much better prognosis in terms of survival, but the group being analyzed was small.

SURGICAL APPROACH TO SOFT PART SARCOMAS OF THE EXTREMITY

The standard surgical approach to extremity sarcomas has long been defined. In approaching any of the deeply seated sarcomas arising within the extremity, the amount of skin around the biopsy site and the amount of muscle and subcutaneous tissue to be resected are important considerations when planning an operation. An elliptical incision is made about the site of any previous biopsy that may have been taken. Thick skin flaps may be raised so long as the tumor does not appear to extend to or infiltrate the subcutaneous tissues. Under such circumstances of freedom, 2 to 4 cm of normal skin should be removed with the underlying subcutaneous tissue. One must constantly palpate the lesion—as dissection progresses and the more deeply it goes, the more important it becomes that margins be carefully palpated so that adequate areas of resection be taken. This can be confirmed later by examining frozen sections obtained during the operative procedure. One may find the tumor mass extending into planes not appreciated by the superficial examination alone. The extent of deeper structures to be included can then be modified. Normal muscles should surround the lesion as it is removed. If the tumor mass is greater than 5 cm in diameter, those muscle groups should be traced to their origins and insertions, with division performed as close to those sites as possible. Occasionally, the tumor mass will cross muscle planes, requiring that additional groups be included in the dissection. Complete control of the blood supply is essential, with isolation of perforating tumor vessels at their origin on the main femoral artery. When dissecting a lesion of the midthigh, it may be necessary to identify the femoral artery by extending the incision superiorly toward the groin. Once defined, the artery can be dissected inferiorly toward the tumor's mass to insure that the lesion can be freed from its primary blood supply with normal surrounding tissue intervening between the vessel and the tumor mass. As the perforating vessels enter the tumors, hemoclips can be used to secure them at their origin; then these structures can be transected. In most instances, if an angiogram and CT scan suggest that the vessel is free of tumor, then adequate dissection to expose the vessels and retract them away from the tumor site can usually be accomplished fairly easily. If there is evidence of tumor invasion of the vessels and dissection cannot be adequately accomplished, then muscle group dissection with removal of the main arterial blood supply can be accomplished with insertion of a vascular graft. The removal of suspicious bone and replacement by prosthesis has already been mentioned.

Vascular Replacement

Fortner et al.[34] reported seven cases of en-bloc resection of tumor with excision of segments of the iliac and femoral vessels. Ischemic loss of the extremity did not occur. By employing both arterial and venous reconstruction, best results with minimal associated edema resulted. Imparato[43] described 13 patients undergoing major vascular resection with reconstruction to allow limb preservation for both soft tissue and primary osseous lesions. Six procedures were for soft part lesions of the thigh. The feasibility of performing en-bloc resections was determined preoperatively from arteriograms taken in at least two planes. Venograms were performed to assess the extent of tumor invasion and unsuspected invasion of major venous structures. Three patients underwent venous reconstruction, whereas nine had ligation of proximal venous structures. There were no instances of intractable edema. Fortner has suggested that an arteriovenous fistula be created proximal to the venous graft–arterial replacement to guarantee patency. If the size of the fistula is not carefully controlled, however, it is possible to create a steal phenomenon.

Muscle Group Dissection

The operation that we describe as muscle group dissection was first carefully described in detail by Bowden and Booher.[8] At that time, they described the practice of en-bloc excision of muscles at the point of origin and insertion as well as sharp dissection through grossly normal tissue at all points of the procedure. They also described the practice of proximal incision and prompt ligation of venous tributaries early in the operative procedure. A case of rhabdomyosarcoma of the left lateral thigh measuring 10 × 9 × 5 cm was described by Bowden and Booher. They employed a curvilinear longitudinal incision from the left costal arch, extending vertically downward across the inguinal ligament into the anterior thigh to the lateral aspect of the knee. A counter incision extended laterally over the hip and well onto the posterior lateral aspect of the thigh, so that the entire tumor mass was ellipsed by the incision. Both incisions joined over the lateral aspect of the knee. This allowed the biospy site to be contained in the center of the area of resection (Fig. 6–35). In our hands the incision probably would have been more confined to an area around the anterior superior iliac spine that ellipsed the tumor. A superficial inguinal

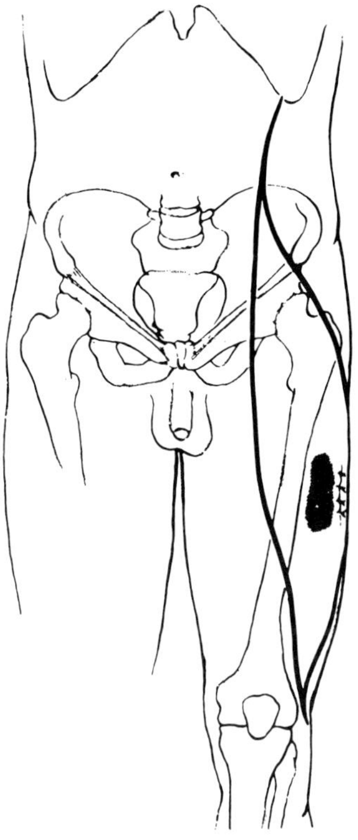

FIGURE 6–35. Classic approach to sarcomas of the extremity.

node dissection was performed in the original procedure, mobilizing subcutaneous tissue over the inguinal canal and reflecting this tissue over Poupart's ligament. A full-thickness incision was then carried through the abdominal musculature to allow the retroperitoneum to be entered and retracted medially. This offered the opportunity for a retroperitoneal node dissection, which currently would not be performed unless there was positive disease in the inguinal region. The incision was then carried over the exposed iliac crest to divide the tensor fascia lata and the gluteus muscles at their points of origin. The anterior border of the gluteus maximus was separated by sharp dissection from the gluteus medius and was retracted posteriorly. The fascia lata was incised along its posterior edge, dividing that portion of the tendon of the gluteus maximus that inserts here; the gluteus medius was again divided on the greater trochanter of the femur. The biceps femoris muscle was retracted posteriorly, and the extensive origin of the vastus lateralis muscle on the lateral surface of the femur was divided. Node-bearing tissue in the femoral triangle was dissected. The quadriceps femoris and the sartorius muscles were exposed throughout for their full length. Remaining fascial attachments were divided, and the specimen was freed from the thigh and removed. As noted by Bowden and Booher, the gluteus muscle could have been spared, but they were unable to determine at the start of dissection how extensive the tumor was. Over the past 25 years, the experience gained in dissections of this type of tumor has allowed us to be somewhat more conservative, attempting limb preservation and maximal extremity function whenever possible. A number of different muscle groups are usually involved in the resection of lower extremity sarcomas. The quadriceps and sartorius are usually taken with tumors in the anterior compartment of the thigh. The adductors are more commonly dissected than the vastus group in completing an en-bloc dissection.[61] Removal of the hamstring is usually necessary for tumors in the posterior aspect of the thigh. For adductor group dissections an elliptical incision is created about the biopsy site. The ellipse should encompass the site of the mass, so that when skin flaps are raised, the entire muscle group to be removed should be exposed. For tumors of the mid-thigh smaller than 10 cm, dissection does not have to include insertion of tendon. The direction of the incision is almost always longitudinal. Muscle bundles can be divided without detaching tendons. Should the tumor approximate the tendon, dissection to the insertion on the pubic tubercle and/or the medial tibial epicondyle is essential. Large flaps must be created to expose the sartorius or the vastus group of muscles if the sartorius is approximated by the tumor. When the tumor encroaches the femoral triangle, the nodes should be removed in the following manner: the femoral vein is identified, the fascia dissected over the external oblique to the inguinal ligaments, and the saphenofemoral junction removed. The femoral artery should then be dissected deeply into the adductor canal of the thigh, raising the adductor group of muscles. The knee is kept slightly flexed and partially abducted during the dissection. When the field is completely exposed, the adductor muscles are divided superiorly on or near the pubic ramus and the profunda femoris artery is ligated. The flexor muscle origins and the quadratus femoris are left intact. Adductor insertions are transected on the femur. By careful dissection, the adductors are then freed from the flexor group and the sciatic nerve.

In a review of cases from the National Cancer Institute, in which adductor muscle group dissection was employed,[61] a relatively high postoperative morbidity was noted. This was attributed to the concomitant lymph node dissection that was part of the operative procedure. We have not encountered an unusual incidence of morbidity with this procedure. For bulky lesions that have a high incidence of spread to regional nodes, or when palpable disease is present in the groin at the time of surgery, we usually employ dissection of the groin lymph nodes rather than just exposure of the vessels. Postoperative elevation in the leg seems to reduce groin and leg edema.

Once a tumor mass has been resected, primary closure of the skin should be planned. Retention-type sutures (pulley-type), using a far-to-near and near-to-far approach, may be necessary, depending on the amount of skin removed over a lesion and the amount of tension on the skin edges. This is particularly true when tension is excessive, a situation that would result in vascular compromise due to compression of skin vessels with resulting avascular necrosis. To obviate this problem, relaxing parallel incisions made peripheral to the resection site will allow closure without undue tension. These relaxing incisions can be left to granulate and require at most daily treatment with antibiotic ointment. In some instances, a skin graft or pedicle flap closure may be necessary because of the extent of the defect. If lymph nodes are palpated and felt to be affected clinically or if the tumor that approximates the node-bearing area is very large, then lymphatic dissection should be considered. There are several advantages to the use of a groin dissection in selected cases of lower extremity neoplasms. The tumor can be staged for possible regional metastasis and the removal of nodes may in itself be therapeutic. The femoral vessels that are identified can be traced and retracted from the operative field, so that the tumor can be easily removed without compromising major blood supply to the extremity. Arterial infusion or perfusion with chemotherapeutic agents can be performed since the femoral vessels are exposed and easy cross-clamping can be achieved at the time of surgery. Stehlin, et al.[83] reported experience with 37 patients having soft part sarcomas of the extremities who were treated with a multidisciplinary approach using hyperthermic perfusion and, when possible, external radiation combined with radical local excision. The ability to carry out the perfusion was based on exposure attained at the time of removal of the extremity tumor; femoral vessels could easily be isolated and prepared for catheterization. The original concept of such regional intra-arterial chemotherapy was initially suggested by Klopp in 1950. Specific techniques for isolation perfusion of extremities, however, was introduced by Kreech, in 1957. Stehlin's modification of this perfusion technique was altered to include heated blood, a modification that resulted in marked improvement for both melanomas and sarcomas.

Experimental data on the use of hyperthermic perfusion was based on the fact that normal fibroblasts were found to survive to a greater degree than fibrosarcoma cells when both were exposed for the same length of time to a temperature of 42.5°C. In experiments with nude mice, it was also found that normal striated muscle cells survived more often than rhabdomyosarcoma or leiomyosarcoma cells when both were exposed to temperatures of 43°C. Stehlin's group of patients undergoing hyperthermic perfusion included nine with liposarcoma, seven with synovioma, six with rhabdomyosarcomas, and four with fibrosarcoma; the remainder of the lesions treated were leiomyosarcoma, alveolar soft part sarcoma, and schwannomas. Once a diagnosis was confirmed, hyperthermic perfusion was applied internally by raising the temperature of the perfused blood to 43°C and the extremities were warmed using Aquamatic K-Pads. When the temperature of the skin and muscle reached 38 to 40° C, cytoxic agents were injected into the venous line in combination with actinomycin C. The incidence of injury to the normal tissues was found to be directly proportional to the amount of drug employed, the temperatures reached in the tissues, and the duration of perfusion. An upper limit of 2.5 hours of tourniquet compression was utilized to avoid damage to nerves. Approximately 1 week after perfusion, radiation therapy was begun. The tumor was left intact until completion of the radiation therapy, i.e., approximately 300 R given in 3 weeks to parallel opposing ports. This was then followed by wide resection of the tumor mass. Among the 37 patients, the 60-month survival rate was 61.9%.

The use of radiation therapy and chemotherapy depend entirely on the tumor type, grade, size, and position of the lesion. Simon and Enneking[80] reported a local recurrence rate of 25% and a distant metastasis rate of 50% using muscle group dissection alone.

As noted previously, we have found it useful to extend dissection of the operative field to the region of the groin, where vessels can be identified and traced inferiorly. This allows separation of the tumor from the major vessels in a manner that is more direct than blind dissection of vessels under the tumor.

There is no question that lymph node dissection may have a beneficial effect when performed as part of the muscle group dissection for sarcoma. Kearney[46] of the Mayo Clinic reported that of 11 patients with malignant fibrous histiocytoma and clinically involved nodes, that five had prolonged survival when lymphadenectomy was performed. In other instances, lymph node metastasis was associated with the presence of disseminated disease. In 1105 cases reviewed by Russel, only 4% had suspected lymph node metastasis in the absence of distant disease. Other data have suggested that distant metastasis is essentially present once lymph node involvement has been defined. Should work-up indicate that the patient is free of metastatic disease, then nodal removal may not only be an effective therapeutic procedure for clinical lymph node disease in the groin, but may avoid the complication of development of an ulcerating tumor in the groin. In this instance, the use of radiation therapy for clinical nodal disease may result not only in flexion contracture at the hip joint due to fibrosis but also tumor growth in the presence of irradiated tissue. The extent of dissection should be marked, when indicated, for radiotherapy with metal clips. If there is a complete muscle mass situated between tumor and margin of resection, radiation may not be necessary. When radiation is planned, ports must extend above and below the resected fields.

Several large series reported the result of surgical resection for lower extremity sarcomas. In each, the lower extremity has appeared to be the most prevalent site for the occurrence of tumor. In a review of 297 cases seen at Memorial Hospital between 1949 and 1968, Shiu[76] described what appears to be the well-founded experience of most surgeons: "Local inadequate resection has resulted in the highest rate of local recurrence." In terms of the distribution of tumors within the lower extremity, the thigh was the most common location (211 cases), followed by the leg itself (60 cases) and the foot (16 cases). One might anticipate such a distribution in terms of the extent of soft tissue present at each site that is potentially at risk. Even though tissue volume was greatest in thigh and normal muscle mass surrounded the tumor to the greatest degree, poor survival rates occurred in the thigh. This was possibly due to the thigh's proximity to the pelvis and a somewhat greater delay in diagnosis.

The bulky normal tissue surrounding the tumor in the thigh may also have led to a longer delay in clinical recognition, especially when the tumor arose in the deeper muscle planes. In terms of tumor size, the largest lesions to be treated occurred in the thigh, both in the anterior and the posterior muscle compartments. We have noted similar findings when treatment was delayed: many tumors expanded subtly within the thigh and the diagnosis of malignancy was not initially entertained. On the other hand, the lesions in some were extremely bulky and we were faced with the decision of doing surgery in borderline situations. These patients had been offered hemiplevectomy as the only treatment. Many of these large bulky tumors did not initially appear to metastasize but had seeded vascular and fascial planes early. Such tumors tend to grow, reaching enormous proportions prior to the onset of therapy. Even at this time, wide muscle group dissection was possible for many of these patients.

The array of tumors most commonly found, as noted previously, includes liposarcoma, fibrosarcoma, rhabdomyosarcoma, and synovioma, appearing in this descending order of frequency. Fibrosarcoma has been the predominant tumor in the leg and synovioma in the foot. Shiu noted that the size of these tumors was important in determining prognosis: small lesions had an overall survival of 63% compared with 46% for larger tumors. Histologic type was also important: fibrosarcomas had an overall survival of 70% versus 45% for rhabdomyosarcomas and synoviomas. In the Memorial Hospital series, 150 patients underwent soft part resection and 139 patients major amputation. The overall survival rate for the resection group was 63% compared with 45% for amputation group, possibly because those lesions that were amputated were considered to be more aggressive.

It is our belief that amputation is not frequently required in the management of lower extremity neoplasms, especially for low-grade primary tumors. For the desmoid tumors and tumors such as chordoid chondrosarcoma, the lesions have been virtually peeled off neurovascular bundles and periosteum; we relied on cryosurgery, radiation therapy, and chemotherapy to delay or obviate recurrence. With large anaplastic lesions, recurrence and metastases are the rule and amputation may have to be considered.

The importance of grade and stage in the prognosis of soft tissue sarcomas has been well documented. In Devereux's study of 19 patients with low-grade sarcomas,[22] 15 had undergone resection without the addition of radiation therapy or chemotherapy. Four had postoperative radiation therapy because the physician was unsure about the adequacy of surgical control; three of these, receiving 6700 R, had recurrence of their lesion at a mean of 38 months. The appearance of local recurrence is frequently associated with a later development of distant metastasis. Since many sarcomas infiltrate fascial planes, it is important not only to have wide margins of resection but also to plan the dissection to encompass muscle groups. If the tumor is of low grade and smaller than 5 cm, it would probably not be important to remove muscle groups from origin to insertion. This series of cases is important also in that the development of microscopic disease could not be prevented with 6750 R postoperatively.

Markhede et al.[56] reviewed a series of 97 patients with soft part sarcomas, 91 cases of which were found in the extremities (12 upper and 79 lower). Malignant fibrous histiocytoma was the most common malignancy seen in their series. When a tumor was found to be highly vascular and was considered malignant on angiography, incisional biopsy was not performed since it was believed that one could reduce the necessary margin of transection in the transverse plane and thus preserve a greater degree of function. For laterally placed lesions in the region of the vastus lateralis or the vastus intermedius, removal could be accomplished from origin to insertion with good margins if the primary procedure was employed without biopsy. In the presence of an incisional biopsy, the rectus femoris and vastus medialis muscles would have to be included in the dissection. All attempts at performing complete but conservative resections with limb preservation were made. The term "radical" was used for the performance of an "adequate" resection. Marginal resections, when performed, were considered "inadequate." Radical local excision was carried out in 63 patients. Tumor-bearing regions were removed en-bloc with a margin of at least one anatomic structure (muscle or fascial plane). Fibrous structures, such as normal fascia and involved periosteum, constituted adequate margins in the transverse planes. In our experience the resection of one fascial plane from the pseudocapsule does not constitute a sufficient margin. Also stripping the periosteum to make one fascial margin from a pseudocapsule is not enough to prevent recurrence. Tumors in Markhede's study were graded from I to IV. Thirty-five percent of the cases were malignant fibrous histiocytoma, 16% liposarcoma, 11% myxoid fibrosarcomas, 9.3% leiomyosarcoma, 7.2% schwannoma, and 5.2% fibrosarcoma. Eighty percent of the tumors were graded from II to IV.The overall rate of recurrence was 21.7%, representing 21 of 97 cases. Seventy percent recurred within 2 years, 80% within 3 years. Local recurrence was noted in 6.6% when a radical procedure was used compared with 76.2% when the operation was considered marginal. The adequacy of surgical resection seemed to be the most important factor influencing the local recurrence rate. Recurrence was about the same in different histologic types, with liposarcoma having both the lowest rate of recurrence and the lower proportion of high-grade tumor. Histologic grading had significant influence. Recurrence was significantly lower in the thigh. The size was of surprisingly little influence. The factors that had significant influence on recurrence were surgical procedure, tumor growth, site (such as thigh), and histologic grading. Distant metastases occurred in 46 of 97 cases (46%): 38 spread to the lung and 8 occurred in the viscera and retroperitoneum. The metastatic rate was 43% for the

76 undergoing radical surgery and 62% for the 21 undergoing marginal resection.

Metastasis developed in 41% who were free of local recurrence versus 71% with local reappearance of disease. The grading of malignancy significantly influenced the risk for metastasis. Tumors of the upper extremity tended to metastasize more often than the lower extremity (67% versus 46%); the lowest rate occurred in the thigh (34%). The absolute 5-year survival for the 97 patients was 59.3%, and the 10-year survival 43.5%.

The surgical management of soft tissue sarcomas depends more on the anatomic location of the tumor than on its histologic type, grade of malignancy, or size. Amputation does not guarantee successful outcome, so most surgeons prefer adequate en-bloc resection with a goal of functional preservation (e.g., the two-finger hand following rejection for synovioma). The major growth phase of most soft tissue sarcomas occurs in a longitudinal direction, staying within the anatomic confines of the muscle group fascial planes. Provided that the planes are not next to the pseudocapsule or invaded by the surgeon, they may serve as boundaries for surgical extirpation. Incisional biopsy, if incorrectly performed, may serve to spread the tumor beyond the normal fascial planes, requiring that wider resection be performed as part of the en-bloc resection. Markhede and Nister[57] and Markhede and Stener[58] evaluated functional impairment as a result of resection of the lower extremity muscle groups and found that in most instances the functional impairment was not a major problem. Amputation was performed in 18.7% of patients with extremity lesions. Shui[76] reported an amputation rate of 42% in previously untreated cases. Simon and Enneking[80] reported an amputation rate of 54%. With more radical local excision and the use of intraoperative chemotherapy, postoperative radiation therapy, and en-bloc bone resection with prosthesis, the primary amputation rate should probably be further diminished, and even lower in thigh tumors than in lesions approximating the knee or the inguinal ligament.

The control of the primary tumor appears important in the prognosis. Cantin[12] found that in two thirds of the patients with metastatic disease, metastases were concomitant with or followed local recurrence and that the earlier the recurrence from the time of surgery, the poorer the prognosis. It appears that the possibility of surviving to 5 years is twice as good in patients in whom tumor recurs in the 21- to 24-month period from surgery than in the patients in whom recurrence appears from 2 to 10 months following surgery.

The grading of tumors, as well as the staging, was important in Markhede's series, in which no patient with grade I or II tumor died of neoplastic disease. The 5-year survival rate was found to be significantly higher for grade III than for grade IV tumors.

Careful follow-up of patients undergoing both en-bloc muscle group dissection and amputation has revealed that the rate of local recurrence is approximately 15%, whereas in patients with amputaton stumps, the incidence of reappearance of the lesion is approximately 7%. Local recurrence treated by amputation will further increase the survival rate. However, a second local radical excision may be preferred over amputation for managing such local reappearance of disease.

REFERENCES

1. Ackerman L. V.: Extraosseous localized non-neoplastic bone and cartilage formation (so-called myositis ossificans): Clinical and pathologic confusion with malignant neoplasms. J. Bone Joint Surg. 40-A:279, 1958
2. Allen P. W., Enzinger F. M.: Hemangioma of skeletal muscle: An analysis of 89 cases. Cancer 29:8–22, 1972
3. Ariel I. M., Pack G. T.: Synovial sarcoma. N. Engl. J. Med. 268:1272, 1963
4. Austin R. M., Mack G. R., Townsend C. M., Lack E. E.: Infiltrating (intramuscular lipomas and angiolipomas). Arch. Surg. 115:281–284, 1980
5. Barone D. A.: Neurofibromatosis: A clinical overview. Postgrad. Med. 66:73–80, 1979
6. Berger P. E., Kuhn J. P.: Computed tomography of tumors of the musculoskeletal system in children: Clinical applications. Radiology 127:171–175, 1978
7. Bizer L. S.: Fibrosarcoma: Report of 64 cases. Am. J. Surg. 121:586–587, 1971
8. Bowden L., Booher R. J.: The principles and techniques of resection of soft parts for sarcoma. Surgery 44:963–977, 1958
9. Brasfield R. D., Das Gupta T. K.: Von Recklinghausen's disease: A clinicopathological study. Ann. Surg. 175:86–104, 1972
10. Brennhovd I. Q.: The treatment of soft tissue sarcomas; A plea for a more urgent and aggressive approach. Acta Chir. Scand. 131:438–442, 1966
11. Cadman N. L., Soule E. H., Kelly P. J.: Synovial sarcomas: Analysis of 134 tumors. Cancer 18:613–627, 1965
12. Cantin J., McNeer G. P., Chu F. C., Booher R. J.: The problem of local recurrence after treatment of soft tissue sarcomas. Ann. Surg. 168:47–53, 1968

13. Carabell S. C., Goodman R. L.: Radiation therapy for soft tissue sarcoma. Semin. Oncol. 8:201–206, 1981
14. Castro E. B., Hajdu S. I., Forther J. G.: Surgical therapy of fibrosarcoma of the extremities: A reappraisal. Arch. Surg. 107:284, 1973
15. Chung E. B., Enzinger F. M.: Benign lipoblastomatosis: An analysis of 35 cases. Cancer 32:482–492, 1973
16. Cohen A. J., Clagett G. P., Nadolo L.: Intramuscular hemangioma. J.A.M.A. 249:2680–2682, 1983
17. Craig R. M., Dugh D. G., Soule E. H.: The roentgenologic manifestations of synovial sarcoma. Radiology 65:837–846, 1955
18. D'Agostino A. N., Coule E. H., Miller R. H.: Sarcomas of peripheral nerves and somatic soft tissues associated with multiple neurofibromatosis. Cancer 16:1015–1027, 1963
19. Denton J. W., Dunham W. R., Salter M., et al: Preoperative regional chemotherapy and rapid fractional irradiation for sarcomas of soft tissue and bone. 158:545–551, 1984
20. deSantos L. A., Goldstein H. M., Murray J. A., Wallace S.: Computed tomography in the evaluation of musculoskeletal neoplasms. Radiology 128:89–94, 1978
21. deSantos L. A., Linaldis, Wallace S.: Computed tomography in liposarcoma. Cancer 47:46–54, 1981
22. Devereux D. F., Wilson R. E., Corson J. M., et al: Surgical treatment of low grade soft tissue sarcomas. Am. J. Surg. 143:490–494, 1982
23. DiMaio S. M., Mackay B., Smith J., DiChersin G. R.: Neurosarcomatous transformation in malignant melanoma. Cancer 50:2345–2354, 1982
24. Eglund N., Ekelund F., Sako M., Perssom B.: CT of soft tissue tumors. Am. J. Roentgenol. 137:725–729, 1981
25. Eilber F. R., Mirra J. J., Grant T. T., et al.: Is amputation necessary for sarcomas. Ann. Surg. 192:431–438, 1980
26. Eilber F. R., Morton D. L., Eckart J., et al.: Limb salvage for skeletal and soft tissue sarcomas. Cancer 53:2579–2584, 1984
27. Ekfors T. O., Rantakokko V.: An analysis of 38 malignant fibrous histiocytomas in the extremities. Acta Pathol. Microbiol. Scand. (A) 86:25–35, 1978
28. Enterline H. T., Culberson J. D., Rochlin D. B., Brady L. W.: Liposarcoma: A clinical and pathological study of 53 cases. Cancer 13:932–950, 1960
29. Enzinger F. M., Dulcey F.: Proliferative myositis: Report of 33 cases. Cancer 20:2213, 1967
30. Enzinger F. M., Winslow D. L.: Liposarcoma: A study of 103 cases. Virchows Arch. (Pathol. Anat.) 335:367–388, 1962
31. Fields J. P., Helwig E. B.: Leiomyosarcoma of the skin and subcutaneous tissue. Cancer 47:156, 1981
32. Fisher M. G., Gelb A. M., Nyssbaum M., et al.: Primary smooth muscle tumors of venous origin. Ann. Surg. 196:720–724, 1982
33. Forrestor D. M., Bechor T. J.: The radiology of bone and soft tissue sarcomas. Orthop. Clin. North Am. 8:973–998, 1977
34. Fortner J. G., Kim P. J., Shiu M. H.: Limb preserving vascular surgery for malignant tumors of the lower extremity. Arch. Surg. 112:394, 1977
35. Gilbert H. A., Kagan R. A., Winkley J.: Soft tissue sarcomas of the extremities: Their natural history, treatment, and radiation sensitivity. J. Surg. Oncol. 7:303–317, 1975
36. Goldman A. B.: Myositis ossificans circumscripta: A benign lesion with a malignant differential diagnosis. Am. J. Roentgenol. 126:32–40, 1976
37. Hachisuga T., Hashimoto H., Enjoji M.: Angioleiomyoma: A clinicopathologic reappraisal of 562 cases. Cancer 54:126–130, 1984
38. Hadju S. I., Shiu M. H., Fortner J. G.: Tendosynovial sarcoma: A clinico-pathologic study of 136 cases. Cancer 39:1201–1217, 1977
39. Hays D. M., Sutow W. W., Lawrence W. Jr., et al.: Rhabdomyosarcoma: Surgical therapy in extremity lesions in children. Orthop. Clin. North Am. 8:883–902, 1977
40. Heelan R. T., Watson R. C., Smith J.: Computed tomography of lower extremity tumors. Am. J. Roentgenol. 132:933–937, 1979
41. Hudson T., Hass G., Enneking, W., et al.: Angiography in the management of musculoskeletal tumors. Surg. Gynecol. Obstet. 141:11–21, 1975
42. Hutton I.: Liposarcoma of the thigh: Management. Proc. Roy. Soc. Med. 67:655–656, 1974
43. Imparato A. M., Roses D. F., Frances K. C., Lewis M. M.: Major vascular reconstruction for limb salvage in patients with soft tissue and skeletal sarcomas of the extremities. Surg. Gynecol. Obstet. 147:891–896, 1978
44. Inoshita T., Youngberg G. A.: Malignant fibrous histiocytoma arising in previous surgical sites. Cancer 53:176–183, 1984
45. Ireland D. C. R., Soule E. H., Ivins J. C.: Myxoma of somatic soft tissues. Mayo Clin. Proc. 48:401, 1973
46. Kearney M. M., Soule E. H., Ivins J. C.: Malignant fibrous histiocytoma: A retrospective study of 167 cases. Cancer 29:961–976, 1972
47. Krementz E. T., Carter R. D., Sutherland C. M., Hutton I.: Chemotherapy of sarcomas of the limbs by regional perfusion. Ann. Surg. 185:555–564, 1977
48. Kyriakos M., Kempson R. L.: Inflammatory fibrous histiocytoma: An aggressive and lethal lesion. Cancer 37:1584–1606, 1976
49. Leibel S. A., Tranbough R. F., Wara W. M., et al.: Soft tissue sarcomas of the extremities. Cancer 50:1076–1083, 1982
50. Lindberg R. D., Martin R. G., Ronsdahl M. D.: Surgery and post-operative radiotherapy in the treatment of soft tissue sarcomas in adults. Am. J. Roentgenol. 123:123–129, 1975
51. Lindell M. M., Wallace S., deSantos L. A., Bernardino M. E.: Diagnostic techniques for the evaluation of the soft tissue sarcoma. Semin. Oncol. 8:160–170, 1981
52. Mackenzie D. H.: Synovial sarcoma—a review of 56 cases. Cancer 19:1695, 1966
53. Marcove R. C., Abou-Zahr K.: En-bloc surgery for osteogenic sarcoma. Bull. N.Y. Acad. Med. 60:748–758, 1984
54. Marcove R. C., Khafagy M. M.: Total femur and knee replacement using a metallic prosthesis. Clin. Bull. Mem. Hosp. 4:69–71, 1974
55. Markel S. F., Enzinger F. M.: Neuromuscular hamartoma—a benign "triton tumor" composed of mature neural and striated muscle elements. Cancer 49:140–144, 1982
56. Markhede G., Angervall L., Stener B.: A multivariate analysis of the prognosis after surgical treatment of malignant soft tissue tumors. Cancer 49:1721–1733, 1982

57. Markhede G., Nister L.: Strength of plantar flexion and function after resection of various parts of the triceps surae. Acta Orthop. Scand. 50:693–697, 1979
58. Markhede G., Stener B.: Function after removal of various hip and thigh muscles for extirpation of tumors. Acta Orthop. Scand. 52:373–395, 1981
59. Masdeu J. C., Rubino F. A.: Traumatic myopathy: A benign cause of pseudohypertrophy of the calves. J.A.M.A. 249:2641, 1983
60. McBride C. M.: Sarcoma of the limbs: Results of adjuvant chemotherapy using isolation perfusion. Arch. Surg. 109:304–307, 1974
61. Mentzer S. J., Sugarbaker P. H.: Adductor muscle group excision. Surgery 91:662–668, 1982
62. Neifeld J. P., Walsh J. W., Lawrence W., Jr.: Computed tomography in the management of soft tissue tumors. Surg. Gynecol. Obstet. 155:535–540, 1982
63. Nesbit R. B., Rob C.: Leiomyosarcoma of a vein. Arch. Surg. 110:118, 1975
64. Pack G. T., Pierson J. C.: Liposarcoma: A study of 105 cases. Surgery 36:687–712, 1954
65. Park J. J., Park H. G., Choi S. H.: Leiomyosarcomas of the extremities. J. Surg. Oncol. 10:407–411, 1978
66. Pratilis V., Arlen M.: Primary myxosarcoma of leg. N.Y. State J. Med. 70:309–311, 1970
67. Pritchard D. J.: Fibrosarcoma of bone and soft tissues of the trunk and extremities. Orthop. Clin. North Am. 8:869, 1977
68. Rajpal S., Moore R. H., Karakousis C. P.: Synovial sarcoma: A review of treatment and survival in 52 patients. N.Y. State J. Med. 84:17–19, 1984
69. Rancey R. B., Christ W. M., Maurer H. M., et al.: Prognosis of children with soft tissue sarcoma who relapse after achieving a complete response. Cancer 52:44–50, 1983
70. Reszel. P. A., Soule, E. H., Coventry M. B.: Liposarcoma of the extremities and limb girdles: A study of 222 cases. J. Bone Joint Surg. 48-A:229–244, 1966
71. Riccardi V M.: Von Recklinghausen neurofibromatosis. N. Engl. J. Med. 305:1617–1627, 1981
72. Rosenberg S. A., Glatstein E. J.: Perspectives on the role of surgery and radiation therapy in the treatment of soft tissue sarcomas of the extremities. Semin. Oncol. 8:1981
73. Rosenberg S. A., Kent H., Costa J.: Prospective randomized evaluation of the role of limb sparing surgery, R>T>, and adjuvant chemoimmunotherapy in the treatment of adult soft tissue sarcoma. Surgery 84:62–69, 1978
74. Ross L. S., Eckstein M. R., et al.: Calcified leiomyoma. N.Y. State J. Med. 83:747–749, 1983
75. Salm R.: The nature of the so-called postmastectomy lymphangiosarcoma. J Pathol. Bacterial. 85:445, 1963
76. Shiu M. N., Castro E. G., Hajdu S. I., Forther J. G.: Surgical treatment of 297 soft tissue sarcomas of the lower extremity. Ann. Surg. 182:597–602, 1975
77. Shiu M. H., McCormick P. M., Hajdu S. I., et al.: Surgical treatment of tendosynovial sarcoma. Cancer 43:889–897, 1979
78. Shiu M. H., Turnbull A. D., Dattaheyudu N., et al.: Control of locally advanced extremity soft tissue sarcomas by function saving resection and brachytherapy. Cancer 53:45–53, 1984
79. Shmookler B. M., Enzinger F. M.: Liposarcoma occurring in children: An analysis of the literature and review of the literature. Cancer 52:567–574, 1983
80. Simon M. A., Enneking W. F.: The management of soft tissue sarcomas of the extremities. Orthop. Clin. North Am. 8:869, 1977
81. Soule E. H., Geitz M., Henderson E. D.: Embryonal rhabdomyosarcoma of the limbs and limb girdles: A clinicopathological study of 61 cases. Cancer 23:1336–1346, 1969
82. Spitle M. F., Newton K. A., Mackenzie D. H.: Liposarcoma: A review of 60 cases. Br. J. Cancer 24:696, 1971
83. Stehlin J., Delpolyi P. D., Giovanella B. C.: Soft tissue sarcomas of the extremity: Multidisciplinary therapy employing hyperthermic perfusion. Am. J. Surg. 130:643–646, 1975
84. Stewart F. W., Treves N.: Lymphangiosarcoma in postmastectomy lymphedema. Cancer 1:64–81, 1948
85. Storm F. K., Eilber F. R., Mirra J., Morton D. L.: Neurofibrosarcoma. Cancer 45:126–129, 1980
86. Stout A. D.: Fibrosarcoma. Cancer 1:30–63, 1948
87. Stout A. P., Hill W. T.: Leiomyosarcoma of the skin and subcutaneous tissue. Cancer 11:844, 1964
88. Suit H. D., Russel W. O., Martin R. G.: Management of patients with sarcoma of soft tissue in an extremity. Cancer 31:1247–1255, 1973
89. Suit H. D., Russel W. O.: Radiation therapy of soft tissue sarcomas. Cancer 36:759–764, 1975
90. Vellios F., Baez T. M., Shumacker H. B.: Lipoblastomatosis: A tumor of fetal fat different from hibernoma. Am. J. Pathol. 34:1149–1159, 1958
91. Weinberger G., Lewinsohn E. M.: Computed tomography in the evaluation of sarcomatous tumors of the thigh. Am. J. Roentgenol. 130:115–118, 1978
92. Weiss S. W., Enzinger F. M.: Malignant fibrous histiocytoma: An analysis of 200 cases. Cancer 41:2250–2266, 1978
93. Woodruff J. M., Chernil N. L., Smith M. C., et al.: Peripheral nerve tumors with rhabdomyosarcomatous differentiation (malignant "triton tumors"). Cancer 32:426–438, 1973
94. Woodward, A. H., Ivins, I. C., Soule, E. H.: Lymphangeosarcoma arising in chronic lymphedematous extremities. Cancer 30:562, 1972.

CHAPTER

7

Tumors of the Hands and Feet

Lesions of the hands and feet occur infrequently and are rarely included in any analysis of sarcomatous lesions of the extremities. As such, there are few reviews of these lesions in the literature. Owens et al.[14] evaluated experience in the management of such cases at Memorial Hospital over a 24-year period. Ninety-eight patients had been seen, 82 of whom were evaluable in terms of treatment response, with a follow-up of 5 to 30 years. Fifty underwent their primary treatment at that institution; 34 (68%) were alive at 5 years. Seventeen of the tumors were found in the hand and 33 involved the feet. Most of the tumors were of high-grade malignancy; 5 of the tumors in the hand and 5 in the feet were of low-grade malignancy. Among the patients with high-grade sarcomas, 36% of those with tumors in the hands survived for 10 or more years, whereas 45% of those with tumors arising in the feet survived for 10 years. In this series, synovioma was the most common tumor: 9 appeared in the hands and 23 in the feet. The second most common tumor reported was fibrosarcoma, with three cases each in the hands and feet. Epithelioid sarcoma, another important lesion to be considered, was not reported in this series. In 1978 22 cases of epithelioid sarcomas (with 10 in the hands) were reviewed by Prat et al.[17] at Memorial Hospital. Because of the proximity of important neurovascular, tendinous, and osseous structures in proximity to tumor, early invasion into these structures must be considered when planning the treatment to be undertaken. Seven patients in this study had local recurrence as the first sign of treatment failure. Nodal metastasis was defined in 12% of the group; 16 of 22 who died succumbed to pulmonary metastasis.

HAND LESIONS

Most tumors that arise in the hands are benign. The most common of these soft tissue tumors is the ganglion, a relatively soft, circumscribed mass frequently localized to the dorsal portion of the wrist. Aspiration usually reveals the characteristic gelatinous material. These lesions may occur in several other areas of the hand, including the volar carpal ligament on the radial side of the hand. Occasionally ganglia can be found in the area of the flexor retinaculum at the base of the digits. Although aspiration with injections of steroids has been used in attempting to control the lesions, their recurrence rate can be high and pathologic confirmation in these cases is absent. Many of the lesions that had been called ganglion were diagnosed late in the course of development and later were proved to be synovioma or epithelioid sarcoma. Aspiration should be used only by experienced individuals in selected cases.

When excising a ganglion, every effort should be made to trace it down to the carpal ligaments in the wrist. When ganglia occur in the region of the radius, the radial artery may pose a problem. An Allen test must be done before surgery in the event that the artery requires ligation, although all efforts should be made to attempt preservation of this vascular structure. In the extensor region of the wrist, the retinaculum does not require repair except in the case of the retinaculum of the extensor pollicis longus. Ganglia at the volar retinaculum, at the level of the metacarpal phalangeal joints, often are palpated as bony hard and may be misinterpreted as osteophytes or osteochondromas. Incomplete surgical resection can result in a high recurrence rate. Certainly, any lesion that recurs after surgical resection must be considered to have had inadequate surgical treatment or to be worrisome because of its malignant potential, even when a previous benign pathologic report exists. The burden of proof lies with the surgeon, who should be aware of dangerous clinical presentations and misinterpretations. Previous pathology should be reviewed. New pathologic specimens should be considered, as previous slide sections may have been taken only from the sites of the benign components, which may have been derived from areas such as secondary bursal tissue.

Clear Cell Sarcoma. Malignant sarcomas of the tendons and aponeuroses have been reported only rarely. In 1965 Enzinger[8] first defined the clear cell sarcoma of tendons and aponeuroses, a tumor that commonly presents as a painless mass or swelling usually on the distal portions of the extremities. Histologically all of the tumors have a nodular pattern and are composed of round and fusiform cells arranged in nests and fascicles separated by fine connective tissue septa. They may be of synovial origin or neural crest derivation; it has been suggested that the tumor is an atypical form of malignant melanoma. The incidence of local recurrence following primary surgical resection is very high. Metastases are said to be in the range of 60 to 70%.

Lipomatous Tumors. Simple lipomas may occur in the hands as bilateral tumor masses, usually on the external surface of the tendon sheaths of the digits. Occasionally, a deep subfascial lipoma may occur under the palmar fascia; because of the resulting closed space, firmness may be noted and considered to clinically represent a malignant process. When the subfascial planes are entered during resection, the benign nature of the lesion expanding from its closed space is readily identified. We have had no experience with liposarcomas arising in the hands. Booher[5] has described lipoblastic tumors arising in the hands and feet.

The glomus tumor is a benign soft part tumor that is characterized by its marked sensitivity to temperature and pressure. In 1924 Masson presented a thesis on the origin and histologic appearance of this tumor. The classic unit was described as consisting of an arteriole, a venule, and a directly anastomosing vessel connecting the arteriole and venule without an intervening capillary bed. These particular vessels were found to be encompassed by longitudinal and circular smooth muscle cells interspersed with epithelioid (glomus) cells that contained oval or globular nuclei. This tumor can be exquisitely sensitive to changes in temperature or pressure. Characteristically the glomus appears as a brownish discoloration at the base of the nail bed (Fig. 7–1), more often affecting the hands than the feet. Of the 35 cases reported by Mullis et al.,[13] 24 were in the upper extremity and 8 in the lower; 13 of the 24 upper extremity lesions were subungual. Other sites were the nose, stomach, and hip region. Pain was the most common complaint for the subungual and forearm lesions. Removal of the nail and surgical

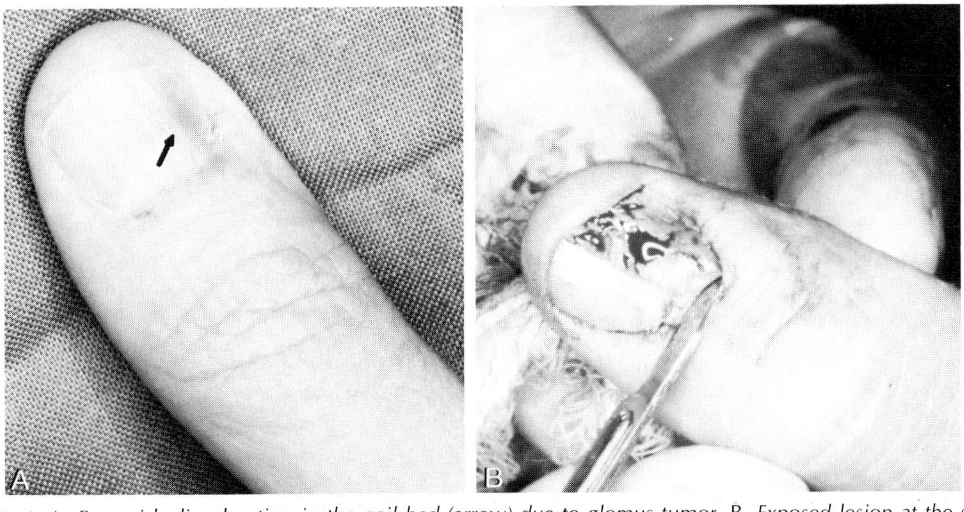

FIGURE 7–1. A, *Brownish discoloration in the nail bed* (arrow) *due to glomus tumor.* B, *Exposed lesion at the site of the resected nail.*

resection of the underlying lesion is the treatment of choice and usually results in immediate relief of symptoms.

Villonodular Tenosynovitis. Another common lesion is benign pigmented villonodular tenosynovitis, often called xanthomatous giant cell tumor of tendon sheath.[19] In tight fascial planes this lesion can grow extensively and erode bone, even extending within the bone tissue. Here it may continue to grow and secondarily expand the bone explosively, appearing like a primary osseous malignant tumor on the x-ray film. This lesion can be so extensive that surgery cannot remove all tumorous tissue. At that point, decisions have to be made as to whether radiation therapy should be added. It is our opinion that surgery should be repeated where symptomatically needed, with attempts made to withhold x-ray therapy for this benign lesion because of the possibility of a later malignant conversion induced by the radiation. Furthermore, skin subjected to radiotherapy becomes thickened, thereby impeding the detection of recurrent disease. We have at times seen spontaneous regression and involution of the expanding lesion when the patient has been treated conservatively or with limited surgery. Benign xanthomatous giant cell tumors tend to occur in the flexor tendons of the hands in women during the third and fourth decades (Fig. 7–2). At times these lesions may be seen arising from the extensor aspect of the fingers or they may develop from the synovium of an interphalangeal joint. Here the lesion is usually pea-sized and quite cellular. Groups of syncytial cells with large oval nuclei are seen along with giant cells, which may number up to 30 per high-power field. Occasionally, these tumors may enlarge to become disfiguring and are often part of hypercholesterolemic xanthomatosis. Fibrosis may develop at sites of tumor degeneration. Furthermore, villous areas may be found, which can coalesce into larger nodular lesions.

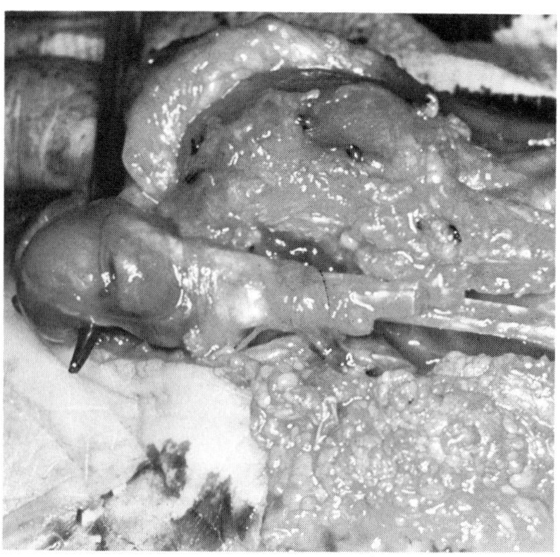

FIGURE 7–2. Clamp under tendon demonstrating a benign xanthomatous giant cell tumor.

Occasionally, when villonodular lesions occur near a joint, secondary degenerative arthritis can result. This arthritis can be treated by a variety of conservative or aggressive means, according to the needs of the patient: synoviectomy (removal of joint debris), surface replacement or arthroplasty, and joint resections or joint fusions. For example, the first metacarpal phalangeal joint and the proximal interphalangeal or distal interphalangeal joints may be amenable to joint fusion in order to increase hand strength in a functional position, especially if mobility at these sites is already limited. The second to fifth metacarpal phalangeal joints may be resected or arthroplasty may be tried. Mobility of the first carpometacarpal joint should usually be preserved. The choice is usually between fusion procedures and methods to preserve mobility; fusion procedures offer increased strength.

Other benign lesions arising in the region of the distal ulna may interfere with pronation and supination. This situation can be resolved by using the Darrach procedure (removal of the distal ulna) in the adult patient. We have observed that this resection performed in children results in a growth deformity (ulnar deviation of the hand) paralleling similar growth disturbances resulting from radial head resections in childhood.

In approaching a lesion deep within the hand, where neurovascular bundles must be mobilized and retracted, it may be necessary to abandon the preferred method for management of soft tissue tumors, i.e., to perform a small biopsy, obtain pathologic confirmation, then do a secondary radical resection. Rather, it may be necessary to perform the definitive extirpation at the time of the initial approach, rather than risk spillage of the biopsy tissue into vital nearby structures. Good judgment coupled with experience is important in these cases.

Fibrous Tumors. Dupuytren's fasciitis, representing the initial phase in the spectrum of fibromatosis, may often present early in the disease process as localized nodular masses rather than the contracting scars within the palmar fascia that appear later in the course of disease.[7] When excised, the histologic appearance of these early nodules may be cause for concern as they can be easily confused with frank sarcoma, even though they are benign and will undergo involution with fibrous contractures. One of the clues to their benign nature is that on section of the entire nodule, the inner nuclear details look worse than the peripheral cytology. The distribution of worrisome cells is much the same as in myositis ossificans. The excision of contracted metacarpal phalangeal joint areas secondary to Dupuytren's contracture may necessitate the use of a skin graft. If possible, skin with little dermis should be carefully dissected off the lesion. This may allow approximation of flap edges without grafting. Severely flexed proximal interphalangeal and distal interphalangeal joints often are said to require amputations rather than soft tissue work. However, we have found that by shortening the bones with necessary joint fusion to match the degree of soft tissue flexure contracture, the severe flexion and contracture will often be relieved and the finger saved even though it may be severely shortened. The fusion can be done in the position of function.

Primary fibrous tumors of the hands arising in childhood may sometimes be interpreted as malignant.[12] Reye[18] described a group of recurring digital fibrous tumors seen over a period of 20 years. Eighteen small fibrous tumors were removed from the fingers and toes of 12 children. These lesions showed a clear propensity for local recurrence, especially when incompletely removed, and initially were considered to be fibrosarcomas. It is possible to distinguish these lesions by inclusion bodies found within the cytoplasm after staining with iron hematoxylin. Expansion into the tendon and periosteum can make total resection difficult, and amputation may be necessary after repeated episodes of tumor regrowth have followed adequate surgical procedures.

Surgical Considerations

Problems related to the management of sarcomas involving the hand are primarily related to the type and grade of tumor and the size of the lesion in relationship to metacarpals, nerves, tendons, and vascular supply. Another important consideration is whether there is involvement of the thumb or little finger and whether the lesion is positioned centrally in the hand. When a large tumor occurs in the region of the thumb, consideration must be given to patterns of spread to the third ray along the adductor muscle. The third ray may be saved by dorsally splitting its extensor tendon, exposing the third metacarpal, and with a dental drill making a dorsal longitudinal trough and freezing the ray with liquid nitrogen. The long adductor muscle attachment can then be separated subperiosteally, thereby salvaging this ray. At a later date, pollicization can be considered. The digital nerve can be saved on the third ray; then with radical excision, a large tumor of the thumb can be removed with the loss of the first two fingers, but not the third.

In the region of the small finger the ulnar nerve is best explored by direct surgery along the route of the ulnar artery. The nerve can be followed as it runs deep to the flexor carpi ulnaris, then dips through the hypothenar area over the flexor retinaculum into the deep palmar space of the metacarpals. It then runs medial to the flexor digiti minimi and the abductor digiti minimi to pierce the opponens digiti minimi as it rounds the hooked bone (os hamatum) and follows the deep palmar arch under the long flexor tendons at the level of the base of the metacarpal bones. In the deep palmar space this neurovascular bundle is often best tracked by using a longitudinal incision made to explore the median nerve across the carpal ligament. The flexor retinaculum is split and the median nerve and long flexor tendons are retracted, as already mentioned. At the base of the metacarpals, one can pick up the deep branches of the ulnar nerve and the ulnar artery. Along this area of the deep arch, for example, surgery for removal of a hemangioma can be performed by tying off the small distal branches from the ulnar artery feeding this lesion (i.e., a lesion of the fifth and fourth fingers). It is important in the hand and finger region to save sensory fibers, particularly of the median nerve, since a hand that moves without sensation will be quite useless to the patient.

When angiograms are performed for hand lesions, the dye should be injected proximally into the brachial artery. The injection should be performed high enough above the digital radial and ulnar arteries to prevent small vessel thrombosis. An Allen test done before surgery is important to define the adequacy of vascular anastomosis in the hand. The radial artery and then the ulnar artery should be compressed and released individually in order to define the pattern of blood flow. This is essential before any radical surgery is undertaken. The restoration of the basic hand functions of grasp and pinch is important in contemplating radical resection. Should the thumb be resected, the resulting function is like using a digital "chopstick" motion to grasp objects. In planning the original procedure, then, one must consider restoration of function. However, the primary purpose of this surgery in the case of malignancy is to save the patient's life, and this cannot be compromised in an effort to restore function.

A number of interesting problems have been encountered during resection of tumors in this region. One case involved a patient with a hemangioma of the hand and necrosis of skin in the region of the fifth finger, which occurred following blockage of the radial artery in the performance of a distal radial arteriogram. Figure 7–3*A* shows the x-ray appearance of the soft tissue swelling around

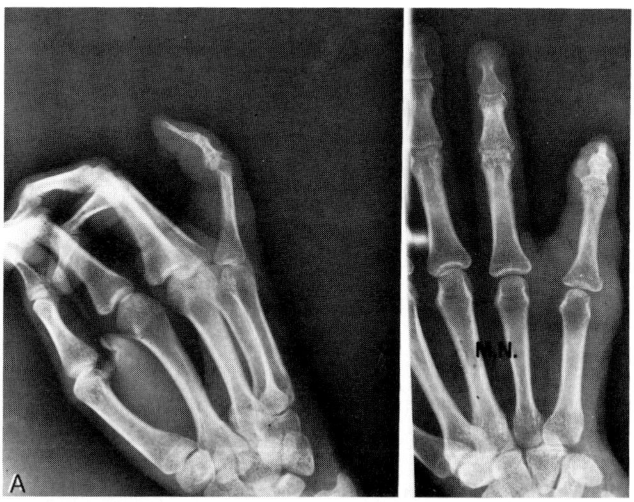

FIGURE 7–3. *A, Hemangiomatous lesion around the fifth finger seen on x-ray film of the hand. B, Appearance after resection of the gangrenous fifth finger. C and D, Recurrence of the angiomatous lesion. E, Angiography shows the residual hemangiomatous lesion and the absence of the radial artery.*

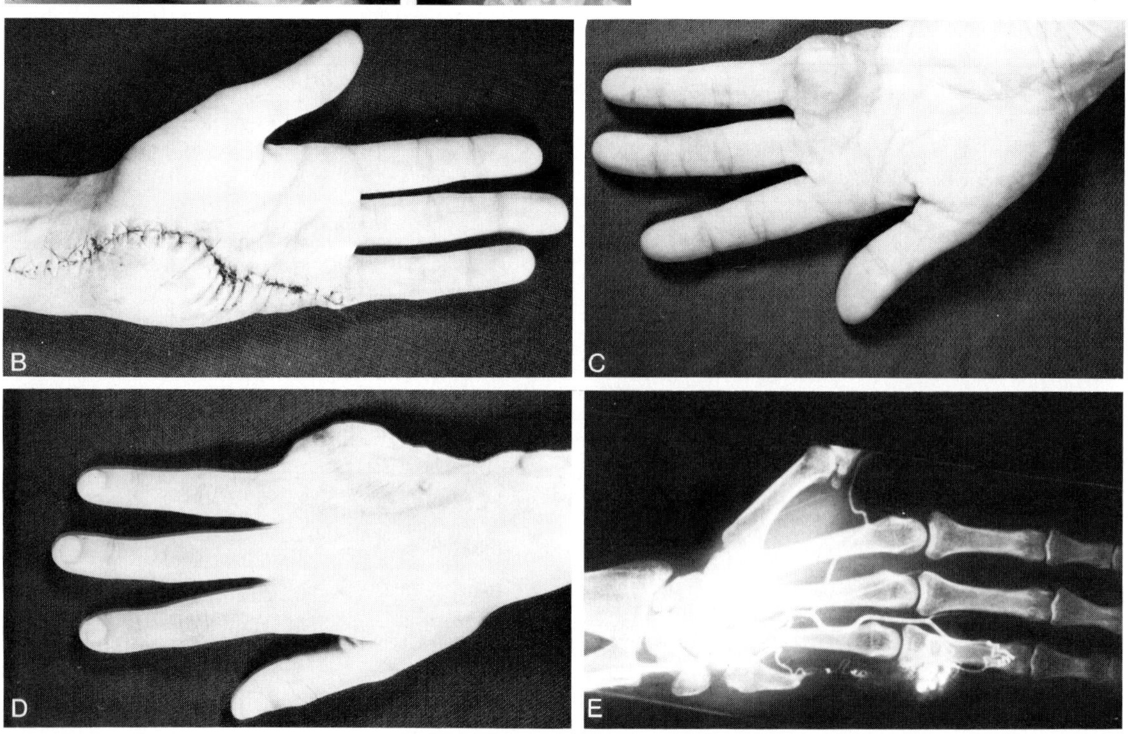

the fifth finger. The gangrenous fifth finger was removed (Fig. 7–3*B*). Postoperatively a new lesion developed at the site of resection (Fig. 7–3*C* and *D*). The arteriogram (Fig. 7–3*E*) shows residual hemangioma and absence of the radial artery. The recurrent hemangioma was controlled by local resection. Two similar cases, one involving pleomorphic rhabdomyosarcoma of the thumb and another, giant cell tumor of the thumb, were managed by preservation of the third ray.

A more interesting problem involved a patient with spindle cell sarcoma of the hand, where only the first two fingers could be saved. The arteriogram (Fig. 7–4*A*) revealed a biphasic synovioma involving the third, fourth, and fifth metacarpals. During resection of the third to fifth rays, the digital nerve to the index finger was preserved, splitting off the digital nerve of the third finger distally to proximally. The second ray was fused at the metacarpophalangeal and carpal joints, and was fixed with an intramedullary wire (Fig. 7–4*B*) in order to preserve its function as a firm post against which the thumb could pinch. Figure 7–4C shows an x-ray film of the hand after removal of the wire. Resection of the distal ulna was performed at the same time. The patient has been free of disease for more than 10 years and has use of the pinching function of the thumb (Fig. 7–4*D* and *E*).

Synovioma. The most common malignant tumor of the soft tissue of the hand is the malignant synovioma, which often presents as a painless mass usually on the palmar surface, but it may occur anywhere in the hand.[10] It is usually a slow-growing tumor, and metastases may not be evident for as

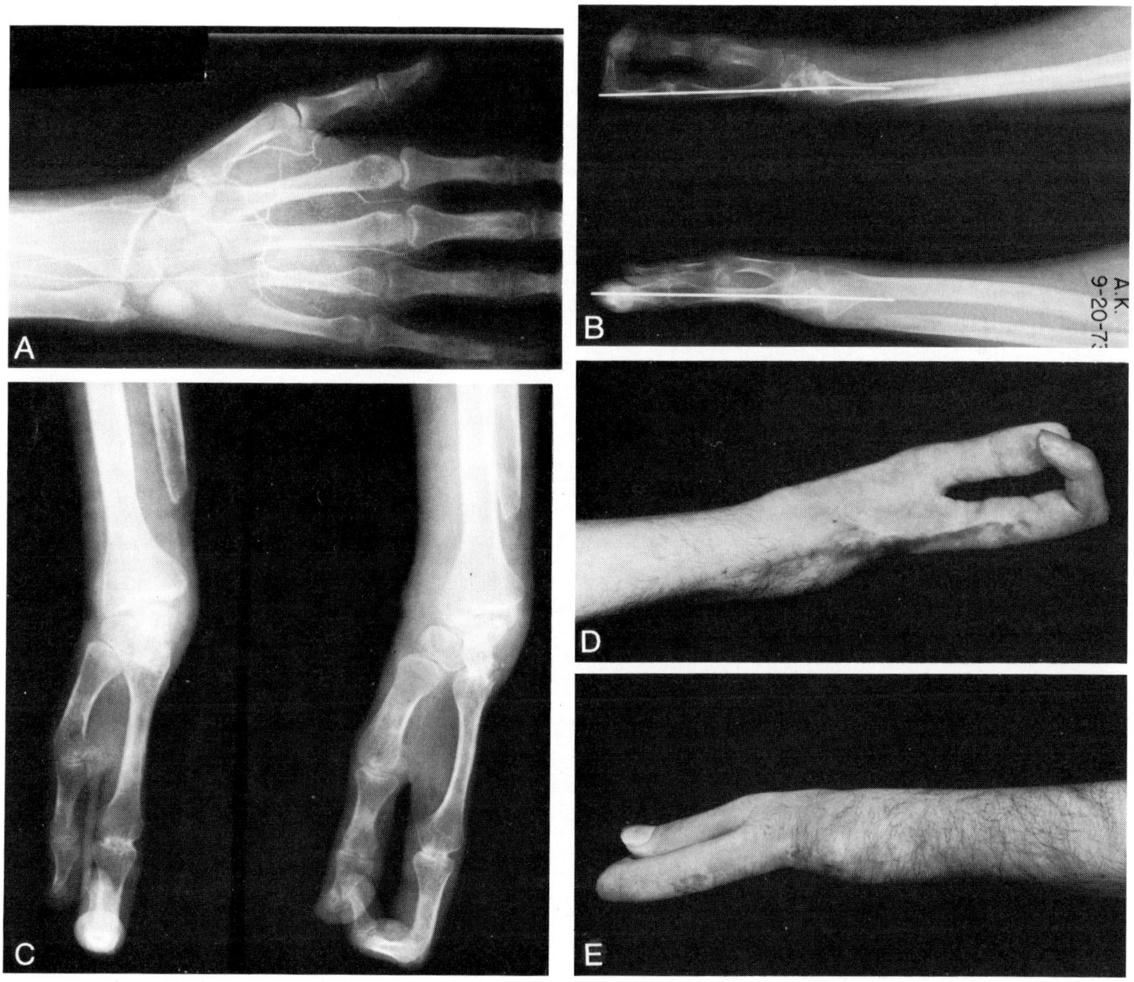

FIGURE 7–4. *A, Biphasic synovioma involving the third through fifth metacarpals on angiography. B, Hand after amputation of the third through fifth metacarpals. C, X-ray film of hand showing pinching function. D and E, Appearance of a two-finger hand.*

long as 10 years. X-ray films show calcification in 20% of cases; these calcifications may be fine, stippled amorphous lesions or coarse and nodular. Figure 7–5 shows the x-ray appearance of a monophasic synovioma occurring about the wrist with calcification in the lesion. Treatment consisted of local resection of the lesion and the distal ulna. Histologically, these lesions may be monophasic or biphasic, i.e., with spindle and synovial elements or with loose spindle or cuboidal elements. Sometimes a specimen has to be recut and slides reviewed many times before the biphasic malignant synovial pattern can be found. We have found that an arteriogram may show a hyperemic pattern even after large doses of radiation therapy have been given for the primary treatment of synovioma. Because this is a radioresistant lesion, radiotherapy is not usually advised.

Epithelioid Sarcoma. Epithelioid sarcoma, another extremely malignant lesion, must be separated from synovioma.[4, 6] This tumor is often confused with synovioma histologically and at times with fasciitis. Epithelioid sarcoma tends to spread extensively in a wide distant pattern through the fascial planes of the hand and wrist. Nodal and vascular invasion occurs within a short time. During surgery for the primary lesion if the distant portions of the limb are found to be unduly swollen, one can assume that epithelioid sarcoma has invaded and blocked the veins and lymphatics. One of our patients was seen with small infiltrating nodular lesions in the hand at a distant site from the primary lesion, which had been excised. Before preparing for amputation for what appeared to be localized disease within the hand, we performed a prophylactic axillary dissection. Microscopic evidence of tumor was noted in grossly negative nodes and in both the subcapsular and the lymphatic vessels. A forequarter amputation was therefore performed, but in a short while recurrent disease was noted in the amputation site (Fig. 7–6*A*). Following this, the tumor burst out in localized areas of the neck and in the anteroposterior chest wall (Fig. 7–6*B*). The patient did not respond to radiation and chemotherapy but survived for several years before pulmonary metastasis appeared. With this sarcoma, pulmonary resection or re-

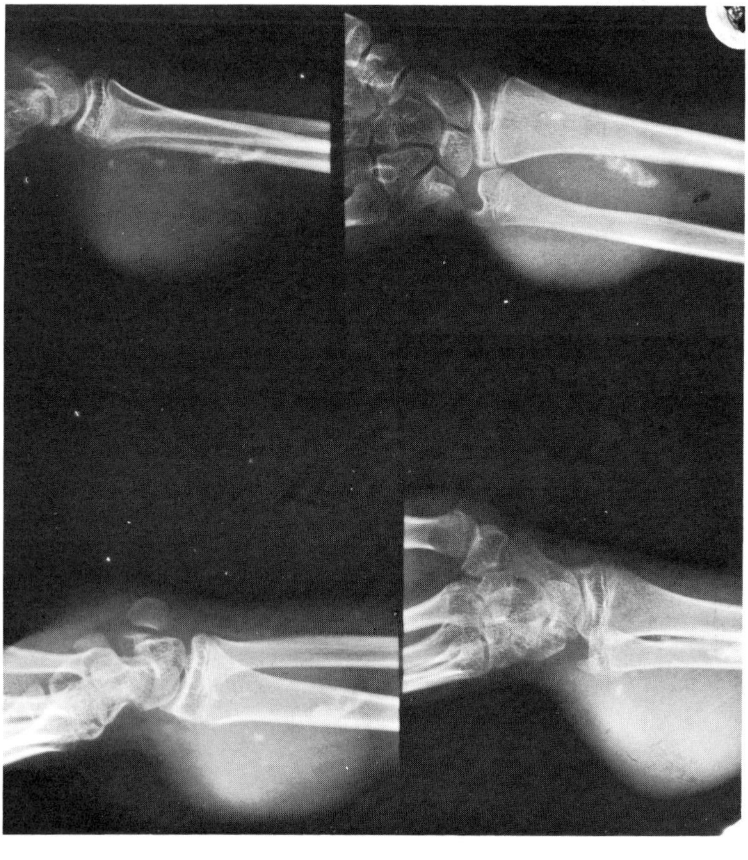

FIGURE 7–5. *X-ray film of a monophasic synovioma about the wrist with microcalcification present.*

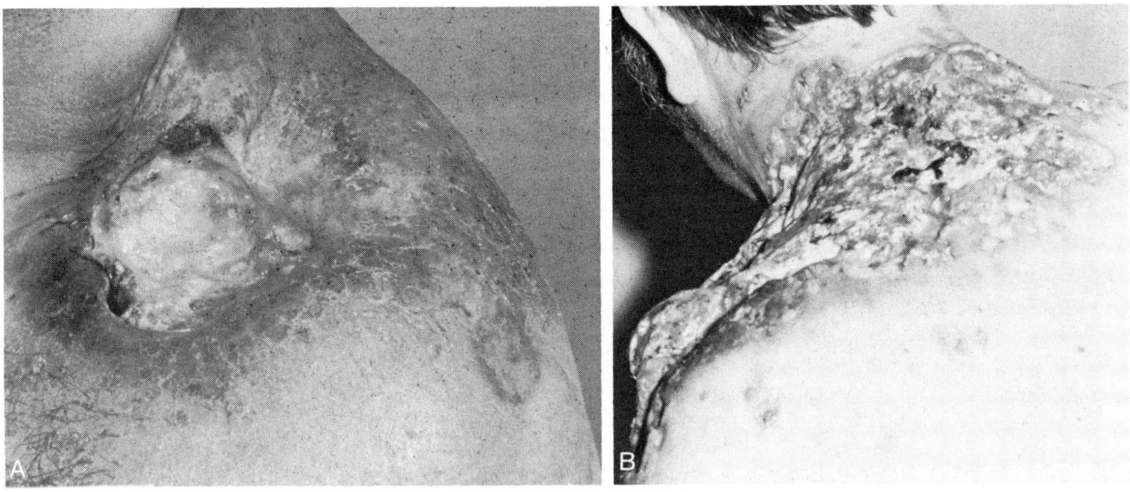

FIGURE 7–6. A, Metastatic lesions from an epithelioid sarcoma. B, Rapid progression of disease.

moval of isolated nodules has not been beneficial because the tumor had infiltrated the lymphatic channels of the amputative and pulmonary sites long before, making cure impossible at this stage of disease. This lesion should never be treated except by the most radical procedure. The cure rates are extremely low, even though distant disease may take over 5 to 10 years to appear. Even metastatic pulmonary nodules exhibit this pattern of lymphatic spread. Here one finds the most diffuse involvement of both local and distant sites when compared to the other sarcomas. This lesion is therefore the least amenable to pulmonary resection.

The epithelioid sarcoma should be considered in the diagnosis of any aggressive subcutaneous extremity neoplasm. It most frequently affects males, is likely to involve the palmar structures, and infiltrates the fascia and tendons. With Enzinger's[9] report of 62 cases, the tumor was reclassified as distinct from synovial sarcoma. Among 22 cases seen at Memorial Hospital, 15 were in the upper extremity and 6 in the lower; one case was reported to appear in the neck. Half the patients presented with a firm, nodular hand lesion of less than 2.5 cm. These lesions tend to grow slowly for several months to years, averaging approximately 3 years before therapy is initiated. Mild pain to ulceration can be noted. Surgeons may be tempted to do multiple local simple nodular excisions, especially if the pathologist cannot readily identify the true nature of this lesion, but this is often a fatal error. The palmar tumors may diffusely infiltrate the soft tissues of the hand, obliterating the adductor and mid-palmar spaces (Fig. 7–7*A*). They may encase the flexor tendons, following along the synovial sheaths (Fig. 7–7*B* and *C*) and extending to the extensor dorsal structures (Fig. 7–7*D*). Recurrent tumors are capable of destroying the carpal and metacarpal bones and can be found to metastasize early to the axilla, invading the brachial plexus and the axillary nodes. Even after forequarter amputation, recurrence has been seen. Cells are oval to polyhedral and contain densely eosinophilic cytoplasm; some areas have the characteristics of spindle cell sarcoma. In general, superficial tumors display less pleomorphism than do the deeply situated lesions. Vascular and neural invasion is common. Recurrence appears in more than 63% of patients, if they are followed long enough. Vascular and regional lymph node metastasis are common. Death occurs by the fifth year in 67% of the patients and by the eighth year in 89%. Radical treatment is required because of the high rate of recurrence following local excision. Extra-wide radical local excision appears to be the minimal procedure for the small cutaneous lesion and should be performed only rarely; local recurrence would necessitate forearm amputation. We believe that an axillary node dissection is always indicated with any high level of amputation. Unexplained swelling in a stump would probably require four-quarter amputation, but even then, control of disease cannot be assured.

Another rare but aggressive lesion, which is somewhat indolent but whose pattern of spread is similar to that of epithelioid sarcoma, is the sweat gland tumor. Embryonal

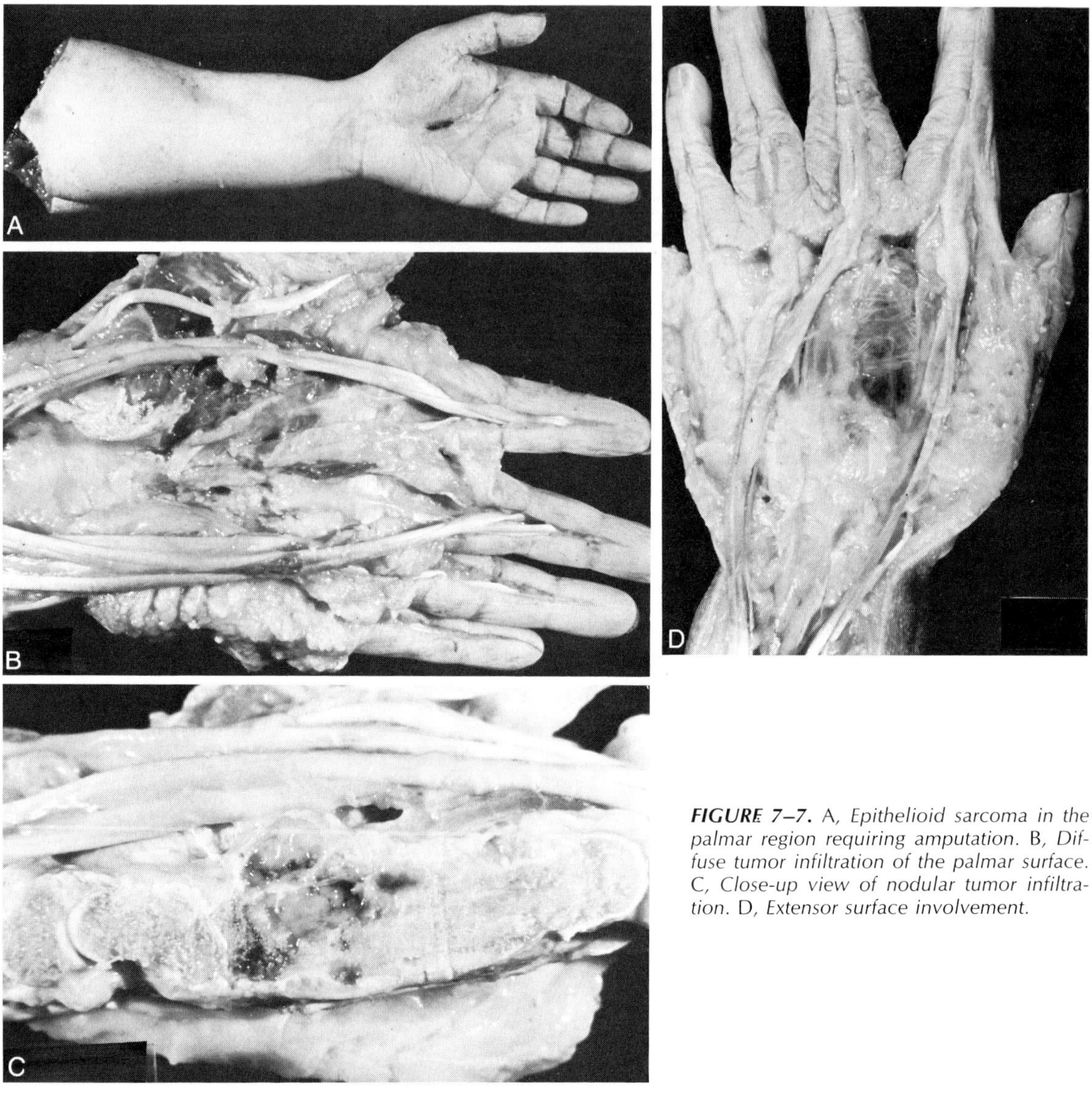

FIGURE 7–7. A, Epithelioid sarcoma in the palmar region requiring amputation. B, Diffuse tumor infiltration of the palmar surface. C, Close-up view of nodular tumor infiltration. D, Extensor surface involvement.

rhabdomyosarcoma, melanoma, and sweat gland tumors may arise within the hand. With these tumors, lymph node metastasis is highly likely. Therefore, lymph node dissection is indicated, even if only for prognostic purposes. Because these tumors spread in a retrograde and centripetal direction, regional node dissection at a higher level should be considered—e.g., if the axilla is thought to be involved, look at neck and mediastinum; for lesions of the groin, look at the retroperitoneum. Sweat gland carcinoma may present subungually and may be confused with paronychia, in which case treatment will be mistakenly delayed as with melanoma.

Before surgery is attempted for many of the malignant lesions, arteriography should be considered. Figure 7–8*A* shows a soft tissue lesion invading and essentially destroying the fifth phalanx. The arteriogram clearly outlines vascular and soft tissue involvement, which is helpful in planning the extent of the surgical resection (Fig. 7–8*B*). CT scan, bone scan, and routine films will provide additional information.

Other tumors that must be considered in the diagnosis of primary tumors of the hand include the myxoliposarcoma, neurogenic sarcoma, and vascular sarcoma. Rarely, tumors of the wrist can spread to involve the hand. Jolly[11] presented a unique case of a giant cell tumor of the distal epiphysis of the radius that spread to the soft tissue of

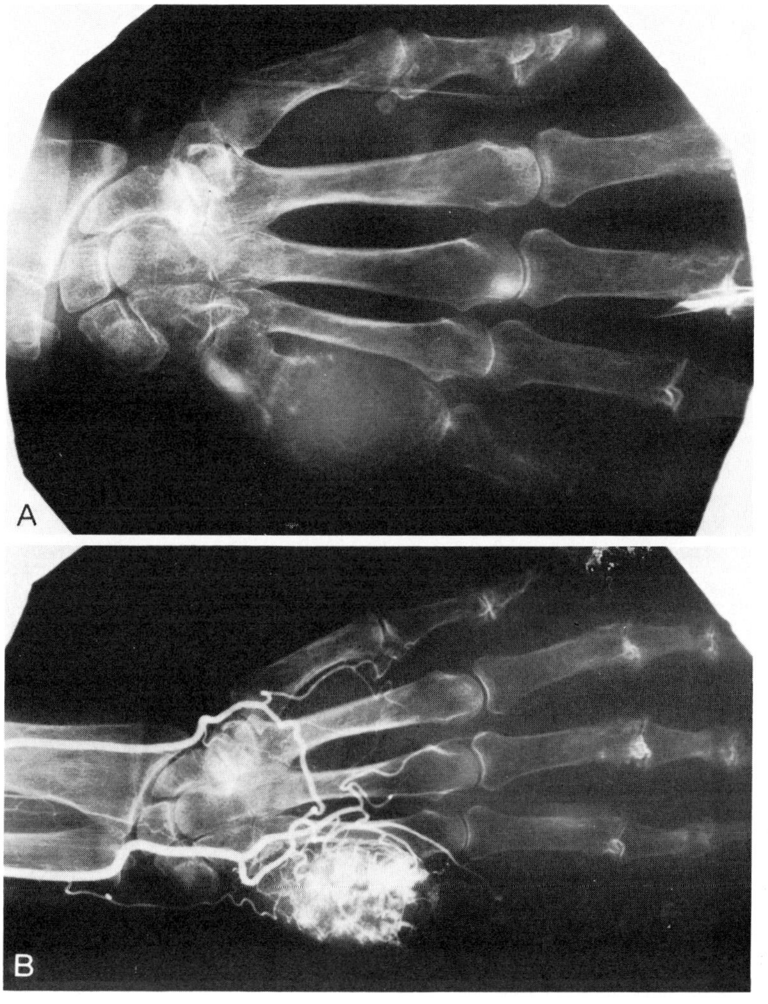

FIGURE 7–8. *A, Destruction of the fifth metacarpal by a soft tissue lesion. B, Angiogram shows the vascular lesion of the fifth metacarpal.*

the hand. Three months after an en-bloc resection, numerous subcutaneous tumor nodules were seen spreading from the wrist to the fingers on both aspects of the hand. It was believed that multiple tumor emboli spread to the hand through a process of retrograde venous embolization.

TUMORS OF THE FOOT

The distal tibia, ankle, and foot present special problems with regard to developing lesions when compared with similar lesions arising in the leg. One must consider that when skin and neurovascular bundles are in close approximation to a malignant tumor in this region, good surgical margins of resection are difficult, if not impossible, to achieve. Of course, each case must be individualized, but in general the occasional use of cryosurgery for selected malignant or benign tumors in these tightly enveloped areas may obviate the need for amputation. In malignant tumors of the ankle, limb salvage procedures have not been successful. Amputation is usually performed when cryosurgery has not been attempted or has proved to be unsuccessful. The forefoot, however, can be successfully amputated as described by Chopart. This operation, although discarded by many because of residual equinus deformity of the ankle, has been valuable for management of forefoot tumors and has resulted in good function. The equinus deformity is easily prevented by Steinmann pin fixation through the heel and ankle at 90°. This pin fixation gives the cut anterior tibial muscle an opportunity to heal if it is sewn into a transfer site at the neck of the talus. Figure 7–9 illustrates the commonly employed operations for osseous resection through the foot. Amputation of the rays on the medial and lateral sides of the foot yield little disability and are preferable

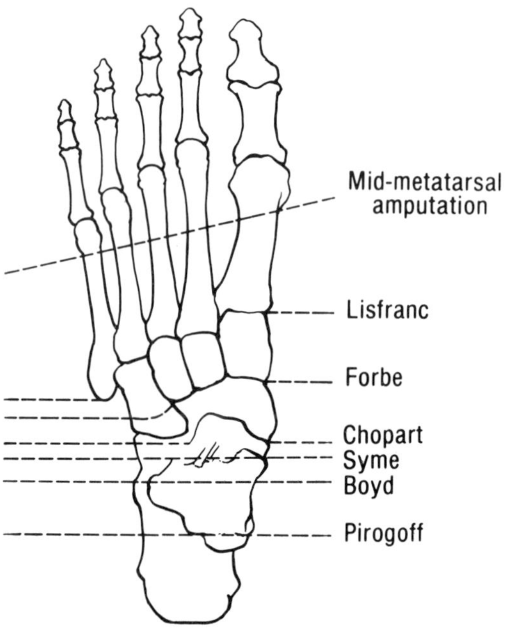

FIGURE 7–9. Common amputation procedures used for the foot.

over amputation of the foot. The Syme amputation is preferred over the below-the-knee amputation unless the skin flaps and fascia are too close to the malignant tumor.

Fibrous Tumors. The presence of a nodular lesion on the plantar surface of the foot may at times represent a fibrous tumor neoplasm. Even if biopsy suggests the possibility of malignancy, the tumor is probably benign. Fibromatosis is more common in this region than are malignant tumors. The first group of these tumors reported were considered malignant, so the patients underwent amputation. It is now recognized that such tumors are entirely benign and that recurrences are merely a matter of having failed to achieve complete resection.[2] Figure 7–10*A* shows the appearance of the soles of the feet of a patient who had a nodular mass present on the right and a scar on the left, representing the site of previous resection of a similar lesion that had been interpreted as malignant. The resected lesion and the microscopic appearance of the tumor are shown in Figure 7–10*B* and *C*. Excision of the tumor of the right foot proved it to be plantar fibromatosis.

In a review of 22 patients seen at Memorial Hospital, 12 cases of plantar fibromatosis appeared on the left foot and 5 on the right; 5 cases were bilateral. At least three cases involved amputation when the benign nature of the condition was not recognized. True fibrosarcoma in the plantar aponeurosis is extremely rare; two cases have been reported by Pack and Ariel.[15]

Simple excision appears to be a poor method of treatment. Allen et al.[1] noted recurrences in 15 of 28 patients treated by simple excision. In the Memorial Hospital series, patients who underwent local excision had a 57% incidence of recurrence at the excision site, whereas those who underwent wide excision (fasciectomy) with or without skin graft had a more favorable result (8% recurrence).

Because incomplete removal of the plantar fascia for treatment of plantar fibromatosis is associated with a high recurrence rate, there is little doubt that wide excision is essential. Skin grafting in the plantar area has not interfered with walking or weight bearing, and the type of incision used can be directed to avoid those sites of weight bearing that underlie the bony prominences. In general, we have been concerned with grafting of the foot not only in terms of the effect on the weightbearing surface, but also when grafts are needed for coverage over tendons such as on the dorsum of the foot. We recently resected a malignant fibrous tumor down to the extensors of the foot, including tendon sheath, and used a graft directly over the tendons. Despite the application of a cast, a major portion of the graft was lost, but normal epithelialization took place and the function of the tendon was good.

Figure 7–11*A* shows the appearance of a desmoid tumor arising on the medial aspect of the foot with extension around the first metatarsal. Because of the low-grade nature of the tumor it was possible to resect it locally along with the metatarsal bone (Fig. 7–11*B*) and to use a rib graft with pin fixation for reconstruction (Fig. 7–11*C*). The specimen obtained by local resection must be carefully studied. We have seen many cases in which the borders of resection were marginal, with the result that the patients were forced to return for a higher level of resection once it was clear that the tumor would recur.

We had the opportunity to examine a 14-year-old boy with a mass of the soft tissues and bones of the left foot (Fig. 7–12*A*), which proved to be a fibrosarcoma. X-ray films (Fig. 7–12*B*) show a peculiar tubulation and curvature of the distal fibula. After a Syme's amputation (Fig. 7–12*C*) the lesion recurred in the calf and was subsequently

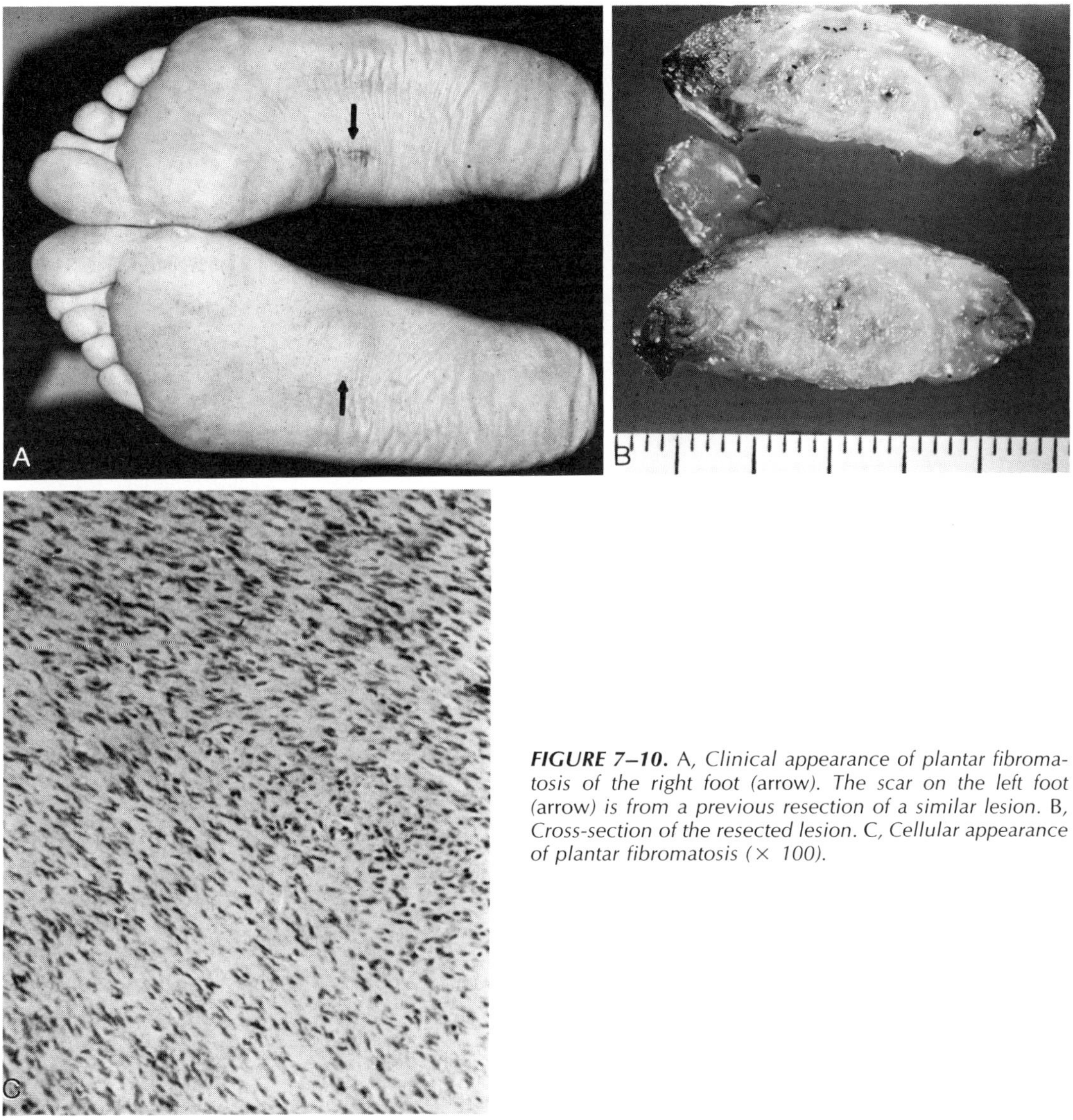

FIGURE 7–10. *A, Clinical appearance of plantar fibromatosis of the right foot (arrow). The scar on the left foot (arrow) is from a previous resection of a similar lesion. B, Cross-section of the resected lesion. C, Cellular appearance of plantar fibromatosis (× 100).*

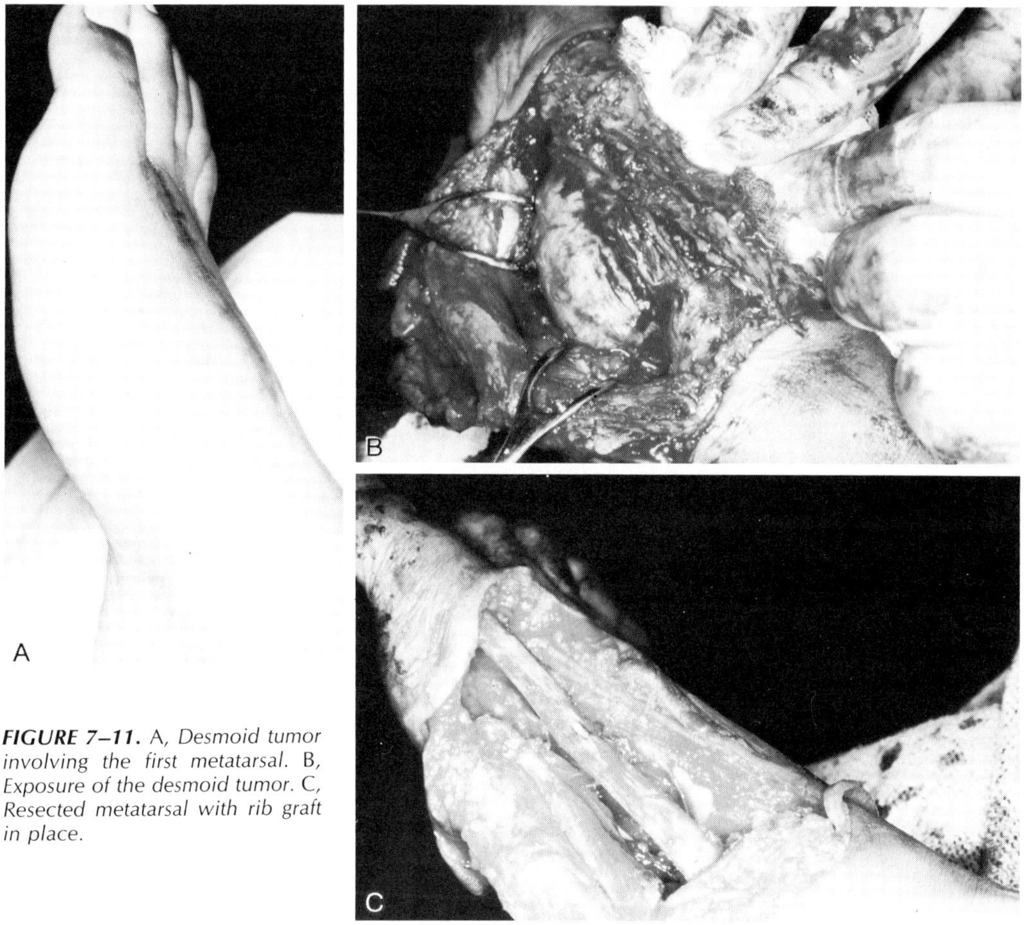

FIGURE 7–11. *A, Desmoid tumor involving the first metatarsal. B, Exposure of the desmoid tumor. C, Resected metatarsal with rib graft in place.*

excised. The lesion then appeared on the thigh. Hemipelvectomy was eventually required, and the patient has remained free of disease. He has since married and has a child. There was no evidence of intestinal polyposis and no family history of related disease such as Gardner's syndrome, which has occasionally been known to present with similar findings of soft part fibrous tumors and peculiar tubulation of bone. Failure of tubulation of the forearm or leg bones has been noted to be an ominous sign for multifocal desmoids, and subsequent follow-up has necessitated progressively higher and higher amputation.

Another patient presented with a mass of the dorsal foot (Fig. 7–13) that had been present for more than 6 years. Biopsy proved the lesion to be a biphasic synovioma, and below-the-knee amputation was performed. A similar lesion in another patient was treated by local resection. The tumor reappeared locally 14 years later at the level of the metatarsal head. Bilateral pulmonary nodules were found at this time and managed by median sternotomy and wedge resections of the lung lesions. A Chopart amputation was performed by making drill holes in the neck of the talus and sewing the anterior tibial muscle through and back on itself (Fig. 7–14). The foot and ankle were stabilized at 90° with a Steinmann pin through the heel into the tibia. The pin was removed in 8 weeks after good positioning of the foot was demonstrated. The patient had normal mobility of the foot with dorsal and plantar flexion, walked without a limp, and has remained well for the past 14 years. One of our patients had a synovioma of the foot that had been treated initially by a Chopart amputation (Fig. 7–15*A*). Breakdown of the skin occurred, but the wound healed well by granulation and secondary epithelialization (Fig. 7–15*B*).

Other tumors such as rhabdomyosarcoma may be encountered. Any of the fully malignant sarcomas rapidly infiltrate the tendons and then bone, requiring amputation, usu-

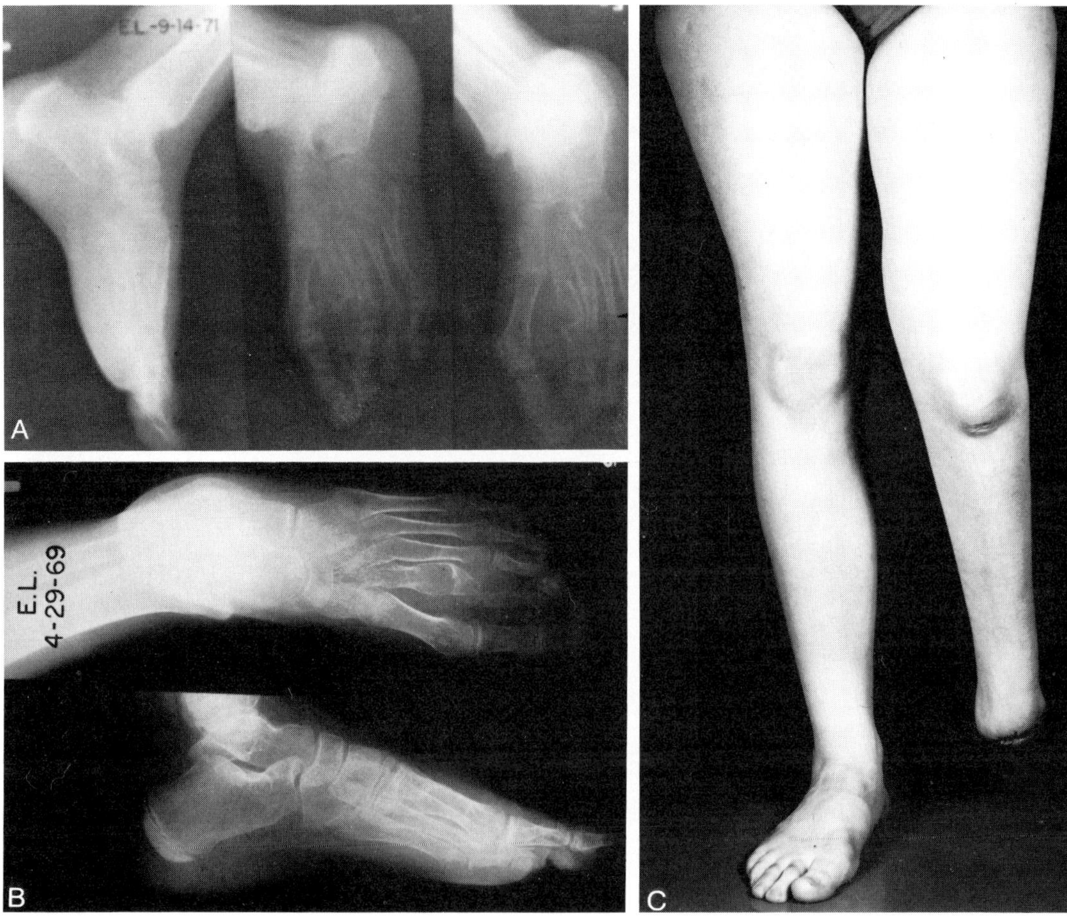

FIGURE 7–12. *A, Mass involving soft tissue of the foot. B, Tubulation and curvature of the distal fibula. C, Syme's amputation.*

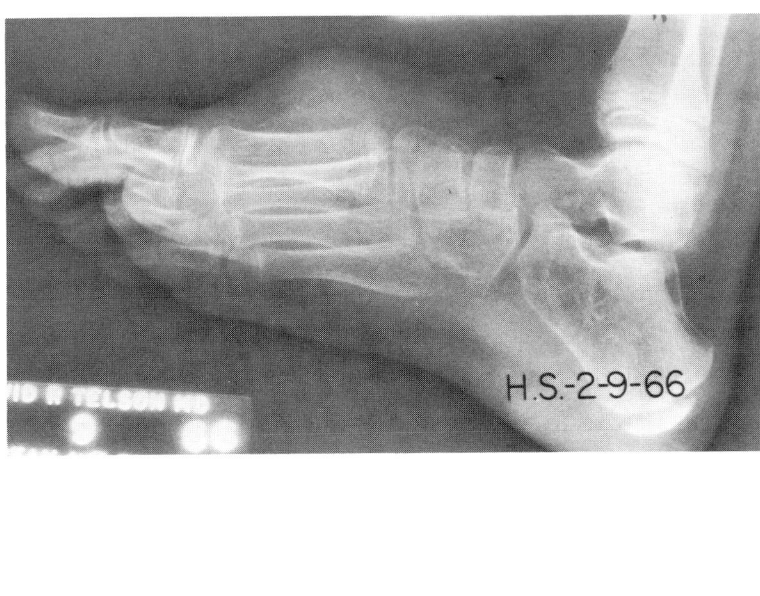

FIGURE 7–13. *Synovioma involving the dorsal foot.*

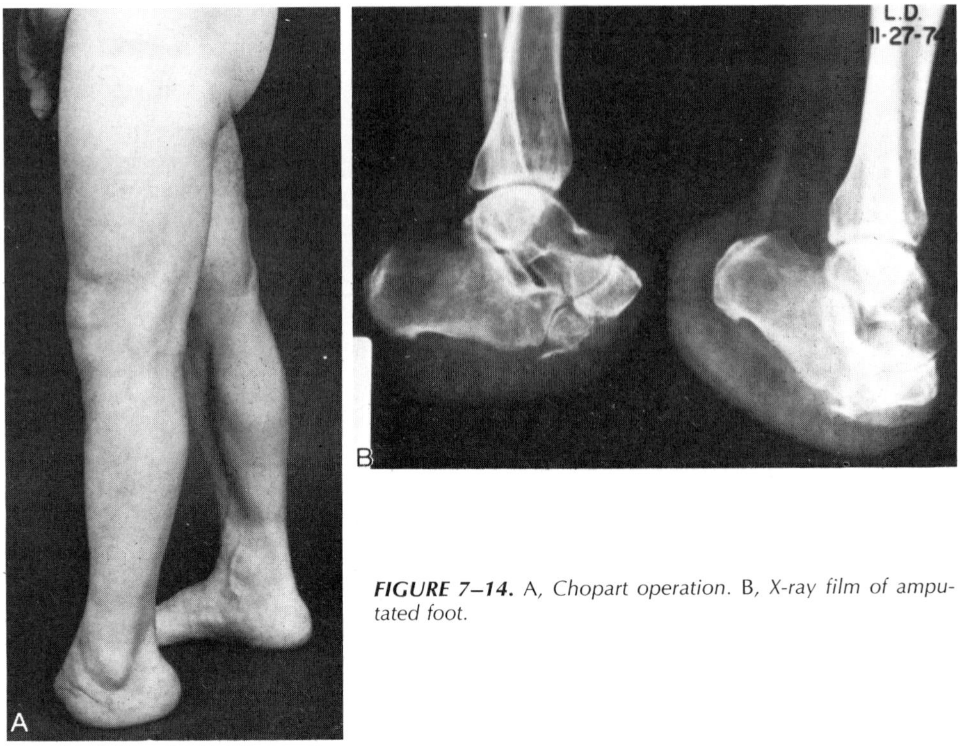

FIGURE 7–14. A, Chopart operation. B, X-ray film of amputated foot.

ally below-the-knee. Figure 7–16 shows the extensive involvement of the osseous structures of the foot by rhabdomyosarcoma.

In rare circumstances, primary sarcomas can be found within the tendinous structures of the foot. Clear cell sarcoma of tendinous origin represents such a lesion and is characterized as a rare form of malignant degeneration of the tendons and aponeuroses.[8] Commonly presenting as a painless mass or swelling, it has a predilection for the distal portion of the extremities. The tumor has a high incidence of local recurrence and distant metastasis.[3, 16]

Vascular lesions of skin can also be found in this region. Figure 7–16 shows the appearance of Kaposi's sarcoma, an endothelial sarcoma that is frequently seen starting on the feet and eventually spreading upward on the lower leg. If control of the initial small primary tumor is lost after local resection, radiation therapy and possibly isolation perfusion with chemotherapy can be offered.

Foot Amputations

Many tumors around the foot are usually seen as small nodular masses and can be handled by wide resection, but when they appear to invade the bones, the Chopart amputation is most frequently employed. Amputation of the toes usually causes minimal gait disturbance in slow, ordinary ambulation and only moderate disability during rapid gait and squatting. A shoe filler rather than a prosthesis is all that is usually required. Amputations through the metatarsals cause moderate disturbances in gait because stability in the ball of the foot and the ability to push off or take off are lost. Again, only a shoe filler is required. However, amputations through the foot in or above the tarsals cause considerable disturbances in walking because of loss of support and push-off ability.

For functional use of the foot, the Lisfranc metatarsal joint amputation is considered the most proximal procedure permitted by most surgeons, as any procedures involving higher levels usually result in an equinus deformity. The Chopart procedure is considered useless by many surgeons because amputation at that level usually results in a severe equinovalgus deformity due to overpull of the Achilles tendon. However, we have successfully modified our Chopart amputations to leave a functional stump, resulting in a gait that is quite satisfactory.

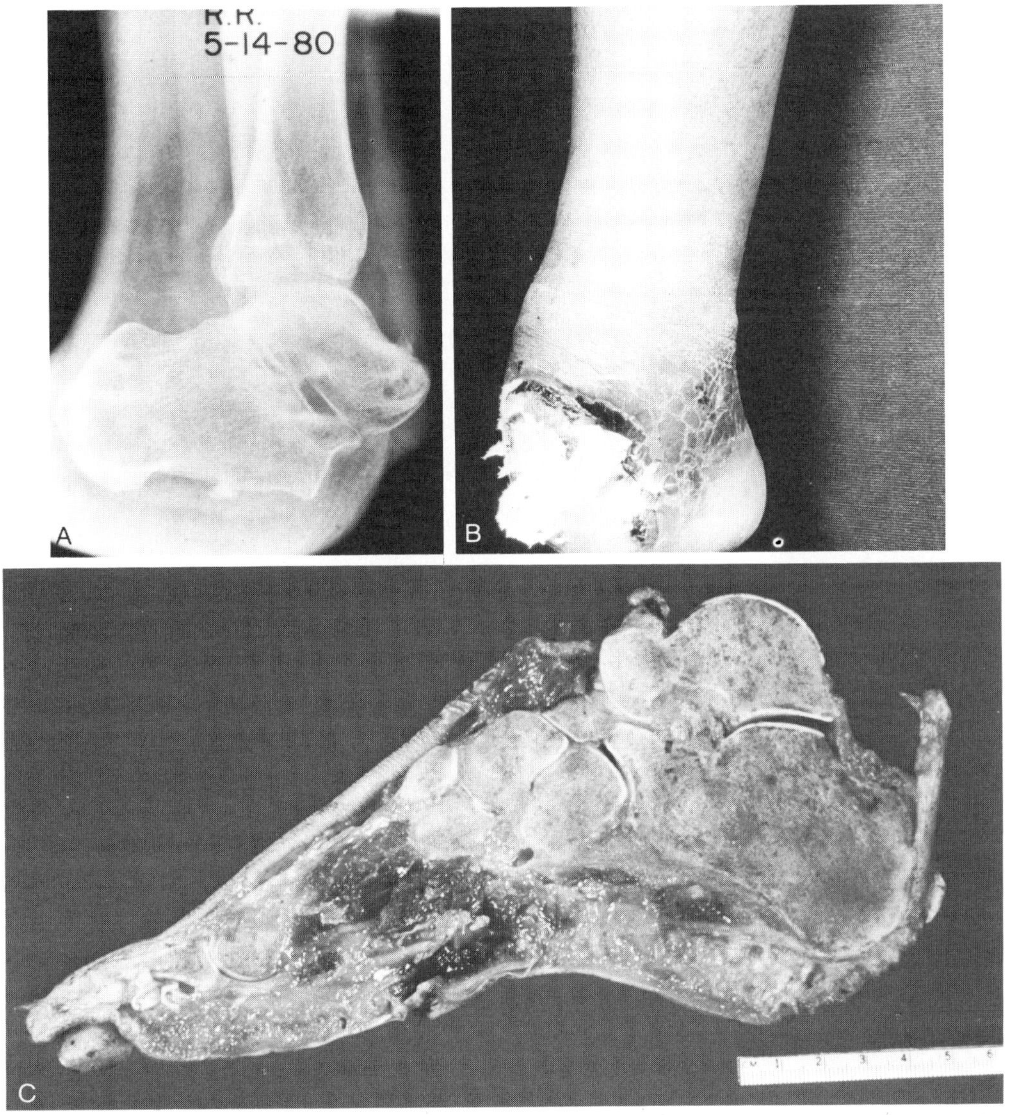

FIGURE 7–15. *A, Chopart amputation for synovioma. B, Breakdown of the amputation site. C, Involvement of osseous structures of the foot by rhabdomyosarcoma.*

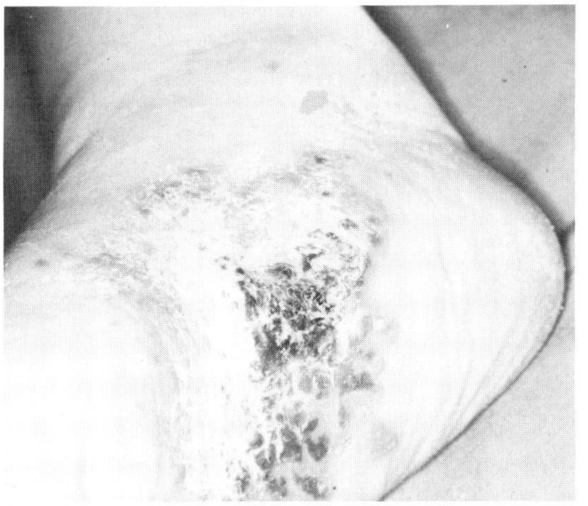

FIGURE 7–16. *Kaposi's sarcoma of the foot.*

Modification of the Chopart procedure is performed by transferring the anterior tibial tendon through a drill hole in the distal talus and suturing it to the posterior tibial tendon or back on itself. Kirschner wires or Steinmann pins are inserted to the calcaneus and distal tibia to hold the ankle in dorsiflexion for 8 to 10 weeks. This allows healing of the anterior tibialis tendon and prevents plantar flexion of ankle because of the stronger gastrocnemius muscle and the strength of the posterior tibialis tendon.

The operation is performed by making an incision over the talonavicular joint on the dorsum of the tumorous foot; the incision is continued on the sole of the foot distally to allow a horseshoe-shaped flap to be raised to meet on the dorsum of the foot. Flaps, of course, are always modified according to the location of the tumor. The incision is carried subcutaneously, and the anterior tibial tendon is identified, retracted, and cut distally. The talonavicular joint is incised and the mid-tarsal joints are separated. The lateral plantar, medial plantar, and anterior tibial arteries are clamped and ligated. A hole is drilled through the superior distal end to the talus. The anterior tibial tendon is passed through the drill hole and sutured to the posterior tibial tendon to insure enough strength for dorsiflexion of the remaining portion of the foot. The foot is held in dorsiflexion.

At this point, heavy Kirschner wires or Steinmann pins are inserted through the calcaneus into the distal end of the tibia to hold the ankle in dorsiflexion and to allow healing of the tibialis anterior tendon. A 3-cm length of Kirschner wire is left extending from the heel of the foot for approximately 8 to 10 weeks postoperatively. Good hemostasis is obtained, and the wound is thoroughly irrigated with antibiotic solution and closed in layers. Usually no drains are employed in surgery of the foot itself.

REFERENCES

1. Allen R. A., Wooner L. B., Ghormly R. K.: Soft tissue tumors of the sole. J. Bone Joint Surg. 37-A:14, 1955
2. Aviles E., Arlen M., Miller T.: Plantar fibromatosis. Surgery 69:117, 1971
3. Bliss B. O., Reed R. J.: Large cell sarcomas of tendon sheath: Malignant giant cell tumors of tendon sheath. Am. J. Clin. Pathol. 49:776–781, 1968
4. Bloustein P. A., Silverberg S. G., Waddell W. R.: Epithelioid sarcoma. Cancer 38:2390–2400, 1976
5. Booher R. J.: Lipoblastic tumors of the hands and feet: Review of the literature and report of 33 cases. J. Bone Joint Surg. 47:727–740, 1965
6. Bryan R. S., Soule E. H., Dobyns J. H., et al.: Primary epithelioid sarcoma of the hand and forearm: A review of 13 cases. J. Bone Joint Surg. 56-A:458–465, 1974
7. Clay R. C.: Dupuytren's contracture. Ann. Surg. 120:224, 1944
8. Enzinger F. M.: Clear cell sarcoma of tendons and aponeuroses. Cancer 18:1163, 1965
9. Enzinger F. M.: Epithelioid sarcoma: A sarcoma simulating a granuloma or a carcinoma. Cancer 26:1029, 1970
10. Hajdu S. I., Shiu M. H., Fortner J.: Tendosynovial sarcoma: A clinicopathologic study of 136 cases. Cancer 39:1201, 1977
11. Jolly M. A., Vazquez J., Martinez A., Guillen F.: Blood-borne spread of a benign giant cell tumor from the radius to the soft tissue of the hand. Cancer 54:2564–2567, 1984
12. Keasbey L. E.: Juvenile aponeurotic fibroma (calcifying fibroma): A distinctive tumor arising in the palms and soles of young children. Cancer 6:338, 1953
13. Mullis W. F., Rosato F. E., Rosato E. F., et al.: The glomus tumor. Surg. Gynecol. Obstet. 135:705–707, 1972
14. Owens J. C., Shiu M. H., Smith R., Hajdu S. I.: Soft tissue sarcoma of the hand and foot. Cancer 55:2010–2018, 1985
15. Pack G., Ariel I.: Tumors of Soft Somatic Tissue. New York, Hoeber Medical, 1958
16. Palvides N. A., Fisher C., Wiltshaw E.: Clear cell sarcoma of tendons and aponeuroses: A clinicopathologic study. Cancer 54:1412–1417, 1984
17. Prat J., Woodruff J. M., Marcove R. C.: Epithelioid sarcoma. Cancer 41:1472–1487, 1978
18. Reye R. D. K.: Recurring digital fibrous tumors of childhood. Arch. Pathol. 80:228–231, 1965
19. Stern R. E., Gauger D. W.: Pigmented villonodular tenosynovitis. J. Bone Joint Surg. 59-A:560, 1977.

CHAPTER

8

Major Amputative Procedures

The role of the neoplastic surgeon in managing a patient with a sarcoma of the extremity is to attempt to remove all tumor in a curative fashion and to preserve the extremity and its functions as far as possible. Occasionally, in spite of aggressive resection and preservation of blood supply by means of vascular grafting, amputation is still indicated.

Amputation represents one on the most ancient of all surgical procedures. Before the use of antiseptics, amputations were the most frequently performed operations. The development of modern surgical techniques, including anesthesia, and improved prosthetic devices have resulted in vast improvement in the techniques of amputation. Thus the most appropriate level of amputation can be chosen in those situations in which a malignancy cannot be removed without sacrificing the limb.

Amputations are most frequently used in treating malignant bone tumors (without evidence of metastasis) and for extensive soft part sarcomas in proximity to periosteum of bone. This is especially true when other surgical procedures or modalities of therapy have been contraindicated or have not been effective in controlling neoplastic growth. Benign tumors rarely require amputation unless the lesion is so massive that en-bloc excision is impossible, or wound healing hopeless because of massive blood loss. The main reason for performing amputation is to remove a malignancy before it metastasizes, although amputations are occasionally performed even after metastasis has been confirmed in order to relieve severe pain in the extremity. Amputations should not be performed unless the surgeon is convinced that there is no other method of therapy that can produce the desired result. Figure 8–1 shows the appearance of a late, extensive, ulcerating rhabdomyosarcoma of the lower leg in the region just below the knee. Although limb preservation is sometimes an option with primary sarcomas, radical resection with or without preoperative radiation-chemotherapy did not apply to this case and mid-thigh amputation was required.

The level of amputation chosen should always be sufficiently proximal to prevent local recurrence of the tumor. We have seen many instances of recurrent rhabdomyosarcoma at the site of a midthigh amputation when the primary was localized below the knee. Such recurrences may even be seen in the hemipelvectomy stump and represent residual tumor just above the site of amputation or neoplastic infiltration of the lymphatic vessels of the surgical wound. While adequate work-up including angiography and CT scan may define what is thought to be the limit of tumor extension, microscopic "skip" areas may be found. This is especially true with fibrous malignancies, where extension along the fascial planes can occur and may not be defined during diagnostic and therapeutic work-up. Distant nodal involvement may occasionally be seen with tumors such as liposarcoma and rhabdomyosarcoma. Even when proper levels of amputation are clinically defined, recurrence in the stump or above the stump may develop at a later date. When the tumor approximates an adjacent joint, several centimeters of the bone above should be removed. The general tendency is to save as much of the affected limb as possible.

Nerves must be severed several centimeters proximal to the amputation site so that they do not become incorporated within the wound scar. One of the major problems with the transected nerve is the development of

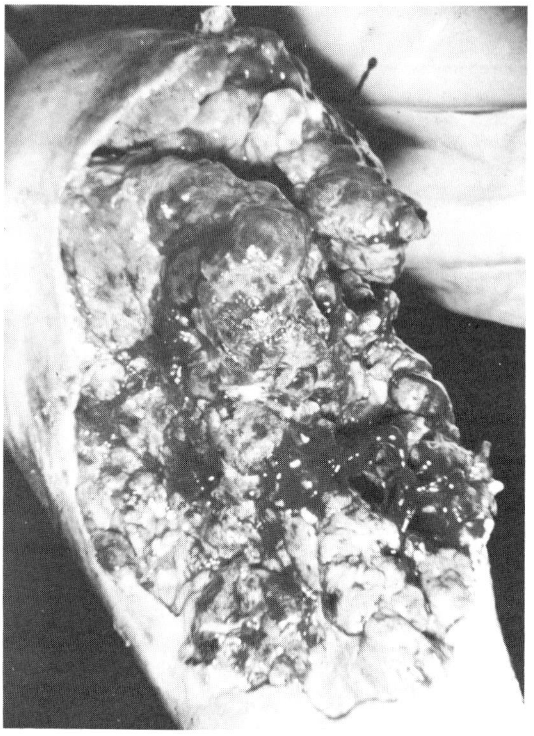

FIGURE 8–1. Extensive rhabdomyosarcoma of the pretibial region.

neuromas, which frequently become large enough to be palpated within the amputation site and so can be confused with tumor. This has been particularly true with hemipelvectomy wounds, especially at the site of the divided roots of the sciatic nerve. We have seen similar problems following neck dissection, where neuroma of the cervical plexus can mimic a recurrent tumor or nodal mass. Only exquisite tenderness on deep palpation alerts one to its true nature. When amputation neuromas are extremely close to the distal wound scar, they can press against the stump site, causing extreme pain and decreased tolerance for weight bearing on a prosthesis. One of the associated complications of amputation neuromas is the additional but unrelated form of pain secondary to the phantom limb. Sugarbaker et al.[48] have described two cases of such pain, progressively increasing over an extended period of time and representing the first indication of recurrent tumor. In a series of amputations reviewed by the National Cancer Institute, 98% of patients described nonpainful sensations following loss of an extremity. Phantom limb pain, on the other hand, is a relentless, potentially debilitating problem that occurs in about 68% of hemipelvectomy patients, 30% of whom complain of continuous, severe symptoms. The incidence of clinically significant phantom pain increases as the amputation level moves proximally: 0% is found below the knee, 19% above the knee, 40% with hip disarticulations, and 68% with hemipelvectomies.

The salvaged muscles in an amputation procedure should be securely attached by myodesis to the bone and used to cover the end of the bone. This will insure that the stump tapers rather than appears bulbous. Before closing any amputation wound, good hemostasis should always be obtained. We frequently employ Hemovac drains, which are inserted into the open wound. They are usually removed 48 to 72 hours postoperatively after evacuation of any hematoma. Covering the stump with normal, healthy, and neurologically sensitive skin is of the utmost importance. Tightly stretched skin flaps are not advised, as extreme dermal tension is highly prone to break down. Skin flaps must contain enough subcutaneous fat so that a cushion is formed, producing a protective barrier between the deep tissue and the outer layer of the dermis.

AMPUTATION OF THE UPPER EXTREMITY

There is a wide choice of procedures for managing tumors on and about the shoulder girdle. Because of proximity to bone the large tumor masses that develop in this region can rarely be removed by muscle group dissection and are therefore primarily treated by amputation. Figure 8–2 illustrates the surgical procedures available; usually forequarter (interscapulothoracic) amputation or shoulder disarticulation has been employed and resulted in pronounced functional disability. One of the alternative procedures is the use of the en-bloc upper humeral interscapulothoracic resection, also known as the Tikhoff-Linberg procedure and popularized by Marcove.[15, 25]

Tikhoff-Linberg Resection

The first report of such an en-bloc upper humeral interscapulothoracic resection was by the Russian surgeon Linberg. In 1922 this procedure was credited to Tikhoff, but it

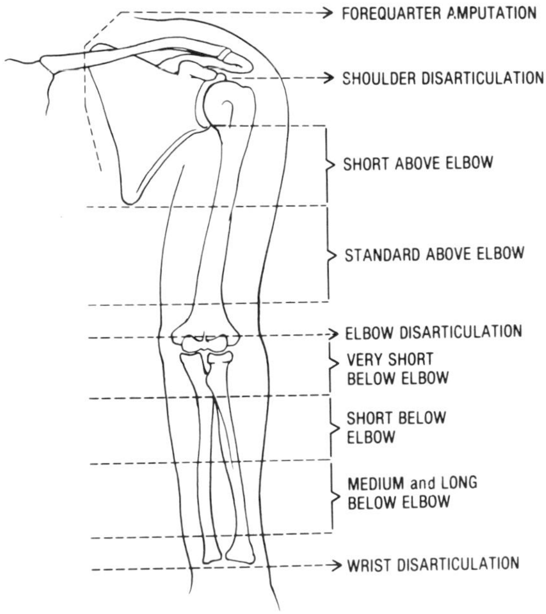

FIGURE 8–2. *Levels of amputation of the upper extremity.*

was Linberg who had described the procedure more fully. Although this operation is more beneficial than forequarter amputation in selective cases, very few of these procedures have been performed to date.[15, 27, 36] We have found that more en-bloc resections can be carried out successfully. One really does not consider this operation to be an amputation of the shoulder girdle but rather an en-bloc radical resection aimed at the definitive treatment of neoplasms found on or about the shoulder girdle. This form of en-bloc resection should be used instead of amputation in the following situations: (1) where contents of the axilla, such as brachial plexus and axillary artery, are not involved by tumor; (2) where there is no fixation of tumor to the chest wall; and (3) where tumor of the shoulder girdle does not involve a major portion of the humeral shaft. Here a part of the arm and some of its function (particularly forearm-hand function) can be preserved. With the use of newer prostheses, elbow function has improved. Primary bone tumors as well as soft tissue tumors adjacent to bone often can be treated by this method, leaving the patient a fairly functional arm and hand (Fig. 8–3). Extensive lymph node involvement in the axilla may require a more definitive type of procedure. Here, either en-bloc radical axillary dissection can be performed as part of the Tikhoff-Linberg procedure, or forequarter amputation may be used and probably will prove to be more useful, since it does remove the entire lymphatic content of the axilla. The forequarter amputation is especially useful for high-grade sarcomas, where local recurrence can be anticipated. On the other hand, one must understand that the presence of isolated node groups may yield to adequate nodal dissection performed along with the Tikhoff-Linberg procedure, since most of the node-bearing tissue exists inferior to the axillary vein and can be encompassed easily by sharp dissection and careful isolation of vessels and nerves that course to the tumor mass.

When the tumor about the shoulder girdle proves to be metastatic, there are probably more effective ways to treat them, using radiotherapy, chemotherapy, or even cryosurgery. With many of these lesions the survival rate is fairly limited, and here one is attempting only palliative treatment. However, where radioresistant lesions are present, the Tikhoff-Linberg resection may still be indicated.

Work-up of the patient usually includes a detailed history and physical examination as well as the standard laboratory tests, skeletal survey, intravenous pyelogram, bone

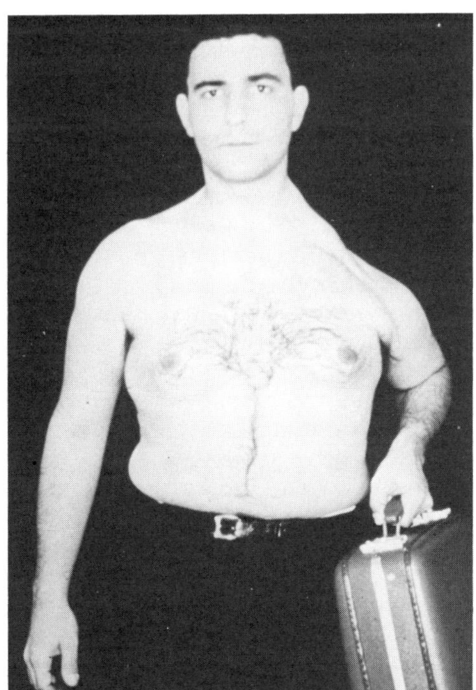

FIGURE 8–3. *Use of the forearm after Tikhoff-Linberg resection.*

scan, tomography, and possibly CT scanning of the chest. Arteriography, both in the posteroanterior and tangential projections, is essential to enable the surgeon to evaluate the extent of soft tissue involvement by the tumor and its potential for resectability in terms of relationship to major axillary vessels. CT scan may also prove to be of benefit in determining the extent of tumor involvement and thus the degree of resectability.

The site of biopsy is carefully chosen so that it will not interfere with any subsequent resection that must be performed. When performing this operation it is an important point to include existing biopsy scar and tract with the specimen in order to properly clear the operative field of tumor seeding and to minimize recurrence in the neurovascular bundle. It is frequently possible to resect the proximal humerus for scapular lesions or to do a mid-humeral osteotomy for lower lesions in the humerus. When levels of humeral division are chosen, it is important not to enter the tumor or to visualize the pseudocapsule. The best way to guarantee a wide margin of resection is to perform multiple frozen section biopsies at the periphery of the excision. When a large portion of the humerus must be resected with the proximal specimen, stability of arm and avoidance of excessive shortening can be obtained by the insertion of a humeral prosthesis such as the Küntscher nail with fixation into the second rib or clavicular stump or to the upper insertion of the serratus anterior fibers. In one patient we observed that a metal ring used to hold the arm to the rib cage resulted in erosion through the rib. Whitehall et al.[50] have described a metallic interpositional device to be used to affix the humerus to the second rib, therby increasing stability and function. The device consisted of a Küntscher nail with multiple holes placed at 3-cm intervals along its length to attach to remaining muscles. A stainless steel V-shaped flange was fashioned to serve as the articulating process between the second rib and a ring that had been attached to the end of the rod. This improved method of fixation appears to allow greater stability to develop at the elbow region and limits random motion at the shoulder joint.

Technique

The initial incision for the Tikhoff-Linberg-Marcove procedure is made overlying the inner two thirds of the clavicle. It is then extended from the region of the coracoid distally along the medial border of the arm, overlying the neurovascular bundle. Posteriorly, the incision extends longitudinally to the midscapular region. The incision is made so that the biopsy scar and tract are excised with the specimen. The deltoid, pectoralis major, and pectoralis minor are incised inferiorly to the clavicle and medially to the coracoid. The clavipectoral fascia is identified and the cephalic vein ligated. The axillary artery and the trunks of the brachial plexus are identified and traced distally. If the neurovascular bundle is free of tumor, the mobilization continues. The anterior and posterior humeral circumflex vessels must be ligated in order to retract the axillary artery medially. Musculocutaneous and radial nerves can easily be identified and are usually preserved. However, if the lesion involves soft tissues in the vicinity of the nerve of the proximal humerus, the radial nerve may be sacrificed along with the musculocutaneous nerve. In one case even the ulnar nerve was removed, the hand having only median nerve function. The site of the humeral osteotomy is then planned and, for primary scapular lesions, is usually made just distal to the capsule of the joint. If the lesion occurs in the proximal humerus, the osteotomy should be made at a distance away from the tumor. By using a humeral prosthesis or a Küntscher nail replacement, excessive shortening can be avoided and better elbow power and stability for flexion provided. Either the prosthesis or the nail should be fixed into the second rib or the clavicular stump. After the neurovascular bundle has been mobilized, the coracobrachialis, biceps, triceps, teres major, and latissimus dorsi muscles are transected away from the tumor. The medial portion of the clavicle is then isolated and osteotomized. At this time, attention is paid to the second part of the skin incision, which originates at the lateral third of the clavicular line and is carried posteriorly and longitudinally along the midscapular plane to the angle of the scapula. The inferior angle of the scapula is mobilized, and the entire vertebral border is resected from the chest wall in a manner similar to that in which the plane is developed in the forequarter amputation. For lesions of the scapula, care must be given to maintaining a wide soft tissue margin. If the lesion involves the head of the humerus or is adjacent to it, a scapular osteotomy can be done at the level of the coracoid process. The skin from the initial incision is raised as a flap over the proximal humerus, leaving the deltoid intact with the specimen in lesions of the upper humerus. Final mobilization of the scapula is completed by transecting the omohyoid and the serratus anterior fibers, with ligation of the suprascapular, subscapular, and transverse cervical arteries. The humerus is then osteotomized at the previously determined level. If this is distal to the deltoid tubercle, the tubercle is removed as part of the specimen. Otherwise, if the osteotomy is proximal to the deltoid tubercle, part of the deltoid is transected. The specimen is then removed. Any questionable tissue from the margins of resection is sent for pathologic examination by frozen section. The wound is copiously irrigated, and the hanging humerus can then be given greater stability by attaching the residual resected ends of the biceps and triceps to the trapezius, cut portions of pectoralis major, and the latissimus dorsi. Another stabilizing aid is to place an intramedullary prosthesis or a Küntscher nail in the remaining portion of the humerus and to secure it to the periosteum of the second rib or the end of the clavicle. Some patients are more comfortable if a greater residual amount of clavicle is removed and if nail fixation is accomplished into the rib. Hemovacs are placed into the open wound fields and closure is accomplished in a routine fashion, usually using subcutaneous chromic sutures and nylon sutures for the skin. A postoperative sling and swath or a Velpeau dressing is employed. Hand and elbow range of motion is tested early in the postoperative period.

When en-bloc resection by Tikhoff-Linberg or forequarter amputation is considered for tumors of the shoulder girdle, the vascular supply to the operative field is identified under the bed of the clavicle. The clavicle is exposed and freed with a periosteal elevator. A Gigli saw is used to divide the outer two thirds from the medial one third of the clavicle. No attempt is made to enter the sternoclavicular junction primarily, as one can inadvertently traumatize the subclavian or innominate vessels. Rather, after removal of the outer two thirds of the clavicle, the underlying vein is freed and the medial one third of the clavicle removed. The axillary artery and vein and the brachial plexus are then exposed and, depending on the procedure anticipated, divided or mobilized.

The Tikhoff-Linberg operation is an excellent modification of the scapulectomy procedure in that it allows additional margins of resection to be obtained about a tumor without resorting to interscapulothoracic amputation. Figure 8–4 shows the anterior skin incision; biopsy for a lesion near or in the head of the upper humerus has been taken. Part of the incision allows removal of the clavicle to expose the neurovascular bundle; another section offers exposure of the muscles of the upper arm so that by dividing them while preserving neurovascular integrity, a portion of the humerus can be preserved with full forearm and hand function, similar to the outcome with scap-

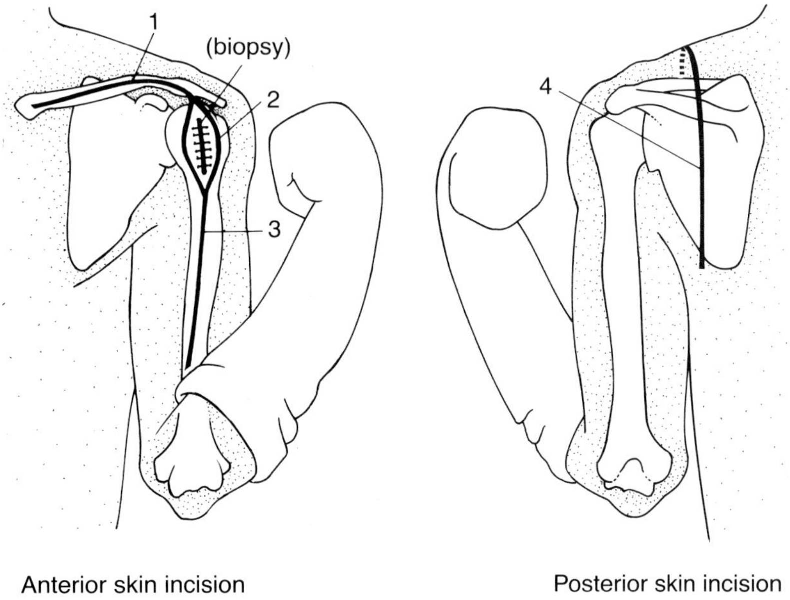

FIGURE 8–4. *Incisions used for Tikhoff-Linberg resection.*

ulectomy. The posterior incision is made as shown in Figure 8–4 or is created on a bias from the acromion to the wing of the scapula, with the biopsy performed for posterior lesions situated over the scapular spine or the region of the posterior shoulder joint. In either instance, the posterior extension of the incision allows definition of the muscles of the scapula (Fig. 8–5). Here the trapezius, levator scapulae, rhomboids, and teres major and minor are divided so that the wing of the scapula can be elevated off the chest wall. Figure 8–6 shows exposure obtained after removal of the clavicle to expose the neurovascular bundle and allow visualization of muscles of the arm. Figure 8–7 shows that the biceps, triceps, deltoid, and coracobrachialis muscles have been divided; the neurovascular bundle is preserved with a tape around it, and preparation is made for division of the humerus and removal of the specimen. If, at any point, the margins of resection, especially in terms of extension into the neurovascular bundle, were considered to be compromised, then high division of the axillary vessels and brachial plexus would convert the operation to the forequarter amputation. Figure 8–8*A* shows the site of biopsy performed on a lesion that proved to be hemangiopericytoma of the scapula adjacent to the glenoid fossa; a bulging mass in the lateral aspect of the scapula can be noted. The scapula was initially mobilized off the posterior rib cage (Fig. 8–8*B*). The head and neck of the humerus are exposed posteriorly (Fig. 8–8*C*), resulting in an operative defect with the upper end of the humeral prosthesis seen in place (Fig. 8–8*D*). Figure 8–8*E* shows tumor in proximity to head of humerus, and Figure 8–8*F* and *G*, the histologic characteristics of the tumor. This lesion is made up of sheets of cells arranged around endothelial-lined vascular channels, ranging from small capillaries to large sinusoid spaces. The individual nuclei are oval to round with moderate amounts of cytoplasm and a high mitotic index. A cosmetically acceptable operative defect and relatively good arm function were achieved so that the patient could return to

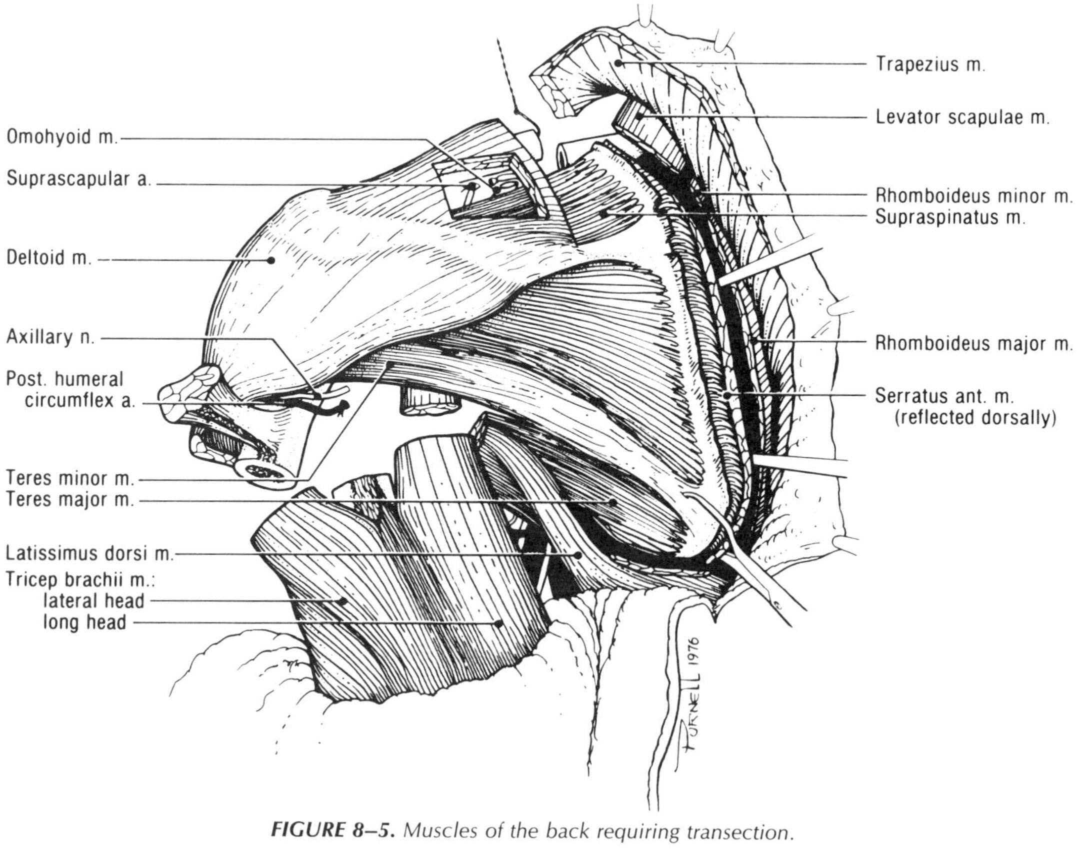

FIGURE 8–5. *Muscles of the back requiring transection.*

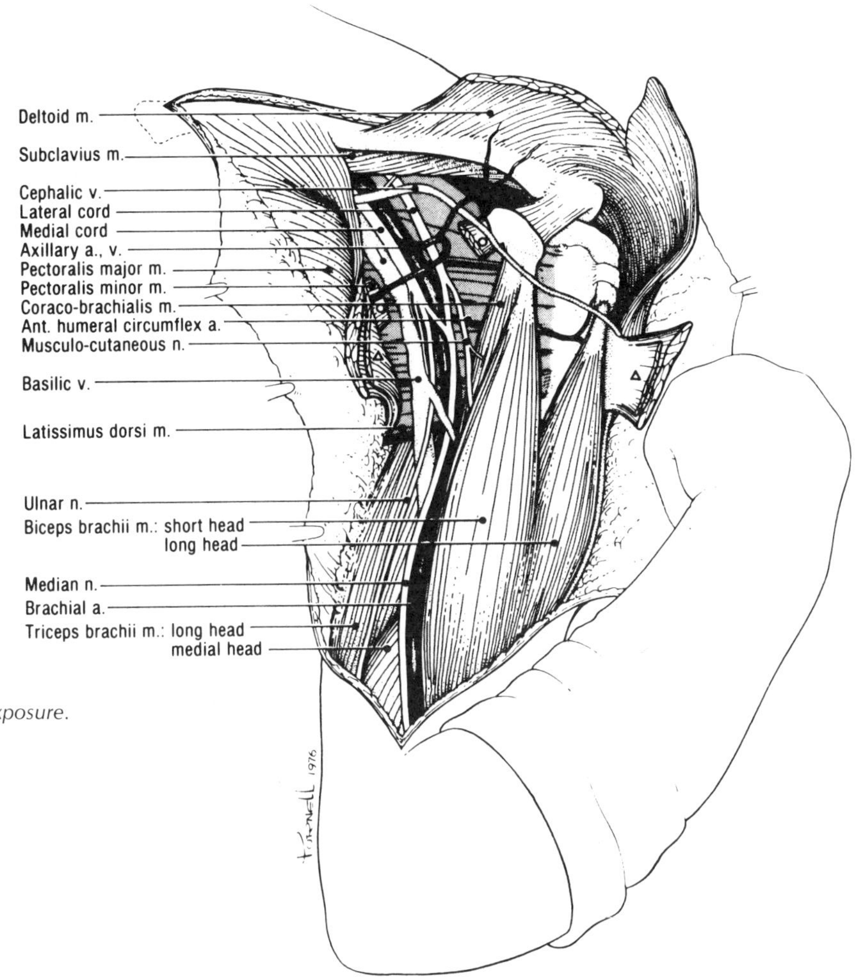

FIGURE 8–6. *Neurovascular exposure.*

work as a piano tuner. A lateral view of the patient is seen one week after surgery. Sutures are still in place (Fig. 8–8*H*).

Hand and elbow motion must be encouraged early in the postoperative period. However, more rapid recovery is found when the elbow is kept in full extension during the immediate postoperative phase and brought into more functional flexion at a later date. Failure to obtain full extension of the elbow causes undue strain on the shoulder by gravity-leverage action.

When this operation is undertaken for a tumor around the upper end of the humerus, the radial nerve may be too close to the tumor to be spared. Should this nerve be excised the patient will develop radial nerve palsy. The resulting wrist drop can easily be eliminated by performing a flexor tendon transfer at a later date. The tendons of the flexor carpi ulnaris and the flexor carpi radialis can be used to achieve wrist extension. The flexor carpi ulnaris is brought through a subcutaneous tunnel around the ulnar aspect of the distal forearm and sutured to the extensor digiti communis or tendon of the finger. The flexor carpi radialis is then brought through another subcutaneous tissue tunnel around the radial aspect of the distal forearm and sutured to the extensor pollicis longus tendon displaced laterally. The tunnel should be wide enough to permit the tendons to glide without obstruction. All superficial fascia should be excised from the tendon attachment areas. The tendons that are transferred should be sutured with more attention than usual because the strong flexors have a tendency to stretch the transferred muscle. A small amount of shoulder padding in clothes usually corrects any surgical de-

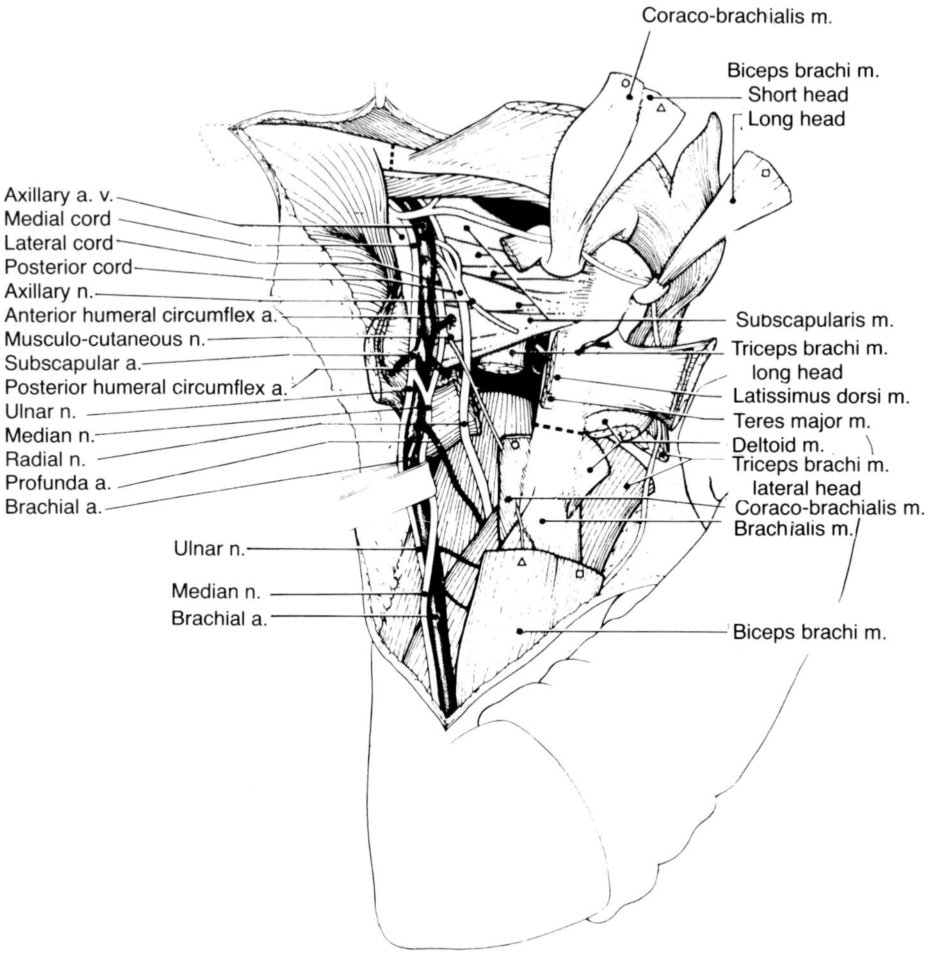

FIGURE 8–7. *Anatomic structures at the time of division of the humerus.*

formity. Hand sensation and function are usually good, and the benefits of performing the Tikhoff-Linberg operation are usually appreciated by the patient when compared with the results of a radical amputation at the shoulder girdle.

The Tikhoff-Linberg resection should be viewed as a significant tumor operation when the proper criteria of selection are employed. This is especially true in evaluating the extent of involvement within the axillary structures, since neurovascular invasion is one of the major contraindications to this procedure. In the presence of isolated pulmonary lesions, one might consider that thoracotomy and resection of the pulmonary lesions should be performed after this resection; as such, there is no actual major contraindication to performing this operation. Strict adherence to concepts of radical tumor surgery must be maintained. During surgery the tumor should not be visualized but identified only by palpation through the normal muscular structures. We routinely use antibiotic prophylaxis because of the large flaps that are raised. Again, one must decide on the need for radical lymph node dissection along with the Tikhoff-Linberg resection or the use of forequarter amputation as the alternative. It is well known that when adequate sharp dissection of axillary structures is performed, one can minimize the degree of recurrence of disease in the axilla. If tumor nodes are not matted or not directly fixed to the neural or vascular sheaths, one should attempt to sharply dissect the lymph nodes from the axillary vein as part of the arm-preserving procedure.

The obvious benefit of this surgical procedure is that hand function and elbow function are preserved. This is quite valuable even with a flail painless shoulder. Furthermore, stabilizing the humeral shaft to the clavicle or rib helps give better elbow function. In our experience, even when the radial nerve has been sacrificed, the hand can func-

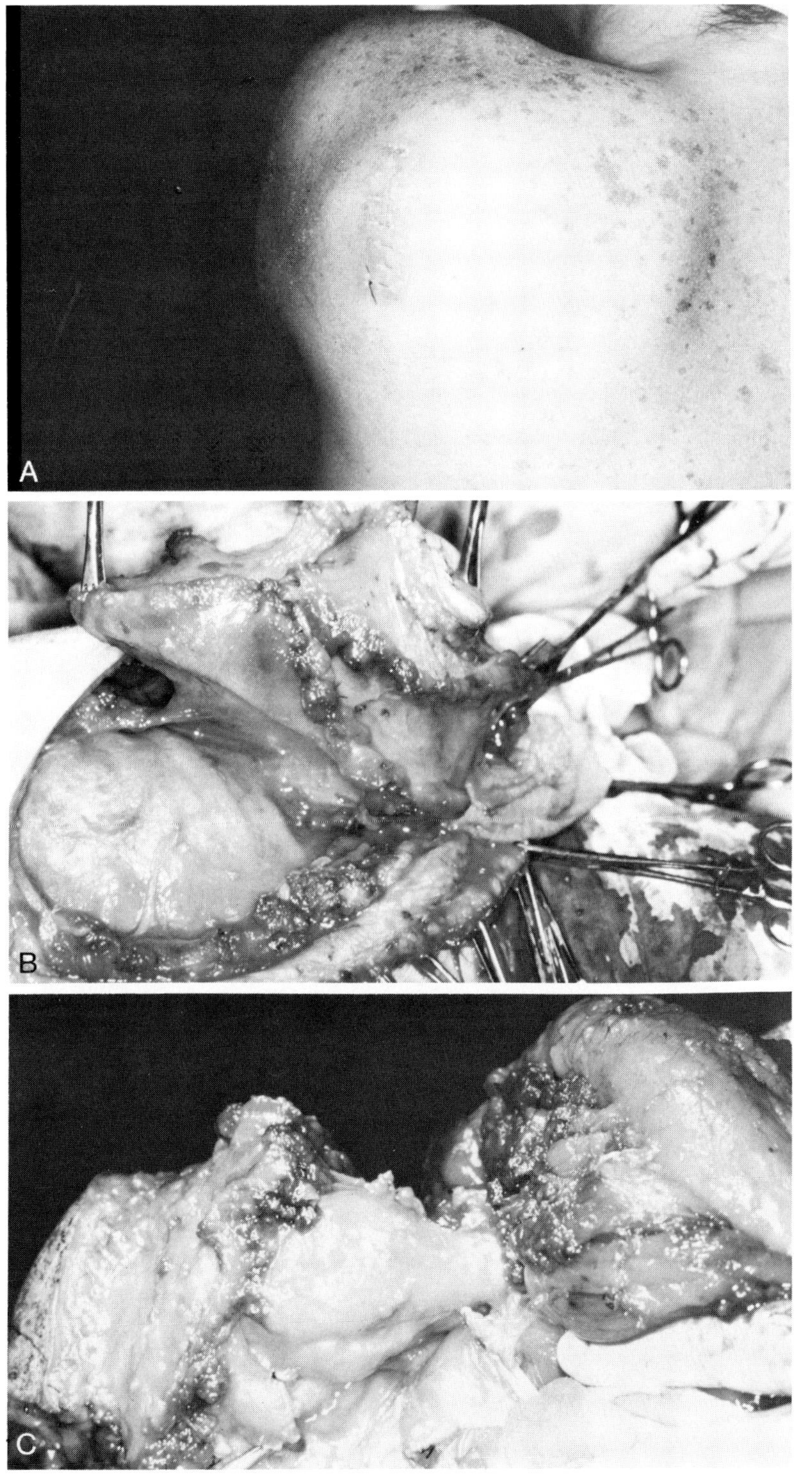

FIGURE 8–8. A, *Biopsy site over the scapula.* B, *Mobilization of the scapula with tumor from the posterior chest wall.* C, *Exposure of the upper humerus just prior to division.*

Illustration continued on opposite page

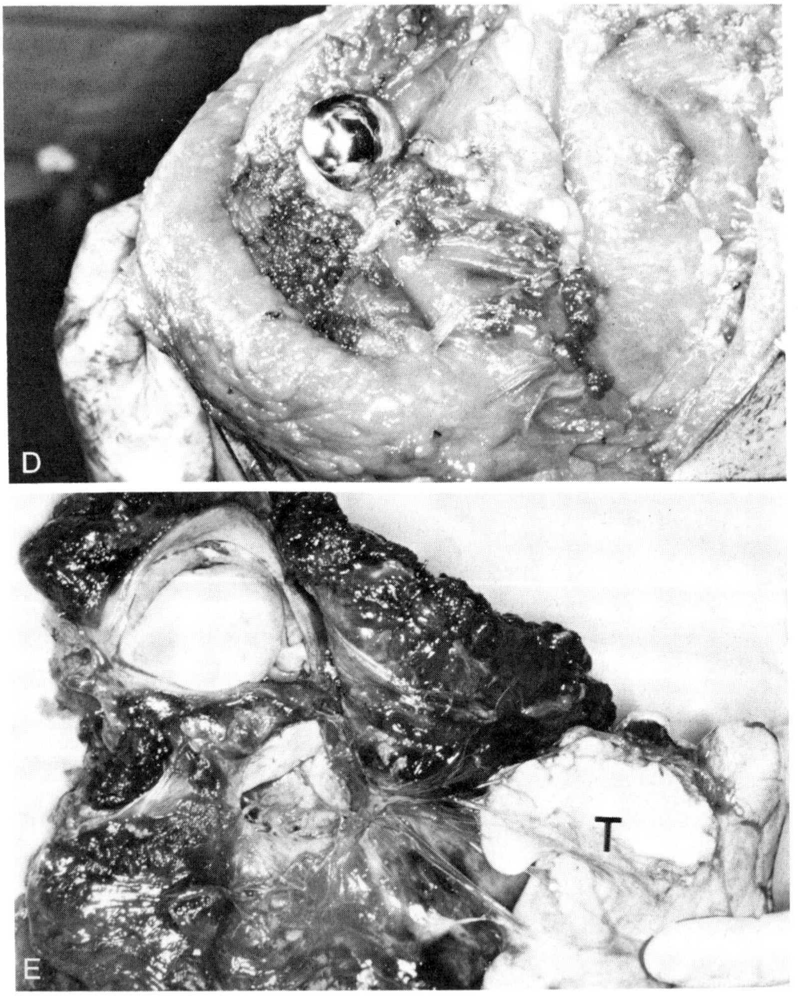

FIGURE 8–8 Continued D, *Completed dissection with humeral prosthesis in place.* E, *Specimen with exposed humeral head and tumor (T).*

Illustration continued on opposite page

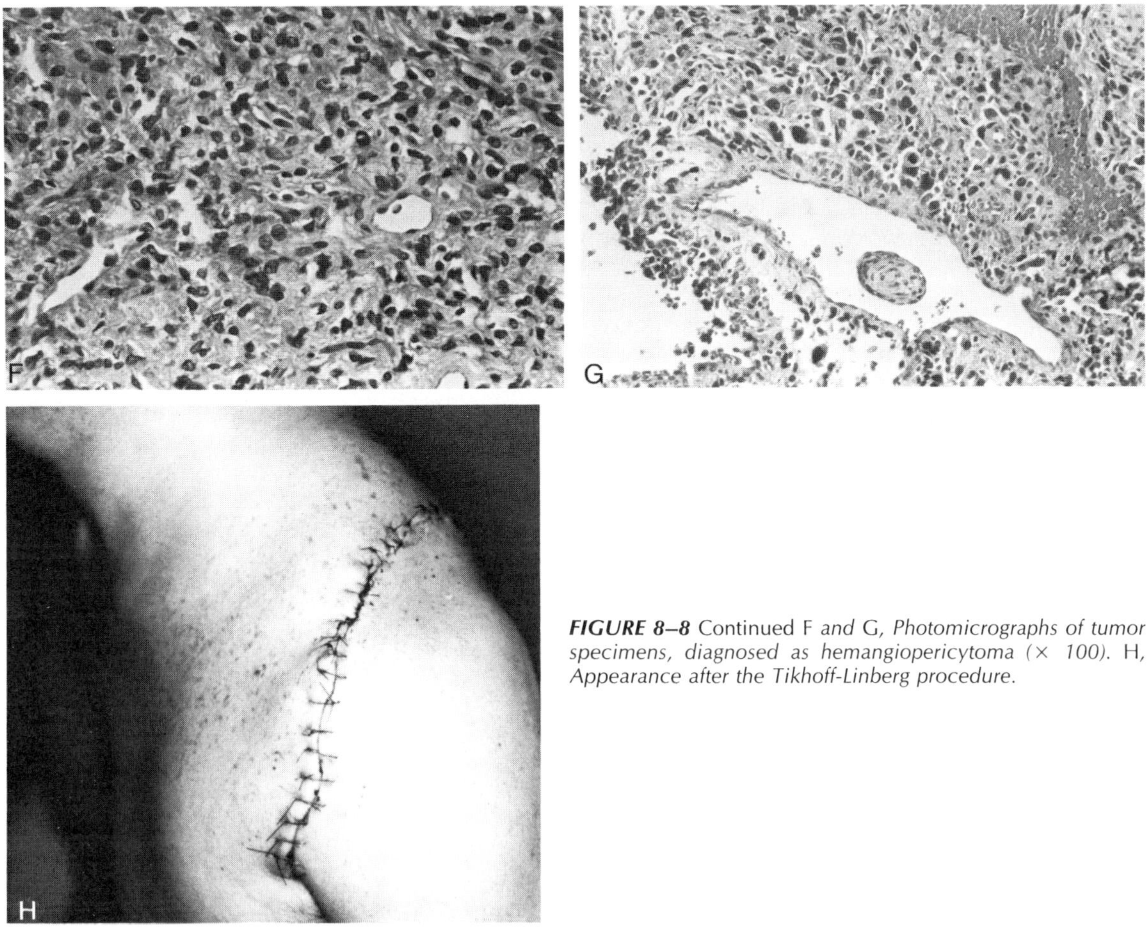

FIGURE 8–8 Continued F *and* G, *Photomicrographs of tumor specimens, diagnosed as hemangiopericytoma (× 100).* H, *Appearance after the Tikhoff-Linberg procedure.*

tion effectively by splinting, and the flexor tendon transfers can be performed later if the patient survives the neoplastic condition. Furthermore, from recent encouraging reports of patients treated with aggressive pulmonary resection and chemotherapy, this operation can be performed with prolongation of the survival rate even in the face of minimal pulmonary involvement.

Forequarter Amputation

Forequarter amputation is the traditional reliable surgical procedure employed for excision of primary bone tumors as well as soft part tumors that extend into or through the shoulder joint.[32, 42] This type of amputation removes margins of normal tissue around the neoplasm as well as the axillary contents included with the specimen. The arm—including the scapula, all or most of the clavicle, associated muscles, axillary adipose tissue and glands, as well as axillary neurovascular structures—is removed en-bloc.[8, 11, 33] Owing to the nature of the tumor to be resected, atypical skin flaps are sometimes necessary. Forequarter amputation may be used as a palliative measure to alleviate severe pain, swelling, ulcerations, or paralysis in metastatic tumors. This type of radical surgery should not be underestimated for palliative purposes in selected cases of metastatic neoplasms.

Because shoulder joint disarticulation fails to remove the axillary contents involved by tumor, we have come to prefer the forequarter amputation for primary lesions of the upper arm. The extent of the disability caused by the forequarter amputation is only slightly greater than that produced by shoulder disarticulation, although there may be some minor difficulty in wearing clothes and filling out a jacket following the forequarter amputation. This is easily compensated for by the use of a shoulder pad. When the axillary contents are free of tumor, the Tikhoff-Linberg operation is the preferred procedure.

A forequarter amputation can be performed either by employing an anterior approach to the neurovascular bundle (Berger approach) or a posterior approach to the neurovascular bundle (Littlewood technique).[23] With the Berger technique, the axillary dissection carried along the chest wall facilitates securing of the neurovascular bundle and excision of the tumor. When a large scapular tumor is present, the Littlewood method more easily preserves the origin of the serratus anterior muscle; excision of the scapular mass by this method provides easy access down along the chest wall to the neurovascular bundle without inadvertently entering the malignant scapular tumor. Both surgical approaches may be used simultaneously in some cases.[8, 11]

Technique

Anterior (Berger) Approach. The patient is positioned on the operating table with the affected side facing up. The entire affected arm, shoulder axilla, and chest are prepped and draped in a sterile manner. The curved incision is begun at the lateral border of the sternocleidomastoid muscle and extended laterally along the anterior aspect of the clavicle to the acromioclavicular joint.

The incision is then carried over the shoulder to the scapular spine and continued inferiorly along the medial scapular border to the inferior angle. At the middle third of the clavicle, the incision is extended inferiorly between the groove of the deltoid and pectoral muscles, curved into the axilla, and continued posteriorly to connect with the inferior scapular incision.

The anterior clavicular incision is deepened to expose the periosteum. The pectoralis major insertion and the lateral edge of the sternocleidomastoid muscle are incised. The clavicle is osteomotized at the lateral border of the sternocleidomastoid and the middle third of the clavicle (approximately 8 cm) and is removed. The pectoralis major and minor are freed and incised to expose the subclavian axillary vessels, which are traced proximally, ligated, and severed. As much as possible of the remainder of the anterior incision is dissected and reflected inferiorly and medially. The brachial plexus is exposed and ligated, and each cord is severed separately. The anterior inferior incision is deepened and the axillary adipose tissue, lymph nodes, and fascia are dissected away from the body. The lateral thoracic and perforating vessels are ligated. The arm may be extended and abducted slightly to facilitate easier dissection between the thoracic cavity wall and the subscapular surface.

The latissimus dorsi is incised along with the remaining fascia so that the shoulder girdle is released from the anterior chest wall. The limb is then adducted across the chest and gentle downward traction is applied. The remaining musculature that attaches the scapula to the shoulder is dissected. The musculature attaching the scapula to the thoracic cavity—the trapezius, omohyoid, levator scapulae, and rhomboids—is incised next. The limb is then removed en bloc.

Adequate hemostasis is obtained and the remaining musculature is sutured to the chest. The wound is copiously washed with antibiotic solution, Hemovac drains are inserted, and routine closure is accomplished.

Posterior (Littlewood) Approach. The same structures are dissected, ligated, and incised in the Littlewood approach as in the Berger approach, but in a different sequence. Two incisions are required, the posterior around the neck and scapula and the anterior around the pectoral region and axilla. The posterior skin flap is made first, beginning at the sternoclavicular joint and extending laterally along the clavicle, over the acromion process to the posterior axillary fold. The incision is continued along the axillary border of the scapula, then curved medially to end 5 cm from the midline of the back.

The entire full-thickness skin flap is lifted off the scapular musculature at the medial scapular border. The trapezius and latissimus dorsi muscles are identified and divided parallel to the scapula. The levator scapulae, rhomboids, and scapular attachments of the omohyoid and serratus anterior muscles are severed. The transverse cervical and scapular arteries are ligated as the dissection deepens. The clavicular musculature and fascia are severed, and the clavicle is osteotomized, allowing the entire limb to fall away from the trunk, exposing the brachial plexus and subclavian vessels. The brachial plexus cords are severed close to their origins, exposing the subclavian vessels, which are ligated.

The anterior skin flap begins at the middle clavicle, continues close to the deltopectoral groove, and joins the posterior incision in the axilla. The pectoralis muscles are severed, allowing the extremity to be removed en bloc. The wound is washed and closed with Hemovac drains, as described for the Berger method.

If a malignant tumor is encountered at the medial portion of the clavicle, a modification of the forequarter amputation can be used. To clear the tumor, the second intercostal space may be entered anteromedially, extending the incision further medially, splitting the sternum upward, and removing the area en bloc. This approach also enables exposure and ligation of the great vessels that enter the arm.

Forequarter amputation can be further modified or expanded to permit excision of neoplasms in the neck, pectoral, or thoracic region. Neck dissection, pectoral muscle resection, radical mastectomies, and thoracic wall resections of proximal rib can easily be performed simultaneously.

The extended forequarter amputation has been employed to encompass those tumors extending beyond the limits of the shoulder girdle.[34] The technical approach to interscapulothoracic or forequarter amputation follows that described in the preceding paragraphs. When tumor spreads beyond the limits described, however, the indications for extending the operation are not clear, especially when tumor spreads through the chest wall. In 1958 Stafford and Williams[43] described the radical transthoracic forequarter amputation, which permitted control of the subclavian vein and artery from within the chest and allowed an initial assessment of intrathoracic involvement. Enbloc chest wall resection can be performed when indicated.[24] Wurlitzer[52] reported a variation of this procedure for recurrent sarcoma, in which examination of the upper chest wall and upper sternum and left upper lobectomy were performed. A recurrent liposarcoma was found to involve the left upper lung and apex of the chest wall, extending through the left posterior chest wall to involve the scapula. A left posterolateral thoracotomy was employed, in which the fifth rib was resected. Forequarter amputation and lung resection, radical chest wall resection, and claviculectomy were performed along with removal of tumor. Wurlitzer's approach has the added advantage of easier and more thorough tumor exposure. A one-piece shoulder and breast prosthesis was used and held in place with a bra.

Total Scapulectomy

Total scapulectomy, a relatively rare procedure, was first described by Syme in 1856. Its primary use is for disease arising within the scapula; however, it has also been employed for tumors sitting over the scapular region.[7, 41] Under such circumstances, wide resection of the tumor with partial scapulectomy, total scapulectomy, or total scapulectomy and chest wall resection has been reported. Ramirez et al.[39] described two cases of soft tissue tumors invading the area of the scapula, one arising from a soft part fibrosarcoma and the other a metastasis of a colon carcinoma. In both cases, scapulectomy allowed for wide margins of resection, and excellent physical rehabilitation in spite of removal of a major portion of the shoulder girdle.

TECHNIQUE

The patient is placed in the lateral decubitus position with the involved extremity draped freely for easy access to the shoulder joint and the area about the scapula. An elliptical incision is made around the tumor in the direction of the long axis of the scapula. A second perpendicular, or T, incision is made to the acromion process. The skin flaps are developed posteriorly to the transverse process and superiorly and inferiorly over the acromion and angle of the scapula. The underlying tumor and scapula are exposed. A cutting current is frequently used to raise the skin flaps and divide muscle. The trapezius muscle is cut near its origin at the vertebral column and from its attachments at the lateral end of the clavicle and at the angle of the scapula. The rhomboideus major and minor and the latissimus dorsi are then divided near the vertebral column, enabling the scapula to be lifted from the chest wall posteriorly by placing the hand under the scapula (see Fig. 8–5). This maneuver facilitates the cutting of the serratus anterior muscle from its insertion at the costal surface of the vertebral border of the scapula. The clavicular origins of the deltoid, the levator scapulae, and the supraspinatous muscles are then transected near their insertions. The descending scapular artery and the suprascapular artery and nerve are encountered in this region. With the free medial superior borders of the scapula, the lateral border can easily be detached from its muscular attachments. The acromioclavicular ligament and coracoacromal ligaments are cut, and the scapula is removed. The remaining muscular tendinous insertions of the humerus are sutured to the residual muscles of the chest wall, forming a site for pseudarthrosis. The clavicle is shortened, the skin flaps are closed, and suction catheters are applied under the skin.

AMPUTATION OF THE LOWER EXTREMITY

Hip Joint Disarticulation

Depending on the site of the tumor, a number of procedures for amputation can be employed (Fig. 8–9). For tumors located high in the thigh in close proximity to bone, yet not invading the hip joint or approximating the inguinal ligament, hip joint disarticulation is the procedure of choice over hemipelvectomy.[4] The operation is simple to perform, complications are minimal, and patients are able to function better.

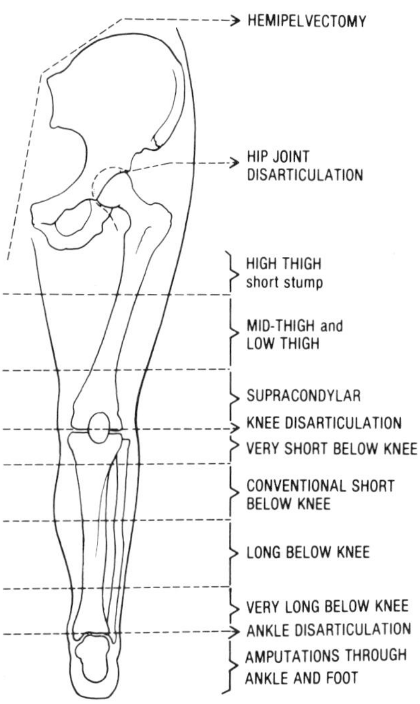

FIGURE 8–9. *Levels of amputation of the lower extremity.*

After the patient is anterolaterally positioned, the entire affected leg, hip, and hemipelvis are prepped and draped in the routine sterile manner. Following the draping, a C-shaped flap is created transversely across the upper thigh, with the C-incision convexly placed anteriorly and posteriorly approximately 6 cm below the anterior superior iliac spine; laterally it is positioned near the greater trochanter and posteromedially approximately 4 cm below the ischial tuberosity. The cross-sectional anatomy of the upper thigh is shown in Figure 8–10.

The dissection is deepened anteriorly through the fascia, and the saphenous vein and its tributaries are identified, ligated, and transected. Deeper dissection will reveal the common femoral vein and artery; these are ligated and severed, and the femoral nerve permitted to retract proximally. Starting anteriorly, the musculature is dissected and transected systematically while all the bleeders are separated, clamped, and ligated. We prefer to use the Bovie cutting and coagulating current to divide the isolated muscle groups. The anterior capsule of the hip is then opened, and at this point in the dissection the medial and lateral muscles are identified and prepared for division. A frozen section of the lymph nodes in the groin is examined now to assure the surgeon that there is no evidence of tumorous tissue in the area being sampled. If the lymph nodes show tumor, hemipelvectomy is usually preferred, since disease can be anticipated above the inguinal ligament at this point. The obturator nerve and the obturator artery and its branches are identified, exposed, ligated, and dissected. After this the joint capsule is entered. The hip is disarticulated by entering the capsule anteriorly and cutting the ligamentum teres (Fig. 8–11). Finally the posterior muscles and sciatic nerve are incised. The complete specimen is sent to the pathology laboratory for analysis. The wound is copiously irrigated and checked for hemostasis, then carefully closed in layers, with Hemovac drains inserted in the deep base of the stump and exteriorized anteriorly. The acetabulum is not filled and the articular cartilage is not curetted.

Modified Hip Joint Disarticulation

A hip joint disarticulation procedure can be modified so that a stump, to be used for

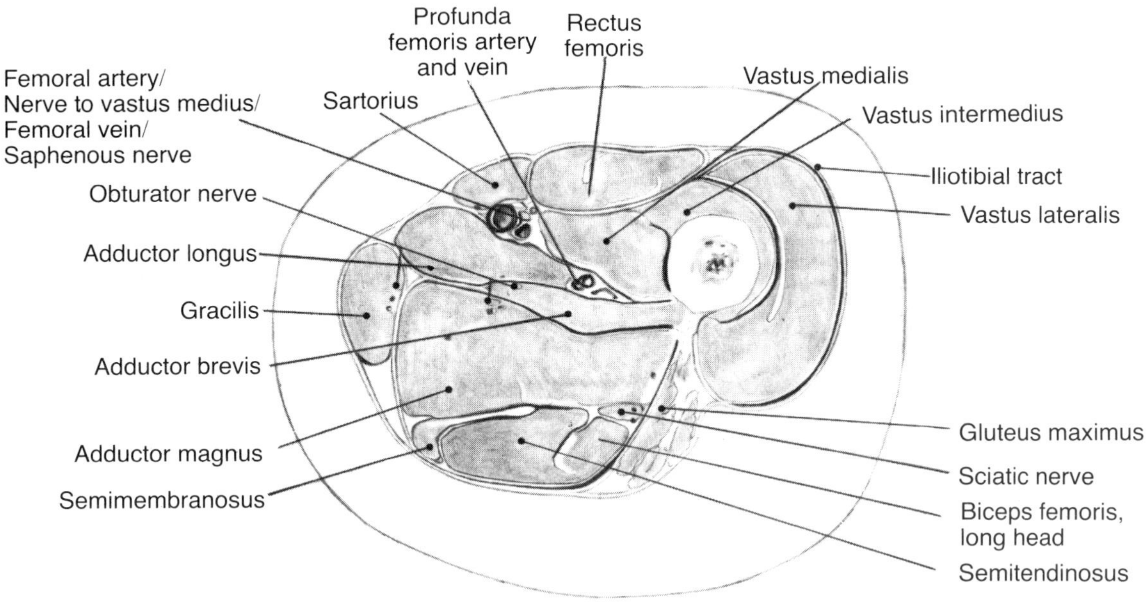

FIGURE 8–10. *Cross-sectional anatomy of the upper thigh.*

a prosthetic fitting, can be created by insertion of a short-stemmed Austin Moore prosthesis.[28] The patient is positioned, prepped, and draped in the same manner as for hip joint disarticulation surgery. Anteriorly, a long lateral incision is made extending through the greater trochanter to a point approximately 10 cm above the knee joint. The incision is swung laterally to the medial portion of the thigh and is continued proximally to the pubic tubercle. The dissection is deepened and the anterior and posterior distal musculature is incised to be removed en bloc with the entire femur, calf, and foot. As much as possible of the proximal musculature, fascia, and neurovascular vessels are salvaged to be later sutured to a drill hole in the distal end of the prosthesis.

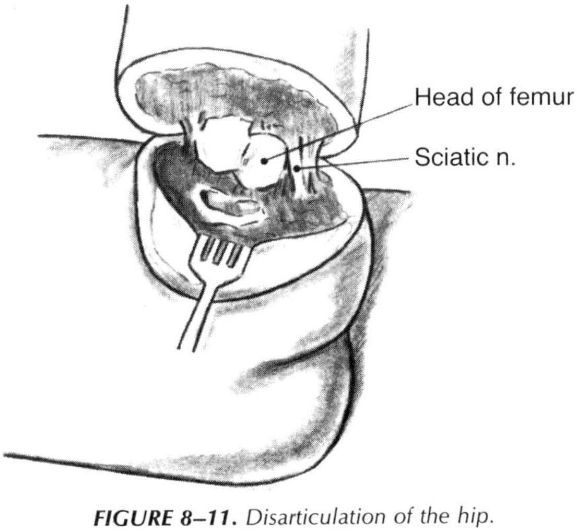

FIGURE 8–11. *Disarticulation of the hip.*

Posteriorly, the same procedure is followed. The posterior skin flaps are made from the distal anterior, lateral, and medial longitudinal incisions. Following en-bloc excision of the entire femur, surrounding distal tissue, knee, calf, ankle, and foot, the wound is copiously irrigated with antibiotic solution. The short-stemmed Austin Moore prosthesis is inserted into the acetabulum. The salvaged proximal thigh musculature with the neurovascular bundles and tendons of the hip musculature are sutured distally to the prosthesis through a previously drilled hole in the distal end of the prosthesis. The remaining skin and fascia are closed routinely with heavy chromic sutures for the subcutaneous layers and 3-0 nylon for the skin. More recently we have begun using skin clips for the final skin closure.

Hemipelvectomy

Hemipelvectomy is used for tumors that approach the hip joint or region of the inguinal ligament and femoral canal, where amputation through the hip joint (hip disarticulation) would fail to achieve adequate margins of resection.[9, 17, 40] While the operation has been designed as a curative form of amputation, it occasionally is employed to relieve severe pain and tissue destruction secondary to massive tumor involvement in the lower pelvic region or region of the groin.[19] Many patients have extensive tumor destruction of the upper thigh, iliac, or inguinal region, resulting in the potential for femoral or iliac artery blowout. This has been and remains the indication for hemipelvectomy in spite of the fact that the patient would not be undergoing a curative procedure. Terms such as "sacroiliac disarticulation" and "interilioabdominal amputation" (hindquarter amputation) more aptly define what the surgical procedure entails. Though we at one time utilized hemipelvectomy for osseous neoplasms of the femur and soft part sarcomas involving vascular structures high in the limb, new and more aggressive surgical procedures employing vascular grafting prosthetic replacement coupled with radiation therapy and chemotherapy have almost eliminated, or at least diminished, the frequency of hemipelvectomy in the treatment of soft tissue sarcomas of the extremity. Where margins of resection are in question, however, any alternative short of hemipelvectomy will prove to be ineffective. One must therefore consider using hemipelvectomy in any case in which muscle group dissection has failed or necessary margins cannot be achieved. In essence, the hemipelvectomy is a high amputation of the lower extremity used for those tumors that are in proximity to the inguinal ligament, obturator fossa, and hip joint. Most surgeons experienced in handling fully malignant extremity sarcomas will agree with these principles. This procedure is also employed for those soft part sarcomas of the gluteal region that infiltrate iliac bone and cannot be encompassed by the muscle group dissection (the radical gluteal resection of Bowden).

The management of most extremity sarcomas involves resection of the lesion by means of muscle group dissection when feasible. Miller[31] has defined the characteristic patterns of behavior for many of the extremity tumors with which we are concerned; these are useful in selecting the surgical procedures that may be of value. Should these principles indicate that conservative surgery cannot be adhered to, then hemipelvectomy is to be considered.

1. Rhabdomyosarcomas may be multicentric, necessitating that the involved muscle groups be removed in their entirety. If this is not possible, then amputation may be required.
2. Most sarcomas infiltrate along fascial planes and extend far superior to the palpable limits of the tumor. The groin may be reached in this way by tumor extension.
3. Fascial fibrosarcomas may be diffuse in their growth pattern so that the entire fascial sheath must be removed to the periosteal attachment.
4. Tumors such as malignant neurilemmomas tend to have central extension along the nerve sheath, occasionally reaching into the pelvis.
5. Invasion of bone by sarcomas is associated with periosteal and intramedullary extension of tumor along the bone shafts.

A soft part tumor extending to the uppermost part of the thigh can be evaluated by needle or open biopsy followed by angiography, CT scan, and NMR. These procedures may help to define the histologic nature of the tumor and the extent of vascular and periosteal involvement, approximation to the innominate bone, and infiltation or extension directly into the pelvis. In the CT scan shown in Figure 8–12, an extensive soft part sarcoma of the upper thigh is seen to extend into the groin. The lesion was found to infiltrate the femoral vessels and groin, making any procedure short of hemipelvectomy impossible. When those alternatives

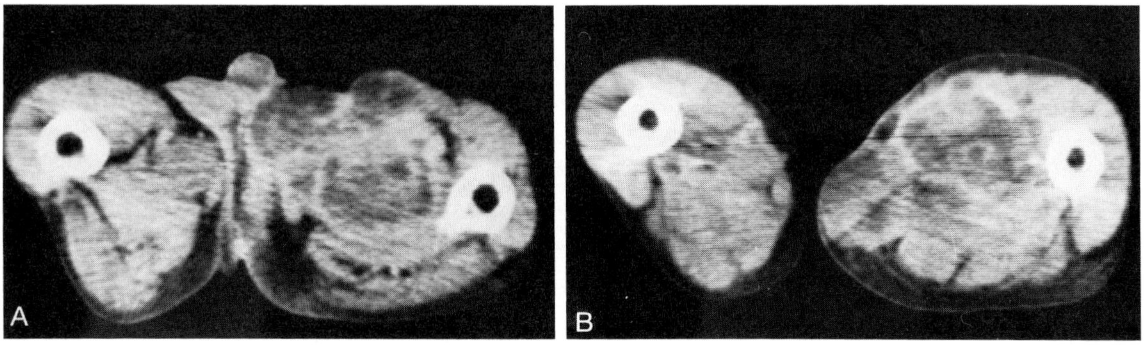

FIGURE 8–12. *A, CT scan of sarcoma invading the right groin. B, Sarcoma in the right upper thigh.*

for removal of tumor by wide resection or muscle group dissection have been ruled out, hemipelvectomy must be contemplated and can usually be achieved with a complication rate not much greater than that seen for hip disarticulation. We usually employ a bowel preparation for the occasional instance in which, on completion of the retroperitoneal dissection of tumor, the lesion is found to adhere to or infiltrate the periosteum or viscera. The average blood loss for this procedure is approximately 1500–2000 cc and is usually due to oozing from the pelvic veins, as the arterial supply is usually brought under control early in the procedure. Hemoclips applied to the sacral branches of the hypogastric venous plexus, as the sacroiliac joint is separated, usually stem this source of blood loss.

Technique

Numerous descriptions of this procedure have appeared in the literature.[2, 3, 16, 17, 38, 51] We adhere to many of the basic approaches but have modified them somewhat to shorten the operating time and decrease morbidity. After the involved leg is prepped and draped to the knee or midthigh, the patient is placed in a supine or modified lateral position, depending on the site of the tumor. The primary area for exposure is the region where the posterior buttock flap incision is carried around the gluteal fold, close to the midline sacrum. When the tumor involves the posterior thigh, the posterior buttock flap, necessary for closure of the wound, cannot be used. Under normal circumstances a buttock flap is mobilized, with dissection carried to the region of the posterior sacroiliac joint. Proper planning of the flap is essential since closure of the primary defect for most thigh sarcomas and those of the pelvic bones usually is accomplished by rotation of the full-thickness skin flap derived from the buttock. For posterior thigh tumors and extensive soft tissue buttock sarcomas, the flap is created from the anterior thigh. It is important that the incision be properly planned, especially when dealing with an ulcerated lesion that may compromise flap closure. Adequate exposure must be obtained at all times in terms of the anterior pelvic exposure and posterior buttock-perianal exposure. This explains why some surgeons employ various degrees of prone or lateral positioning rather than the purely supine position, which, in actuality, can offer all the exposure needed. The knee can be flexed and internally rotated at the hip joint when needed; this allows the buttock to be brought up 180°, giving the necessary field for dissection. The supine position also allows for easy entry into the retroperitoneum and offers adequate and rapid exposure of the major retroperitoneal blood vessels, which must be ligated early in the procedure.

The incision begins at the iliac crest and parallels the inguinal ligament to the midline pubis (Fig. 8–13). This incision allows for entry into the retroperitoneum and offers an opportunity for wide exposure of the iliac vessels and psoas muscle, which must be divided, and for retraction of the retroperitoneum away from the iliac fossa. The remaining incision is outlined in two steps: The knee is flexed and rotated internally to expose the buttock. An upper iliac incision is carried out in a convex direction over the insertion of the gluteus on the trochanter, ending just over the ischial tuberosity (Fig. 8–14). The flexed knee is then rotated externally at the hip joint and the groin incision that has been brought to the pubis now joins the incision at the ischial tuberosity, being carried just lateral to the scrotum or vulva. This latter incision allows for later entry into the ischiorectal fossa and the supralevator space. Dissection here allows the rectum to be mobilized away from the operative field and insures that adequate exposure of those ligaments inserting on the ischial tuberosity can be easily divided.

With the leg now extended and returned to a modified or full supine position, the

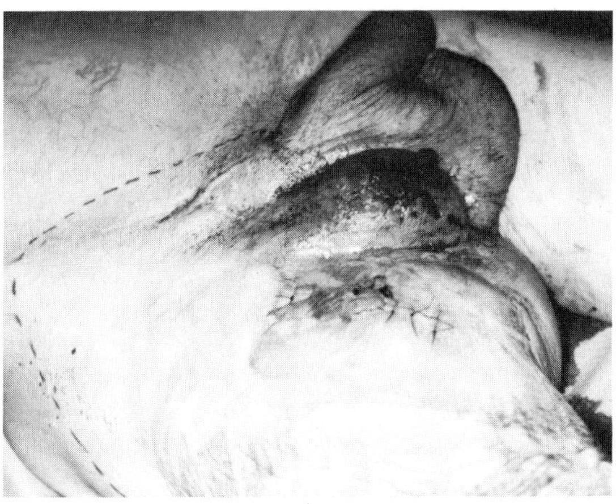

FIGURE 8–13. *Initial hemipelvectomy incision.*

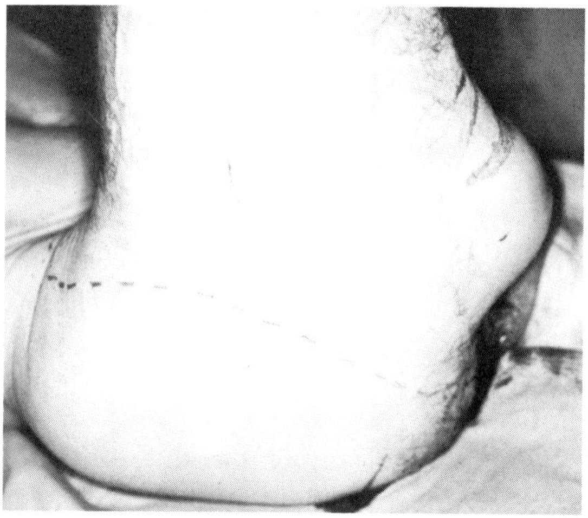

FIGURE 8–14. Incision around the thigh used for raising the buttock flap.

initial inguinal portion of the incision is carried to the external oblique fascia and internal oblique muscles (Fig. 8–15). The inferior epigastric vessels are identified and ligated, and the retroperitoneum is exposed. The round ligament in female patients and the spermatic cord in males is mobilized superiorly with the abdominal flap. With careful dissection to avoid entry into the peritoneal cavity, the peritoneal sac is mobilized superiorly above the bifurcation of the iliac vesssels and is retracted somewhat superiorly and medially across the midline structures to give exposure of midline pubis. Should the tumor have entered the peritoneal cavity, an extended hemipelvectomy must be considered, in which case the visceral contents of the pelvis or abdomen are included with the operative specimen.

Retraction of the peritoneal sac superiorly and medially exposes the ureter against the retracted bladder. Further exposure of the retroperitoneum can be achieved by dividing the internal and external oblique attachments at the iliac crest in preparation for creating the buttock flap. Retraction is next carried in a line over the common iliac vessels, affording complete exposure of this region. A Deaver retractor holds the peritoneum superiorly while a Richardson retractor is placed over the external iliac vessels and retracted inferiorly to the femoral canal. Complete exposure of the ipsilateral vessels is obtained and the vessels can be divided (Fig. 8–16). It is usually advantageous to divide the common iliac artery and vein just above the bifurcation of the internal vessels. At times, ligation of the external rather than

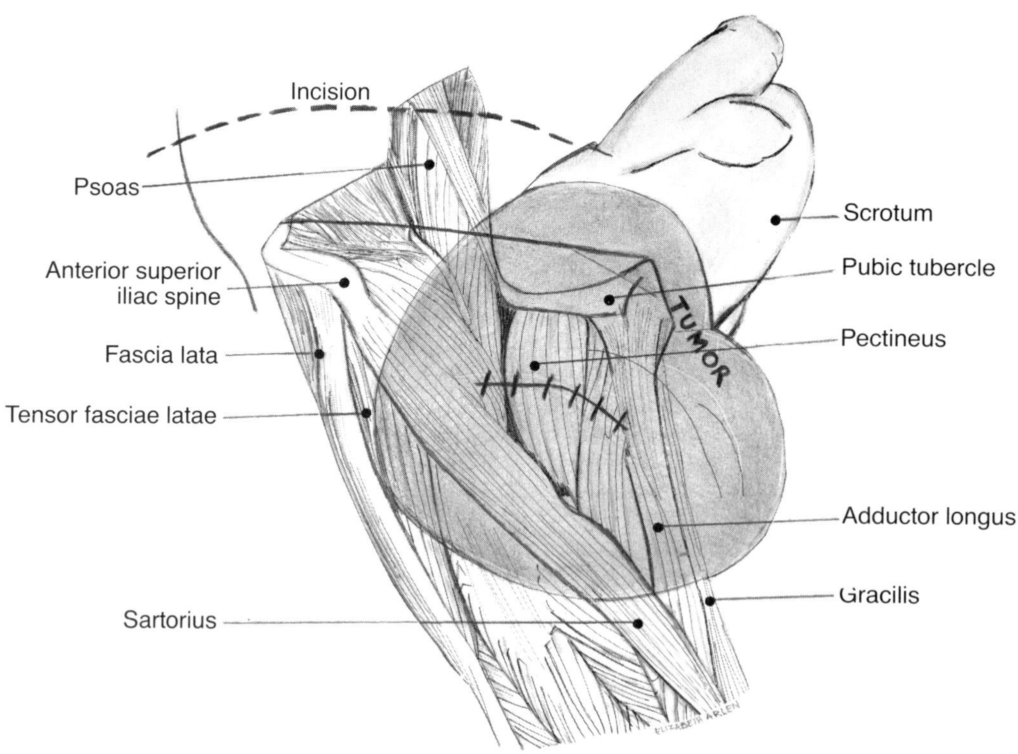

FIGURE 8–15. Incision approaching the retroperitoneum.

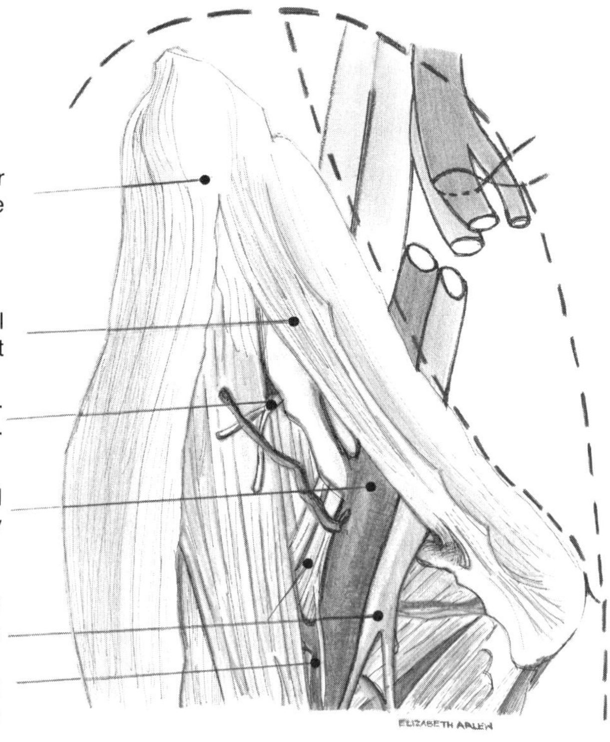

FIGURE 8–16. *Exposure and ligation of the retroperitoneal vessels.*

the common iliac vein below the hypogastric vein take off allows the return collaterals from the venous drainage of the pelvis to remain open and minimizes venous engorgement in the pelvis. Rarely does this compromise circulation to the buttock flap. Pack originally described the resection of a V-shaped wedge from the mid-buttock flap to minimize the degree of possible skin necrosis. Should tumor be found to extend to or infiltrate bladder or rectum, the decision can be made to include these structures as part of the operation or to terminate the operation before vessel ligation is performed.

The ligated distal iliac artery and distal veins are mobilized with the surrounding fat and nodes swept inferiorly (Fig. 8–17) as part of the specimen. Fine oozing from venous and arterial branches to the pelvic wall is controlled with vascular clips or by direct pressure with warm lap pads until completion of the pelvic dissection, at which time final vascular control is carried out prior to the flap closure. Next the psoas muscle is divided with a Bovie cutting current down to the anterior aspect of the sacroiliac joint, which is found just inferolateral to the L5 vertebra. The femoral nerve, which can be defined in the belly of the psoas muscle, is divided. Fine oozing in the muscle is controlled by electrocoagulation. Retraction of the divided edges of the psoas muscle at the anterior aspect of the sacroiliac joint allows exposure of the sacroiliac joint and prepares for later division of this joint; an osteotome is placed into the joint for leverage.

The site of pelvic dissection is now packed in preparation for raising the buttock flap. A

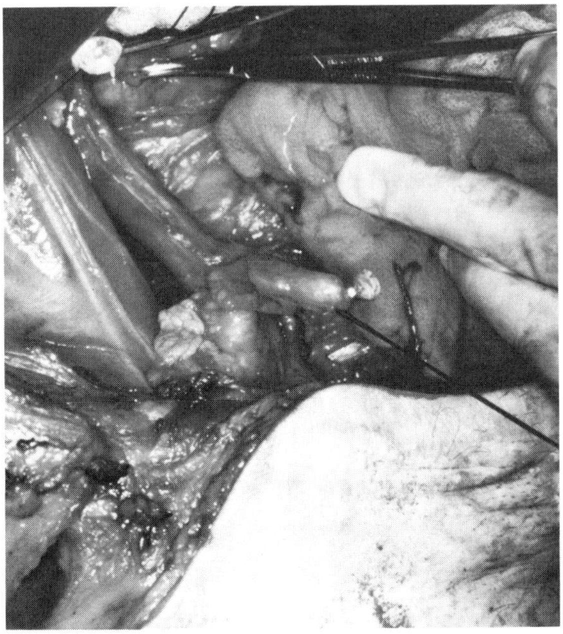

FIGURE 8–17. *Ligated and divided external iliac artery.*

full-thickness cutaneous buttock flap is raised, with muscle left on the side of the specimen. We use electrosurgical cutting current to raise many flaps. Exposure of this region is accomplished by flexing the thigh on the abdomen and internally rotating the hip to expose the entire buttock to the midline. The flap is raised from a lateral to posterior midline direction while palpating for a well-defined ridge near midline, which represents the dorsal aspect of the sacroiliac joint. On identifying this area, the posterior limit of flap dissection has been reached. The subcutaneous gluteal surface, both flap and specimen side, is controlled hemostatically and then packed. The leg is now repositioned to expose the pubis. The space of Retzius is entered and the bladder is mobilized inferiorly, in a posterior direction, away from the pubic symphysis. Finger dissection on the underside of the pubis usually guarantees that the urethra has been freed from the site of the bone to be divided. The presence of a Foley catheter in the bladder usually allows easy palpation of urethra. If the lesion is laterally placed on the ipsilateral side, the midline pubis can be divided by manipulating an osteotome in the pubic symphysis or by using a Gigli saw placed around the symphysis. A blunt clamp is placed from the pelvic side under the pubis to the external side. The Gigli saw is then passed under the midline symphysis, and pubic division is carried from underneath the symphysis in an upward direction, avoiding the urethra. Should tumor approach the symphysis, then the opposite side of the pubis can be divided. Here, one must be careful to insure that the position of the contralateral femoral artery has been defined.

After division of the pubis, the knee and thigh are again flexed at the hip joint and the hip is externally rotated. The ligamentous attachments to the ischial tuberosity are exposed and divided. The pelvic diaphragm is dissected and the supralevator space entered. A heavy Mayo scissors is usually needed to divide the ligaments. Rectum is mobilized away from the operative field, and the sacrotuberous and sacrospinous ligaments are next divided so that the pelvis is essentially attached only by sacroiliac joint, where dense interosseous sacroiliac ligaments hold the sacrum and iliac bone together. The sacrotuberous and sacrospinous ligaments convert the greater and lesser sciatic notches into foramina, where neurovascular structures are identified. As the coccygeus muscle is divided, the pudendal vessels, inferior gluteal artery, and sciatic nerve are seen and transected. Pelvic packing previously inserted into the operative field is removed to expose the anterior aspect of the sacroiliac joint.

Pressure is now placed on the flexed knee in a posterior lateral direction to begin separating ligaments in the sacroiliac joint. At times an osteotome can be placed into the joint space to allow complete cleavage. Rocking the hip at the anterior superior iliac spine usually helps to separate the joint. The division of the remaining muscles and ligamentous attachments is now completed. Nerves and fine vessels that remain are clipped, and the extremity and hemipelvis are completely removed. Figure 8–18 shows the operative field with the divided pubis and the buttock flap, which will be used to close the defect. Should tumor approach the sacroiliac joint, the sacrum can be cleaved closer to the midline with the osteotome. When hemostasis has been assured, a suction catheter is placed into the wound and the buttock flap is turned up to close the defect (Fig. 8–19). For a primary buttock lesion, the previously created anterior thigh flap is turned to close the defect.

In one case, an extensive pelvic tumor crossed the bifurcation of the aorta, which was mistakenly clamped when we thought we were dealing with an external iliac vessel. Figure 8–20*A* shows the barium enema of this patient with an extensive pelvic mass arising off the medial wall of ilium and extending to the sacroiliac joint. Examination of pulses in the opposite leg identified the problem (Fig. 8–20*B*), which required dissection of tumor away from the site of bifurcation so that the actual region of aortic separation into the iliac vessels could be identified. This dissection allowed proper identification of the common iliac vessels, which were then ligated in their proper position.

Blood loss during any of these procedures is usually in the range of 3 to 5 units and should not be a major consideration when all steps are properly observed and performed. The exact amount used depends on the size and position of the lesion as well as its vascularity. This is one of the major reasons for performing an angiogram preoperatively. One may unexpectedly be dealing

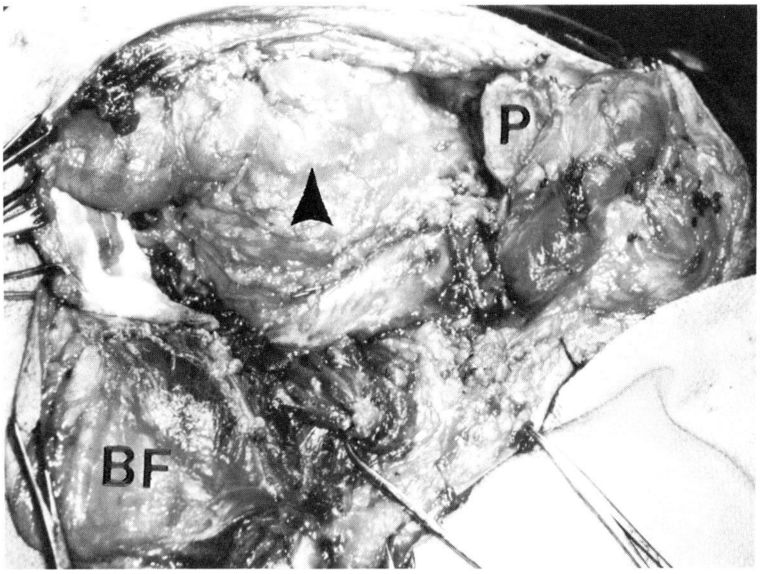

FIGURE 8–18. *Completed operation: BF shows the buttock flap just before closure of the wound and P the divided pubis. The arrow points to the peritoneal sac.*

with a metastatic tumor with no obvious primary tumor focus. We recently saw a patient with a large soft part pelvic mass eroding into the region of the sacroiliac joint. Work-up was entirely negative in terms of defining the possible origin of the tumor, and needle biopsy showed tumor cells that could not be classified. An open biopsy revealed that the tumor mass was pulsatile, suggesting a highly vascular neoplasm. Two units of blood were needed for the biopsy. Postbiopsy studies of the kidney were normal. Thyroid work-up indicated a small lesion that proved to be a sclerosing carcinoma. The dilemma over the treatment to be offered was resolved when we realized that the pelvic mass was metastatic from the thyroid lesion. Chemotherapy with adria-

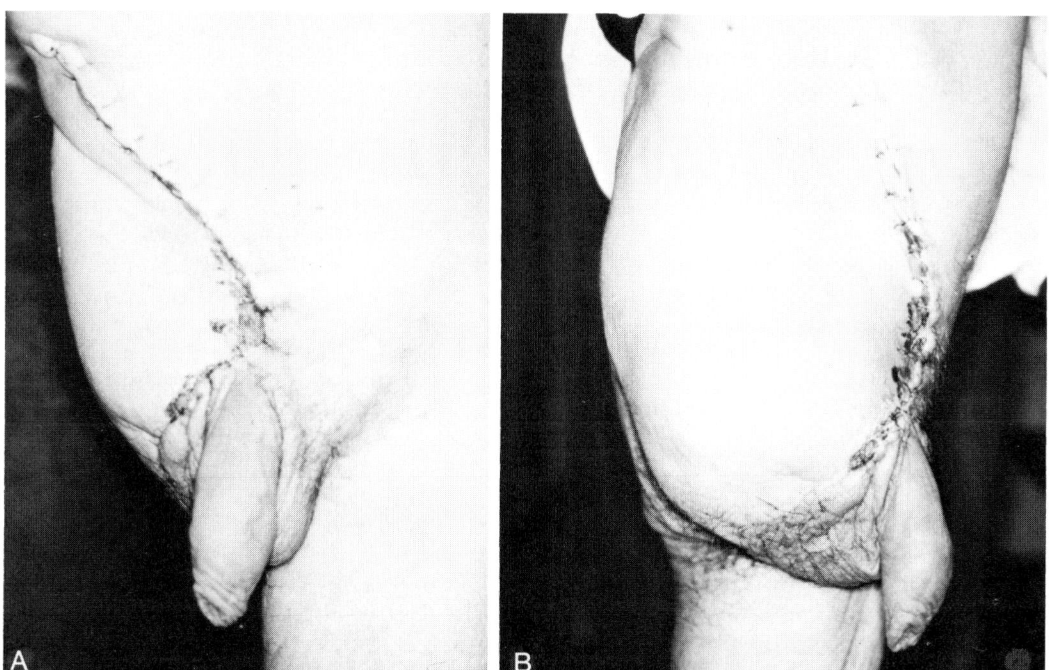

FIGURE 8–19. *A and B, Appearance of the patient 1 week after surgery.*

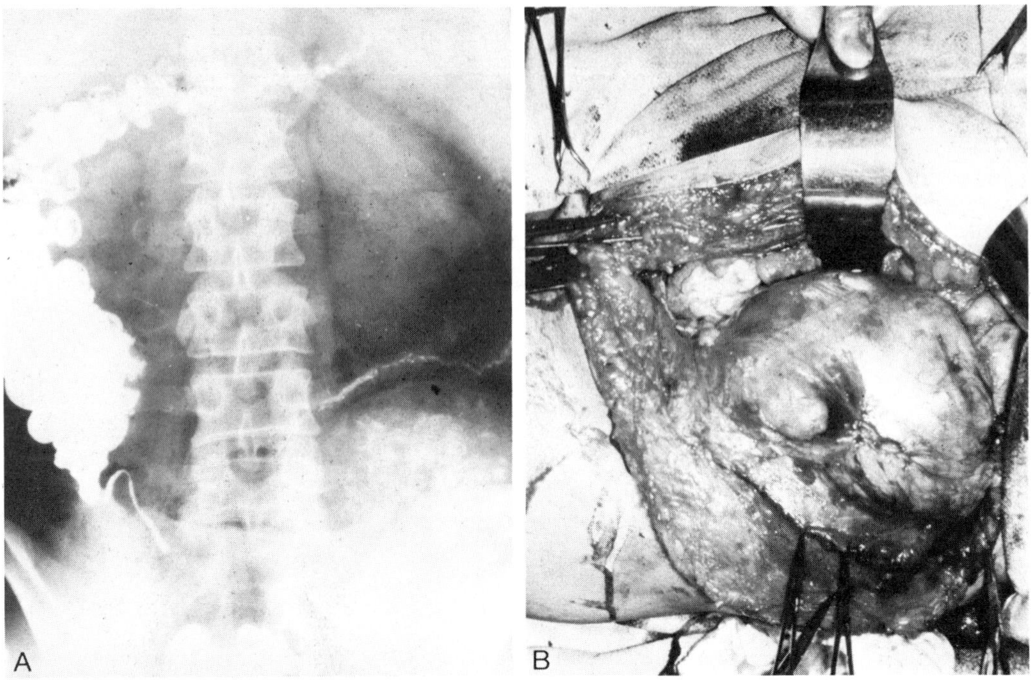

FIGURE 8–20. *A, Barium enema showing displacement of the retroperitoneal colon by tumor. B, Exposure of the tumor, which sits over the bifurcation of the aorta.*

mycin was initiated, followed by almost complete regression of the tumor. If surgery were to be entertained, failure to recognize the degree as well as the patterns of vascularity could have resulted in unnecessary complications. If such a vascular lesion proved to be primary and surgical resection were contemplated, angiographic thrombosis would be required prior to the attempted surgery.

The classic operation that we currently perform was first attempted by Billroth in 1891 for a soft part sarcoma but was later successfully performed by Girard in 1895. The operation has been considered by many to be one of the most colossal mutilations practiced on the human frame. In actuality, it is really nothing more than an extension of a high-thigh amputation. In the present era of vascular surgery employed for preserving limbs diseased by arterial insufficiency, failure of the graft may require amputation just short of hemipelvectomy. On the other hand, our more aggressive local surgical approaches to extremity sarcoma have limited our indications and, therefore, our use of the hemipelvectomy.

In the standard procedure the skin and underlying subcutaneous tissue of the buttock is utilized as the posterior flap for closure. When the skin of the buttock is involved by tumor, an alternative site for deriving the pedicle flap must be chosen.[22] In such instances, a thigh skin flap from the anterior thigh is created. After this flap has been raised, the incision can be extended to just above the inguinal ligament to allow for entry into the retroperitoneum. The ligament and rectus abdominis muscle are divided at the pubic insertion, and the procedure is completed as usual. Temple et al.[49] described the problem of flap closure using well-vascularized flaps, especially in the presence of extensive tumors for which the classic closure could not be employed. They described the total thigh and the rectus abdominis myocutaneous flaps, which significantly decreased morbidity and increased resectability of unusual pelvic and thigh tumors.

Depending on the position and type of tumor, when planning and performing a hemipelvectomy several modifications should be considered: (1) partial or conservative hemipelvectomy, internal hemipelvectomy, and (2) extended hemipelvectomy with exenteration. Many of these modifications of the hemipelvectomy—e.g., preservation of the iliac crest or division of the hemipelvis just above the acetabulum—have been devised in an attempt to preserve the lower extremity. These modifications are of value only for managing extensive soft part tumors situated above the sciatic notch area.

Conservative Hemipelvectomy. Conservative hemipelvectomy involves the complete resection of the lower extremity combined with partial resection of innominate bone. In contrast to the standard hemipelvectomy, sacroiliac disarticulation is not performed. The sacroiliac synchondrosis, including the upper portion of the iliac bone, remains intact. Bony transection is accomplished by severing the ilium through the greater sciatic notch. In certain soft tissue sarcomas of upper thigh the lesion may extend along fascial planes to attachments on the osseous structures of the pelvis. In such cases, disarticulation would be inappropriate since disease would remain proximally. Such reports of recurrences after disarticulation have been noted by Higinbotham.[19] Here conservative hemipelvectomy allows for better prosthetic rehabilitation.

In performing this procedure, the retroperitoneum is entered, as described for the standard procedure. The vessels are divided, and the psoas and iliacus muscles are separated off the ilium by blunt finger dissection, passing from the anterior superior iliac spine medially along the inner aspect of the ilium to the sciatic notch. Similar blunt dissection separates the gluteal muscle from the ilium on its posterior aspect, and a Gigli saw is run through the greater sciatic notch below the inferior origin of the gluteus minimus. Bone is divided at the appropriate level, and the pubis transected through the symphysis. As the extremity separates away, the remaining muscles and vessels with the sciatic nerve are divided and hemostasis is assured.

Internal Hemipelvectomy. The necessary element for controlling any primary tumor is adequate excision with proper margins of resection. In the case of pelvic-sacral tumors, freedom at the acetabulum could set the stage for modification of the classic hemipelvectomy. Eilber et al.[10] described their experience with five patients who underwent internal hemipelvectomy, involving excision of the hemipelvis, ilium, ischium, and pubis along with contiguous sacral alae and proximal femoral head; in all cases a functionally intact distal extremity was preserved.

The patients were placed in a supine position and turned obliquely to elevate the hemipelvis approximately 45°. A downward incision was begun at the posterior iliac crest and curved at the anterior superior iliac spine to the upper third of the lateral aspect of the thigh. Flaps were raised, the retroperitoneum entered, and the hypogastric vessels isolated, ligated, and divided. A plane was developed between the psoas and iliacus muscles, and the psoas muscle was retracted medially with the femoral nerve. The rectus femoris muscle was divided and dissection carried to the capsule of the hip joint, allowing for division of the femoral neck. The medial hamstrings and adductors were amputated, leaving a cuff attached to the pubis and ischium. The gluteal muscles were divided laterally and the sciatic nerve moved posteriorly and medially. Division of the pubic symphysis was followed by an osteotomy through the sacral alae just lateral to the neural foramina. Division of the levator ani allowed removal of the specimen. Nonweightbearing ambulation was begun at 6 weeks. An average of 3.5 cm was lost in leg length.

Karakousis[21] described a similar procedure wherein the pubic symphysis was divided. The femoral nerve and psoas muscle were preserved, and the adductor muscles were divided near their origin from the pubic bone. The origins of the sartorius, tensor fasciae latae, and rectus femoris, as well as the gluteal insertions on the greater trochanter, were divided to allow entry into the hip joint for division of the femoral neck. The procedure may be modified to allow preservation of the uninvolved portions of innominate bone. If the pubic bone is left intact, this permits preservation of the adductor group of muscles and nerve. When the acetabulum can be preserved, minimal or no functional impairments can be expected. Other attempts at conservative procedures as well as preserving portions of the pelvis have been described.[1, 12, 13, 30, 44, 45, 46, 49] In addition to preservation of portions of the pelvis depending on extent of tumor involvement, prosthetic devices as well as allografts have been utilized in an effort to preserve the lower extremity.[25, 26, 29, 37]

Hemipelvectomy for Buttock Tumors. For the most part, many sarcomas of the buttock can be managed by the radical gluteal resection. When hemipelvectomy is found to be necessary, a procedure is advocated in which the buttock skin flap can be partially sacrificed with specimen. An anterior skin flap is raised, containing the external iliac vessels and a small portion of the superficial femoral vessels, which are necessary for nourishing the flap. Sugarbaker and Chretien[47] described a modified technique using a myocutaneous quadriceps flap fed by superficial femoral vessels. This procedure was essentially employed in patients in whom, after dissection of the gluteus, extension of tumor to the pelvic bone or to the femoral or sciatic nerve was noted, suggesting that the margins for resection were not adequate.

In certain instances, we have safely attempted to shave tumor off the nerve or bone. We have found this to be possible in many cases of desmoid tumor and chordoid chondrosarcoma, where minimal margins of resection have sufficed and where the operative field then received radiation therapy. If recurrence were noted, amputation would be necessary.

Should biopsy indicate an aggressive, fully malignant lesion requiring hemipelvectomy, the patient would be placed in a lateral decubitus position. Instead of preserving the buttock flap, it is included as part of the specimen, in the same manner described for cases requiring an anterior thigh flap.

Extended Hemipelvectomy. Extended hemipelvectomy and exenteration have been utilized in the past in those rare instances in which the operative procedure appears to be potentially curative. We have utilized this operation for occasional tumors crossing the sacroiliac joint or when pelvic visceral involvement is found. We performed our first procedure of this kind on a young woman with recurrent osteogenic sarcoma that had been managed by disarticulation. Recurrence had developed in the hypogastric fossa invading the urinary bladder. The amputation was converted to hemipelvectomy with cystectomy. Brunschwig[6] was known to have performed several cases of total exenteration-hemipelvectomy for advanced cervical carcinoma invading the lateral pelvic bone. The operation has also included nephrectomy. Figure 8–21 shows a hemipelvectomy specimen containing the contents of a total pelvic exenteration performed by Brunschwig. Such surgery has limited value but defines the extent of surgery that can be performed for pelvic lesions short of hemicorporectomy.

Douglas et al.[9] reviewed the experience with hemipelvectomy at Roswell Park. Among the 50 patients in the study, there was a wide array of neoplasms including rhabdomyosarcoma (7 cases), liposarcoma (7), chondrosarcoma (6), osteosarcoma (3), fibrosarcoma (3), and synovioma (3). The levels of vascular ligation varied from the common iliac artery at the bifurcation of aorta to the common femoral artery, with the lower levels of ligation more commonly utilized for posterior tumors. On occasion

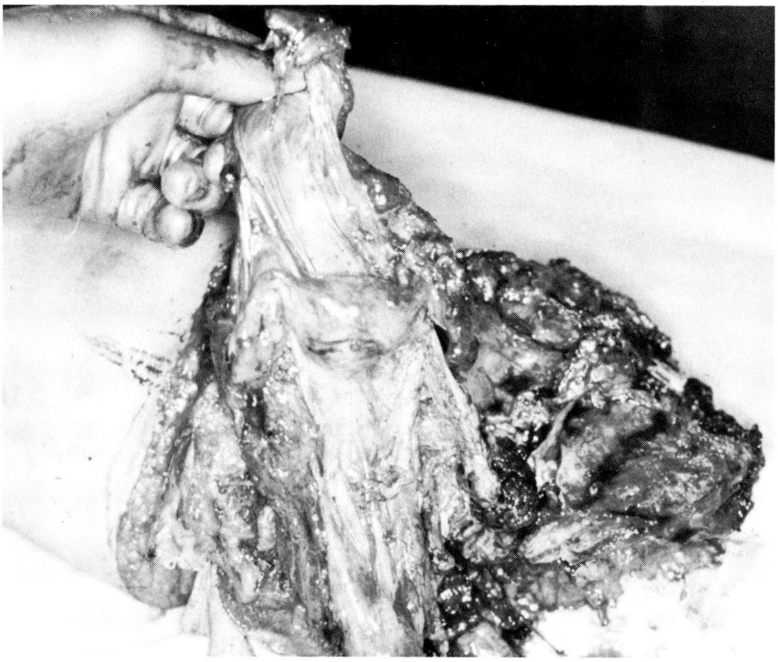

FIGURE 8–21. Extended hemipelvectomy with contents of total pelvic exenteration.

the peritoneum was opened to permit extension of the procedure to include resection of intraperitoneal organs. When the tumor was located anteriorly, retroperitoneal dissection was less extensive and a segment of ilium was often left on the sacrum to support a belt or prosthesis. Blood loss averaged 8 units.

Avascular slough of skin flaps occurred in 40 (80%). This phenomenon was originally described by Pack, who advocated resecting a wedge of potentially devascularized skin in the center of the flap. Ten patients in the Douglas series required skin grafting. Recently, fluorescein injected intravenously at the conclusion of the procedure allowed visualization of the degree of vascularization and modification of the flaps to account for any flap necrosis.

Urethral injuries occurred in two patients and were repaired over a Foley catheter. When the pubis was divided, the symphysis was initially entered with a scalpel with a clamp placed under the symphysis. The remainder of the division was carried out with an osteotome. Six of the liposarcomas treated arose in the upper thigh, the seventh in the buttock; two of the patients died of metastasis. Of the seven patients operated on for rhabdomyosarcoma, four died of pulmonary metastasis within 18 months of the surgery. None of the synovioma patients were cured by the operative procedure. The three fibrosarcoma patients did well. Seven of the hemipelvectomies were performed for palliation. Six of these patients had uncontrollable severe pain that could not be managed by medication or surgical neurolysis. Independent walking on crutches should be accomplished in the majority of patients within 1 week of surgery. Limb prostheses are cosmetic and usually not functional in the older patient. Physiologically most patients function normally except for the possibility of bowel herniation at the site of pedicle (buttock) flap closure. This may cause some difficulty in bearing down and may lead to bowel problems that can be managed conservatively. Brockunier[5] reported that in spite of such problems, normal delivery can be expected in the occasional female patient of child-bearing age.

REFERENCES

1. Ariel I. M., Shaw J. P.: The conservative hemipelvectomy. Surg. Gynecol. Obstet. 144:407–413, 1977
2. Bailey R. W., Steven D. B.: Radical exarticulation of the extremities for the curative and palliative treatment of malignant neoplasms. J. Bone Joint Surg. 43-A:845–854, 1961
3. Banks S. W., Coleman S.: Hemipelvectomy: Surgical techniques. J. Bone Joint Surg. 38:1147–1155, 1956
4. Boyd G. B.: Anatomic disarticulation of the hip. Surg. Gynecol. Obstet. 84:346, 1947
5. Brockunier A., Jr.: Vaginal delivery following hemipelvectomy for malignant neoplasm of the bone and soft parts. Obstet. Gynecol. 23:67–71, 1964
6. Brunschwig A.: Hemipelvectomy in combination with partial pelvic exenteration for uncontrolled recurrent and metastatic carcinoma of the cervix. Surgery 52:299–304, 1962
7. Burnel H. N.: Resection of the shoulder with humeral suspension for sarcoma involving the scapula. J. Bone Joint Surg. 47-B:300–303, 1965
8. Byron R. L., Cronemiller P. D., Bierman H. R., Yonomoto R. H.: Interscapulo-thoracic amputation and sacroiliac disarticulation with adjuvant arterial chemotherapy. Surg. Gynecol. Obstet. 111:457–463, 1960
9. Douglas H. O., Razack M., Holyoke D.: Hemipelvectomy. Arch. Surg. 110:82–85, 1975
10. Eilber F. R., Grant T. T., Skai D., Morton D. L.: Internal hemipelvectomy: Excision of the hemipelvis with limb preservation—an alternative to hemipelvectomy. Cancer 43:806–809, 1979
11. El-Domeri A. A., Miller T. R.: The role of interscapulothoracic amputation in the treatment of malignant tumors. Surg. Gynecol. Obstet. 129:1203–1206, 1969
12. Enneking W. F.: Local resection of malignant lesions of the hip and pelvis. J. Bone Joint Surg. 48-A:991–1007, 1966
13. Evans J. E., Harvey J. P., Jr., Nickel V. L.: A nineteen-year follow-up of chondrosarcoma of the proximal portion of the femur treated by resection, autoclaving and bone replacement. J. Bone Joint Surg. 51-A:598–600, 1969
14. Fanous M., Dildolkar M., Holyoke E. D., Elias E. G.: Evaluation of forequarter amputation in malignant diseases. Surg. Gynecol. Obstet. 142:381–384, 1976
15. Francis K. C., Worcester J. M.: Radical resection for tumors of the shoulder with preservation of a functional extremity. J. Bone Joint Surg. 44-A:1426–1430, 1962
16. Frey C., Matthews L. S., Fidler W. J.: A new technique for hemipelvectomy surgery. Gynecol. Obstet. 143:753–756, 1976
17. Gordon-Taylor G.: The technique and management of the "hind quarter" amputation. Br. J. Surg. 39: 536–541, 1952
18. Hall C. B., Bechtol C. O.: Modern amputation technique in the upper extremity. J. Bone Joint Surg. 45-A:1717–1722, 1963
19. Higinbotham M. L., Marcove R. C., Casson P.: Hemipelvectomy: A clinical study of 100 cases with five-year follow-up on 60 patients. Surgery 59:706–708, 1966
20. Janeciz C. J., Nelson C. L.: En-bloc resection of the shoulder girdle: Technique and indications. J. Bone Joint Surg. 54-A:1754–1758, 1972
21. Karakousis C. P.: Internal hemipelvectomy. Surg. Gynecol. Obstet. 158:279–282, 1984
22. Karakousis C. P., Vezeridis M. P.: Variants of hemipelvectomy. Am. J. Surg. 145:273–277, 1983
23. Littlewood H.: Amputation at the shoulder and at the hip. Br. Med. J. 1:381–383, 1922

24. Mansour K. A., Powell R. W.: Modified technique for radical transmediastinal forequarter amputation and chest wall resection. J. Thorac. Cardiovasc. Surg. 76:358–363, 1978
25. Marcove R. C., Lewis M. M., Huvos A. G.: En-bloc upper humeral interscapulothoracic resection: The Tikhoff-Linberg procedure. Clin. Orthop. 124:219–227, 1977
26. Marcove R. C., Lewis M. M., Rosen G., et al.: Total femoral replacement. Comp. Ther. 3:13–19, 1977
27. Marcove R. C., Lewis M. M., Rosen G., Huvos A. G.: Total femur and knee replacement. Clin. Orthop. 126:147–152, 1977
28. Marcove R. C., McMillan R. D., Naste E.: Preservation of the functional above-knee stump following hip disarticulation by means of an Austin-Moore prosthesis. Clin. Orthop. 141:217–222, 1979
29. Marcove R. C., Rosen G.: En-bloc resections for osteogenic sarcoma. NCI Monograph No. 56:165–168, 1981
30. Milch H.: Partial resection of the ischium: The operative procedure. J. Bone Joint Surg. 17:166–179, 1935
31. Miller T. R.: Hemipelvectomy in lower extremity tumors. Orthop. Clin. North Am. 8: 903–919, 1977
32. Mosely H. F.: The forequarter amputation. Edinburgh, E. S. Livingston, 1957
33. Nadler S. H., Phelan J. T.: A technique of interscapulothoracic amputation. Surg. Gynecol. Obstet. 22:359–364, 1966
34. Pack G. T., McGraw T. A.: Interscapulo-mammothoracic amputation for malignant melanoma. Arch. Surg. 83:694–699, 1961
35. Pack G. T., McNeer G., Coley B. L.: Interscapulothoracic amputation for malignant tumors of the upper extremity. Surg. Gynecol. Obstet. 74:161–174, 1942
36. Paciz G. T., Bladwin J. C.: The Tikhoff-Linberg resection of the shoulder girdle. Surgery 38:753–757, 1955
37. Parrish F. F.: Allograft replacement of all or part of the end of a long bone following excision of a tumor: Report of 21 cases. J. Bone Joint Surg. 55-A: 1–22, 1973
38. Phelan J. T., Nadler S. H.: A technique of hemipelvectomy. Surg. Gynecol. Obstet. 119:311–318, 1964
39. Ramirez J., Arlen M., Jourdain L. M.: Total scapulectomy for soft part tumors of the shoulder girdle. Surgery 69:271, 1971
40. Ravitch M. M.: Hemipelvectomy. Surgery 26:99–107, 1949
41. Ryerson E. W.: Excision of the scapula. J.A.M.A. 113:1958, 1939
42. Sim F. H., Pritchard D. J., Ivins J. C.: Forequarter amputation. Orthop. Clin. North Am. 8:921–931, 1977
43. Stafford E. S., Williams G. R., Jr.: Radical transthoracic forequarter amputation. Ann. Surg. 148:699–703, 1958
44. Steel H. H.: Partial or complete resection of the hemipelvis. J. Bone Joint Surg. 60-A:719–730, 1978
45. Steel H. H.: Resection of the hemipelvis for malignant disease: An alternative to hindquarter amputation for periacetabular chondrosarcoma of the pelvis. Semin. Oncol. 8:222–228, 1981
46. Stener B., Gutenberg B.: High amputation of the sacrum for extirpation of tumors: Principles and technique. Spine 3:351–366, 1978
47. Sugarbaker P. W., Chretien P. A.: Hemipelvectomy for buttock tumors utilizing an anterior myocutaneous flap of quadriceps femoris muscle. Ann. Surg. 197:106–115, 1983
48. Sugarbaker P. W., Weiss C. M., Davidson D. D., Roth Y. F.: Increasing phantom limb pain as a symptom of cancer recurrence. Cancer 54:373–375, 1984
49. Temple W. J., Mnaymneh W., Ketcham A. S.: The total thigh and rectus abdominis myocutaneous flap for closure of extensive hemipelvectomy defects. Cancer 50:2524–2528, 1982
50. Whitehall R., Wanebo H. J., Mabie K. H., et al.: Reconstruction after the Tikhoff-Linberg procedure. Arch. Surg. 117:1248–1249, 1982
51. Wu K. K., Guise E. R., Frost H. M., Mitchell C. L.: The surgical technique for hindquarter amputation. Acta Orthop. Scand. 48:479–486, 1977
52. Wurlitzer F. D.: Improved techniques for radical transthoracic forequarter amputation. Ann. Surg. 177:467–471, 1973

CHAPTER

9

The Effect of Structural Loss on the Extremities

During any major muscle group dissection, certain neurovascular and muscle structures must be sacrificed as part of the procedure. The effects that may be expected from such surgery are described here.

LOWER EXTREMITY OSSEOUS STRUCTURES

Ilium and Adjacent Sacrum. These bones are removed during the internal hemipelvectomy. Replacements, including cadaver bone (autograft), have been used. Bone struts have been taken from cut ilium distally and placed across the pubic symphysis to offer improved stability. This may help to prevent shortening of the lower extremity, especially in younger children. The greater stability helps to reduce secondary scoliosis.

Whole Innominate and Upper Femur. A prosthesis can be attached to replace these missing pelvic structures. If no upper prosthesis is used, the remaining upper femur and surrounding region will scar and show evidence of limb shortening. Spontaneous fusion may occur later between the residual bones. The resulting gait can be improved with an ischial weightbearing brace (if the ischium is present), and a pelvic band with a drop-lock hip joint should be used.

Upper Femur. When the upper femur is removed it should be replaced with an equivalent metallic segment with an intermedullary stem. A total or bicentric hip joint must also be used. When the whole femoral shaft is removed, a total or bicentric hip should be snapped onto a metallic shaft (35-mm inner diameter) and Guepar knee prosthesis with an intermedullary tibial stem.

Knee. The entire knee with wide areas adjacent to the femur, tibia and fibula may need to be resected. A small-diameter Guepar knee prosthesis is preferred with long shaft replacement and strong intermedullary pin fixation.

Ankle Joint Resection. The distal fibula can be resected in growing children. A valgus deformity may follow, in which case stapling of the distal tibial epiphysis prevents such a deformity. Malignancies around the heel may respond to cryosurgery when the lesion is low-grade. Circumduction fusions shifting weight to the fibula may allow major large bone resection of the tibia. Midfoot lesions may be treated with cryosurgery. If the lesion is high-grade a Syme amputation can be used. A forefoot tumor may be treated with the Chopart amputation. The foot must be fixed at 90° with a Steinmann pin and the anterior tibial tendon transferred into the talus.

LOWER EXTREMITY MUSCLE LOSS

Quadriceps. Large areas of quadriceps are easily sacrificed with little disturbance in gait. If the knee loses extension it can be braced. Scar contracture with the knee in full extension is encouraged. The knee will be prevented from giving out if the ankle is fused in an equinus position, which locks the knee when stepping (Hibbs). For massive loss of quadriceps the hamstrings can be transferred.

Hamstrings. Loss of these muscles results in only minor gait disturbance. The patient may complain that he is unable to run as fast as previously.

Adductors. Extensive loss of these muscles gives a circumduction gait to the pattern of walking.

Abductors. Loss of these muscles results in gluteus medius lurch. When scar tissue develops and fixes the gluteus medius firmly, the gait disturbance becomes significantly minimized.

Triceps Surae Group. Loss of this group results in a calcaneal gait of minimal significance.

Anterior Tibial Muscle. Resection of this muscle causes the development of a drop-foot gait. This may be helped by a Klensac brace or just the use of high-heeled shoes in a woman to avoid steppage gait. An ankle fusion can be performed, but few patients opt for this procedure. With a drop-foot gait the posterior tibial muscle may be transferred to the anterior compartment.

Intrinsic Muscles. Loss of these muscles may produce painful calluses.

LOWER EXTREMITY NERVE LOSS

Femoral Nerve. When damaged there is a resultant loss of knee extension. A hamstring transfer may be needed, but unless some original strength is already present, the transfer will fail. Knee fusion is rarely preferred over use of a brace with knee locked in extension.

Sciatic Nerve. The loss of this nerve does not obligate one to do a hemipelvectomy, as some have recommended. Foot numbness that develops must be treated in much the same way as with diabetic neuropathy. Ulcers must be observed and treated by limiting trauma to the feet. Motor loss can be managed by using a drop-foot splint to avoid steppage gait. Posterior tibial muscle transfer may be utilized, or a Lambrinudi operation or total ankle fusion may avoid the drop-foot gait. A malignant tumor too close to the line of resection can first be treated by cryosurgery, then dissected off the nerve; this can still be curative.

UPPER EXTREMITY OSSEOUS STRUCTURES

Humerus. In general, the loss of bone length in the upper extremity is not so critical a problem as in the lower extremity. Patients accept shortening without major difficulty. Loss of the scapula and upper humerus (Tikhoff-Linberg procedure) will still result in good elbow flexion, provided that the humerus is well fixed superiorly. A prosthesis for the upper humerus cannot possibly function if the rotator cuff has been removed with the tumor, which is usually the case. It sometimes will cosmetically fill in the shoulder when the prosthesis is properly positioned. Nails as prostheses help to lengthen the humerus and aid in its superior fixation, which will also help to strengthen elbow flexion. Total humerus removal yields a weak elbow.

The elbow can be resected and, if allowed to stiffen mediolaterally while mobilizing in an anteroposterior position, may yield satisfactory function. Prostheses for such replacement are not yet available. If resection is required beyond the radial head-capitulum area, cryosurgery is preferred in that the lesion will be destroyed while good elbow function is maintained.

Radius and Ulna. Forearm resection can best be managed by filling any bone gap with fragments of iliac crest skewed on an intramedullary pin and the conversion of one massive forearm bone into a fused upper ulnar–distal radius, also called the "one-bone forearm" (Fig. 9–1). The upper end of the radius and distal ulna is therefore easily sacrificed.

UPPER EXTREMITY MUSCLE LOSS

Shoulder Muscles. As already mentioned, the shoulder rotator cuff, as well as the deltoid, is essential for elevation of the humerus. Triceps function (with high radial nerve loss) may not be missed, as gravity can extend the elbow (except in the case of crutch walking). Flexion is lost without the musculocutaneous nerve, or with removal of the brachialis muscle unless a Steindler procedure–brachioradialis muscle origin transfer is done to increase elbow strength.

Long Flexors. Long flexors give strength to the distal phalanges: the sublimis to flex the mid-phalanges and the intrinsic muscles to flex the metacarpophalangeal joints. Joint fusion and the Brand procedure will increase some of these losses.

Long Extensors. The long extensors will extend the metacarpophalangeal joints and help the intrinsic muscles extend the more distal joints. Interphalangeal fusions have

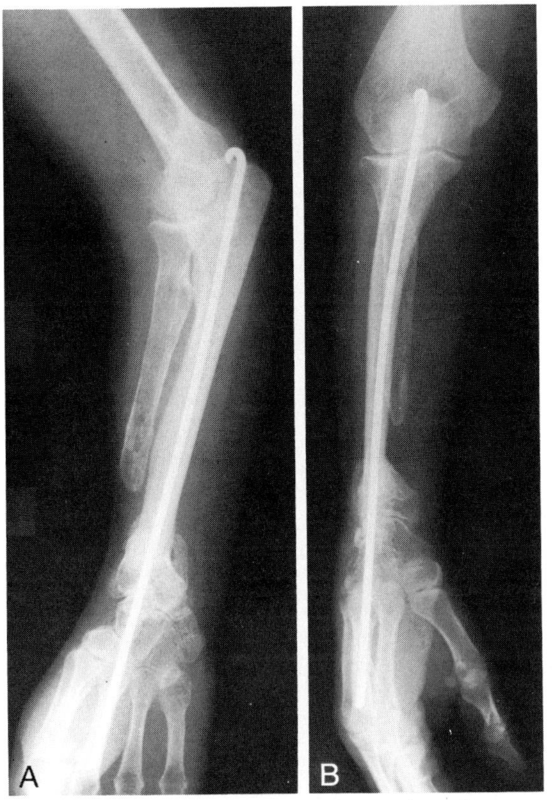

FIGURE 9–1. X-ray appearance of a one-bone forearm.

already been mentioned as aids in overcoming these joint losses. A wrist fusion can help to improve weak hand strength and will allow residual tendons to be freed up for transfer.

UPPER EXTREMITY NERVE LOSS

Musculocutaneous Nerve. Musculocutaneous nerve loss will result in inability to flex.

Radial Nerve. With radial nerve loss it is recommended that flexion transfer (the Jones procedure) be done.

Median Nerve. The worst disability can result with median nerve loss since the patients may complain of extreme numbness in their fingers. However, we all know of cases in which nerve damage has resulted in few side effects, since there has been an overlapping nerve distribution. When nerve loss is total, nerve grafting can be attempted.

Ulnar Nerve. The disability caused by ulnar nerve loss can be somewhat relieved with the Brand procedure, which will substitute for intrinsic muscle function.

In those instances in which it is necessary to resect bone, it has become apparent that prosthetic replacement may be feasible as a means for improving the potential for preserving the extremity.

EN-BLOC SURGERY

Total Femur Replacement

This procedure was originally performed by Marcove for a 65-year-old man with chondrosarcoma of the left femur that involved a major portion of the shaft and both metaphyses. It is now available for use in any patient in whom a large soft part sarcoma of the thigh occurs in proximity to femur. In the original case, because of the apparent low-grade nature of the malignancy and because the patient refused amputation, cryosurgery with curettage was attempted, first on the soft tissue mass and then on the bone itself. At re-exploration 3 months later persistent tumor was found in both metaphyses, away from the area of the earlier cryosurgery. However, the soft tissue mass originally encountered at the midshaft had been eliminated. The procedure was judged unsatisfactory because of the massive extent of tumor throughout the shaft of the femur. The patient still refused amputation. At this time, it was decided that the entire femur should be resected and that total femur and knee replacement would be provided. As a standard part of the work-up, anterior, posterior, and lateral x-ray films of the involved area, as well as a skeletal survey, bone scan, and chest tomography, were performed and is routinely recommended. In addition, biplane femoral arteriography is now performed. All data are evaluated to determine the size, location, and resectability of the tumor, particularly with regard to the degree of soft tissue involvement as well as the presence or absence of metastatic disease. In children, whose epiphyses are still open, the degree of skeletal maturity and projected growth must be evaluated prior to bone replacement.

The objectives and potential risks of this protocol as well as the difficulties in terms of wound healing are carefully explained to the patients and their families. The presence of pulmonary metastasis is not necessarily a contraindication so long as the lesions appear surgically resectable or responsive to chemotherapy. Once a patient has been accepted, scanograms of the right and left femurs are done and are used as the model for construction of the total femur prosthesis with a hinged Guepar knee.

Construction of the prosthesis takes approximately 8 weeks. During this time, chemotherapy is initiated. When the prosthesis is ready, the patient is reevaluated. If the protocol criteria are still valid, the lesion is resected and total femur replacement performed. Figure 9–2 shows the total femur prosthesis with hinged knee and tibial stem that was used for replacement. A Guepar knee is now used with a bicentric hip (Hexcel). The appearance of one of the first patients to undergo total femur replacement is shown in Figure 9–3. A long leg ischial weightbearing brace with pelvic band was originally used. The pelvic band has been eliminated, and the brace is ischial weightbearing only. The appearance of the patient stands in marked contrast to the appearance of a patient who has undergone hemipelvectomy, which requires a bucket prosthesis (Fig. 9–4).

Technique. A lateral biopsy approach is used in previously untreated cases. The Roy-Gibson skin incision is employed; posterior and anterior approaches are made about the

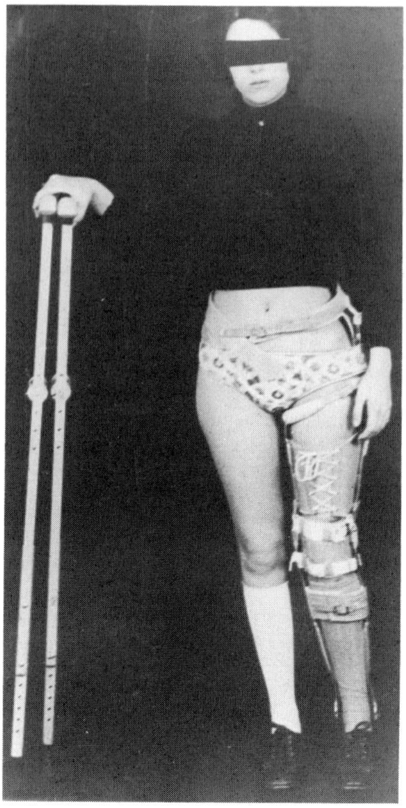

FIGURE 9–3. One of the early patients treated by total femur replacement.

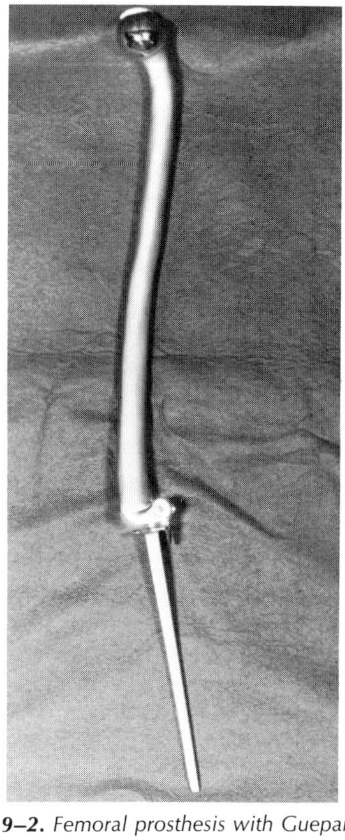

FIGURE 9–2. Femoral prosthesis with Guepar knee.

hip on the affected side. The incision itself is carried along the greater trochanter down to the lateral aspect of the femur distal to the knee, then curved anteriorly over the proximal lateral tibia to extend 4 cm distal to the tibial tubercle. The biopsy scar and tract are usually excised or included in the surgical resection. The incision is carried into the fascia lata and the iliotibial band; the gluteus maximus and femoral attachments are incised and tagged with heavy chromic sutures. The sciatic nerve is identified and isolated, and its branches are protected. The common peroneal nerve and the posterior tibial nerves are also identified and isolated. The popliteal artery and vein are identified at the adductor hiatus and are again checked to ensure that they are free of tumor. These vessels are carefully isolated so that no damage during dissection can occur. The branches supplying the neoplasm are isolated and ligated either with clips or silk ties, and the genicular arteries are likewise ligated at the level of the main vessel.

In the proximal wound, the adductor muscles are divided from the femur as well as the remaining glutei, psoas, and pectineus

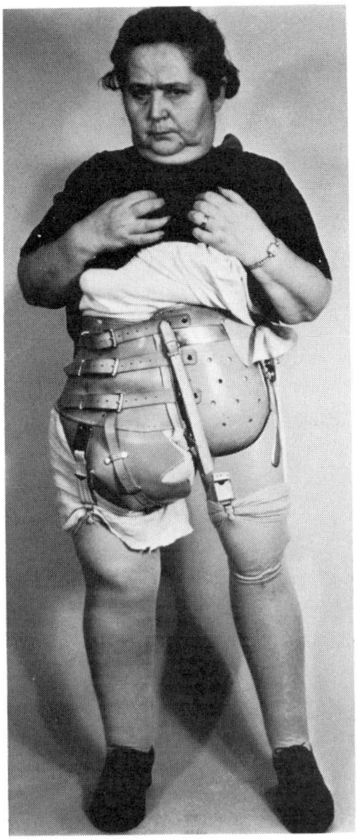

FIGURE 9–4. Hemipelvectomy patient using bucket prosthesis.

muscles. The hip capsule and ligamentum teres are next transected, and the hip is dislocated. The short head of the biceps femoris is transected from the femur. Ample margin is left on the femur, especially as the site of the tumor is approached.

Attention should next be given to controlling hemostasis from perforating vessels. The vastus lateralis and intermedius are separated from their borders remaining on the femoral bone. As the dissection approaches the knee region, the gastrocnemius muscle (both the medial and lateral heads) is separated from bone; the semimembranosis, plantaris, and popliteus muscles are also separated.

The tibia is next osteotomized just proximal to the tibial tubercle, and the insertions of the sartorius, semitendinosus, and gracilis muscles are freed from bone. Collateral ligaments are not cut, as the knee is removed en bloc with the distal femur. The patellar tendon is maintained intact and the patella is split coronally, so that the inner half stays with the specimen and the outer half remains continuous with the retained quadriceps mechanism. The specimen is next reflected proximally and the remaining musculature, especially the vastus medialis and the remnants of the adductors, are separated from the tumor. The tibia is then reamed to accept the stem of the total prosthesis, and methylmethacrylate is placed in the tibia after a trial reduction of the prosthesis. After the tibial component is secured, the prosthesis is set into the acetabulum. The previously tagged glutei are attached with heavy chromic catgut through preformed holes in the proximal prosthetic shaft; the medial and lateral thigh muscles are attached to each other. The distal hamstrings are brought anteriorly to act as knee extensors. The wound is carefully checked for hemostasis, irrigated, and closed with heavy sutures prior to final skin closing. The wound is drained with suction catheters, and the patient is placed on large doses of antibiotics. Following any major resection in the extremity, a drop-foot gait is fairly well tolerated, even from the en-bloc resection, and the gait is usually normal with a Klensac brace. Hamstrings are not necessary for walking, but the patient will say that his leg is sluggish while running. The quadriceps muscles can be absent, but some sort of knee extension brace is necessary to ensure strength and to prevent the patient from falling. Those patients without abductor or extensor (gluteus maximus) hip muscles have characteristic limps: they tend to lean toward their weak side. If the common femoral vein is removed as part of the operation, replacement is usually not necessary, but the legs should be carefully evaluated for several months to ensure only minimal edema formation. In general, a patient with extensive resection of the muscle groups of the thigh associated with total femoral replacement can function quite adequately when normal wound healing occurs.

Total Knee Replacement

En-bloc excision for malignant tumors involving the region of the knee has been performed with good results. The surgery involving the proximal tibia, knee joint, and distal femur with soft tissues in the popliteal space is compensated for by insertion of a Guepar total knee replacement. Figure 9–5 shows the Guepar knee prosthesis with the knee joint bolted and separated. The stems are interchangeable so that appropriate lengths can be chosen in the operating room.

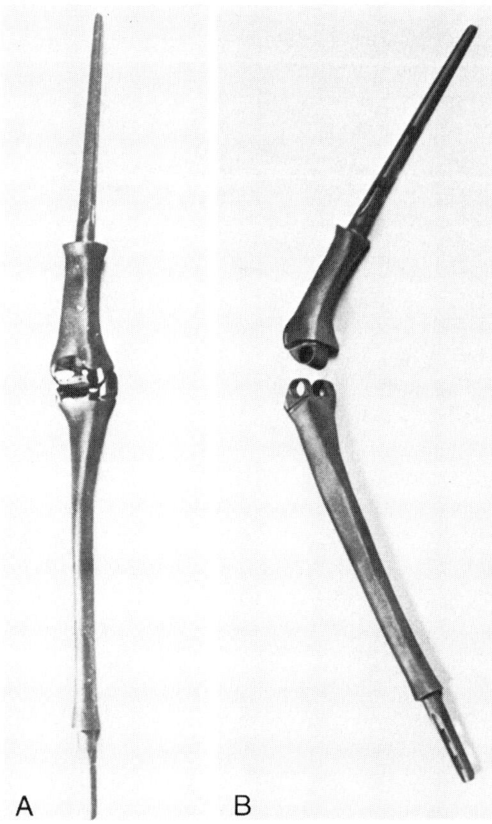

FIGURE 9–5. A and B, Guepar knee prosthesis.

The candidates for this procedure are informed prior to surgery that they will need to use a long-leg ischial weightbearing brace for an extended postoperative period. Other limb-saving alternatives include knee fusion with a long bone graft, and use of the Küntscher nail from the hip to the ankle, a procedure that has been used since 1963. To date, no patient has opted for the knee fusion to avoid wearing a brace.

The operation is performed to include the biopsy site and the tract of the incision. All of the thigh muscles are incised at their insertions at the distal femur, patella, and proximal tibia and fibula, provided that they are clear of the tumor pseudocapsule. Similarly, the muscle origins of the calf that are clear of the tumor site are dissected. As much as possible of the neurovascular system is salvaged. Care must be taken to preserve the cutaneous nerves.

The distal femur, patella, proximal tibia and fibula, and the muscles, nerves, arteries, and veins immediately surrounding the tumor are removed en bloc and sent for pathologic analysis after the bones are osteotomized. If frozen section shows margins of the specimen to be free of tumor, then the rest of the procedure is continued. If any of the marginal areas show tumor, a mid-thigh amputation is usually performed after sterile instruments are supplied. Good hemostasis is obtained. After removal of the en-bloc specimen, the femur and tibia are reamed to accept the Guepar total knee prosthesis. Frozen section readings are obtained to ensure that no tumor is present in the remaining bone marrow. (A Guepar knee prosthesis is preferred since it allows for 160° knee flexion, whereas a Walldius prosthesis only allows for 90° flexion at the knee.)

The prosthesis is inserted to assure proper fitting. It is then removed, and the entire wound (and prosthesis) is cleansed with an antibiotic solution. The femoral components of the prosthesis are inserted and properly aligned, and methyl methacrylate is introduced into the medullary cavity through the previously drilled holes. The same procedure is followed for the tibial component. Then the knee joint is secured with a bolt and washer.

After the cement has hardened, the remaining musculature and neurovascular bundles are attached to the prosthesis. Skin and fascia are closed in layers. Hemovac drains are placed in the wound to allow for drainage. Immediately after closing the wound, sterile dressings and a large knee splint are applied to mobilize the knee.

Total replacement procedures can easily be modified to the desires and needs of the surgeon.[1]

REFERENCE

1. Marcove R. C., Abou-Zahr K.: En-bloc surgery for osteogenic sarcoma: Analysis and review of ninety operative cases. Bull. N.Y. Acad. Med. 60:748–758, 1984

CHAPTER

10

Sarcomas On and About the Abdomen and Chest Wall

Sarcomas arising on and about the superficial structures of the trunk, chest, and abdominal wall are well defined. These lesions, however, are not so frequently encountered as those of the extremities. When they do appear, it is essential that they be identified correctly and be treated promptly and in the proper manner, since failure to do so may result in an uncontrollable situation. Figure 10–1 shows a patient with advanced myxoliposarcoma of the back, treated by local excision and radiation. It illustrates the extent to which an incompletely resected sarcoma can spread to involve surrounding structures. This involvement occurred even though the tumor was initially believed to be low-grade with a high potential for cure. Such tumors require wide resection with adequate margins of normal surrounding tissue for there to be any potential for cure. Resection here may require that dissection be carried to the underlying deep fascial planes and muscles of the chest wall and perhaps even include a portion of the rib cage. Under such circumstances a moderate amount of overlying skin may be lost, so that pedicle flap (cutaneous or myocutaneous) reconstruction may be necessary. Incomplete resection, as in this case, can lead to uncontrollable disease and subsequent fatal hemorrhage. At no time was there evidence of distant metastasis in this patient; rather the problem represented one of failure to control local disease. When an aggressive approach is taken early, even high-grade malignancies can be managed satisfactorily. As an example, rhabdomyosarcoma arising from rib cage of the chest or back can present with difficult management decisions that must often be resolved quickly. One of our patients, a 35-year-old woman, noticed a peculiar lump on her back. In actuality, a mass had arisen from under the wing of the scapula. Biopsy proved the lesion to be rhabdomyosarcoma encompassing the teres and rhomboid muscle groups. Our initial impression was that the lesion had arisen primarily from one of the intrinsic muscle groups of the scapula, but on exploration for resection the lesion proved to arise from the intercostal muscles of the posterior rib cage, secondarily invading the scapula. The lesion grew in an inferior direction, forced by the overlying scapula to follow the path of least resistance. The tumor eventually reached the undersurface of the teres region, then protruded from under the scapula. In preparation for scapulectomy, it was obvious that en-bloc resection with the underlying chest wall was necessary. The rib cage that was resected was replaced by Marlex mesh, and the patient was placed on a course of chemotherapy for approximately 1 year. Five years later she remains free of disease.

That chest wall resection may be necessary is again illustrated in the case of a 55-year-old man who presented with a soft axillary mass that was clinically believed to be a lipoma. The tumor mass was locally resected, and histologic examination revealed it to be a low-grade liposarcoma. Radiation therapy was given externally and by afterloading to a dose of 6000 R. Within 1 year, the tumor had recurred in the radiated field (Fig. 10–2A). On clinical examination and review of the CT scan (Fig. 10–

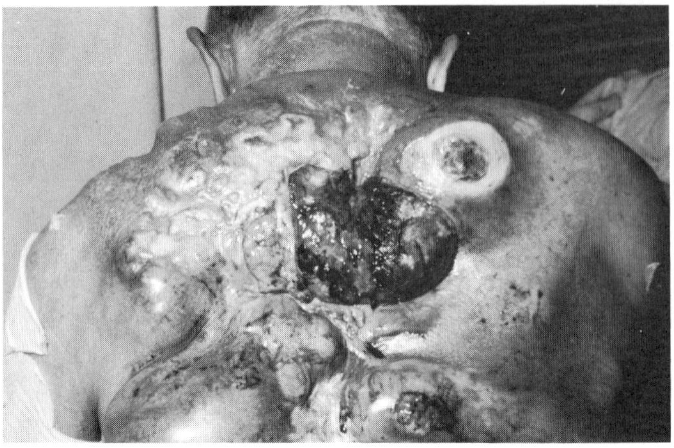

FIGURE 10–1. Extensive myxoliposarcoma of the back.

2*B* and *C*) it was obvious that the tumor had invaded the rib cage and infiltrated close to the neurovascular bundle of the axilla. Wide resection of the tumor with the underlying fourth and fifth ribs along with axillary dissection appeared to provide adequate margins. Figure 10–2*D* shows the defect in the rib cage with exposure of the underlying lung. The chest wall with overlying attached tumor and pleura has been turned laterally off the lung. Marlex mesh was inserted, and sliding pedicle flaps were used to cover the resulting defect.

PLEURAL MESOTHELIOMA

Among the tumors occasionally encountered in the region of the chest wall are

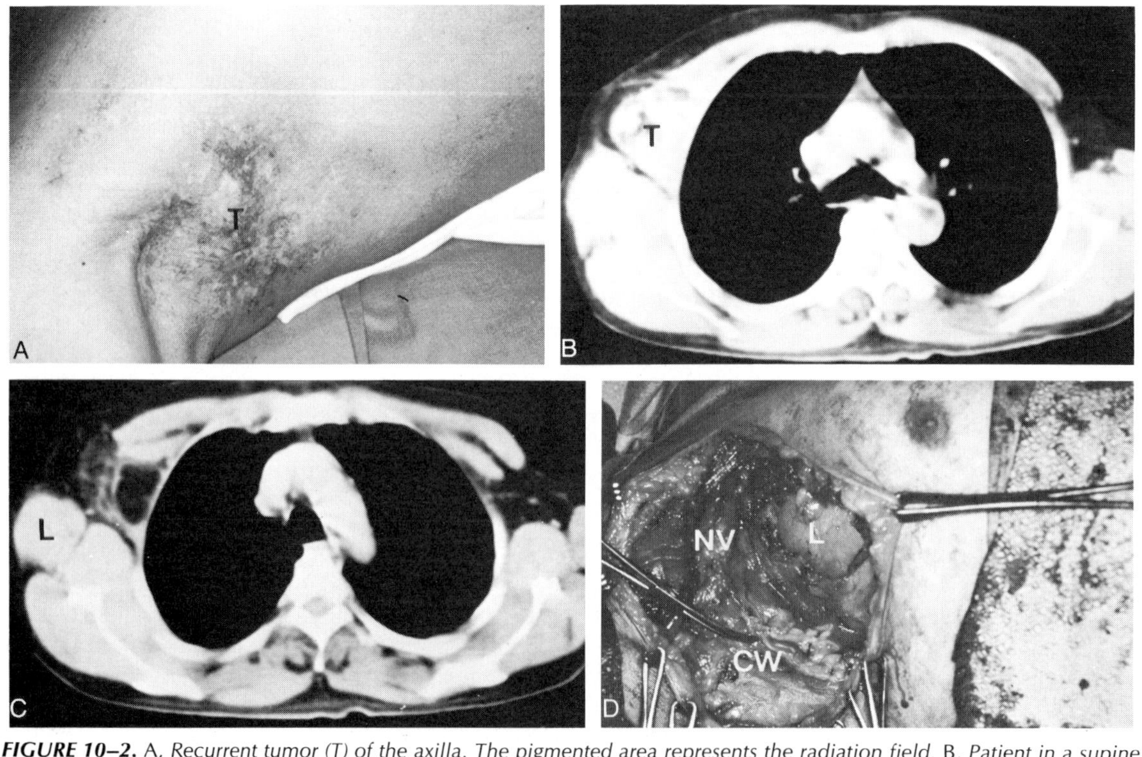

FIGURE 10–2. A, Recurrent tumor (T) of the axilla. The pigmented area represents the radiation field. B, Patient in a supine position with his right arm extended. CT scan of the chest, with tumor (T) arising in the axilla adjacent to the chest wall. C, The recurrent tumor is seen in close relationship to the latissimus (L). D, Chest wall resection of the tumor. The underlying lung (L) has been exposed as a result of mobilizing chest wall (CW) with tumor. The proximity of the site of resection to the neurovascular bundle (NV) can be seen.

sarcomas arising primarily from the pleura and lung parenchyma.[12] Two categories of primary pleural tumors have been defined. The more common, diffuse type, associated with asbestosis, is the malignant mesothelioma. The patients present with chest pain, shortness of breath, and significant weight loss over a short period of time. Pleural effusion usually accumulates rapidly.[25] This tumor is rarely resectable and responds poorly to known chemotherapeutic protocols. Less frequent in occurrence but of importance in terms of management is the solitary type, representing a spectrum of pathologic lesions known as fibrous mesothelioma, benign mesothelioma, and localized fibrous tumor of pleura. Briselli et al.[8] reported eight cases of this tumor seen at the Massachusetts General Hospital and reviewed 360 previously reported cases. None of these patients had been exposed to asbestos. Five of the eight patients were asymptomatic but their lesions had been defined on routine chest x-rays. Two patients complained of chest pains and cough. None had pulmonary osteoarthropathy. Of the 360 cases reviewed 4% had hypoglycemia, a symptom known to be associated with an array of fibrous tissue tumors.

Categorization of the mesotheliomas into localized and diffuse can be attributed to Klemperer and Rabin (1931). The cell of origin is not well defined, but it appears that fibroblasts and mesothelial cells may be related through a common precursor cell or modulation of one cell type to another. Wide resection of the solitary lesion is essential.[20] Although hemorrhage, necrosis, and cellular pleomorphism may be worrisome features, this does not suggest nor has it implied that recurrence will take place. Conversely, lack of cellular atypia and mitosis does not guarantee freedom from recurrence. Pedunculated lesions are less likely to recur. Patients with unresectable tumors, whether primary or recurrent, deteriorate rapidly. At no time does the solitary lesion convert to the diffuse type, and metastasis with this form of mesothelioma is uncommon. We recently encountered a primary abdominal wall tumor thought to be a desmoid. Biopsy proved it to be a solitary mesothelioma arising in abdominal wall (Fig. 10–3). Wide resection with Marlex mesh replacement was performed.

SARCOMAS OF THE LUNGS

Intrathoracic sarcomas arise not only from the pleura and chest wall but also from the pulmonary structures. Nascimento et al.[29] described 18 patients with primary sarcomas of the lung seen at the Mayo Clinic between 1950 and 1978. Such lesions are known to be rare, with only one case appearing for every 500 carcinomas of the lung. Fibrosarcomas and leiomyosarcomas appear to be the most common of these pulmonary lesions, although osteosarcomas, chondrosar-

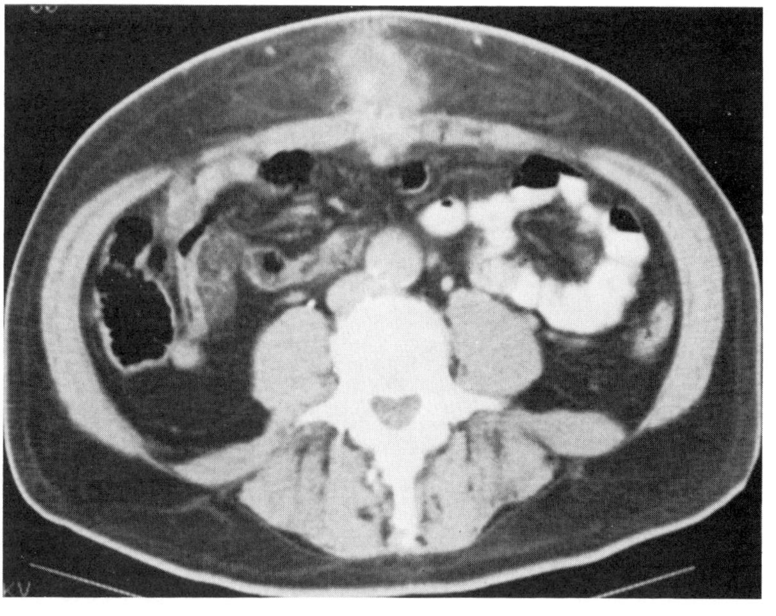

FIGURE 10–3. Solitary mesothelioma of the abdominal wall seen as a midline anterior lesion extending through the rectus to infiltrate the peritoneum.

comas, and hemangiopericytomas have all been described.[39] In 1972 the AFIP reported 32 cases of bronchopulmonary fibrosarcomas and leiomyosarcomas. Among those patients reported in the Mayo Clinic study, chest pain and cough were the most frequent signs. Dyspnea, fatigue, fever, and hypoglycemia were also noted. In one patient, hypoglycemia was corrected when the tumor was removed, but recurred with the reappearance of disease in the mediastinum. The roentgenographic manifestations of primary pulmonary sarcomas have no distinctive characteristics and usually appear as large, well-circumscribed, peripheral mass lesions without cavitation. Several of the tumors have been primarily interbronchial, and here obstructive pneumonitis has dominated the abnormalities seen on x-ray examination. Surgery is the primary treatment to be offered when feasible. Of the nine patients in the Mayo series with fibrosarcoma, seven died of disease 3 months to 18 years after treatment. Two of the patients with leiomyosarcoma have remained free of disease after 5 years. One of the major considerations with resection of such lesions is for one to be fully assured that a primary occult lesion does not exist elswhere, e.g., in the retroperitoneum or extremity. With the use of CT scanning techniques, however, the possibility of missing a primary retroperitoneal sarcoma has been minimized. Three of the four patients in the Mayo Clinic series who survived had undergone lobectomy for their tumor; the fourth had a wedge resection. More extensive surgery was usually associated with the larger lesions, thus carrying a less favorable prognosis.

MEDIASTINAL TUMORS

Intrathoracic Neurogenic Tumors

Soft part tumors of mediastinal origin must also be included among those arising within the confines of the chest wall. For the most part the lesions represent intrathoracic neurogenic tumors.[1] There are few areas of tumor pathology as confusing as neoplasms of the nervous system, and primary intrathoracic neurogenic tumors are no exception. The clinical presentation and management of these patients is fairly uniform, regardless of tumor type. It is common for the lesion to be discovered on a routine or screening chest x-ray film. Symptoms, when present, usually are due to encroachment by the tumor on adjacent structures and include pain, dyspnea, cyanosis, orthopnea, cough, and hemoptysis. Subsequent chest x-ray film usually delineates the lesion. These tumors may manifest an uncommon clinical form in which a portion can be intrathoracic and the other portion intraspinal (dumbbell or hourglass tumor). In these cases symptoms referable to spinal cord compression may be the initial complaint. In almost all cases, these tumors are located in the posterior mediastinum. They are by far the most common tumor in that area. There are, however, rare cases of neurogenic tumors found elsewhere in the thorax. By definition, the paravertebral gutter is considered part of the posterior mediastinum and most of the tumors arise here. Once the presence of a tumor in the posterior mediastinum has been established, the treatment is thoracotomy and adequate excision. This treatment applies in all cases, regardless of the histology of the tumor. The confusion in the nomenclature and classification has prevented uniform reporting of results; therefore, the prognostic evaluation of each lesion is speculative. Three or four decades ago many of the neurogenic tumors were reported as malignant, with figures in many series reaching 40%. With experience in diagnosis of such lesions, the percentage of malignant neurogenic tumors has dropped to about 15%. Primary intrathoracic neurogenic tumors obviously arise from nervous

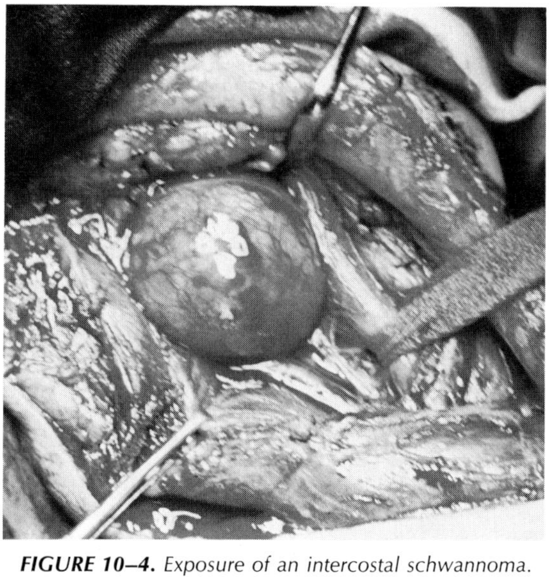

FIGURE 10–4. *Exposure of an intercostal schwannoma.*

tissue found in this region: mainly the intercostal nerves and the sympathetic chain (Fig. 10–4). There have been reports of vagus nerve tumors, tumors of the aortic glands of Zuckerkandl, and tumors of the chromaffin tissue found in sympathetic ganglia (paraganglionic tissue), but they are rare and comprise less than 1% of the total. Their clinical manifestations and subsequent management are the same as the more common ones. Tumors of nerve sheath origin are generally classified into the benign neurilemmoma, neurofibromatosis, and the malignant schwannoma. The variable microscopic patterns seen with both the benign and the malignant forms account for the different classifications applied to nerve tumors such as triton tumor with rhabdomyoblastic differentiation, malignant glandular schwannoma, and malignant epithelioid schwannoma.

The variable microscopic pictures account for the different classifications employed. A careful search of each tumor will reveal some characteristics of all of the known patterns, but the diagnosis depends on the predominant one. Common features include long, slender wire-like fibers with elongated nuclei that have a tendency to be arranged in parallel or palisade fashion. Palisading always suggests nerve sheath origin. In the malignant form, these characteristics tend to be lost. Unencapsulated neurilemmoma (neurofibroma) is often associated with von Recklinghausen's disease, a poorly understood, often familial condition associated with multiple nerve tumors and patchy skin pigmentation. There are many other possible manifestations of this disease, and it is considered to be a generalized connective tissue abnormality. Many malignant neurilemmomas are found in patients with von Recklinghausen's disease, probably secondary to changes in previously benign tumors.

Tumors of sympathetic nervous system origin arise in the sympathetic chain. The ganglioneuroma is composed of mature ganglion cells in the stroma of myelinated and nonmyelinated sheathed nerve fibers. Neuroblastomas consist of undifferentiated small round cells, a few imperfect ganglion cells, and nerve fibrils. The nerve fibrils form a distinctive feature, as the neuroblasts grouped around them form "rosettes," which are highly characteristic of this tumor.

In 1951 Ackerman[1] reported 48 cases of primary neurogenic tumors of the thorax; 31 (65%) were of nerve sheath origin and 17 (35%) originated from the sympathetic nervous system. Four of the nerve sheath tumors were malignant; three of these patients died. The survivor developed a local recurrence 20 months after initial excision and lived for more than 54 months after reexcision. Three of the patients had von Recklinghausen's disease, and one of these was the survivor. Seven (41%) of the 17 sympathetic nervous system tumors were ganglioneuromas, and these patients were well at the time of the report. All patients with malignant tumors of the sympathetic nervous system and of nerve sheath origin had symptoms, the most common of which was pain, usually as a result of involvement of the intercostal or brachial nerve plexus. Spinal cord compression, seen in three cases (two malignant, one benign), was produced by the growth of tumor through the spinal foramina into the spinal canal. Horner's syndrome was present in six cases but had no clinical significance. There may be dyspnea, orthopnea, cyanosis, or dysphagia caused by tracheal or esophageal obstruction.

Practically all of these neoplasms are located in the posterior mediastinum and present a sharply circumscribed round or oval homogeneous mass. There may be local areas of calcification in both benign and malignant masses, but this is rare for mediastinal neuroblastomas. The retroperitoneal neuroblastomas, however, are frequently calcified around the adrenal gland. Erosion of the ribs and spine adjacent to the tumor is usually a consequence of pressure and not of malignant infiltration. Neuroblastomas are rarely discrete and practically always are located superiorly in the posterior mediastinum. In a review of 24 cases from Memorial Hospital, Godwin found only two cases of malignant nerve tumors.[15]

Mediastinal lymph nodes may at times be involved with metastatic sarcoma. We have seen clear cell schwannoma metastatic to the mediastinal nodes and containing triton tumor as part of the histologic diversity of the nodal involvement. Such findings represent end-stage disease, and attempts at therapy have not been fruitful.

Mediastinal Lipomatous Tumors and Liposarcoma

Lipomatous tissue can also found in the mediastinal region and is subject to changes that occur elsewhere in the body. We have

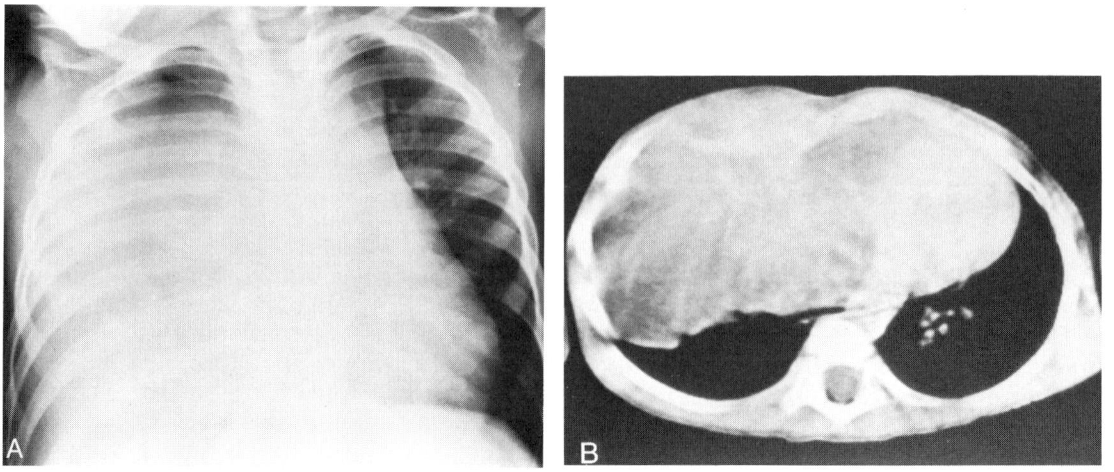

FIGURE 10–5. A, Large intrapleural-mediastinal mass opacifying the right pleural space and displacing the mediastinum to the left. B, CT scan shows displacement of the midline structures to the left.

encountered large mediastinal lipomas but have not dealt with any liposarcomas in this region. We recently examined a 2-year-old child who had been evaluated at Brookdale Hospital by Esteves and Strikoff. The child had been complaining of progressive respiratory distress. Chest x-ray film and CT scan showed a large mass displacing the mediastinum to the left (Fig. 10–5). Resection proved the tumor to be lipoblastomatosis, a fetal fatty tumor that has a grossly lobular pattern. Two forms have been described: (1) a diffuse infiltrating variety and (2) a well-circumscribed noninfiltrating type, the lipoblastoma. The diffuse type has lobules joined by loose connective tissue septa and supplied by an arborized vascular system. Histologically it resembles hibernoma with numerous spindle-shaped cells but contains fewer cells with eosinophilic cytoplasm. Conservative resection of such tumors is believed to yield an excellent response. Cicciarelli et al. reviewed 14 lipomas and liposarcomas of the mediastinum, one of which was a lipoma of the thymus.[11] Castleberry et al.[10] presented a case of a 13-year-old boy with a mediastinal liposarcoma. The patient was noted to have progressive shortness of breath over a 5-month period, and a nonproductive cough that developed over the preceding 2 weeks. Chest x-ray film revealed complete opacification of the right thorax. At thoracotomy a large friable fatty tumor was found arising from the mediastinum. A biopsy was performed and revealed myxoid liposarcoma. Because of airway impingement and the size of the lesion, postoperative radiation therapy was attempted. A regimen of vincristine, adriamycin, and cyclophosphamide was started, and an objective response was apparent on chest films 6 weeks after discharge from the hospital. Four months later sufficient resolution had occurred to allow complete resection of the tumor.

The diagnosis may need to be reevaluated after the clinical behavior of a tumor has been watched over a period of time. Heinman and Lehman[17] treated a 63-year-old woman for a large mediastinal liposarcoma. The tumor eventually metastasized to other parts of the body as a liposarcoma, fibrosarcoma, and chondrosarcoma, proving that they were in reality dealing with a mesenchymal sarcoma.

Mediastinal Leiomyosarcoma

Leiomyosarcoma has also been noted to arise in the mediastinum. Sunderrajan et al.[40] described a patient with associated superior vena cava obstruction. Initially although there was no evidence of metastases, but because of extensive local disease, radiation therapy was administered. Pleural effusion formed rapidly, and biopsy showed leiomyosarcoma with negative esophageal studies. The lesion was consistent with vena caval origin, the most common origin for such tumors invading the mediastinum. In terms of venous disorders resulting in an x-ray diagnosis of a mediastinal mass one must consider mediastinal pseudotumor. In patients with cirrhosis and portal hypertension, aneurysmal dilatation of the azygos vein, hemiazygos vein, or esophageal varices has been reported and confused with malignant neoplasm.[18]

TUMORS OF CHEST WALL

With respect to the external region of the chest and abdominal wall, size and clinical appearance of the tumor do not always characterize the behavior of the neoplasm in question. A common lesion of the trunk is the lipoma; less common is its malignant counterpart, the liposarcoma. At times an unusual variation will present as a painless, circumscribed subcutaneous mass that resembles an ordinary lipoma on gross examination. Microscopically, however, this neoplasm is characterized by an intimate admixture of variably sized fat cells and bizarre, pleomorphic, multinucleated giant cells. This tumor, the pleomorphic lipoma, occurs principally in men (83%) during the fifth to seventh decade and shows a predilection for the posterior neck, shoulder, and back. Despite its usual pleomorphic picture, which not infrequently leads to a misdiagnosis of liposarcoma, follow-up data obtained for 34 patients (Shmookler et al.[37]) establish the invariably benign nature of this tumor.

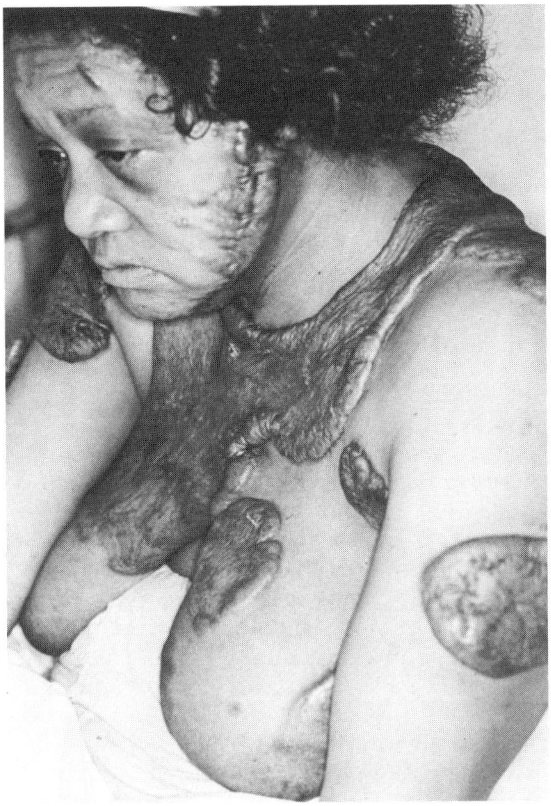

FIGURE 10–6. *Extensive keloids of the chest wall.*

Fibrous Tumors

Figure 10–6 shows the appearance of extensive tumor masses of the anterior chest wall resulting from minor skin irritation duc to mosquito bites. While such cutaneous fibrous tumors (keloids) are atypical when compared with what can normally be seen as a result of surgery or trauma, they do represent the extent to which fibroblastic proliferation can take place. In considering the clinical behavior of such lesions, it is apparent that there is a wide spectrum for such tumors of fibrous tissue origin, beginning with the well-known keloid, progressing to plantar and palmar fibromatosis, then to the desmoid tumor and dermatofibrosarcoma protuberans, a tumor commonly involving chest wall. Eventually the fully malignant fibrosarcomas are seen at the other end of the spectrum of such tumors. The clinical pattern set by any of these lesions does not appear to be wholly related to any existing microscopic pattern; rather the behavior of such tumors tends to be associated with the relative position it occupies within this spectrum of fibrous tissue responses.[2] Knowledge, therefore, of the relationship that exists within this spectrum is important in predicting the clinical behavior and deciding treatment.

In the past, the significance of cellular activity among the fibrous tissue tumors has often been misinterpreted, with early invasiveness or metastasis predicted yet never occurring. Similarly, a lesion that appears to be histologically benign may have already either invaded locally or metastasized. In a case reported by Prior and Sisson,[34] a thumb was amputated because of a fibroma. A lung lesion subsequently was removed by pneumonectomy and proved to be a fibroma similar to that on the thumb.

The simplest and least reactive of the fibrous tissue tumors occurs at the lower end of a spectrum of fibrous tumors and is represented by the keloid; the other end is the fully malignant fibrosarcoma. The keloid is characterized by an overproduction of fibrous tissue, usually as the result of trauma to the skin. In the aforementioned patient who presented with extensive cutaneous lesions of the chest wall, a mosquito bite was sufficiently traumatic to induce the proliferative fibrous response. While this response may vary, most keloids remain confined to the site of injury and produce, at minimum, a cosmetic problem. Microscopically, a large amount of collagen characterizes the lesion. In rare instances, massive proliferation of tumor tissue can occur; such lesions may fail to respond to the classic treatment with intralesional steroids or to the use of post-resection radiation therapy (800 R).

More commonly, among the large nodular masses found on the anterior abdominal and chest walls, desmoids are of prime consideration.[7,13,31,36] These growths, which denote the presence of a tendinous tumor, were described by Mueller in 1938. That these tumors have a tendency for local recurrence after resection has long been recognized (Bennett, Paget). In 1923 Hartman reported 16 cases of tumor arising from the anterior abdominal wall. Brasfield and DasGupta[7] described a series of 38 cases seen at Memorial Hospital. The ratio of females to males was high, 3 to 1. The mean age for the group was 30 years, with two patients younger than 10. Eighteen of the tumors in this series occurred in the rectus abdominis muscle and the external oblique muscle of the abdominal wall; two were in the internal oblique and transverse muscles and two in the transverse abdominis muscle. The majority presented with a painless anterior abdominal wall mass. Only four patients complained of any abdominal symptoms. Pregnancy could be directly linked to the tumor in six patients; the pregnancy was usually a second one, and the tumor usually arose in the anterior rectus sheath. The origin of tumors arising at this site may represent the effect of stretching of muscle fibers or the effect of trauma. Cases of abdominal desmoids have been seen after repeated traumatic episodes to the anterior abdominal wall. Surgical scars were definitely associated with the development of tumor in six patients. The differential diagnosis of the abdominal wall masses should include the following: (1) fibrosarcoma, the most important tumor to be considered; (2) neurilemomma, a softer lesion, more commonly seen with von Recklinghausen's disease; (3) dermatofibrosarcoma, which usually presents as a more nodular lesion; and (4) lipoma, a tumor frequently of subfascial origin. The findings of an abdominal wall mass in a patient recently pregnant usually signifies the presence of an abdominal desmoid tumor. There is little question that these tumors are under the influence of hormones and that the pregnant state offers the optimal milieu for the growth of this tumor. Kinzbrunner et al. described the remission of rapidly growing desmoid tumors after therapy with the antiestrogen tamoxifen.[21] While metastases are essentially never seen, wide resection must be performed to prevent local recurrence. Only four patients in Brasfield's[7] series developed such local recurrence after curative resection; three presented with recurrence when first seen. Adequate surgical management may necessitate resection of a considerable portion of abdominal musculature, underlying the parietal peritoneum and periosteum of pelvic bones when necessary. In certain instances, large tumors may actually penetrate through the peritoneum, necessitating inclusion of the visceral contents with the resection. The defect that remains is usually reconstructed by inserting Marlex mesh and sliding skin flaps over the inserted plastic prosthesis. Because the desmoid tumor is considered by many to represent a low-grade fibrosarcoma, wide resection (Fig. 10–7) with adequate margins of resection (at

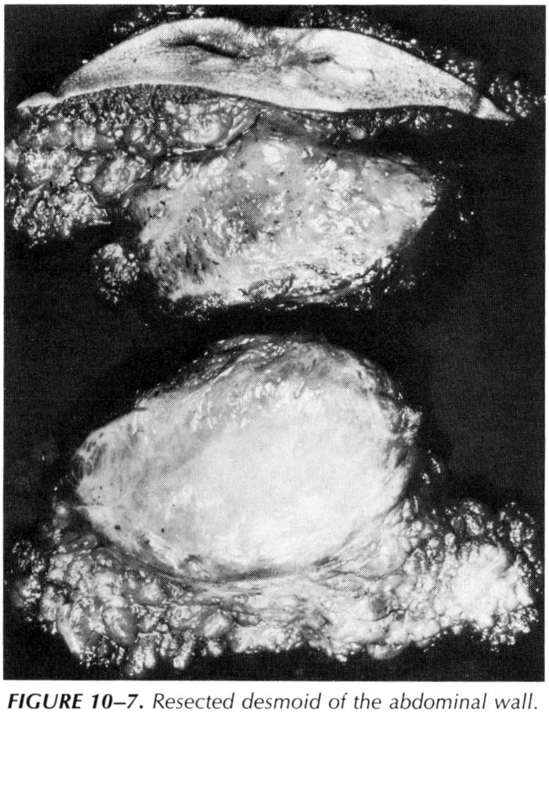

FIGURE 10–7. *Resected desmoid of the abdominal wall.*

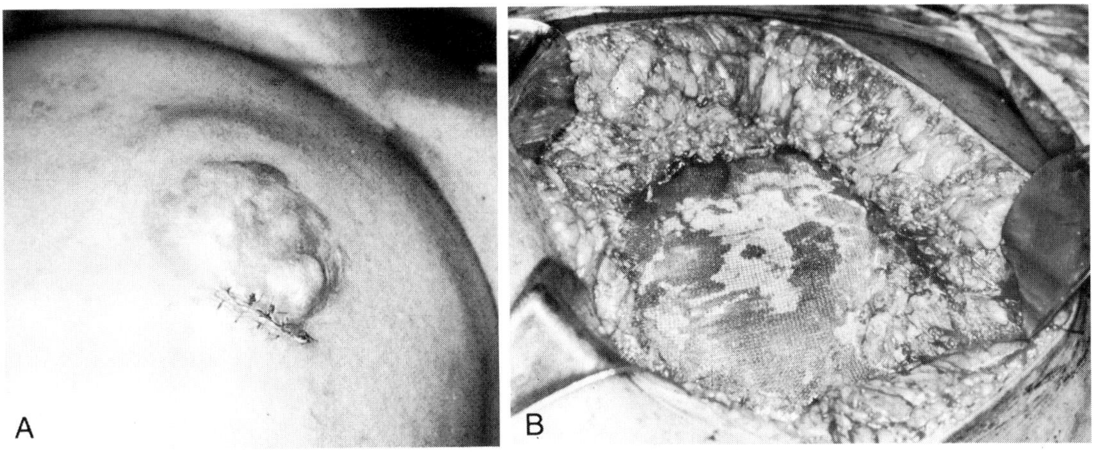

FIGURE 10–8. A, Desmoid of the abdominal wall. Sutures represent the site of biopsy. B, Operative field showing Marlex mesh used for replacement.

least 4 to 5 cm) is needed to prevent the typical patterns of local recurrence seen. The treatment, in general, is well defined and follows the principles established for essentially all sarcomas. This tumor, in particular, tends to infiltrate through its pseudocapsule and into the adjacent fascial planes, making margins of resection difficult to define even by frozen section. The finding of giant cells in the periphery of the tumor and in the surrounding tissue usually represents coalesced muscle nuclei destroyed by tumor invasion. Adequate resection usually requires that the underlying fascia be resected along with the tumor mass; Marlex mesh is most often used for replacement of musculofascial defects, though other synthetic meshes, ox fascia, and tensor fasciae latae have also been used. Figure 10–8*A* shows the clinical appearance of such a lesion and the defect as it was being repaired with mesh (Fig. 10–8*B*). A variant of this tumor may be found in the extra-abdominal position.[13] These tumors appear to be somewhat more aggressive and travel centripetally, frequently invading the pleural cavity when the primary has appeared on the shoulder girdle. Figure 10–9 shows a resected desmoid of the chest wall, which appeared in the second interspace adjacent to the clavicle and sternum. The specimen consisted of the lateral half of the clavicle, the sternum, and the ribs, with tumor well contained in the resected material. Marlex was used to close the defect and achieve chest wall stability.

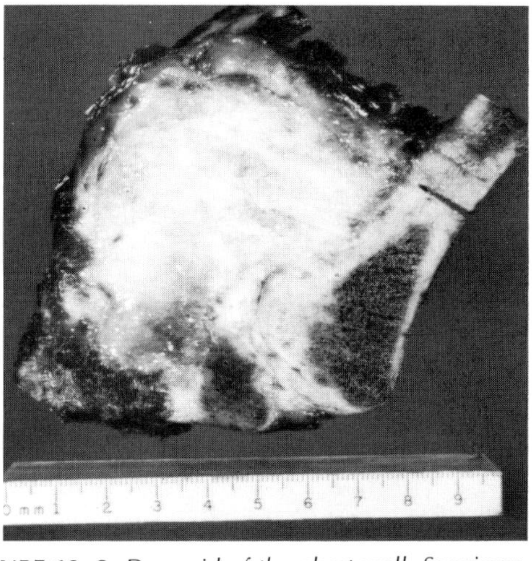

FIGURE 10–9. Desmoid of the chest wall. Specimen contains resected medial clavicle and a portion of the sternum.

Desmoids may affect all age groups, including children. The first case reported in a young child was by Temain, in 1893. His patient, a 2-year-old, presented with a markedly enlarged abdominal wall lesion that weighed 1400 gm. The tumor was removed when the child was 14 years of age. Greeg, in 1915, reported the occurrence of a desmoid tumor in the sheath of the rectus abdominis muscle in a 20-month-old female child. Wausch, in 1940, described a case of a 5-year-old who had injured his abdominal wall by falling from a bed. Within 1 month of this trauma, a small tumor had developed and by 4 months it had measured 7 by 10 cm. Pathogenesis was probably related to a disturbance in the organization of the hematoma that resulted from the fall. Booher and Pack[6] described three additional cases of desmoid tumors in children. It was believed that every relatively cellular fibroma, no matter how indolent the clinical or his-

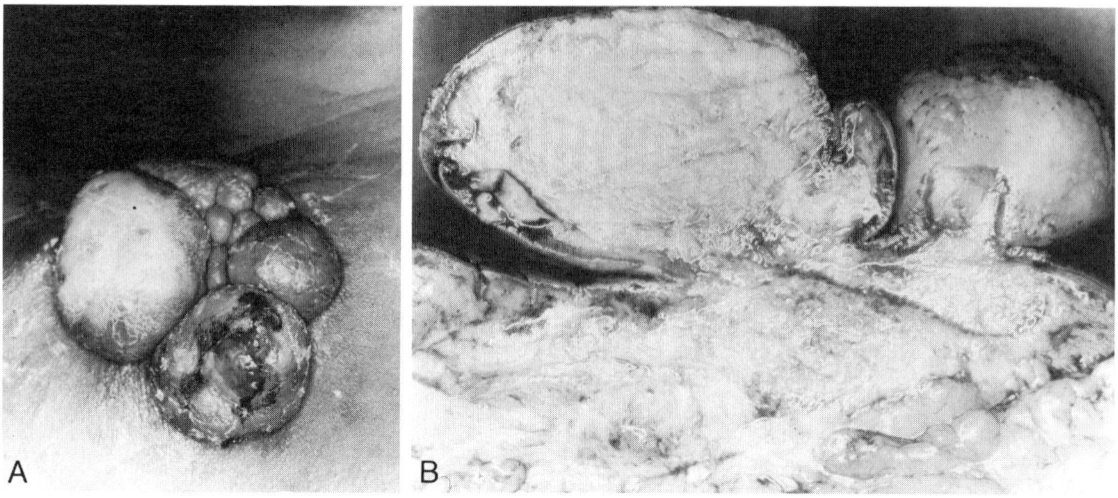

FIGURE 10–10. *A, Large dermatofibrosarcoma protuberans of upper midline back. B, Section taken through tumor.*

tologic appearance, should be considered malignant until the subsequent behavior of the tumor is established.

The problem of dealing with recurrence of desmoids is quite common, because all too often the lesion has not been considered malignant and adequate resection is not performed. When this tumor reappears it requires further resection beyond what was initially performed, even if a major portion of the abdominal wall or chest wall is to be removed. Replacement by means of mesh and use of a rotation pedicle flap for skin coverage is always necessary. Adequate resection is usually curative. Recurrence developed in only 4 of 35 patients among the patients with desmoid treated at Memorial Hospital.[7, 36] Distant metastasis is unusual. The more common patterns for recurrence are with those lesions that are classified higher in the spectrum of fibrous tissue tumors, such as dermatofibrosarcoma protuberans. Figure 10–10*A* shows the appearance of dermatofibrosarcoma of the back, which had been present since the patient was a teenager. He stated that he had been repeatedly struck on his back with a stick and that the initial lesion developed at the site of trauma. The lesion continued to enlarge slowly. This growth pattern persisted until the time of surgical intervention. The lesion was completely resected and the defect closed with a split-thickness graft because of the size of the base of the tumor. Figure 10–10*B* shows the transected specimen.

Dermatofibrosarcoma frequently recurs locally. Figure 10–11*A* shows a recurrence on the chest wall. Wide resection to the periosteum of the sternum and ribs was performed and closure carried out with an abdominal rotation pedicle flap. Should the underlying chest wall need to be resected, stability can be achieved with Marlex mesh. The mesh should be folded over at its edges (doubled) and sutured first with interrupted Marlex or prolene sutures placed into the bone or periosteum. A second layer of running sutures is used for approximation of the edges of the prosthesis to the surrounding fascia, which results in a taut, firm layer of mesh. In the abdominal wall, stability with Marlex alone is easily achieved and hernias are obviated. To prevent paradoxical motion in the chest wall, methyl methacrylate can be applied between layers of Marlex to achieve rigidity. Figure 10–11*B* shows the site of primary resection of the large recurrent dermatofibrosarcoma of the chest wall seen in Figure 10–11*A*. The pedicle was mobilized and folded adjacent to the nipple. The pedicle was then turned into the defect and the abdominal wall edges approximated to fill in the donor site (Fig. 10–11*C*). This patient has remained free of recurrence for more than 5 years.

The term "dermatofibrosarcoma protuberans" was first used by Hoffman, in 1925, to describe the characteristic lesion he noted. In 1951 Pack and Tabah[32] reported the first series of these tumors; this has been followed by more recent studies that indicate a more aggressive potential for metastases

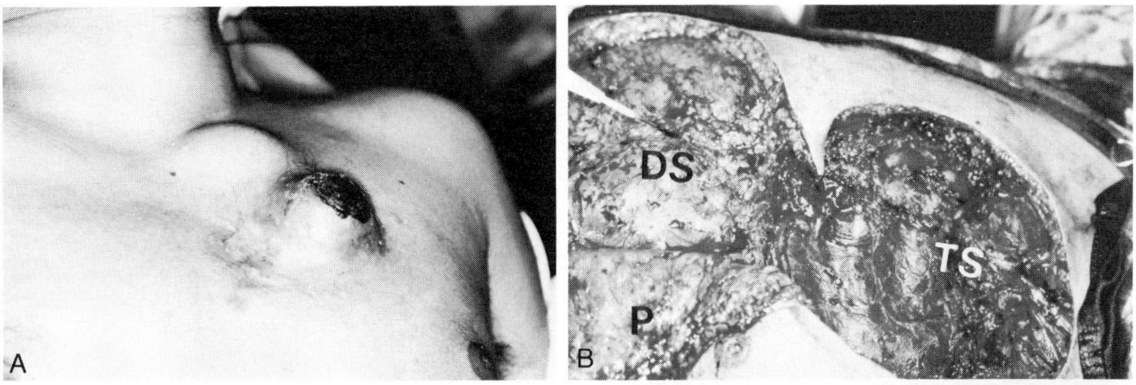

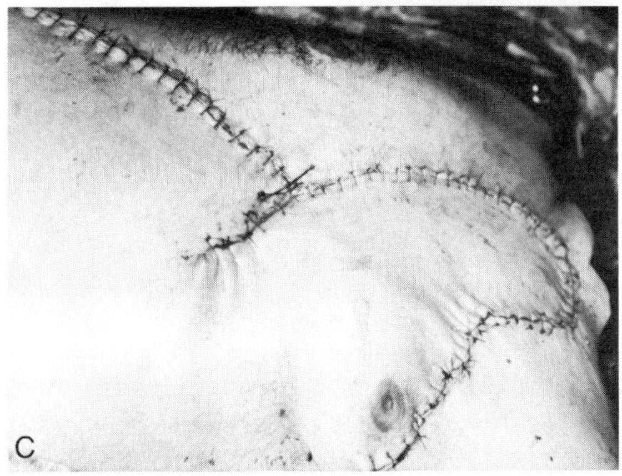

FIGURE 10–11. A, Recurrent dermatofibrosarcoma of the chest wall. B, Operative field following resection of tumor. TS represents the site of tumor resection and DS the donor site from which the pedicle P was raised. The pedicle is seen turned on itself adjacent to the areola in preparation for placement into TS. C, The appearance of the chest wall after the pedicle flap has been turned into position (TS). The defect (DS) was closed by mobilizing wound edges and approximating them in a verticle line.

than was originally realized. One of the initial reports of metastatic spread from this tumor was described by Bezency in 1933. Among the more than 100 cases seen at Memorial Sloan-Kettering Cancer Center, the abdominal wall has been the most common site, followed by the chest, back, and shoulder.[13]

Microscopically the lesion is composed of plump fibroblasts arranged in whorls around an inconspicuous vasculature. Mitosis and nuclear pleomorphism are rare. In spite of a circumscribed clinical appearance, tumor cells tend to diffusely infiltrate the dermis, requiring wide margins of resection for cure. A nodule usually enlarges and eventually erodes the skin. Over a prolonged period, satellite nodules will appear, tending to coalesce and eventually become more protuberant. As the overlying skin stretches, it tends to be more susceptible to ulceration from trauma.[41] Twenty-three of the patients among 86 reported by McPeak et al.[28] were evaluated within 1 year of the appearance of their lesions. Twenty-five others had evidence of disease for over 10 years before their referral for treatment. Five of the patients in McPeak's series presented with hematogenous metastasis. The clinical and gross pathologic findings were typical for dermatofibrosarcoma in each of these patients; in three, however, the tumor had more than eight mitotic figures per high-power field. This would suggest that in certain instances increased cellular activity may define a more aggressive subpopulation.[33] One of our patients underwent wide resection of a recurrent supraclavicular dermatofibrosarcoma with pedicle flap closure derived from the chest wall. Three years later he presented with a large pleural mass that infiltrated the lung and chest wall. The site of the primary lesion remained free of recurrence. Chest wall resection with partial pneumonectomy was performed, but brain metastasis developed 1 year later. In each phase of recurrence the tumor had become more aggressive.

At times, spindle cell melanoma may take on the clinical appearance of dermatofibrosarcoma protuberans and microscopically show a classic cartwheel pattern. We have treated two such patients, whose lesions arose on the lower extremity, and more recently, one on the back that had the classic appearance of an extensive, neglected der-

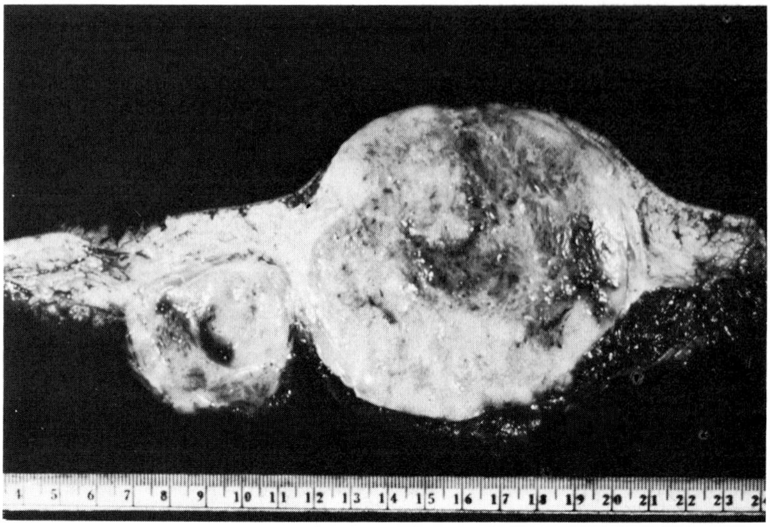

FIGURE 10–12. Large resected fibrosarcoma of the abdominal wall. Satellite nodules are characteristic of many of the fibrous tumors.

matofibrosarcoma. When dermatofibrosarcoma does metastasize, there have been occasional instances in which biopsy of the metastatic lesions have been said to resemble Hodgkin's disease or histiocystic lymphoma.[14] It is essential that an experienced pathologist review the slides in such an instance so that proper therapy can be instituted. Frequently, electron microscopy and cell surface markers can be used to define tumor characteristics not identifiable by light microscopy.

Certain patterns typifying the tumors to be treated may be noted. Resected fibrosarcoma of the abdominal wall has a characteristic circumscribed sclerotic appearance or may demonstrate nodular satellitosis spreading from the primary lesion (Fig. 10–12). At a farther distance, tumor cells blend into the fascial planes adjacent to the tumor.[35] When rhabdomyosarcoma appears, it may have the characteristics of a hemorrhagic mass. Biopsy can produce extensive bleeding without evidence of an underlying tumor mass being appreciated by the surgeon. Most adult pleomorphic rhabdomyosarcomas tend to appear in the muscle groups of the anterior thigh, with only an occasional primary developing on the trunk. When extensive vascularity and necrosis are among the initial features of the tumor, it becomes apparent that cure is only theoretical and that clinical management is essential, but only for obviating potential problems. Radiation and chemotherapy must be considered in the overall management of this condition. Extensive hemorrhage can also be seen in other tumors, such as the hemangiopericytoma arising on the abdominal wall. Under such circumstances, adequate tissue sampling is mandatory for proper diagnosis.

ABDOMINAL WALL TUMORS

In a review of abdominal wall tumors, Shiu et al.[36] evaluated the experience at Memorial Sloan-Kettering and found 10 desmoids and 22 other lesions which were fully malignant. Among the fully malignant sarcomas were five rhabdomyosarcomas, four fibrosarcomas, four leiomyosarcomas, three liposarcomas, and two synoviomas. While occasionally seen arising on the abdominal wall, the liposarcomas more frequently appear on the back. Figure 10–13 shows the usual appearance of a liposarcoma resected from the back. The specimen is surrounded by wide margins of muscle and fascial tissue.

Among the abdominal wall tumors one can find lesions that appear to be clinically benign. Diagnostic acumen here is of the utmost importance. One of our patients, a 30-year-old woman, presented with a mass in the anterior rectus sheath at the site of a previous incision for cholecystectomy. The initial interpretation was that we were probably dealing with an incisional hernia. (CT scanning was not yet available.) A biopsy proved the lesion to be a hemangiopericytoma. Wide resection of the abdominal wall was accomplished with Marlex mesh replacement of the abdominal wall defect. By the time of discharge we noted a metastatic

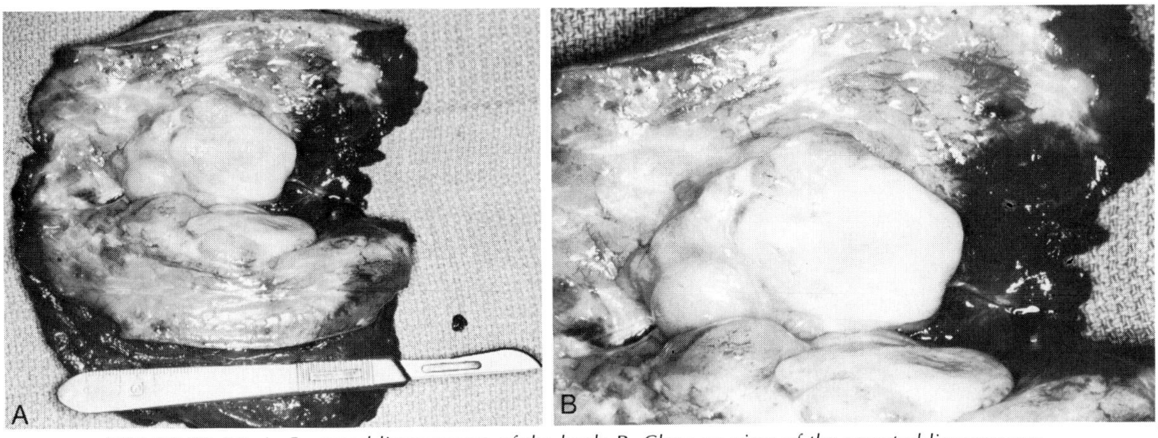

FIGURE 10–13. *A, Resected liposarcoma of the back. B, Close-up view of the resected liposarcoma.*

lesion in the right upper lung field. Resection of this lesion and subsequent chemotherapy failed to control further progression of disease.

The abdominal wall tumors in the Memorial Hospital series ranged in size from 1.5 to more than 35 cm in diameter, with the majority measuring approximately 5 to 15 cm. Direct extension to the lower ribs, pubis, and iliac crest was found in three patients. Extension through the abdominal wall with tumor invading the underlying viscera was noted in two of seven patients who were previously untreated and in eight of 15 who had recurrent tumor. This pattern of tumor extension, with invasion through the chest and abdominal walls to encroach and invade the underlying viscera, is frequently seen with sweat gland carcinoma as well as the more aggressive, fully malignant sarcomas. Twelve of 22 patients in this series had undifferentiated high-grade malignancies.

Malignant Fibrous Histiocytoma

Malignant fibrous histiocytoma, a common sarcomatous lesion of the extremity, may also be found as a primary tumor mass on the chest and abdominal wall. Occasionally it has been reported to arise within mammary tissue. Among the 53 cases described by O'Brien and Stout[30] the breast was the site of origin in five. Langham et al.[22] reported the appearance of a similar lesion in the left breast of a 51-year-old woman. Seven additional cases were reported by others. Three occurred in women with a history of other tumors or after radiation therapy. One tumor developed in association with cystosarcoma phylloides and three arose following radiation therapy for carcinoma of the breast. Histologically these lesions were composed of a storiform pattern of spindle cells with sparse cytoplasm and ovoid nuclei that lacked nucleoli. Some form of modified mastectomy appears in order when these tumors are found in the breast. In the case reported by Tsuneyoshi and Emjoji,[42] the patient had four recurrences over a period of 4 years but was free of disease at 68 months. Metastasis is unusual, and axillary node dissection probably is not indicated unless the nodes are palpable.

Sarcomas of the Breast

Malignant fibrous histiocytic lesions arising in the skin (dermatofibrosarcoma protuberans) have also been reported to involve the breast. More localized resection can be offered for these cases in contrast to the therapy required for the deep malignant fibrous histiocytoma of the breast; McPeak suggested obtaining margins of 3 cm in width and depth and that the underlying fascia of the breast be included with the specimen.[27] Callery et al.[9] reviewed 32 patients with mammary sarcomas (excluding angiosarcomas and lymphomas) treated at Memorial Hospital between 1949 and 1982. Twenty-five were treated as primary tumors (fibrosarcoma, 7; malignant fibrous histiocytoma, 5; desmoid, 3; dermatofibrosarcoma, 2; and leiomyosarcoma, 2) and 7 as recurrences. Overall, 8 of the 32 patients (25%) died of disease. Adverse prognostic factors included high histologic grade and high mitotic index. When total mastectomy was employed, 8% of the patients had local recurrence; with local excision 53% had recurrence. None of the 32 patients had evidence of regional node involvement.

Epithelioid Sarcoma

Epithelioid sarcoma is an additional lesion that has been described as a distinct entity occurring in the abdominal wall.[5] The patient, a 61-year-old woman, was first seen for treatment of a recurrent ventral hernia with abscess and draining sinus tracts. This was not too dissimilar from the patient that we had seen with hemangiopericytoma. Excision of this lesion, however, revealed the tumor to be an epithelioid sarcoma. This was confirmed by review at the AFIP. While most of these tumors have occurred on the extremities, two have been noted on the penis, several on scalp, and one on the vulva. It appeared that the tumor was responsible for destruction of large amounts of abdominal subcutaneous tissue, followed by secondary infection. The treatment of choice appears to be surgical resection. Radiation therapy and chemotherapy have been ineffective with this lesion, but there is some suggestion that cyclophosphamide plus 5-fluorouracil offer some opportunity to control disease.

Surgical Resection and Repair. Wide enbloc resection with adequate margins of normal uninvolved abdominal wall and possibly the underlying viscera is a fundamental principle to follow in resecting abdominal wall sarcomas. Closure of large abdominal defects has been accomplished using ox fascia, fascia lata, or Marlex mesh.[43] In our experience we have found that Marlex mesh appears to give the most satisfactory closure. In most of our patients we have used Marlex by itself. Only when considering the possibility of paradoxical motion in the chest do we occasionally use methacrylate incorporated into the Marlex.

Karakousis[19] has discussed the problem of managing tumors in the lower retroperitoneum and abdominal wall. He described use of a lower abdominal midline incision, extending it in a transverse direction at the inferior end and coming down vertically at the femoral triangle. Ligation and division of the inferior epigastric vessels achieve full exposure of the area for dissection. Lower abdominal wall reconstruction is accomplished with mesh. Ledesma et al.[23] discussed their management of isolated abdominal wall recurrences, emphasizing that radical surgical excision should be considered when the abdominal wall is the only identifiable metastatic site.

Metallic and Polymer Mesh. The need to devise methods for closure of abdominal and thoracic wall defects dates back more than 50 years. For lesions that are not too large, attempts are always made to approximate the edges of the defect directly without undue tension. Brunschwig (1947) stressed this in the 12 cases of visceral cancer that he had resected with a portion of the abdominal wall. The overlapping of the fascia as used in the Mayo repair was considered desirable. Historically when large defects have been encountered, various artificial materials have been tried. Phelps in 1894 first used coiled silver wire to treat abdominal and inguinal hernias. Witzel in 1900 constructed within the site of the defect a rude network of crossed silver wires and suggested the idea of embedding a ready-made filigree. The discomfort to the patient, the high incidence of wound infection, and prolonged drainage caused the technique to fall into disuse. Other metals were used for repair of the abdominal wall defects, but all were abandoned because of poor results. Complications were usually due to the electrochemical phenomenon known as corrosion of metal, which introduces soluble and more or less toxic salts into the body fluids. The use of tantalum mesh, first proposed by Burke in 1940, was widespread at one time. It was woven into a fine monofilament mesh. The material was first developed as a dressing for burns and later for the repair of abdominal wall defects. Koontz was able to demonstrate that there is always a tantalum oxide coating on the outer surface of the metal, which stimulates the growth of normal fibroblasts. While this has been a desirable feature in the repair of abdominal wall defects, it does cause problems when dealing with desmoid or other abdominal wall malignancies. McPeak and Miller[27] advised against the use of tantalum since tumor recurrences can rapidly grow along the latticework of the mesh. The differentiation of scar tissue from fibrous tumor growth was also found to present a problem when such mesh was used for repair. It was also pointed out that metallic material could interfere with radiation therapy should it be necessary to consider this form of therapy for recurrence. In 1952 Cumberland ennumerated certain desirable qualities for use of a foreign body in the repair of a tissue defect. The material should be chemically and biologically inert, easily sterilized, and durable and should provide a supporting framework for a sufficiently long time to allow a firm and stable tissue matrix. Plastics, in general, have had an advantage here since they are easier to handle and have no problem with fragmentation, as seen with the metals. Usher[43] experimentally compared fabrics such as nylon, Orlon, Dacron, Ivalon, Teflon and Marlex. All but Teflon and Marlex had to be removed in the presence of infection. He found that Marlex mesh, a monofilament polyethylene developed in 1958, was the best of the prosthetic materials. The cloth made from this fiber is impervious to water and possesses outstanding chemical resistance; the softening temperature is 260° F, allowing sterilization in an autoclave, and its tensile strength is exceptional. Also the foreign body reaction to it is much less than to the other plastic materials. When Marlex was used in dogs, infection studies showed that after drainage of wounds, granulation would occur without further care and without fragmentation of the material, slough of the graft, or sinus formation. We frequently employ this material in the initial phase of our reconstruction, and follow with coverage with some form of skin pedicle flap.

Pedicle Flap Coverage. We attempt to employ musculo(myo)cutaneous flaps when possible for final coverage. The use of pedicled musculofascial grafts to cover large abdominal wall defects was first described by Farr in 1922. He reported three cases of superior abdominal wall tumor resections in which the defect was covered by pedicle flaps of pectoralis major muscle and fascia. The method was popularized in 1932 by Wangensteen. He and later Hamilton[16] proposed the use of the iliotibial tract of fascia lata to cover the abdominal defects. Techniques of pedicle flap coverage have become popular as new sources of blood supply to the pedicles have been defined. Flaps such as the latissimus dorsi[24, 26] and pectoralis minor[38] have as such become standards in the repair of many defects. Regardless of where the defect is created, however, muscle and skin must usually be employed for final coverage, with such tissues being derived from adjacent areas of the chest and abdomen. The coverage to be obtained must allow reestablishment of proper pulmonary function in the case of the reconstructed chest. Such problems do not occur with abdominal wall defects, in which case viability of coverage is the prime concern. Mobility of the chest wall is needed when chest reconstruction is performed, and permanent coverage is mandatory. In chest wall resections the initial problem of paradoxical motion can be obviated by a strong mesh, double sewn in the surrounding bony framework of the defect. If assisted ventilation is employed the patients can usually be extubated in 3 to 5 days. While some paradoxical motion will remain, the patient will exhibit adequate ventilatory exchange at this time. As mentioned previously, one may obtain greater rigidity from the mesh by spreading methyl methacrylate over its surface. Should too much rigidity develop, adjacent tissues can erode and the prosthesis will be exposed. Loss of the prosthesis over the chest may expose pulmonary and mediastinal contents. In the abdominal region this problem rarely occurs since granulation eventually covers the exposed prosthesis, and because the motion encountered with chest wall grafts does not exist here. Lee and Hines[24] described their experience with chest wall reconstruction using the latissimus dorsi myocutaneous flap. This flap originally described by Tansini at the turn of the century is now considered one of the most reliable and versatile flaps available. For chest wall reconstruction it offers advantages such as reliability, predictable blood supply, great size potential, exceptional range of the arc of rotation, luxury of a single-stage reconstruction without delay, no appreciable functional deficit following extirpation of the muscle, and relatively minimal donor site deformity. Six cases of successful one-stage reconstruction were described.

Arnold and Pairolero[3, 4] described their experience with 100 consecutive patients requiring chest wall reconstruction over a 7-year period; 42 had tumors of the chest wall, 19 had radiation necrosis, 24 had infected median sternotomies, and 15 had combinations of the three. Ninety-two patients underwent 142 muscle flaps: 77 pectoralis major, 29 latissimus dorsi, and 36 of other muscles, including serratus anterior, rectus abdominis, and external oblique muscles.

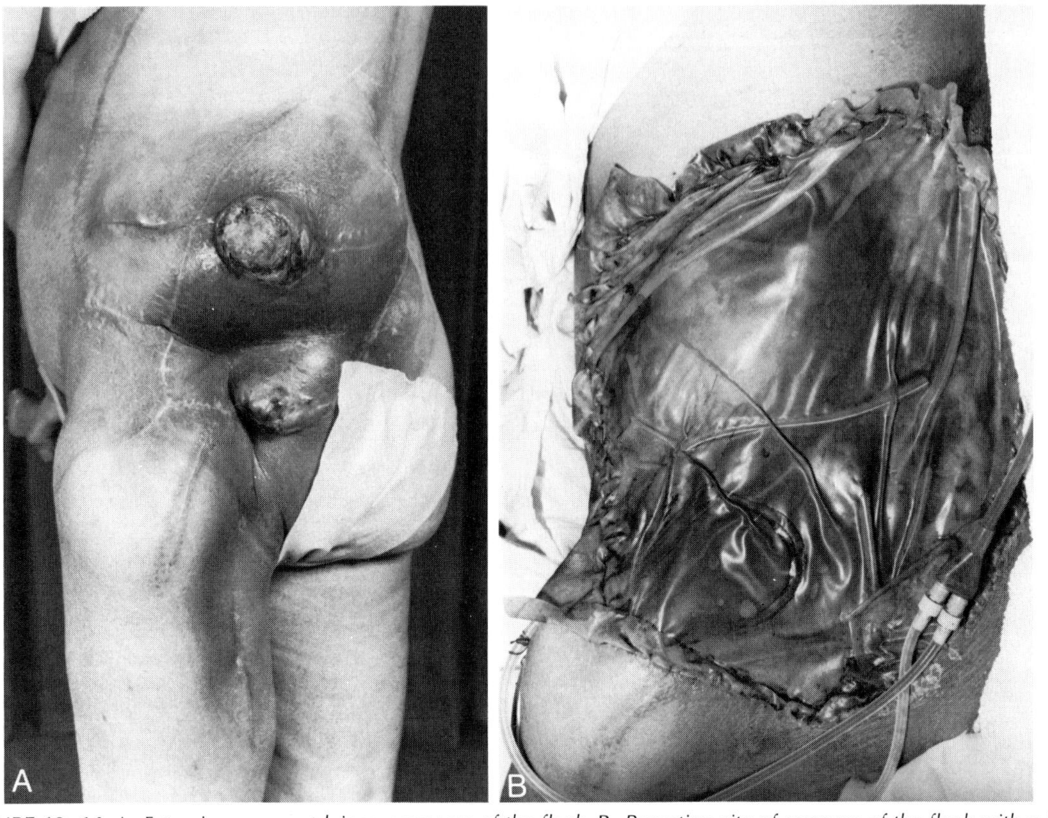

FIGURE 10–14. A, *Extensive recurrent leiomyosarcoma of the flank.* B, *Resection site of sarcoma of the flank with a large rubber dam covering the defect to allow granulation in preparation for grafting.*

Omentum was transposed in ten patients, a technique that has been described to increase vascularity to a region. The 100 patients underwent an average of 2.1 operations, with hospitalization averaging 17.5 days.

In order to provide adequate coverage of any prosthetic mesh, a proper myocutaneous flap should be used and will guarantee thickness and vascularity to the pedicle. The deltopectoral flap is one of the few that can be raised without adherent underlying muscle since it is supplied by direct cutaneous vessels fed from the internal mammary chain. Other flaps such as the pectoralis myocutaneous and the latissimus dorsi flap are fed by large vessels, such as the thoracoacromial and thoracodorsal arteries. The thoracoacromial artery enters the pectoralis flap, leaving the second portion or the axillary artery and entering the muscle 2 cm medial to the coracoid process and 2 cm inferior to the clavicle. A pedicle based at the clavicle and extending just medial to the nipple can be raised with a sizable paddle of skin.

Another useful flap for closing defects and covering synthetic meshes is derived from the latissimus dorsi. Its blood supply, the thoracodorsal artery, is a continuation of the subscapular artery, which arises from the third portion of the axillary artery. Together with the subscapular nerve (routinely identified in the subscapular fossa during mastectomy), it forms a neurovascular pedicle that enters the medial edge of the anterior margin of the muscle 8 to 10 cm from its insertion in the humerus. A long pedicle can be mobilized so that coverage across the chest wall is feasible.

Occasionally the defect created in resecting a neoplasm is so large that none of these approaches for pedicle closure or initial use of mesh are of value. Recently one of us (Marcove) encountered a case of extensive recurrent leiomyosarcoma of the flank involving the ilium (Fig. 10–14*A*). There was no possible chance for resection in the standard manner. Radical extirpation of the lesion was accomplished, leaving a defect that appeared unmanageable. The entire area was covered with a rubber dam sutured in place to contain the viscera and to allow granulation to take place for secondary grafting at a later date (Fig. 10–14*B*).

In the Memorial Hospital series,[36] six patients required resection of the underlying viscera at the time of resecting abdominal wall neoplasms. The necessity for such resection especially holds true where a large lesion has penetrated through the fascia. At this time the aggressiveness of the lesion can be anticipated and one must not only be ready to resect abdominal wall with probable mesh and myocutaneous reconstruction but also to anticipate that intestinal viscera will be involved. Among the 22 lesions that were found to be fully malignant abdominal wall sarcomas in the Memorial series, 12 were eligible for evaluation. Four had been untreated when first seen and eight previously treated. Two of the four patients survived 5 years; 4 of the eight previously treated recurrent tumors reappeared again after an additional surgical attempt. Among the abdominal wall desmoids seen at Memorial Hospital there was local recurrence in one of ten patients. Eight of nine remained free of recurrent tumor 5 to 24 years after definitive surgery.

Survival among those patients treated palliatively ranged from 1 to 18 months, with a median of 7 months. Therapy usually consisted of radiation therapy or chemotherapy, or both. No desmoid tumor in the series metastasized or showed malignant transformation. If local recurrence did appear and was not controlled by more extensive resection, then the continued growth resulted in invasion and obstruction of abdominal and pelvic viscera. Fully malignant lesions were found to grow rapidly, with distant metastases usually found in association with extensive local recurrence.

While biopsy is important in establishing the diagnosis of a recurrent sarcoma, it is essential not to seed the wound at the time of this initial surgery. The biopsy site must be carefully planned so as not to interfere with any further surgery that may be required. When local control is not obtained, the majority of high-grade sarcomas tend to disseminate through the peritoneal surfaces of the abdominal wall into the peritoneal cavity. Once the peritoneum is invaded, the ability to control the disease is problematic. This would suggest that prophylactic chemotherapy be considered in such instances where the potential for response exists.

REFERENCES

1. Ackerman L. V., Taylor F. H.: Neurogenic tumors within the thorax. Cancer 4:669–691, 1951
2. Arlen M.: tumors of fibrous tissue origin. N.Y. State J. Med. 74:344–348, 1974
3. Arnold P. G., Pairolero P. C.: Use of the pectoralis major muscle to repair defects of the anterior chest wall. Plast. Reconstr. Surg. 63:205, 1979
4. Arnold P. G., Pairolero P. C.: Chest wall reconstruction. Ann. Surg. 199:725–732, 1984
5. Bloustein P. A., Silverberg S. G., Waddel W. R.: Epithelioid sarcoma. Cancer 38:2390, 1976
6. Booher R. J., Pack G. T.: Desmomas of the abdominal wall in children. Cancer 4:1052–1063, 1951
7. Brasfield R. D., Das Gupta T. K.: Desmoid tumors of the anterior abdominal wall. Surgery 65:241–246, 1969
8. Briselli M., Mark E. J., Dickersin G. R.: Solitary fibrous tumors of the pleura. Cancer 47:2678–2689, 1981
9. Callery C. D., Rosen P. P., Kinne D. W.: Sarcoma of the breast. Ann. Surg. 202:527–532, 1985
10. Castleberry R. P., Kelly D. R., Wilson E. R., et al.: Childhood lipsarcoma. Cancer 54:579–584, 1984
11. Cicciarelli F. E., Soule E. H., McGoon D. C.: Lipoma and liposarcoma of the mediastinum: A report of 14 tumors including one lipoma of the thymus. J. Thorac. Cardiovasc. Surg. 47:411–429, 1964
12. Dalton W. T., Zolliker A. S., McCaughey W. T. E., et al.: Localized Primary Tumors of the Pleurm. Cancer 44:1465–1475, 1979
13. Das Gupta T. R., Brasfield R. D., O'Hara J.: Extra-abdominal desmoids: A clinicopathological study. Ann. Surg. 170:109, 1969
14. Fisher E. R., Hellstrom H. R.: Dermatofibrosarcoma with metastasis simulating Hodgkin's disease and reticulum cell sarcoma. Cancer 19:1165, 1966
15. Godwin J. T., Watson W. L., Pool J. L., et al.: Primary intrathoracic neurogenic tumors. J. Thorac. Surg. 20:169, 1950
16. Hamilton J. E.: Fascia lata patches in hernia repair. Ann. Surg. 157:925–931, 1963
17. Heinman M. W., Lehman W. L.: Mediastinal mesenchymoma masquerading as liposarcoma. Cancer 4:692–696, 1951
18. Jacobson H. G., Beneventano T. C.: Mediastinal mass in a patient with liver disease. J.A.M.A. 247:1873–1874, 1982
19. Karakousis C. P.: Exposure and reconstruction in the lower portions of the retroperitoneum and abdominal wall. Arch. Surg. 117:840–844, 1982
20. Kerr W. R., Nohl H. C.: Recurrence of "benign" intra-thoracic fibromas. Thorax 16:180–189, 1961
21. Kinzbrunner B., Ritter S., Domingo J., Rosenthal C. J.: Remission of rapidly growing desmoid tumors after tamoxifen therapy. Cancer 52:2201–2204, 1983
22. Langham M. R., Mills A. S., DeMay R. M., et al.: Malignant fibrous histiocytoma of the breast. Cancer 54:558–563, 1984
23. Ledesma E. J., Tseng M., Mittleman A.: Surgical treatment of isolated abdominal wall metastasis in colorectal cancer. Cancer 50:1884–1887, 1982
24. Lee G. W., Hines G. L.: Chest wall reconstruction using a latissimus dorsi myocutaneous flap. N.Y. State J. Med. 83:727–731, 1983
25. Legha S. S., Muggia F. M.: Pleural mesothelioma: Clinical features and therapeutic implications. Ann. Intern. Med. 87:617, 1977

26. McCraw J. B., Penix J. O., Baker J. W.: Repair of major defects of chest wall and spine with the latissimus dorsi myocutaneous flap. Plast. Reconstr. Surg. 62:197, 1978
27. McPeak C. J., Miller T. R.: Abdominal wall replacement. Surgery 47:944–952, 1960
28. McPeak C. J., Cruz T., Nicastri A. D.: Dermatofibrosarcoma protuberans: An analysis of 86 cases, five with metastasis. Ann. Surg. 166:803–816, 1967
29. Nascimento A. G., Unni K. K., Bernatz P. E.: Sarcomas of the lung. Mayo Clin. Proc. 57:355–359, 1982
30. O'Brien J. E., Stout A. P.: Malignant fibrous xanthoma. Cancer 17:1445–1455, 1964
31. Pack G. T., Ehrlich H. E.: Neoplasms of the anterior abdominal wall with special consideration of desmoid tumors. Int. Abstr. Surg. 79:177–198, 1944
32. Pack G. T., Tabah E. J.: Dermatofibrosarcoma protuberans: Report of 39 cases. Arch. Surg. 62:391–411, 1951
33. Penner D. W.: Metastasizing dermatofibrosarcoma protuberans. Cancer 4:1083–1086, 1951
34. Prior S. T., Sisson B. S.: Dermal and fascial fibromas. Ann. Surg. 139:453, 1954
35. Pritchard D. J.: Fibrosarcomas of bone and soft tissues of the trunk and extremities. Orthop. Clin. North Am. 8:869, 1977
36. Shiu M. H., Flamebaum L., Hajdu S. I., Fortner J. G.: Malignant soft tissue tumors of the anterior abdominal wall. Arch. Surg. 115:152–155, 1980
37. Shmookler B. M., Enzinger F. M.: Pleomorphic lipoma: A benign tumor simulating liposarcoma. Cancer 47:126–133, 1981
38. Soyfer A. E., Graeber G. M.: The use of latissimus dorsi and pectoralis major musculocutaneous flaps for chest wall reconstruction. Contemp. Surg. 22:29–39, 1983
39. Sun C. C., Kroll M., Miller J. E.: Primary chondrosarcoma of the lung. Cancer 50:1864–1866, 1982
40. Sunderrajan E. V., Luger A. M., Rosenholtz M. J., Maltby J. D.: Leiomyosarcoma in the mediastinum presenting as superior vena cava syndrome. Cancer 53:2553–2556, 1984
41. Taylor H. B., Helwig E. B.: Dermatofibrosarcoma protuberans: A story of 115 cases. Cancer 15:717–725, 1962
42. Tsuneyoshi M., Emjoji M.: Postirradiation sarcoma (malignant fibrous histiocytoma) following breast carcinoma. Cancer 45:1419–1423, 1979
43. Usher F. C.: New technique for repairing incisional hernias with Marlex mesh. Am. J. Surg. 138:740–741, 1979.

CHAPTER

11

Retroperitoneal Sarcomas

The retroperitoneal sarcomas represent a large array of neoplasms that arise from mesenchymal structures situated between the diaphragm and the pelvic brim. Few are symptomatic, especially during the early stages of their growth. Many patients are usually alerted to the presence of such tumors as a result of the expansion in their abdominal girth resulting from tumor growth and from displacement of viscera.[48] Intermittent episodes of poorly defined pain have been described by approximately 70% of patients presenting with this type of tumor. Symptoms are most often represented by vague discomfort that patients cannot clearly localize. Some patients have given a history of mild abdominal discomfort preceding the clinical diagnosis of tumor by as much as 2 years. It may be that early lumbar nerve compression originating at the beginning of the growth phase of the retroperitoneal tumor may be responsible for such symptoms. Occasionally celiac axis compression gives rise to complaints of high lumbar backache from which the patient gets relief by sitting up and leaning forward. Percussion of the spine in this region may reveal some tenderness.

In general, retroperitoneal tumor masses can be palpated in approximately 90% of patients when careful examination is performed. In 15% of the patients reported by Pack and Tabah[48] the abdominal swelling that had been noted was not due to a mass but occurred secondary to ascites resulting from portal vein compression. This type of ascites can easily be confused by the presence of a large retroperitoneal cyst containing liters of fluid that is mistaken for ascites. An improper diagnosis may be obtained at the time of paracentesis since the abdominal girth becomes smaller.[49]

While such abdominal distention may have been secondary to ascites, this type of swelling is more frequently associated with the presence of a large palpable abdominal mass. The large size of many of these masses results from tumor expansion, with the viscera stretched over their surface (Fig. 11–1). This visceral displacement may help in defining the site of origin of the tumor as well as in determining its size.

The existing tumor mass that has been clinically diagnosed can best be defined by a combination of radiologic studies, including a barium enema, GI series, and intravenous pyelogram. Following identification of the lesion by these basic radiographic techniques, CT scan, selective angiography, and MRI are often used. Definitive diagnosis and attempted treatment (resection) are next undertaken by laparotomy.

DIAGNOSTIC STUDIES

The degree to which the tumor arises from the retroperitoneal and adjacent structures may be defined by the extent of visceral displacement seen on the GI series and barium enema. An intravenous pyelogram is usually of value since it can show ureteral as well as renal displacement, should the retroperitoneal mass impinge on these regions. In Fig. 11–2 there is evidence of a large retroperitoneal mass producing ureteral displacement. In this particular instance, the tumor was not neoplastic, but represented an inflammatory mass secondary to perforation of a diverticulum into

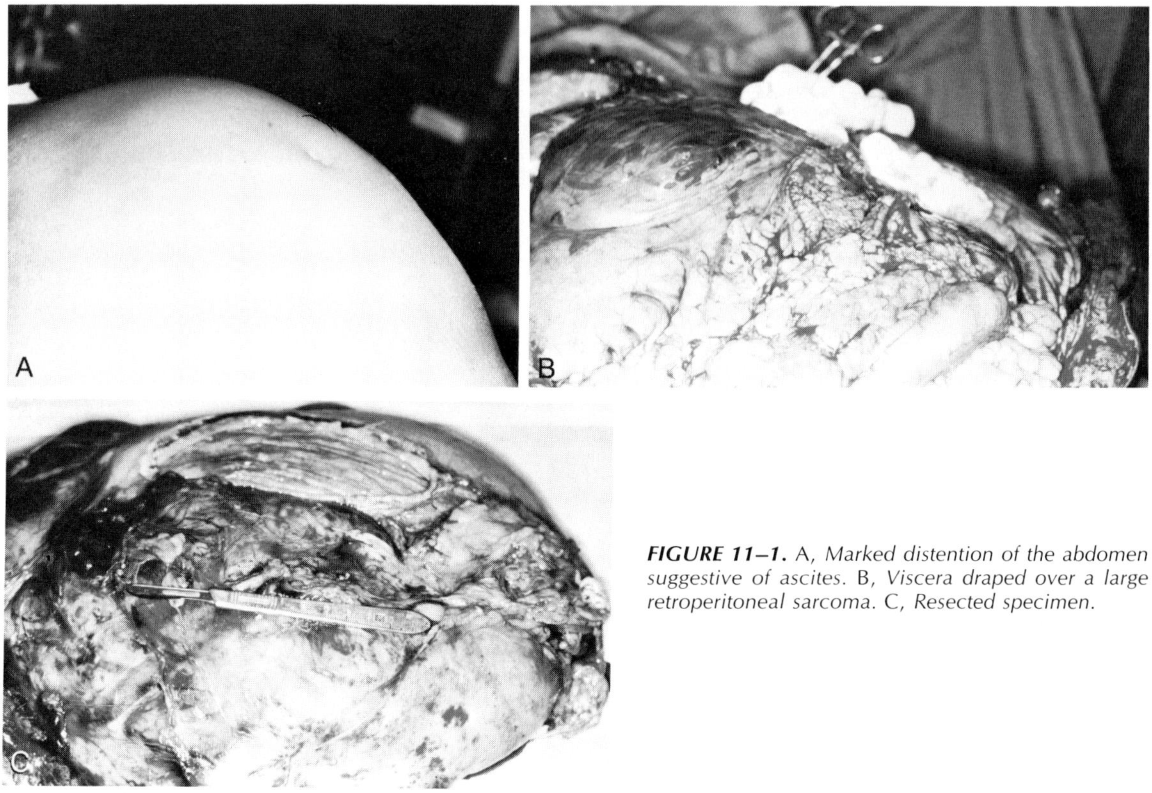

FIGURE 11–1. A, Marked distention of the abdomen suggestive of ascites. B, Viscera draped over a large retroperitoneal sarcoma. C, Resected specimen.

the mesentery of the descending colon. Extension of the inflammatory process reached into the retroperitoneum. This was followed by extensive retroperitoneal abscess formation, which produced a bulge in the patient's left flank. There was some discomfort, which one could attribute to the presence of the retroperitoneal mass; spiking temperatures did not appear until just prior to admission. An intravenous pyelogram showed displacement of the ureter similar to that noted in the presence of many retroperitoneal tumors.

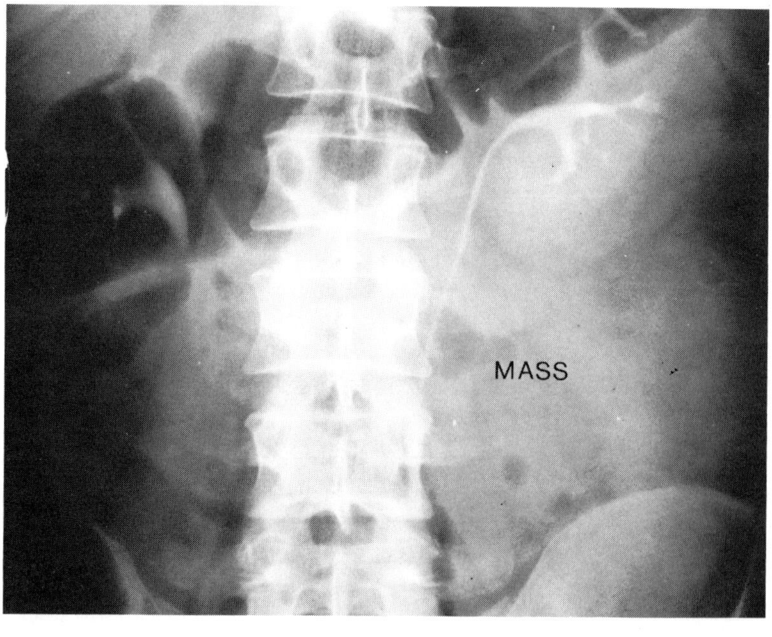

FIGURE 11–2. Abscess presenting as a retroperitoneal tumor. The abscess displaced the ureter medially and bulged from the left flank.

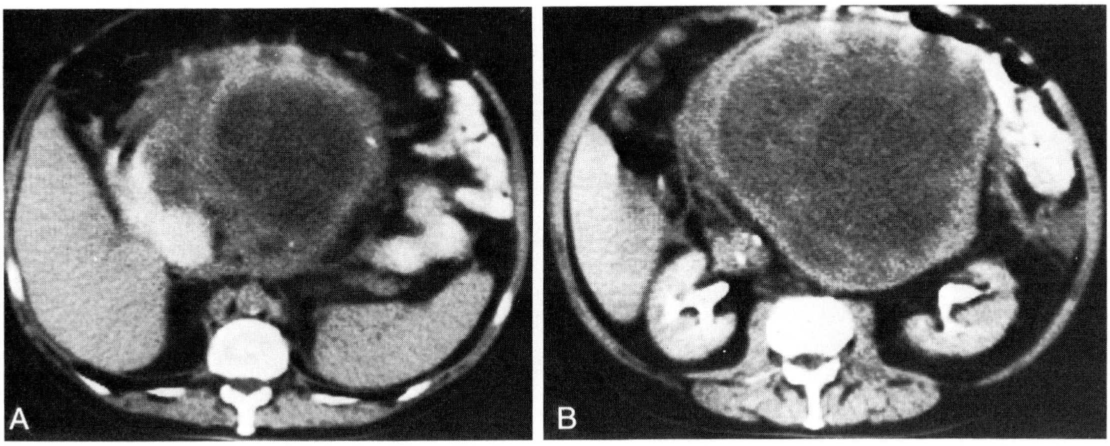

FIGURE 11–3. A and B, Large retroperitoneal tumor mass with central area of necrosis, situated over the aorta.

The intravenous pyelogram may also indicate tumor invasion of the ureter with secondary obstructive uropathy.[9]

Sonography can also be of value in defining the size and position of the retroperitoneal lesion, its consistency, and those structures that may be related to it. CT scanning has, however, become one of the more important tools in evaluating retroperitoneal sarcomas since it may be more specific in depicting the exact dimensions of the lesion, as well as which visceral structures lie adjacent to or are being invaded by the mass. We examined a 67-year-old man with marked abdominal swelling that had developed over a period of one year. At the time that he was examined it was apparent that there was a large abdominal mass and the question arose as to whether this represented fluid (ascites) or a retroperitoneal lesion. A CT scan of the abdomen revealed a markedly enlarged tumor mass, displacing most of the viscera, both anteriorly and inferiorly into the pelvis (Fig. 11–3). This offered most of the information necessary for planning surgery as well as the suggestion that we were dealing with a sarcomatous lesion of probable retroperitoneal origin.

CT Scan

In general, we have found the CT scan to be an exquisite tool for defining the extent to which a primary tumor has grown and those adjacent structures that may be invaded or infiltrated by it.[18, 22, 53] In rare instances, however, there may be exaggerated radiographic findings, which may not be confirmed at the time of laparotomy. We have encountered several such instances in which recurrent tumor was found at a site other than that predicted by the study. In some instances, the report of enlarged para-aortic nodes (suggesting lymphoma) could not be confirmed by exploration. Small masses, however, that are situated directly over the aorta, whether representing metastasis to the nodes or a primary tumor, can easily be distinguished and accurately located in relationship to adjacent structures such as the renal vessels, kidney, and duodenum (Fig. 11–4). In this instance, a nodular mass was found sitting on the aorta and vena cava, just below the renal vessels and extending to the bifurcation of the aorta. At this stage of disease, para-aortic dissection was feasible. For those sarcomas extending around the renal vessels, it is possible to remove the left renal vessels flush with the aorta-cava should criteria for resectability of the lesion exist.

The CT scan is also helpful in that it allows identification of the superior mesenteric vessels as they cross over the fourth portion of the duodenum to pass behind the pancreas. Figure 11–5*A* shows the appearance of a metastatic soft part osteosarcoma to the retrogastric space, invading the anterior surface of the pancreas. On entering the peritoneal cavity the tumor could easily be identified. Early exposure of the lesion was achieved by opening the gastrocolic ligament (Fig. 11–5*B*). The ability to visually identify the superior mesenteric vessels on other views of the scan, and be relatively assured of their freedom from involvement by tumor, suggested the possibility of resect-

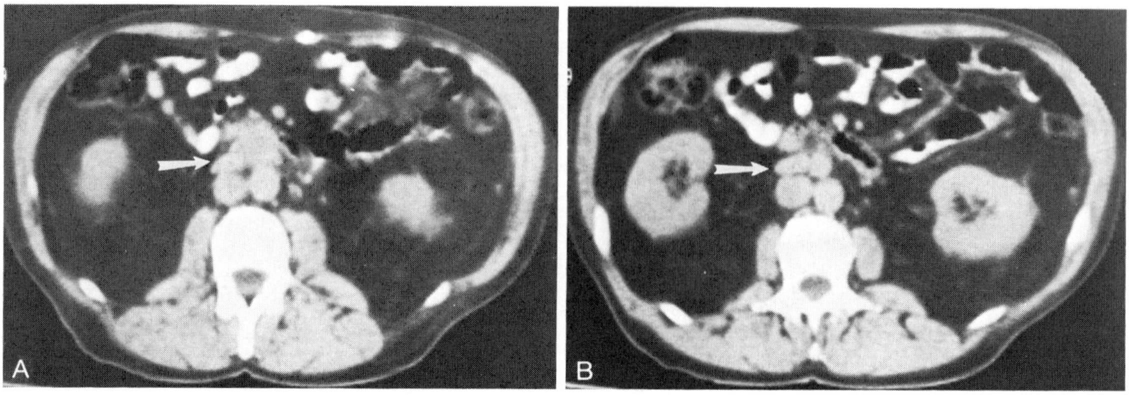

FIGURE 11–4. A *and* B, *Para-aortic tumor masses* (arrow).

ability. It was necessary to mobilize the duodenum to its fourth portion using the Cattell maneuver (mobilizing hepatic flexure over the duodenum) and identify the superior mesenteric vessels to them. This was considered an important step toward achieving resectability since it allowed separation of the pancreatic head from the tumor and ascertained that the biliary tract and portal system were intact. In this part of the procedure we were able to trace the superior mesenteric vein (by splitting the head of the pancreas over the tunnel created by finger dissection on the superior mesenteric vein) to its junction with the splenic vein, where it formed the portal vessel (Fig. 11–5C). Resection of tumor after this maneuver could be accomplished since no vital structures had been invaded.

Neifeld et al.[47] reported results obtained with the use of CT scan for evaluating retroperitoneal lesions. While he asserted that this technique greatly improved the ability to define tumors in this region, the barium

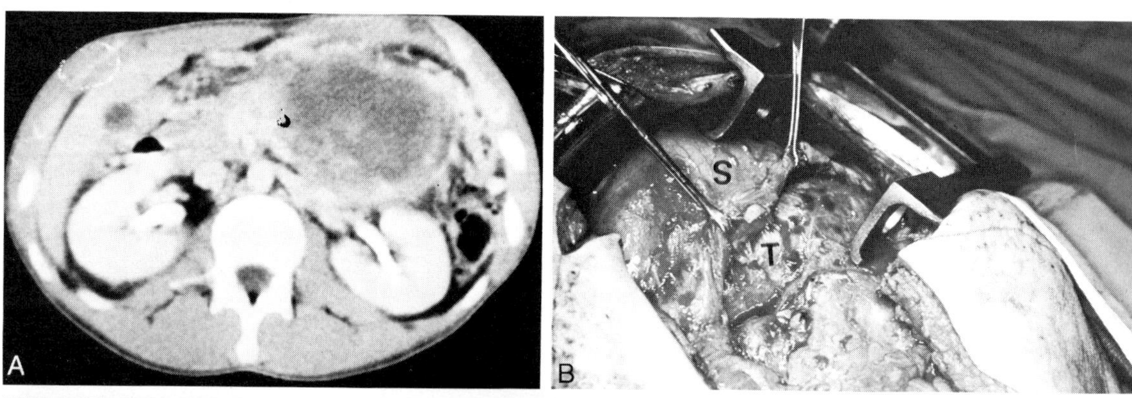

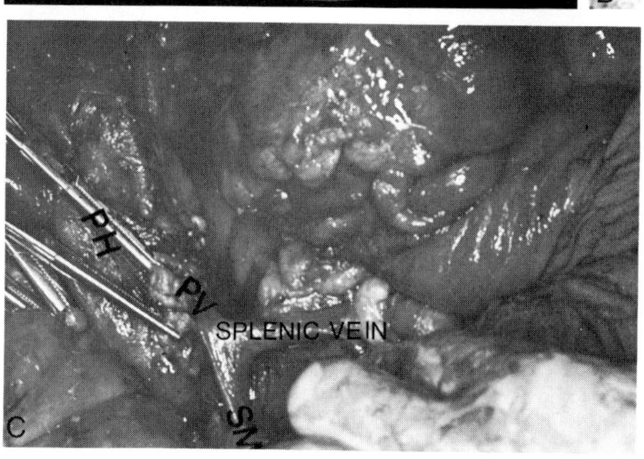

FIGURE 11–5. A, *CT scan showing metastatic osteosarcoma involving the distal pancreas.* B, *Babcock clamps elevating the stomach (S) off the tumor (T).* C, *Transected pancreatic head (P) showing formation of the portal vein (PV) by the joining of the superior mesenteric vein (SM) with the splenic vein.*

enema and GI series were still considered to be important in the complete work-up of the patient with an abdominal or retroperitoneal tumor mass. Information from the CT scan was considered important but did not rule out the need for additional studies, especially for determining the source and extent of the vascular supply to the neoplasm. In Neifeld's series dealing with retroperitoneal tumors, there were five liposarcomas, four malignant fibrous histiocytomas, nine leiomyosarcomas, one fibrosarcoma, and two rhabdomyosarcomas. The CT scan accurately delineated the size, extent of tumor involvement in the retroperitoneum, and contiguity of adjacent structures in 14 of 17 patients studied prior to surgery. At times, the CT scan was found to inadequately demonstrate the true extent of neoplastic involvement. At other times, it was found to define more than was actually noted at laparotomy, in terms of tumor size and potential retroperitoneal node involvement.

One of the major advantages in using this imaging technique has been the use of follow-up scans to detect recurrence following primary surgical resection. A 70-year-old man was initially seen with a large left flank mass which proved on laparotomy to be a retroperitoneal sarcoma (malignant fibrous histiocytoma) situated inferior to the left kidney. At the time of surgery, a large mass, separate and distinct from the kidney, was defined and resected. Six months following re-evaluation of the patient we could not find any evidence of clinical recurrence; the patient was totally asymptomatic at the time. A routine CT scan performed shortly thereafter demonstrated reappearance of the lesion. This was important in that it allowed reexploration when the recurrence was still resectable. One of the major problems with

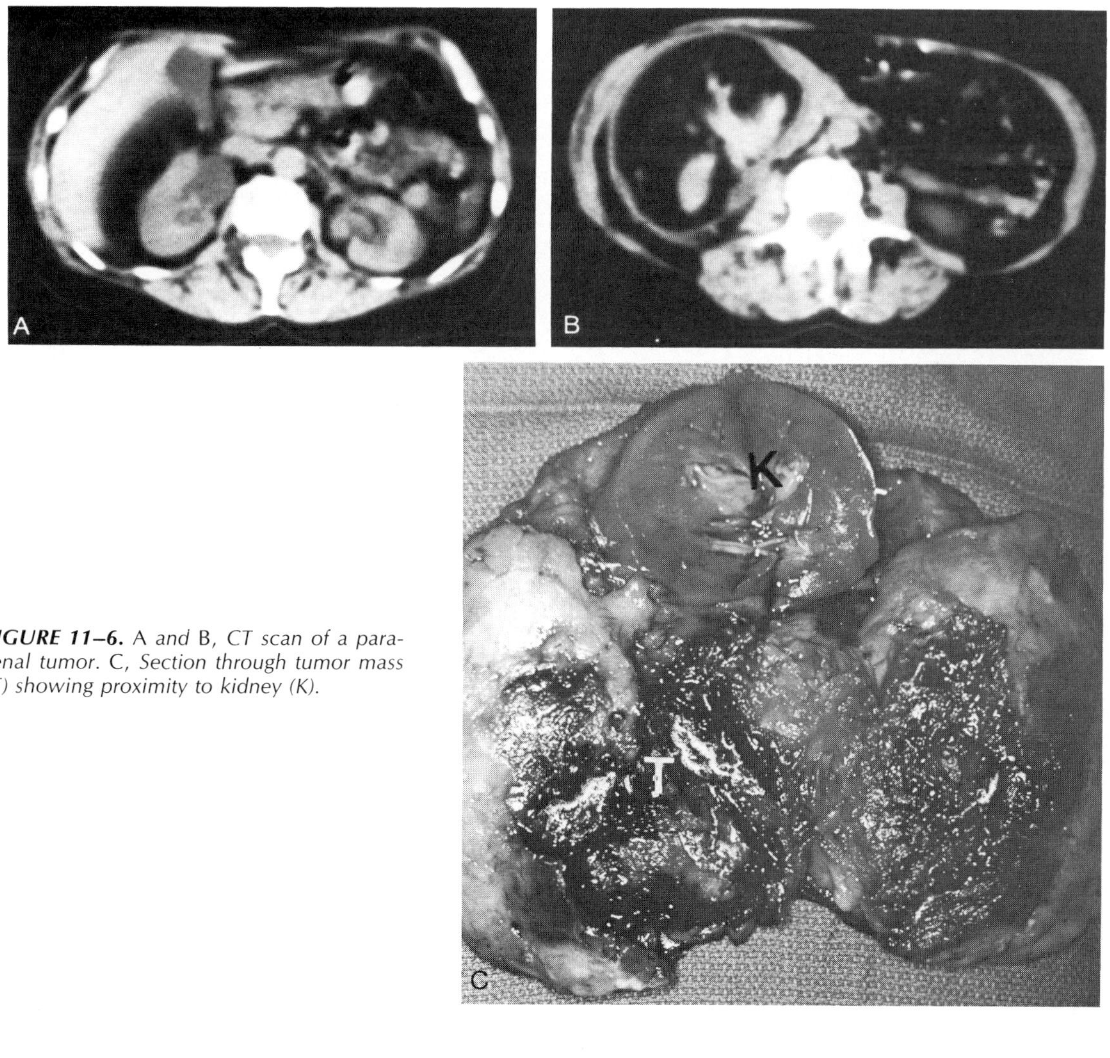

FIGURE 11–6. *A and B, CT scan of a pararenal tumor. C, Section through tumor mass (T) showing proximity to kidney (K).*

follow-up CT scan after surgery is distortion of the image by scarring as well as by the presence of metallic clips. These problems may eventually be resolved with the use of non-metallic clips and better imaging in these circumstances by MRI. We have now successfully employed this technique in defining recurrent hepatic lesions following partial hepatectomy where CT scan imaging was distorted by the metallic clips left at surgery.

It is our opinion that CT scan should be performed every 6 months for at least 3 years after initial resection of large retroperitoneal sarcomas. Following this period of time, yearly CT scans for at least another 3 to 4 years should be performed to define any potential for recurrence of tumor. Compared with sonography, CT scans of the retroperitoneum appear to be more accurate, even in terms of the characterization of internal structures of the tumor. In Figure 11–3, the dark central area of the mass represented cystic degeneration of the tumor. CT scans have been shown to be valuable in certain areas not clinically assessible by palpation or when the lesion is in proximity to the aorta and mesenteric vessels.

Even when the CT scan is used for studying specific tumor types such as the liposarcoma,[18] it should not be used to attempt histologic evaluation. Rather, its importance is in determining the extent of disease, defining adjacent structures that are infiltrated by tumor, locating residual disease, and contributing to radiotherapy planning. Recently we had the opportunity of seeing a patient with a large retroperitoneal sarcoma that had been identified by CT scan and was considered to be liposarcoma by the radiologist. The lesion, located in the right subcostal region just under the liver edge, was clinically palpable by the patient and the examining physician. The patient had pain in this area, and shortly thereafter a large palpable mass was found, extending from the subcostal region to the iliac crest. The CT scan was believed to clearly indicate the presence of a large fatty tumor, consistent with liposarcoma, in proximity to the right kidney (Fig.

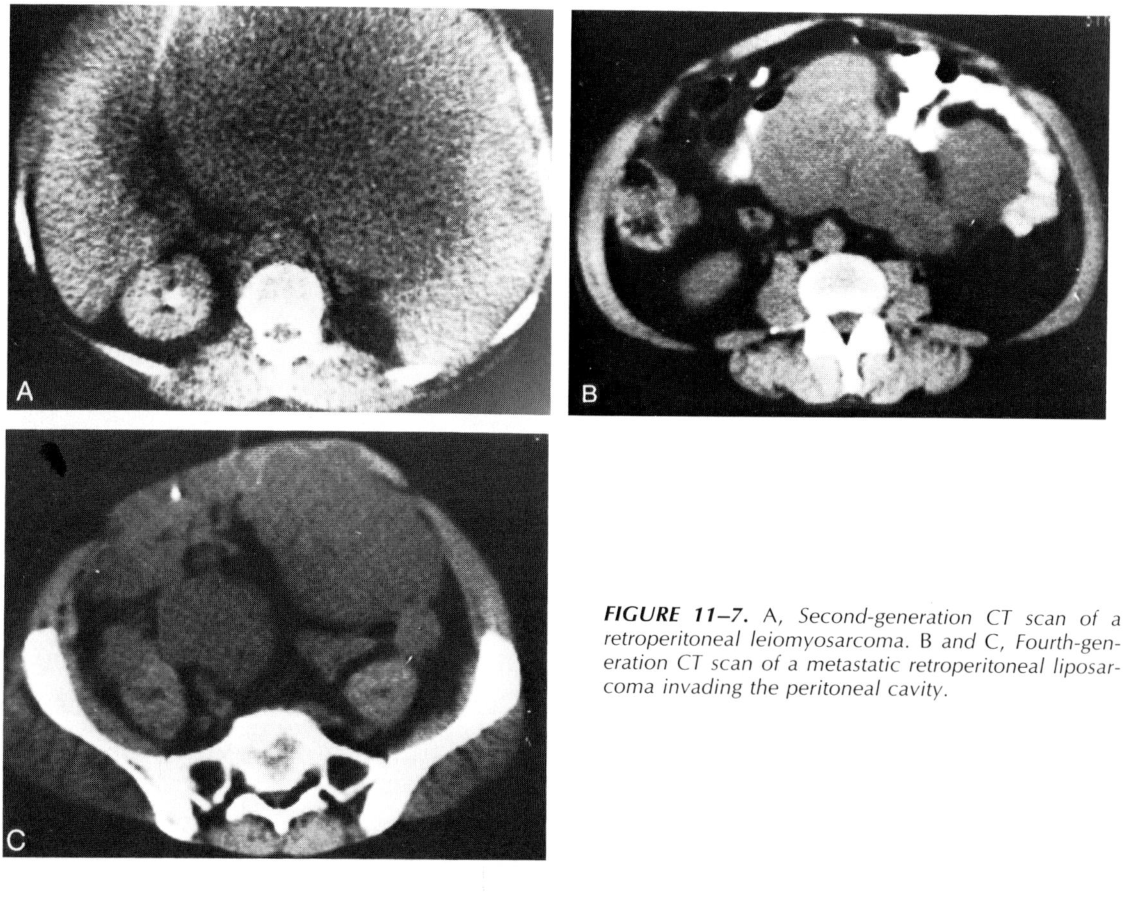

FIGURE 11–7. *A, Second-generation CT scan of a retroperitoneal leiomyosarcoma. B and C, Fourth-generation CT scan of a metastatic retroperitoneal liposarcoma invading the peritoneal cavity.*

11–6*A* and *B*). The tumor was resected through a thoracoabdominal approach; it was found just inferior to the lower renal pole, displacing the kidney superiorly behind the liver. Histologically, this lesion adjacent to the inferior pole of the right kidney was found to be an angiomyolipoma of extrarenal origin (Fig. 11–6*C*).

Angiomyolipoma probably represents a hamartomatous tumor arising in the kidney and, in rare instances, adjacent tissue of the renal bed. It is usually composed of three components: mature adipose tissue, thick-walled vessels, and bundles of smooth muscle. Occasionally, because of its large size and pleomorphic features, it has been mistaken for liposarcoma. This was the impression we had in managing this case at the time of laparotomy and constituted one of the main reasons for performing the radical nephrectomy. In rare instances the malignant form of angiomyolipoma has been seen.[7]

With each new generation of CT scanner (and the usual resultant shortening of the time for the scan), the ability to define the structure and margins of the lesion, extent of tumor growth, and adjacent anatomic structures has improved. Figure 11–7*A* shows the appearance of an early-generation scan compared with more recent ones, as were obtained in the following case. A 46-year-old man was referred for recurrence following initial resection of a retroperitoneal liposarcoma. The multiple lesions representing recurrence are easily defined and the extent of visceral, pelvic, and abdominal disease is readily apparent (Fig. 11–7*B* and *C*). Based on these findings, as well as clinical small bowel obstruction, the patient was reexplored. The tumor was resected and bowel continuity was reestablished. Findings at laparotomy correlated closely with the interpretation of the CT scan. The surgical approach and techniques of resection are described later in this chapter.

We usually scan liver and lung when large tumor masses are present, to assure that there is no disease distant to the primary retroperitoneal sarcoma. The addition of contrast material to the gastrointestinal tract, kidney and ureter, or vascular supply may enhance the relationship of the tumor with the areas that are being differentiated. Soft tissue masses usually have densities ranging from +10 to +60 EMI units, making it difficult to define histologic types unless fat, calcium, or contrast material is present.

Imaging

Attempts at defining the extent of tumor involvement by aortography and selective angiography are also important. Lowman et al.[41] have described lumbar angiography as a useful approach for making decisions about the surgical procedure to be employed. Flush aortography is usually performed first, followed, as indicated, by selective angiography. Certain selected studies of aortic tributaries have occasionally added additional information believed to be of diagnostic importance. Characteristic arching and curving of the lumbar vessels have been described. An increase in abnormal vascular patterns may suggest malignancy. Hypertrophy of the feeding lumbar arterial supply may be the first sign of vessels entering the tumor. Their stretching, elongation, draping, and separation can, however, be found in both benign and malignant neoplasms. If the abnormal vessels arise from the lumbar or upper intercostal system, then the mass is usually retroperitoneal in origin. When the tumor is opacified by feeding vessels that arise from celiac axis, or superior or inferior mesenteric artery, then an intraperitoneal lesion should be suspected. Masses situated adjacent and extrinsic to visceral structures will project distal to terminal branches vascularizing and opacifying the organ.

In contrast to CT scanning techniques, aortography not only may offer a better perspective of the size of the lesion and its vascular supply, but also may aid in visualization of the major vessels that must be ligated before resection of the tumor is attempted. The distribution of vessels within the lesion may offer information on the histologic type of tumor. Many sarcomas parasitize the blood vessels of adjacent viscera, which frequently become hypertrophied as the tumor mass increases in size and could pose major technical problems if they are not isolated and ligated at the beginning of tumor dissection. Angiosarcomas may develop a vascular pattern that is so extensive and derived from so diverse a source that resection becomes impossible. We see such a pattern of extensive vascularity in Figure 11–8, where the tumor blood supply is derived from both the superior and inferior mesenteric vessels. Lymphangiograms occasionally are used in a lateral lumbar view to define the extent of recurrent disease along the para-aortic chain and may prove a useful supplemental study to selective angiography.

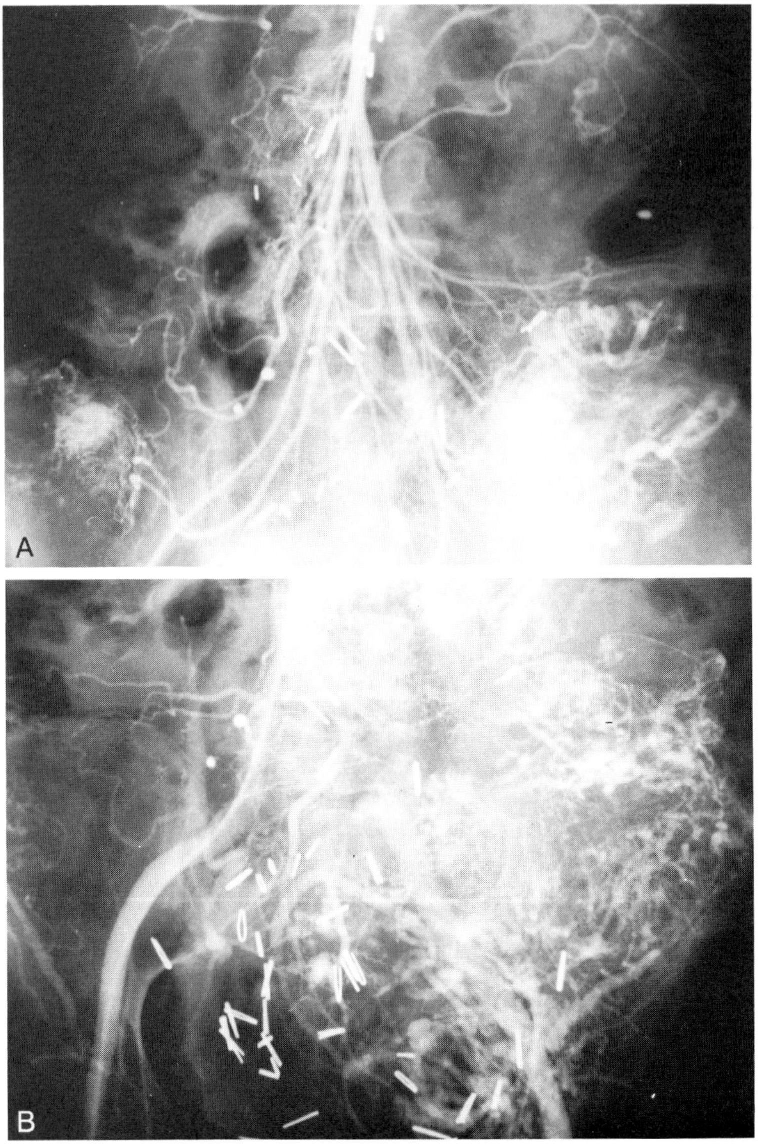

FIGURE 11–8. A and B, *Extensive vascular supply to a pelvic wall sarcoma. Both the superior and inferior mesenteric vessels are seen feeding the tumor.*

SURGICAL TECHNIQUE

One must have a basic concept of the anatomic structures that could be involved by a tumor mass before attempting resection of any large retroperitoneal lesion. This is particularly true in attempting en-bloc resection of the tumor mass and the involved surrounding structures.[2, 28, 45] Flank liposarcomas frequently arise from Gerota's fascia or surrounding retroperitoneal fat and may circumscribe the kidney as they grow. Figure 11–9 shows the extent of such a resected retroperitoneal tumor in relationship to a kidney that has essentially been circumscribed by the lesion. Under such circumstances, nephrectomy is usually necessary to accomplish complete removal, since the tumor tends to infiltrate surrounding fascia and derives a large portion of its blood supply from the renal vessels as well as those vessels that vascularize the kidney bed. It is rare for a tumor such as a liposarcoma to infiltrate the aorta and vena cava early in the disease process, so that dissection can usually be accomplished after appropriate structures are isolated and the tumor dissected away from them. In other instances, one may find it impossible to separate important structures such as the colonic mesentery from the tumor mass. Here, colectomy is required as part of the

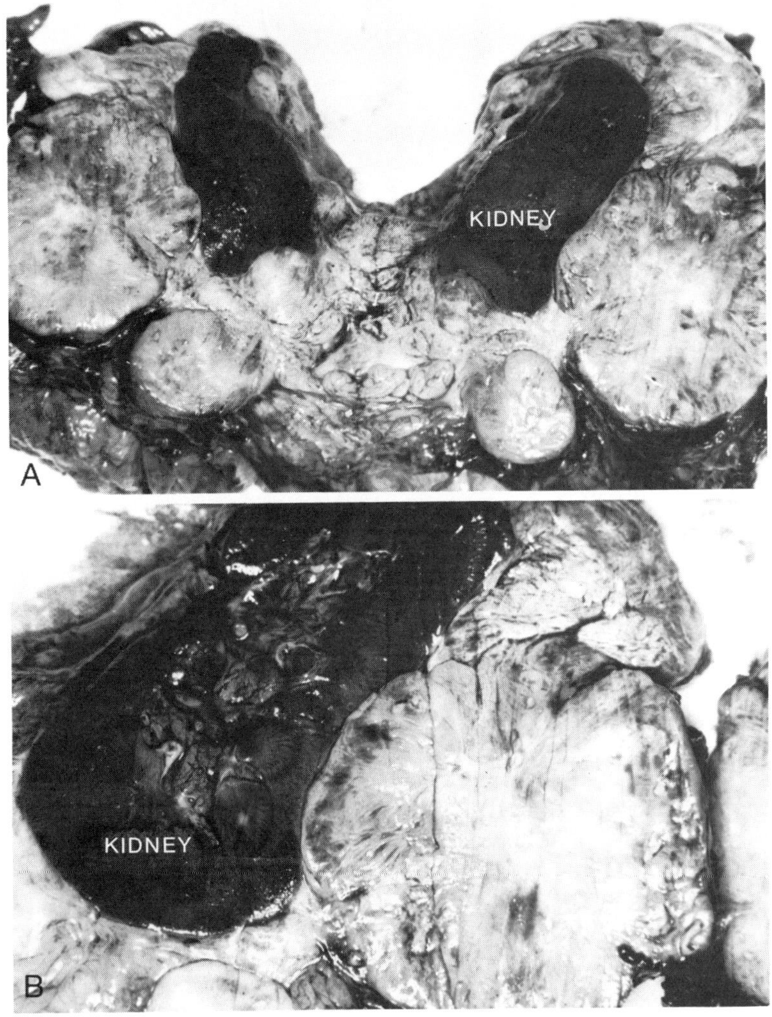

FIGURE 11–9. *A and B, Retroperitoneal sarcoma surrounding the kidney.*

en-bloc resection. The attempt to preserve the overlying colon has occasionally led us to reexplore the patient for necrotic bowel, which would result from failure of the marginal vessels to properly vascularize the remaining bowel. Figure 11–10 shows a tumor adjacent to the left kidney, where branches of the renal vessels perforate into and supply the tumor mass.

When adequate information has been obtained on completion of the diagnostic workup, then proper decisions regarding the type of resection can be made by the surgeon. Such studies may sometimes indicate that the tumor seen in the region of kidney is not invading Gerota's fascia. Under such circumstances, preservation of the kidney may be possible with low-grade tumors but not with fully malignant sarcomas. More frequently, any attempt at limiting the extent of the en-bloc resection can result in early local recurrence of disease, a situation that could necessitate re-exploration at a later date, with one performing that operation which should have been initially planned for.

With proper preoperative planning, we have been able to anticipate the type of incision that must be used to give adequate exposure. The incision must be large enough to deliver the tumor through the wound, as well as allow adequate exposure of all anatomic landmarks about the tumor that may require dissection, especially the vascular supply. For those retroperitoneal masses that are clinically palpable through the anterior abdominal wall, it is usually difficult for us to obtain adequate exposure with the classic midline approach alone. We have found that the initial exploration should be started through a long midline incision extending

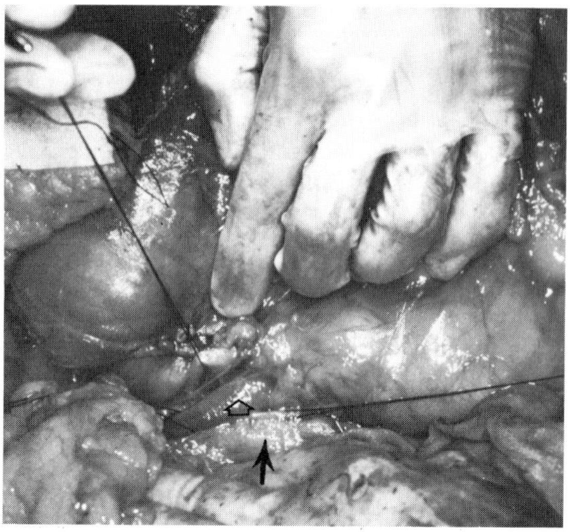

FIGURE 11–10. Tumor surrounding the left kidney. Dark arrow points to the aorta, light arrow to the left renal artery. The upper tie is on the renal vein draining the kidney and tumor; the lower tie is on a vascular branch feeding the tumor.

from the xiphoid to the pubis. With this exposure, moderately sized retroperitoneal sarcomas can easily be defined and resected. We are also able to evaluate whether metastases are present within the abdomen and if more aggressive surgery is indicated. More often, when the tumor mass is easily palpable through the abdominal wall, its size has been underestimated and extension of tumor is often found superiorly under the left diaphragm or liver on the right side. Adequate exposure can be achieved by carrying the upper end of the vertical incision to the left or right of the midline in a T-shaped fashion, usually entering the right or left eighth interspace as needed. A thoracoabdominal incision of this type may be required at any time, so the operative fields should be properly prepped prior to draping and positioning of the patient. In some instances, single or bilateral subcostal incisions have been advocated. We prefer to use a midline incision, as it allows adequate exposure and mobilization of the left and right colon as well as full exposure of the aorta-cava when needed. Figure 11–11 shows the exposure achieved using a thoracoabdominal incision. The tumor was initially considered unresectable through the bilateral subcostal incisions that were used.

The retroperitoneal space wherein surgery is performed reaches from diaphragm superiorly to the levators in the pelvis and from the twelfth vertebra to the coccyx. The psoas and quadratus muscles form the posterior space covered by fascia and peritoneum, investing the aorta and extending laterally. The space extends anteriorly in the leaves of the small bowel mesentery, where many tumors, especially those of lymph node origin, may infiltrate visceral mesentery. The retroperitoneal space containing aorta and inferior vena cava also have other structures of importance such as the portal and renal veins, duodenum, kidney, adrenal glands, ureter, nerve roots, sacral plexus, and extensive nodal chains paralleling the aorta and vena cava. These node groups may be involved by metastatic carcinoma from the

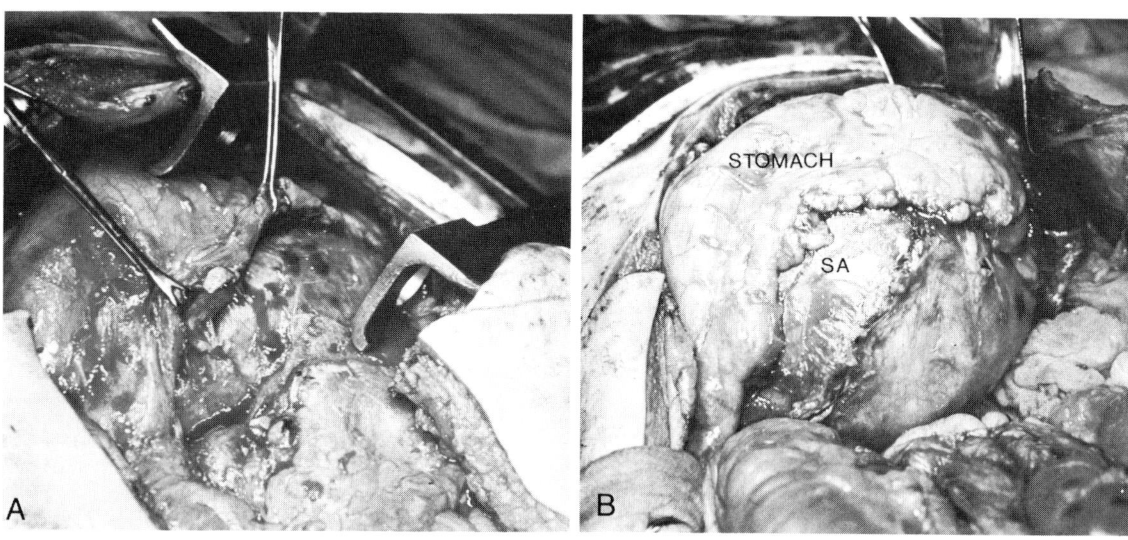

FIGURE 11–11. A, Thoracoabdominal approach for exposing large retroperitoneal masses. Babcock clamps are elevating the stomach off the tumor. B, Retrogastric lesion more clearly defined.

bowel, breast, or testis, as well as by rhabdomyosarcoma or lymphoma. We have all seen large retroperitoneal node masses arising secondary to metastatic testicular lesions or metastatic breast carcinoma, extending along the aorta superiorly to infiltrate the region of the retroperitoneal duodenum. Such infiltration can actually compromise this portion of bowel to produce partial intestinal obstruction.

Fixed portions of bowel such as the retroperitoneal duodenum can also be infiltrated by tumor arising from the kidney and prostrate (extending along the vena cava) as well as by liposarcomas and malignant fibrous histiocytomas. Additional displacement of the retroperitoneal duodenum can be seen before its infiltration by tumor. Attempts at kocherization of the duodenum should be made early in the operation. The lesser curvature of the stomach should then be followed along the first and second portions of the duodenal sweep. The Cattell maneuver (bringing hepatic flexure of colon across the midline abdomen to expose the entire retroperitoneum duodenum) is next performed and the duodenum dissected in its third and fourth portions, where the superior mesenteric vessels are defined. The lesser sac should next be entered along the greater curvature of the stomach after the gastrocolic ligament has been opened. When the posterior wall of the stomach is defined we can be assured that we are in the lesser sac. The retroperitoneal space can now be explored to evaluate tumor infiltration of this region and its proximity to the duodenum and pancreas. The ability to totally expose and then resect tumor here is what is necessary for cure. This holds true for lesions found in younger patients or those with relatively low-grade tumors. One can resect a portion, if not the entire retroperitoneal part of the duodenum, en bloc with the tumor mass itself. In essence, for a patient with sarcoma we would perform an en-bloc pancreaticoduodenectomy (Whipple procedure). We would not consider such surgery in elderly patients, since they are not usually able to withstand such extensive resections. In those situations in which the tumor extends below the transverse mesocolon and impinges on one of the gutters, ureteral displacement may also be seen. Ureteral obstruction is uncommon in the early stages of disease. For those tumors arising low in the abdomen and pelvis, where pelvic bones limit expansion of tumor, the bladder, rectum, and pelvic nerve roots may be compressed. Venous compression with leg edema is also a common finding with large pelvic tumor masses.

As a tumor mass enlarges, the vena cava can become involved. Initially, compression precedes invasion of the cava with development of enough collaterals to allow sacrifice of this structure, if necessary. By the time invasion of the vena cava occurs, exten-

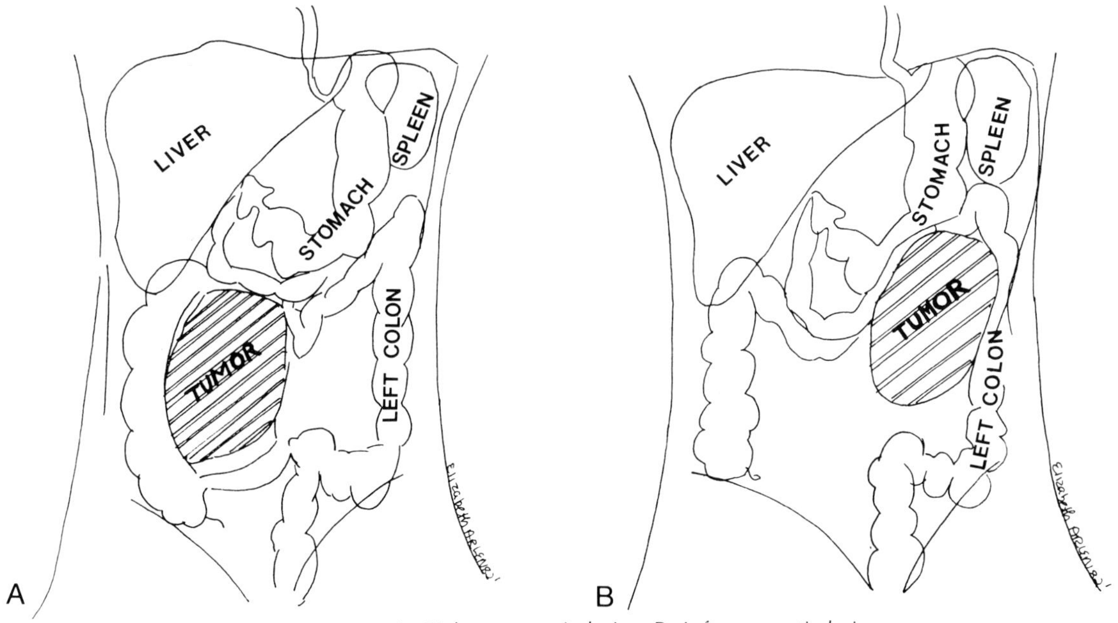

FIGURE 11–12. *A, Right para-aortic lesion. B, Left para-aortic lesion.*

sive abdominal wall and retroperitoneal collaterals have developed via the spermatic and ovarian vessels. This collateral supply allows sacrifice of the cava with minimal complications. When rapid invasion of the cava is seen early in the clinical course of disease and other adjacent structures are extensively infiltrated, such as the liver and abdominal wall, one must consider adrenal carcinoma to be the primary tumor of concern. Under such circumstances, one should be prepared for en-bloc resection to include partial hepatectomy and radical nephrectomy along with sacrifice of the vena cava.

Figure 11–12 shows the typical pattern of retroperitoneal involvement by tumor arising lateral to the aorta or vena cava with impingement on the mesentery of the colon. Retroperitoneal tumors most frequently arise in the gutters under the peritoneal reflection of colon, lateral to the aorta or cava, rather than directly over the midline structures. When found, centrally placed tumors are usually represented by leiomyosarcomas of caval origin, paragangliomas, pheochromocytomas, lymphomas, and fibrosarcomas. The laterally placed tumors most often are found to be liposarcomas and malignant fibrous histiocytomas, although all neoplasms may arise from any of the laterally placed soft part structures.

The ideal surgical approach for most large retroperitoneal sarcomas is, as we have mentioned, a long midline incision with thoracoabdominal extension when needed. This exposure offers an adequate approach for those tumors extending upward behind the spleen to invade the diaphragm, as well as those tracking up behind the liver and displacing the vena cava to the left. Figure 11–13 shows a sketch of the characteristic tumor mass that displaces either the splenic flexure or hepatic flexure inferiorly and the colon medially. Tumors near the splenic flexure require exposure of the kidney, body and tail of the pancreas, transverse mesocolon, and stomach. In the tumor depicted, division of the gastrocolic ligament along the transverse colon is required to allow entry into the lesser sac. We know that we have entered the correct plane when the posterior surface of the stomach is defined. This exposure may indicate that the body of the pancreas is involved by tumor. Similarly, on completion of mobilization of the splenic flexure, we can easily expose the surface of the kidney, where the capsule or vascular pedicle may be found to be invaded by tumor.

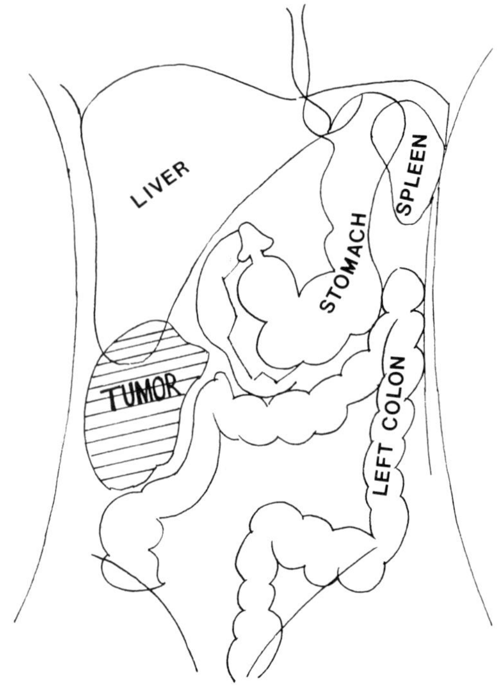

FIGURE 11–13. *Common position for a sarcoma arising in the lateral gutter and usually involving the kidney.*

En-bloc resection of a sarcoma near the splenic flexure would probably necessitate inclusion of a portion of the left colon, kidney, stomach, and distal pancreas. The dissection would be carried out to the left of the superior mesenteric vessels, which are usually isolated after mobilization of the hepatic flexure and dissection of the third and fourth portions of the duodenum to the ligament of Treitz. The vessels can then be palpated as they pass under the body of the pancreas to cross the fourth portion of the duodenum. As in the Whipple procedure, a tunnel is created over the superior mesenteric vessels and under the pancreas, permitting transection of the body of the pancreas (Fig. 11–5C).

Tumors found in the position seen in Figure 11–13 invariably invade the kidney and duodenum and attach to or infiltrate the porta hepatis, mesentery of colon, and possibly the liver. To approach these tumors the right gutter of the colon is mobilized to define the kidney capsule and ureter. After examination of the right colon, it may be necessary to include this part of the bowel with the tumor specimen should resectability be defined. The porta hepatis is evaluated and T-tube drainage of the common duct may be required if extensive dissection is needed here. The mid-transverse and ileocecal portions of the bowel are divided and elevated as a fulcrum on the tumor mass, with mobilization of the retroperitoneal duodenum away from the tumor. The liver edge may even require division as part of the specimen. The peritoneum over the aorta is next opened to the retroperitoneal jejunum exiting from the ligament of Treitz, and dissection is carried inferiorly to the bifurcation of the aorta. In one case, a large mass in the renal bed, which eventually proved to be an adrenal carcinoma, encompassed the kidney and invaded the liver. The above surgical principles were followed. We resected the tumor along with kidney, thrombosed vena cava, right lobe of liver (which had been completely infiltrated), and diaphragm. Marlex mesh was used to replace the diaphragm. The marked edema of the legs noted immediately after surgery resolved prior to discharge.

Exploration of the abdomen must be completed. For laterally placed masses, continuation of the mobilization of the left or right gutter of the colon follows. A small window is created at the site of the left or right peritoneal reflection (gutter) if mobilization has not already taken place. The developing peritoneal window is opened inferiorly for an additional 4 to 5 cm usually at the level of the pelvic brim, and a Richardson retractor is placed on the exposed external iliac artery, catching the inferior edge of the peritoneum and retracting it to the femoral canal. Dissection of the peritoneal gutters can then be carried superiorly with mobilization of the hepatic or splenic flexure, if necessary. The ureters are then defined along the medial peritoneal leaf initially created, and they are dissected deep into the pelvis in the direction of the trigone. We usually place tapes around dissected ureters for traction as they are dissected off tumor. Rarely do we employ ureteral catheters. It is essential that the ureters be dissected into the fibromuscular tunnel (Meig's canal in females) surrounding the ureters as they enter the trigone of the bladder. It is important that a Foley catheter be kept in the bladder for approximately 10 days after ureteral dissection. This allows the dissected ureters to lie against the retroperitoneal bed and become revascularized. Otherwise, as the uncatheterized bladder fills, the ureters are lifted off their retroperitoneal bed and may fail to gain the needed vascularization required for healing. We employ ureteral catheters when there is a question of invasion of these structures by tumor, and dissection of the tumor mass off the ureter is accomplished more easily.

Many retroperitoneal tumors tend to invade mesentery of the large bowel (mesocolon), parasitizing the blood supply and requiring that the overlying colon be included in the specimen. Small bowel is rarely infiltrated since its mobility on a rather free mesentery results in displacement of the small bowel rather than infiltration by sarcoma. The exceptions are when radiation therapy has been employed or when previously performed pelvic surgery has caused the small bowel to drop into the pelvis, resulting in extensive adhesions and fixation.

In one patient, pelvic liposarcoma had recurred in the abdominal cavity, invaded abdominal wall (Fig. 11–7*B* and *C*) and totally encompassed the rectum and sigmoid colon. The small bowel was partially obstructed where it had dropped into the pelvis at the site of previous surgery. We bypassed the obstructed bowel to the ascending colon and performed a sigmoid colostomy, after debulking of the pelvic mass. The patient was discharged and placed on adjuvant therapy.

If mobilization of normal bowel off a tumor invading gutter shows that the kidney is involved by tumor growth, we next attempt to dissect the retrorenal space to separate tumor from the lumbar muscles. The dissection behind the kidney is performed blindly by finger palpation to the aorta on the left and to the vena cava on the right. If these structures are not easily found because of the size and position of the tumor, additional dissection is begun at the bifurcation of the aorta and iliacs and carried superiorly up to and under the tumor mass. For high-lying retroperitoneal masses, the greater curvature of the stomach is mobilized next, so that the lesser sac can be entered. The retroperitoneal duodenum is freed (kocherization), and the transverse mesocolon is evaluated for invasion. In rare instances, it has been necessary to resect the vena cava en bloc with the tumor if it has been invaded by neoplastic tissue. By that time, retroperitoneal collateral circulation, as described above, has usually developed and is clinically apparent prior to surgery as a result of the presence of a caput medusae on the anterior abdominal wall.

On occasion, the lesion is so extensive

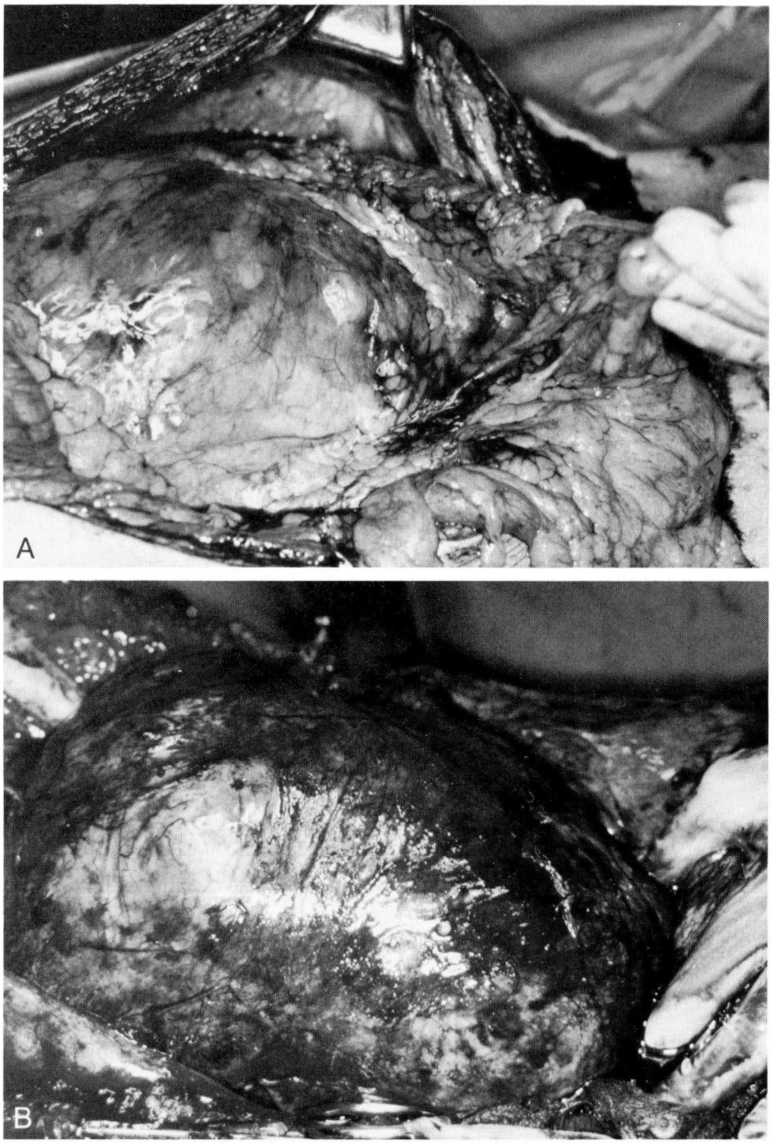

FIGURE 11–14. *A, Exposure of an extensive midline sarcoma displacing the transverse colon inferiorly. B, Initial mobilization of the midline sarcoma.*

(Fig. 11–14) that the aorta-cava cannot be approached in the usual manner, even after lateral gutter dissection has been accomplished and even when one dissects toward the normal iliac vessels. Under such circumstances, the size of the tumor must be reduced by incising the pseudocapsule of the tumor and enucleating a large portion of its mass. With an extremely vascular tumor, such as hemangiopericytoma, such debulking is usually not feasible. The extent of vascularity can usually be anticipated by preoperative angiography, which should be considered prior to resection of all large tumors. Should an abundant vascular supply be defined, thrombosis of the tumor vessels can sometimes be accomplished prior to exploration.[52] Where several major vessels feed the tumor, resection is impossible (see Fig. 11–8).

Should moderate bleeding develop during central cytoreduction, the debulked tumor mass can be packed within its pseudocapsule to control the bleeding, so that exposure of the cava and aorta can be accomplished more easily. In many instances, such debulking improves the chances for completion of a successful dissection. An important rule to follow is that vessel dissection, as well as visceral dissection, should be carried out from a normal to an abnormal plane. Mobilization should not begin in the middle of the tumor field. Rather, it should be begun in a clean plane, moving toward the tumor,

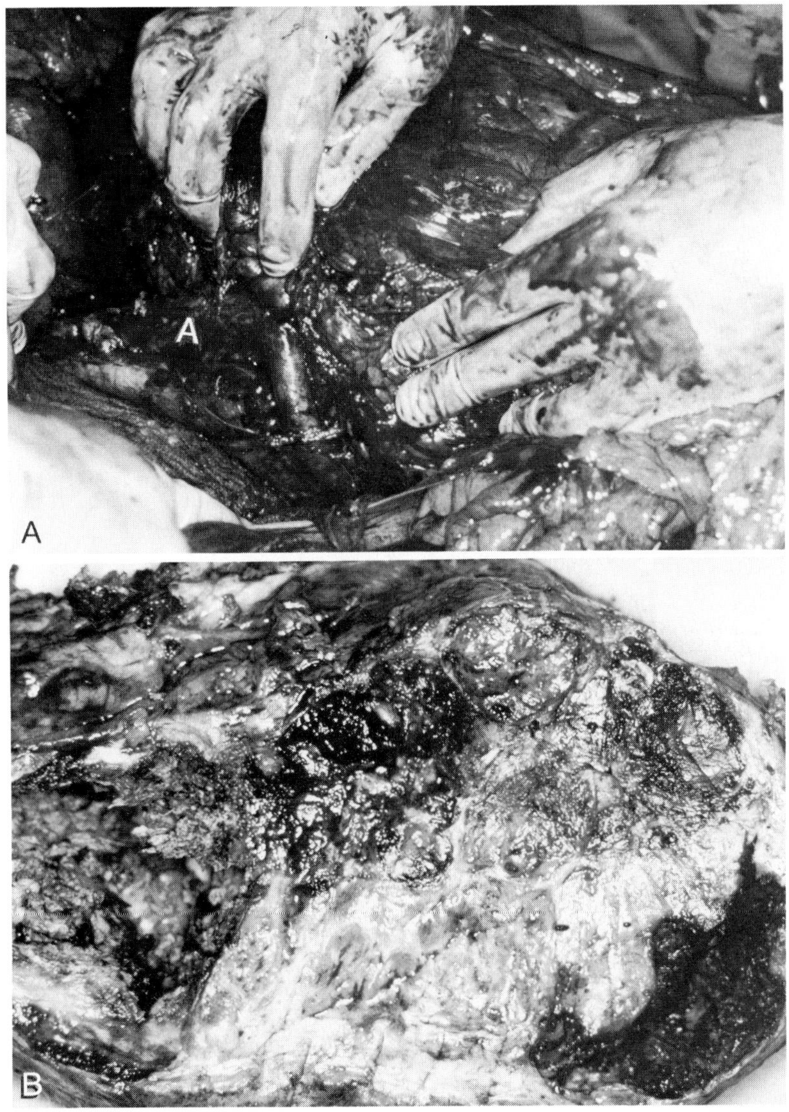

FIGURE 11–15. A, After central debulking, the aorta (A) and cava were identified by tracing the common iliac artery superiorly. B, Bisected specimen.

within boundaries determined prior to initiation of the procedure.

If the tumor mass is sitting in the upper midline abdomen, making definition of the aorta difficult, the iliac vessels are traced up along the cava and aorta until the site of invasion is identified. Sharp scalpel dissection is usually carried out at this time within the vascular (aorta and cava) adventitia, which aids in freeing the tumor mass from its adherence to the great vessels. Figure 11–15*A* shows the bowed aorta-iliac bifurcation caused by tumor extending behind the iliac vessels. Despite the massive size of this lesion, virtually total extirpation was accomplished. The histological diagnosis was retroperitoneal fibrosarcoma. Adjuvant therapy was planned after discharge from the hospital, and the patient has remained free of disease over 4 years after surgery.

For those retroperitoneal tumors extending along the psoas muscle and compromising the iliac vessels and abdominal wall, the approach described by Karakousis can be employed (see Chapter 10). A lower midline incision is brought to the pubis, then "hockey-sticked" across the inguinal ligament to the site of the femoral canal; this incision can then be extended over the femoral vessels to the apex of the femoral triangle. This incision allows for complete exposure of the entire lower retroperitoneum on either the left or the right side.

With a large part of the blood supply of

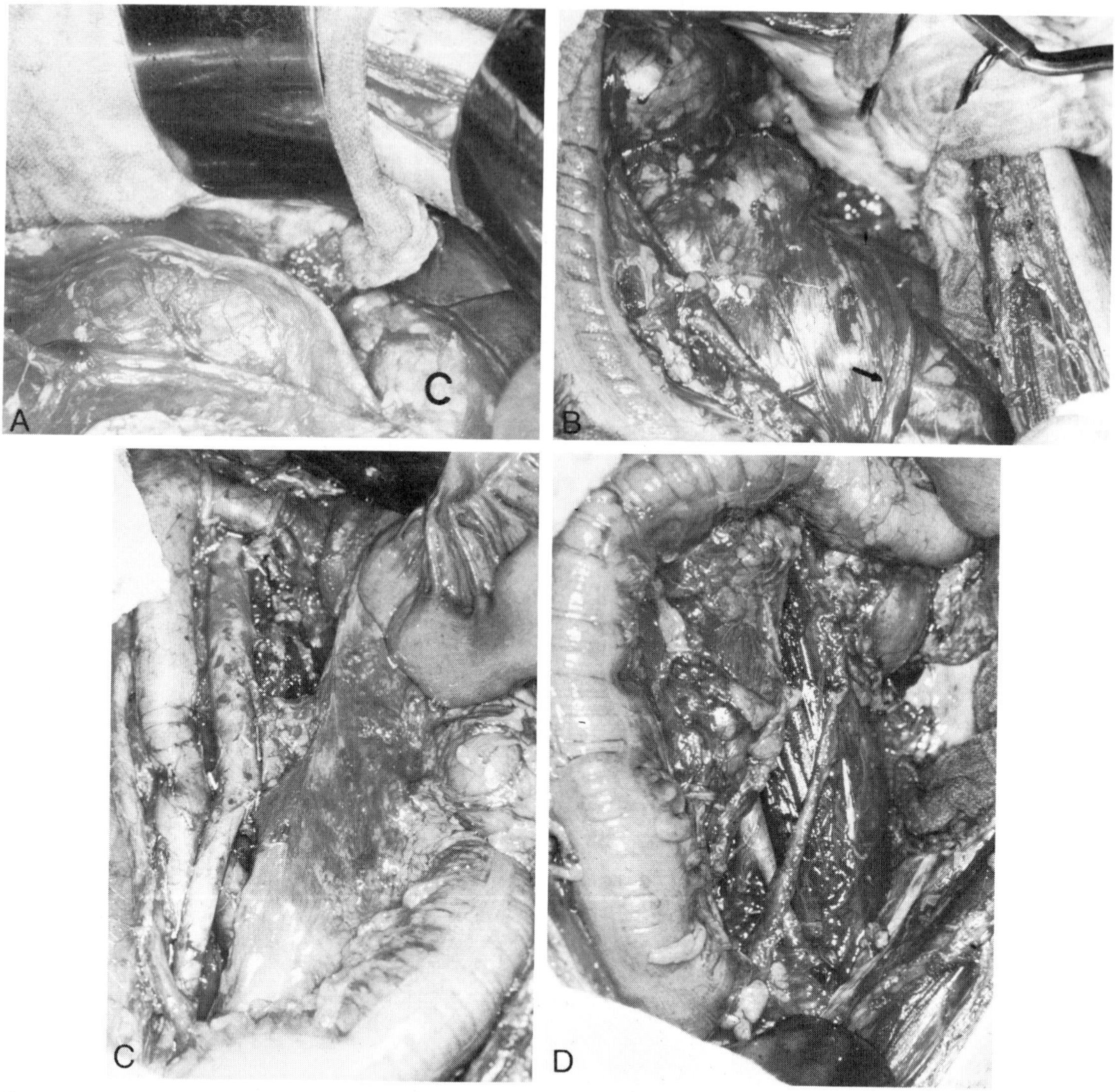

FIGURE 11–16. A, *Para-aortic sarcoma displacing the left colon* (C) *laterally.* B, *Sigmoid colon mobilized medially over the tumor. Ureter* (arrow) *is seen crossing over the tumor.* C, *After the tumor has been resected, mobilization of the colon laterally reveals the dissected aorta-cava. The left renal vein is seen crossing the aorta in the upper field.* D, *Medial displacement of the colon shows the extent of the left gutter dissection. The mobilized ureter crosses pelvic vessels (external iliacs) lower than normally. The ureter is usually seen crossing the hypogastrics.*

the retroperitoneal sarcomas being derived from the lumbar vessels, the ability to approach the aorta-cava in the midline offers the obvious opportunity to control the blood supply to this region. Figure 11–16*A* shows the presence of a large retroperitoneal mass covering the region of the aorta-cava and bulging into the left lateral retroperitoneal region, displacing the left colon and sigmoid laterally. Mobilization of the descending and sigmoid colon medially over the mass allows better definition of the tumor, with the ureter crossing over it (Fig. 11–16*B*). After complete dissection of the bowel to expose the mass and further mobilization of this lesion from the aorta and cava, the resected field was clearly defined. The renal vein and bifurcation of aorta are distinctly seen, and the right iliac artery is noted to pass under the mesentary of the colon (Fig. 11–16*C*). The left renal vein is seen crossing the aorta in the upper field. With the colon next retracted medially, the bifurcation of the iliac artery with the ureter crossing the external iliac artery is well defined (Fig. 11–16*D*). The bladder should remain catheterized in such instances for at least 10 days to allow the ureter to remain against retroperitoneal structures to allow for revascularization.

Sarcomas involving the transverse mesocolon in the region of the ligament of Treitz may have already compromised the superior mesenteric artery. Similarly, invasion of the celiac axis may result in compression of the hepatic vessels. In such instances, we have ligated the celiac axis. These vessels were resected as part of the tumor mass without any undue consequences. Collateral circulation usually develops over the ensuing period of tumor growth, so there is usually sufficient ancillary blood supply. The hepatic artery can be evaluated at the time of dissection and occasionally mobilized free from tumor by clamping and dividing the gastroduodenal artery just above the duodenum. This short vessel can then be used as a lever to elevate the hepatic artery loop that arises from the celiac axis and passes in an arch-like fashion in the direction of the liver bed. At this point, the common hepatic artery can be completely dissected off the porta hepatis prior to its bifurcation into left and right branches. This approach is ideal when planning catheterization of the hepatic artery via the gastroduodenal artery. It allows insertion of the catheter into the hepatic artery at the junction with the gastroduodenal artery. The catheter can be either brought out on the skin or attached to an implantable chemotherapy delivery pump. Hepatic artery angiography should be performed to assure origins of the vessels supplying the liver.

Obstruction of the vena cava by tumor is frequently accompanied by sufficient collateral circulation, so that the cava can be resected in continuity with the tumor mass. In the presence of large sarcomas such as leiomyosarcoma, the potential for metastasis to adjacent viscera and liver is great. If pulmonary metastasis have been ruled out, one can be aggressive and attempt total resection of the tumor mass. One need not, however, limit resection because of multiple pulmonary lesions from sarcoma, especially if the lesion is low-grade and is thought to have been present for a long time.

As a rule, it is not important how large the tumor mass is or how extensive the visceral resection must be; what is important is the quality and function of those structures that are left behind. Inadvertent pinpoint perforation of the bowel or ureter, damage to the lumbar vessels, or failure to control bleeding from the pelvic veins in a poorly planned operation is more of an impediment to achieving proper results than removal of an extensive but localized tumor. Adequate drains should be placed at all gutter sites, liver, and renal bed as well as at areas of anastomosis to protect surrounding structures. The drains are necessary to handle possible extensive lymphatic drainage, anastomotic leaks, or oozing with the potential development of an infected seroma or hematoma. In some patients we have had such extensive retroperitoneal lymphatic drainage that the possibility of ureteral leak had been raised and the use of methylene blue was necessary to confirm that the ureters were intact. When the question of ureteral devascularization is raised, especially after ureters have been dissected over a long distance and the potential for vessel thrombosis becomes great, we have inserted ureteral catheters and left them in place from 5 to 10 days. This assures that some fibrosis around the ureters will occur and that vascularization will follow. Because of the extent of inanition in some patients, we frequently use hyperalimentation for 1 to 2 weeks before surgery. Postoperatively there is always the possibility of poor wound healing. Hyperalimentation should therefore be continued after surgery to ensure continued improvement in protein reserves. In those patients who have undergone extensive retroperitoneal dissections, there is usually prolonged ileus, and postoperative hyperalimentation becomes one of the most important factors in a successful outcome.

PATTERNS OF TUMOR BEHAVIOR

The surgeon dealing with retroperitoneal tumors usually has a fair idea of whether a lesion is malignant or benign from clinical and preoperative findings and gains further insight based on what he observes at the time of laparotomy. This is important, since the pathologist may have difficulty in classifying low-grade lesions on the basis of frozen section alone. At times, classification may be difficult after careful histologic examination of paraffin sections. In the majority of cases, though, most retroperitoneal tumors are malignant.

Lymphomas, which represent a large percentage of the tumors found in the retroperitoneum, tend to involve para-aortic nodes;

as they expand, such nodal masses may present as a large palpable abdominal mass. Most of these tumors, as a result of their growth patterns, do involve midline structures. However, reticulum cell sarcomas (malignant histiocytic sarcomas), in contrast, may attain an even larger size and invade all surrounding structures. In addition, this tumor frequently appears within the retroperitoneal gutter and is known to invade mesentery and bowel.

In rare instances, we have seen pancreatic carcinoma presenting as a retroperitoneal tumor mass extending down the para-aortic nodes. It then progresses along the iliac vessels to appear in the region of the femoral canal. We have not only seen this tumor confused with retroperitoneal sarcoma but have also seen other common tumors presenting in an unusual manner suggestive of the retroperitoneal sarcoma. Prostatic cancer can occasionally present as an extremely small neoplastic process within the prostate and "skip metastasize" along the pelvic lymph nodes, extending up the para-aortic nodes to present as a large retroperitoneal mass. In one case we encountered such a tumor extending along the lumbar gutter to infiltrate the mesocolon and totally surround the sigmoid colon. More often this neoplasm does involve the retroperitoneal bowel by circumscribing the rectum in the region of the levators without penetrating the lumen of the rectum. When such a retroperitoneal tumor is seen compromising the lumen of the bowel, a primary prostatic tumor should be suspected and proper work-up (including acid phosphatase levels and transrectal biopsy) carried out.

Table 11–1 reviews several series of retroperitoneal sarcomas. The maximum percent of benign cases in any of the series was 25%. Lymphoma and lymphosarcomas represented a small but significant percent of the cases managed. The majority of the cases were liposarcoma of fibrosarcoma. In most series of retroperitoneal tumors, the most common lesion to involve flank structures (Pack and Tabah)[48] was the liposarcoma; in this and other series the tumor was frequently found to reach an enormous size. Extensive growth as well as infiltration of surrounding structures readily occurs because of the prolonged period of growth before symptoms develop.

Benign tumors are not commonly found in the retroperitoneum; when they are present they can appear in the form of cysts, which as mentioned previously, could be mistaken for ascites. They may also be seen as benign nerve tumors, lipomas, lymphangiomas, benign histiocytic tumors, or even adrenal cysts. Benign lipomas may invade the entire mesentery of the small bowel in single or multiple areas (Fig. 11–17), causing the surgeon to assume at the time of clinical

TABLE 11–1. Primary Retroperitoneal Tumors

	Donnelly[61] *(1946)*	*Newman and Pinck*[62] *(1950)*	*Mellicow*[63] *(1953)*	*Pack and Tabah*[64] *(1954)*	*Johnson et al.*[65] *(1954)*	*Donhauser and Bigelow*[66] *(1955)*	*Braasch and Mon*[67] *(1967)*	*Felix, Wood, Das Gupta*[68] *(1981)*
Number of cases	91	33	162	120	72	48	101	48
Per cent benign	10	16	23	14	22	23	13	25
Per cent malignant	90	84	77	86	78	77	87	75
Lymphoma and lymphosarcoma	1	10	48	28	27	17	31	
Fibrosarcoma	19	—	11	6	16	2	16	2
Liposarcoma	2	2	14	17		3	6	10
Leiomyosarcoma	—	1	15	5	1	3	6	7
Neurosarcoma	2	5	13	8	7	5	2	3
Hemangiopericytoma	—	—	1	1	—	—	—	5
Rhabdomyosarcoma	—	—	1	22	—	—	—	4
Urogenital tumors	13	1	5	1	3	1	3	—
Undifferentiated sarcoma	37	4	3	8	1	6	7	—
Undifferentiated carcinoma	7	5	10	6	1	—	6	—
Mesenchymal tumors	1	—	3	2	—	—	3	—
Mesothelial tumors	—	—	—	2	—	—	—	—
Synovial tumors	—	—	—	1	—	—	—	1
Other	—	—	—	—	—	—	11	—

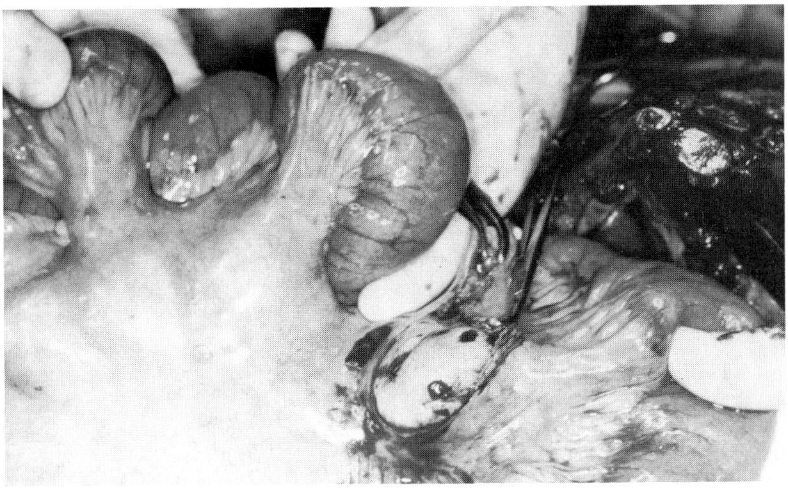

FIGURE 11–17. Nodular lipomatosis.

examination that he is dealing with a large retroperitoneal tumor mass.

Benign extensive retroperitoneal neurilemmomas have been described by Regan et al.[50] Of the five patients reported by him, the tumors found were more than 12 cm in diameter. Three were fixed to the right side of the sacrum and two to the left. Their most striking characteristic was the marked vascularity of the overlying peritoneum and capsule. Tumors were attached to the presacral tissue; they displaced the ureters, colon, and rectum and partially surrounded the pelvic blood vessels. None were invasive.

The primary retroperitoneal cysts that arise in the region of the retroperitoneal fatty tissues have no apparent connection with any adult anatomic structures, except for the loose areolar connective tissue that is found there. They are thought to arise embryologically from mesonephric structures and become symptomatic only by virtue of their size and position. The first major review of such lesions by Handfield Jones in 1924 effectively excluded pancreatic, renal, and adrenal cystic lesions. Embryologically, the ureters, renal pelvis, and collecting tubules have been found to arise from a bud of the mesonephric duct, which fuses with the secretory tubules from the nephrogenic cords to form the kidney. Should the ureteric bud fail to join the developing metanephric mass, it has been postulated that the metanephric mass could undergo normal development and accumulate secretions that result in the cyst. Several reports have reinforced this concept, each describing a large retroperitoneal cyst arising in a persistent metanephros with congenital absence of the ipsilateral kidney and ureter. These cases support the concept of formation of retroperitoneal cysts from anomalies in the progenitors of the kidney, which may at times result in incorporation of functionally active endocrine tissue. Proctor et al.[49] reported a case of a retroperitoneal cyst associated with clinical abnormalities of Cushing's disease and pheochromocytoma. In a series of 32 cases reported by Galloway and Priestly,[29] 28 (87%) had clinical symptoms, among them pain (in 15) and an abdominal mass (in 7). Acute symptoms were also reported and were related to hemorrhage into the cysts. When large, the cysts have been mistaken for ascites, and paracentesis, as well as exploration, of the ascitic fluid has been described. Complete excision is the treatment of choice.

In the CT scan shown in Figure 11–6, the radiologic interpretation of liposarcoma was made. On completion of the resection the histologic diagnosis was changed to angiomyelolipoma arising outside the renal capsule. This was our first experience with the extrarenal form of this disease. Other than for the presence of a mass, the patient was totally asymptomatic and has remained so since surgery. An association of angiomyolipomas with tuberous sclerosis has been reported in the literature; however, in reviewing the experience at Memorial Hospital, Hadju and Foote were able to find only 9 of 53 renal lesions in association with tuberous sclerosis. These tumors are usually sharply demarcated from renal parenchyma and are composed of fat, smooth muscle, and blood vessels. At times, they present with a pleomorphic pattern, confused with liposarcoma or leiomyosarcoma. At least three reported cases of malignant angiomyolipoma have appeared in the literature. While the tumor is usually intrarenal, it may rarely present as a pedunculated mass or a separate lesion in proximity to the kidney within the retroperitoneal structures, as in our case. The clinical course for such tumors is entirely benign.

Since most retroperitoneal tumors are malignant when they are encountered at exploration, one should attempt resection of such a lesion even without definitive pathology confirmation of malignancy. However, when extensive resection with en-bloc removal of adjacent organs is required, or when a partial hepatectomy or pelvic exenteration is needed, one either should have a frozen section read to confirm the nature of the neoplastic process of should reconsider the type of surgery, postponing it for a later time. In anticipation of massive blood loss, all of our patients are brought to the operating room with central venous pressure lines in place and frequently have a Swan-Ganz catheter inserted for pressure measurements.

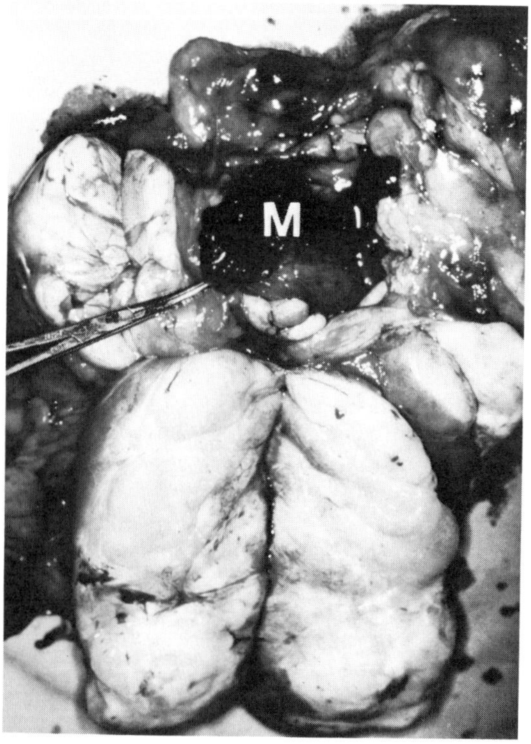

FIGURE 11–18. *Retroperitoneal myxoliposarcoma. M represents the myxomatous component.*

Even when a frozen section is read as benign, the final report does not always confirm benignity. This must be taken into consideration when performing a procedure. The nature of the biopsy must also be considered. This is especially true when a tumor does not have a uniform composition. Large fatty neoplasms are usually heterogeneous, with fully malignant areas in one or more regions and low-grade or benign areas intermittently dispersed. Adequate representative sampling during the biopsy of such tumors is mandatory. Figure 11–18 shows the appearance of a large lipomyxosarcoma. The multinodular areas represent discrete regions of both myxomatous, relatively benign-appearing tissue and fully malignant sarcoma. A small biopsy taken here could be misleading. We are very careful in attempting to obtain a representative sample when sending such biopsies for evaluation.

Neuroblastoma

Embryonal (pediatric) tumors of the retroperitoneum comprise a small but definite portion of the spectrum of retroperitoneal tumors referred for surgical management. Excluding Wilms' tumor, neuroblastomas and embryonal rhabdomyosarcomas are the predominant lesions encountered.[25] Chemotherapy plays a major role in their management. Should the tumor be considered unresectable, it is possible to offer radiation and chemotherapy alone or in combination to reduce the tumor size. Surgery can then be reconsidered if residual disease is found. In other instances, the chemotherapeutic agents available can be made relatively more effective if the tumor mass can be surgically debulked. We usually explore, biopsy, cytoreduce (when feasible), then initiate chemotherapy with or without radiation therapy. The principles of management are the same as for adults, except when the tumor is exceedingly bulky, in which case biopsy is followed by an attempt at chemotherapeutic reduction.

Neurogenic (neuroblastoma) tumors are a common form of retroperitoneal tumor in infancy and childhood and may be found wherever sympathetic ganglia arise,[24] but most often in the retroperitoneum (representing about half of the cases we define clinically). One half of these are of adrenal gland origin. In the retroperitoneum, the tumor usually produces anterolateral and

TABLE 11–2. Staging of Neuroblastomas

Stage I	Tumor confined to the origin or site of origin.
Stage II	Tumor extends beyond the site of origin by contiguity, but not crossing midline.
Stage III	Tumor crosses midline, and regional nodes may be involved bilaterally.
Stage IV	Metastasis exists in the skeletal system or other distant sites.

inferior displacement of the kidney, with the palpable mass frequently crossing midline. Calcification of tumor is seen in approximately 50% of cases. Bone metastases are common at the time of definition of the retroperitoneal mass. The tumor comprises sheets of small rounded cells divided into small lobules by a delicate fibrovascular stroma. Staging of this tumor is based on the effect of the tumor on surrounding structures and whether the midline has been crossed (Table 11–2).

According to Beckwith and Perrin,[4] in-situ forms of neuroblastoma are probably not uncommon and may be present in a far higher proportion of infants (by a factor of 500) then actually is clinically apparent. This would suggest that maturation factors are at play in the neonate, causing such in-situ lesions to regress. This is believed to be related to an immune surveillance phenomenon suggested from lymphocyte studies, where inhibition against the patient's own tumor as well as other neuroblastoma populations can be demonstrated.

Metastic bone lesions secondary to neuroblastoma can frequently be confused with Ewing's sarcoma on biopsy. Children under 1 year of age, when diagnosed, appear to do better than older children, and lesions of the retroperitoneum are considered worse than those above the diaphragm. Complete removal of the tumor without radiation therapy is recommended for stage I disease confined to structures of origin; for stage II disease, demonstrating en-bloc continuity spread that has not crossed midline. Figure 11–19*A* shows a large neuroblastoma in the process of being resected, with the right lobe of the liver elevated to define the tumor that has arisen from the right adrenal gland. Exposure was obtained using a midline incision from the xiphoid to below the umbilicus. The exposure is essentially identical to that used for transabdominal adrenalectomy. The right adrenal, where this tumor arose, sits posterolateral to the vena cava at the site where the cava passes through the crura of the diaphragm. In this situation, the adrenal gland could be separated from the right lobe of the liver. Frequently the tumor invades the posterior capsule of the liver. To obtain adequate exposure the abdominal incision must be curved into the eighth or ninth interspace and the diaphragm divided to allow the partial hepatectomy to encompass the tumor. Cava and aorta must be identified

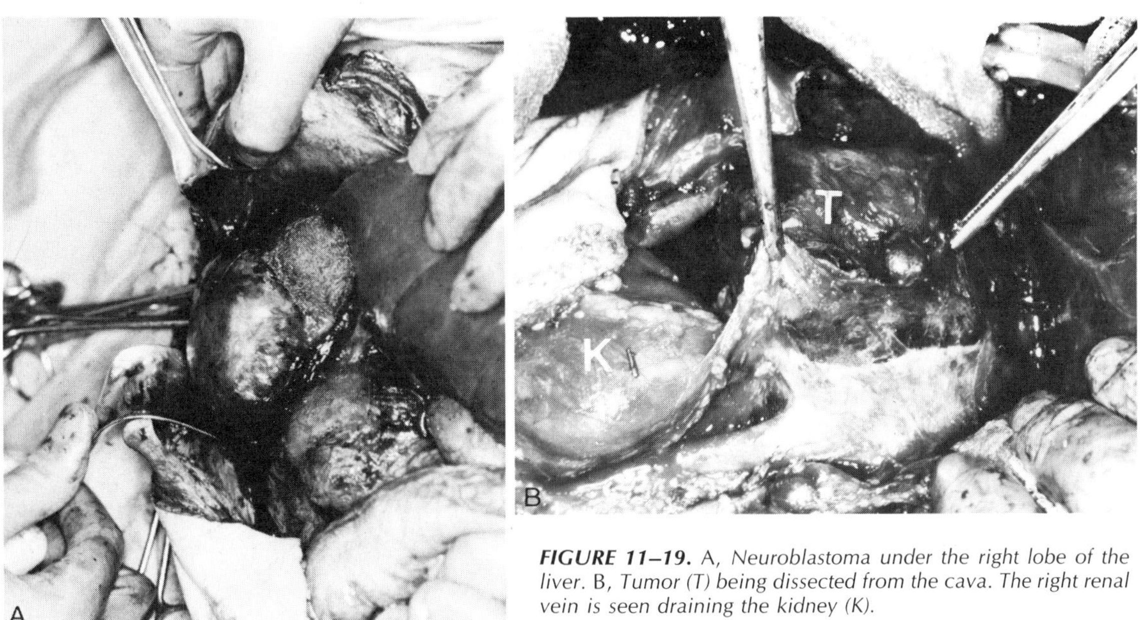

FIGURE 11–19. A, *Neuroblastoma under the right lobe of the liver.* B, *Tumor (T) being dissected from the cava. The right renal vein is seen draining the kidney (K).*

and tumor separated from the cava (Fig. 11–19*B*). This is true for both adult and pediatric forms of adrenal tumor. In the adult forms of carcinoma of the adrenal cortex, the vena cava must at times be sacrificed. As such, one can probably count on the obstructed cava to have developed sufficient retroperitoneal collaterals to allow its sacrifice without compromising venous return.

Approximately 30 cases of non-functioning paragangliomas have been described arising in the retroperitoneum. These tumors are composed of collections of neurosecretory cells closely connected with the ganglia of the autonomic nervous system. The tumors, which may be malignant in 20 to 30% of cases, have a metastatic rate of approximately 15%. They present as large, slow-growing masses with long-term survival. They can be extremely vascular and require angiography to evaluate the extent of their blood supply. Surgery is the only effective therapy.

Neurilemmomas are rare but occasionally present as large retroperitoneal masses. The larger these tumors grow, the more they are associated with degeneration and cyst formation. If they are difficult to remove, enucleation can be attempted.[50]

Liposarcoma

The most common retroperitoneal lesion to be defined at laparotomy is the liposarcoma. Between 12 and 20% of liposarcomas are found to occur in the retroperitoneum. Liposarcomas are more common, however, within the lower extremity. The head and neck region represents one of the less common sites for clinical involvement by this type of tumor.

Liposarcomas of the retroperitoneum characteristically have a less favorable prognosis than those we have treated in the lower extremity (Kinney et al.),[37] probably owing to the prolonged time before their identification and the proximity of the growing tumor to vital structures. Over a 25-year period, 249 cases of liposarcoma have been seen at the Memorial Sloan-Kettering Cancer Center. Thirty-four (13.6%) occurred in the retroperitoneal region. Patients ranged in age from 23 to 72 years (mean, 49.3 years). Three groups of patients were described: (1) those who underwent complete excision with or without the use of radiation therapy (11 patients); (2) those who underwent partial excision of the tumor with radiation therapy (15 patients); and (3) those in whom biopsy proved the tumor to be inoperable (8 patients).

The overall survival rate for this series was 41%. Two late recurrences were found 10 and 12 years after resection, supporting the contention that long-term follow-up with CT scanning is necessary, at least every 6 months during the first and second years and yearly for the next 10 years.[39] Four of the Memorial patients were free of disease 6, 13, 19, and 30 years postoperatively; three had received radiation therapy. Metastatic disease developed in 19 of the 34 patients. When recurrence appeared, the liver and lungs were the most frequent sites of involvement. Two of the patients demonstrated nodal spread of disease. Among the remaining 15 patients, 8 died with extensive local recurrence into the surrounding structures, 3 died in the postoperative period, and 4 remained free of disease. Well-differentiated lipoblastic tumors were seen in 7 patients; myxoliposarcoma was found in the majority of cases (23 of 34 patients). Pleomorphic sarcoma occurred in 4 patients.

What surprised us in the patient whose CT scan is shown in Figure 11–7*B* and *C* was that in spite of massive recurrence, extending upward from the pelvis, the liver was free of disease, the primary site of extension being the muscle planes along the psoas. Extensive muscle infiltration is exceedingly rare and represents a major factor leading to unresectability. In spite of some clear-cut indications that the retroperitoneal sarcoma that has been resected fits into the classification of low-grade liposarcoma, a consensus must be reached in terms of the gross and microscopic presentation. In one of our patients, a bulky sarcoma adherent to the right psoas muscle and extending into femoral nerve was identified (see Chapter 1). The tumor was resected en-bloc with psoas muscle. Nerve repair was accomplished with fine interrupted silk sutures. Based on a predominant myxomatous component with the suggestion of lipoblastic cells, the initial interpretation was low-grade liposarcoma. We were considering use of radiation therapy to the operative field; however, a final diagnosis of low-grade malignant fibrous histiocytoma with a major myxomatous component was finally established.[59]

Farberman,[26] in reviewing his experience

with retroperitoneal tumor size noted that lesions of 7.4 kg to 25.4 kg were among the most common. While extremity lesions had a 5-year survival of 71%, only 39% of patients with tumors in the retroperitoneum were alive at 5 years; this dropped to 4% at 10 years, which appears to be a common finding in most series that have reviewed retroperitoneal sarcomas. Histologic type could not be documented as a major factor in survival; rather, complete excision appeared to be the most important factor, with the extent of resection of adjacent organs when necessary another factor. Partial resection plus radiation and chemotherapy may be of some value when a curative resection cannot be achieved. In Kinney's series, one third of the cases survived for 5 years.[37] Postoperative radiation therapy afforded a disease-free interval of 32 months compared with 16 months when no radiation therapy was employed. McNeer et al.[44] noted that the liposarcomas were among the most sensitive of the soft part tumors to radiation therapy and that survival was enhanced by this adjuvant form of treatment.

When, on the basis of clinical and x-ray studies, a malignant tumor is suspected to be present in the retroperitoneum, multiorgan involvement has probably already occurred. As the lesion enlarges, it spreads along the fascial planes in a multicentric pattern. If a patient has had a history of a primary extremity sarcoma, it is probable that any retroperitoneal mass found represents an active metastatic focus. Many of the patients whom we have treated for large primary lesions of the thigh later were noted to have retroperitoneal tumors, which represented skip patterns along fascial planes, passing either through the femoral canal or the obturator membrane. In one patient with extensive liposarcoma a cerebrovascular accident occurred 2 years after muscle group dissection of the thigh. The cerebrovascular accident was found to be secondary to a hypertensive episode, which was further investigated and found to be associated with renal artery stenosis. In attempting to repair the renal vascular problem, it was noted that vascular compression had resulted from recurrent tumor, which had spread through the retroperitoneum along the fascial planes near the aorta and into the area of the renal vessels. Figure 11–20*A* shows a large recurrent liposarcoma on the psoas muscle in the left hypogastric fossa. This tumor represented metastasis spreading from the thigh along the fascial planes of the femoral artery through the femoral canal into the retroperitoneum. Figure 11–20*B* demonstrates the approach needed to handle the larger retroperitoneal tumor, which has taken its blood supply from the renal vascular bundle. Here the various branches feeding the tumor are ligated. In Figure 11–20*C* the denuded renal fossa can be seen after resection of the large retroperitoneal tumor taken en-bloc with the kidney. The diaphragm is clearly seen, as is the psoas muscle denuded of overlying fascia.

Binder et al.[8] reviewed their experience with retroperitoneal liposarcomas. Between 12 and 40% of these tumors occurred in the retroperitoneum; 35% were found to develop in perirenal fat. Slow-growing, well-differentiated myxoid type of sarcoma was found to be relatively radiosensitive compared with the rapidly growing anaplastic, highly malignant variant. The radiation dose needed to cure extremity liposarcomas was found to range from 5000 to 6000 R, a dose that is difficult to deliver to retroperitoneal structures because of the sensitivity of adjacent viscera. Since radiation therapy is most effective with minimal tumor burden, debulking the liposarcoma should be attempted. Local recurrence more than doubles the probability that the patient will die of disease. Large, bulky, marginally resected tumors may respond to preoperative radiation therapy, and where questionable margins are present, postoperative radiation therapy may also be of value.

Depending on the series reviewed, retroperitoneal liposarcomas have a 20 to 85% rate of local recurrence.[12] The incidence of recurrence for this lesion depends on how adequately the excision has been performed.[19] Survival rates four times that achieved by local resection can be accomplished following radical resection. Over half of the patients with local recurrence will also show signs of concurrent distant metastasis. Primary tumors tend to grow by local expansion with little tendency to invade surrounding tissue in their initial growth phase. Rather, as noted, they grow along fascial planes and tend to produce separate tumor masses. Metastases may occur anywhere in the body but are commonly seen in lungs, liver, and lymph nodes.

When retroperitoneal liposarcoma does recur, the new lesion is usually far more ag-

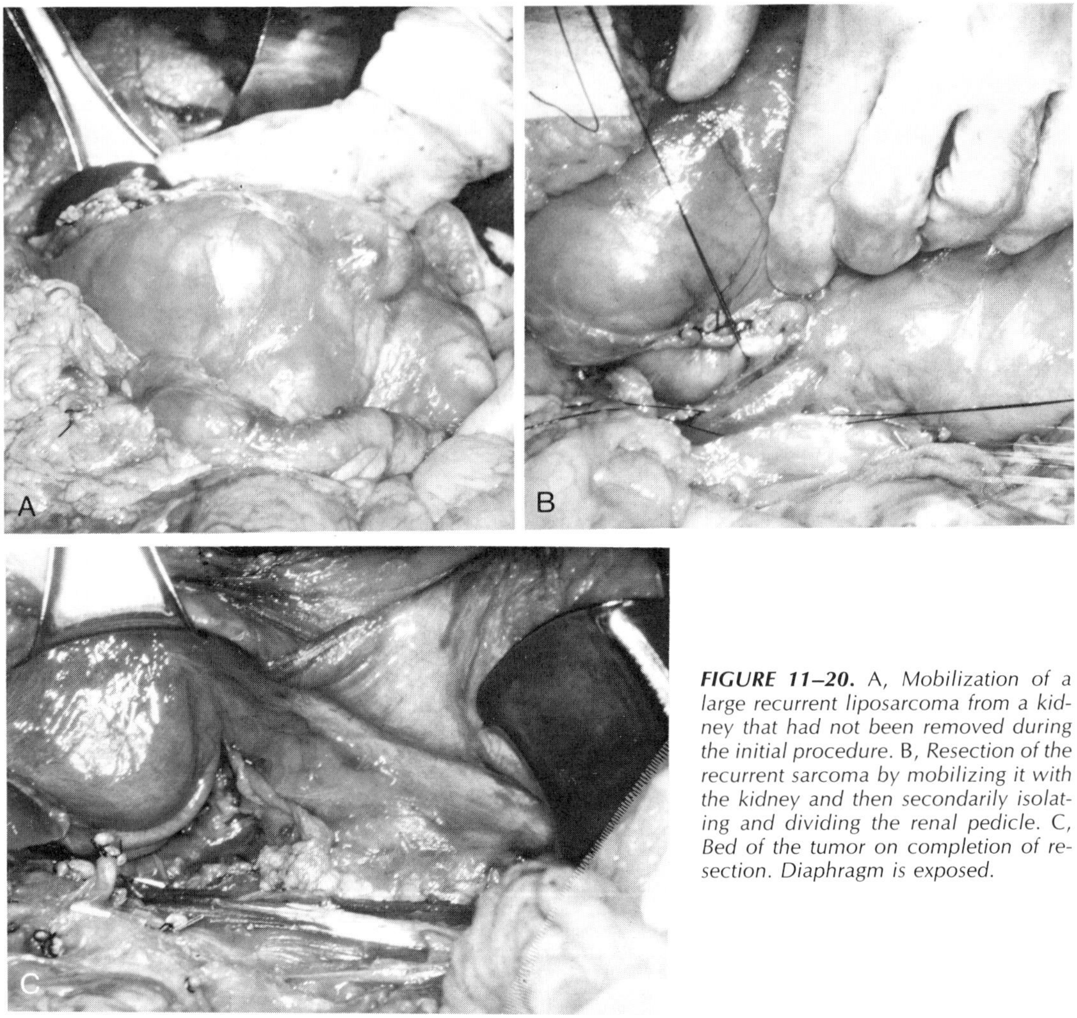

FIGURE 11–20. A, Mobilization of a large recurrent liposarcoma from a kidney that had not been removed during the initial procedure. B, Resection of the recurrent sarcoma by mobilizing it with the kidney and then secondarily isolating and dividing the renal pedicle. C, Bed of the tumor on completion of resection. Diaphragm is exposed.

gressive than the primary one. It may spread widely, going to multiple areas outside the retroperitoneum and abdominal cavity. When a small primary liposarcoma behaves in an unusual fashion, the presence of an unexpected lesion such as mesenchymal sarcoma must be ruled out. In our experience, tumors that have been interpreted as liposarcoma arising in areas such as the buttock have eventually metastasized to the neck, chest wall, and abdominal wall. Here, biopsy of the recurrent lesion has demonstrated patterns suggestive of a mixed histologic form. A diagnosis of mesenchymal sarcoma is usually entertained on review of such primary tumors. Stout coined the term "mesenchymoma" to represent a malignant tumor with two or more unrelated, differentiated tissue types in addition to fibrosarcomatous elements. The term has also been used for a group of myxoid liposarcomas, because of their lipoblastic, myxoid, and vascular components. At the AFIP these neoplasms are divided into two different categories. The first and smaller group is characterized by the coexistence of rhabdomyosarcomatous and liposarcomatous elements. The second and larger group contains a specific sarcoma together with varying foci of malignant lipoblastic and cartilaginous tissue. A majority of these tumors occur in individuals over 55 years but occasionally in young children. The retroperitoneum and thigh are most commonly involved. Prognosis is based on the predominant element, with the liposarcomatous component giving a more favorable prognosis than the rhabdomyosarcomatous element.

Most oncologists agree that when recurrent liposarcoma of the retroperitoneum is defined, an aggressive approach at removal should be made. Response to chemotherapy has been reported. There is also some evidence that hyperthermia in combination with radiation therapy and chemotherapy may reduce the possibility of recurrence.[60] Reduction in the volume of tumor preoperatively will increase the potential for resectability.

Leiomyosarcoma

Sarcomas arising from midline retroperitoneal structures may prove to be of smooth muscle origin arising from adjacent venous structures.[1, 13, 57] In general, when a tumor occurs in the region of the midline retroperitoneum, anywhere from pelvic brim to porta hepatis, leiomyosarcoma of the vena cava should be considered. CT scan and venography of the inferior vena cava may show close association or infiltration of the cava by tumor.[55] Over 80% of the retroperitoneal leiomyosarcomas occur in females, usually in the older age groups. The first case of such a tumor was described at autopsy by Perl in 1881. While most of the lesions attain significant size before becoming symptomatic, when growth does occur near the porta hepatis, Budd-Chiari syndrome can develop, with tumor extending toward or into the heart. Approximately half of the cases reported appeared in the region of the upper cava, causing hepatomegaly, jaundice, ascites, and edema of the lower extremities. Approximately 25% of these tumors will extend up the cava to the right atrium.[33]

In its mid-portion, renal vein involvement by sarcoma can occur, but by that time extensive venous collateral circulation will develop along the lateral retroperitoneal structures as well as abdominal wall. The caput medusae of the abdominal wall with varices connecting epigastric vessels gives a clue to the caval obstruction that can result from renal carcinoma, adrenal carcinoma, or leiomyosarcoma that has infiltrated the vena cava. The mid-third caval lesions are usually associated with renal vein thrombosis and development of the nephrotic syndrome. One case of renal vascular hypertension attributed to the compresssion of the renal artery by neoplasm has been reported. We have seen it more frequently in association with renal artery involvement, secondary to compression from retroperitoneal sarcoma, such as liposarcoma arising from the region of Gerota's fascia.

While resection of lesions arising from the upper cava are not feasible, one can occasionally resect lower lesions by taking the cava just below the hepatic veins to the caval bifurcation, with inclusion of renal veins.[14, 51] The left kidney can survive because of the collaterals that usually develop. Drainage from the right kidney is more tenuous, and not infrequently this structure must be sacrificed. If the right kidney must be preserved, it should be reimplanted to the groin region. Lesions of the lower cava are easily resected since these tumors are fairly well circumscribed and preservation of the kidney makes surgery less complicated. These tumors usually produce varying degrees of lower extremity edema. Marked edema is usually not evident unless secondary venous thrombosis occurs. Since synchronous metastases are not common in encountering a primary tumor, this should lead the surgeon to consider resection. While relatively well defined, these tumors can extend to adjacent retroperitoneal structures to invade the head of pancreas and the celiac axis. As long as the superior mesenteric artery is not involved, resection should be attempted.

Venous leiomyosarcomas that begin in the spermatic cord should be considered in the spectrum of the non-visceral manifestations of this disease. These tumors are usually found high in the scrotum but occasionally appear in the flank, rapidly infiltrating the internal ring to invade the retroperitoneum.

Ackerman[1] noted 29 cases of leiomyosarcoma among 256 patients (11%) with retroperitoneal tumors. Kaye and McNeill[35] reported 13 cases of retroperitoneal leiomyosarcomas. It is essential to rule out visceral origin when a leiomyosarcoma is found. Exophytic gastric leiomyosarcomas of the posterior stomach wall can present with the finding of a retroperitoneal tumor mass. The stomach is usually found stretched over the neoplasm. Complete resection of the tumor with involved viscera will usually allow proper identification. Those tumors that appear to be very low grade may not be recognized until evidence of metastasis appears. At that time, evaluation of recurrence may show a different histologic pattern, making it easier to define the nature of the original lesion. Long-term survivors are generally not the rule when liver and lung are involved by metastasis, regardless of the grade of the original neoplasm. Should one, on examination, visualize a caput medusae or diffuse abdominal wall venous distention, then compression or invasion of the vena cava with extensive retroperitoneal collateralization must be anticipated.

Typical of what has been described with such patients is the case of a 55-year-old woman admitted with intermittent abdominal pain radiating to the right flank. A slightly tender, deep-seated 6 by 8 cm mass was palpable in the mid-epigastric region with signs of fixation to the underlying structures. Sonography showed a solid echo-poor retroperitoneal mass silhouetting the inferior vena cava below the level of the kidneys. An intravenous pyelogram showed lateral displacement of the right ureter, and a GI series showed anterior displacement of bowel. The CT scan showed a large retroperitoneal tumor mass extending from L2 to the upper pelvis. At laparotomy, the mass was found to arise from the anterior wall of the infrarenal inferior vena cava adherent to, but separate from, the aorta. The mass and cava were resected, with the cava defect bridged with a composite autograft fashioned from both saphenous vein trunks. Venography 3 months postoperatively showed complete occlusion of the cava.

Malignant Fibrous Histiocytoma

Among other tumors encountered in the retroperitoneum, malignant fibrous histiocytoma should be considered. Figure 11–

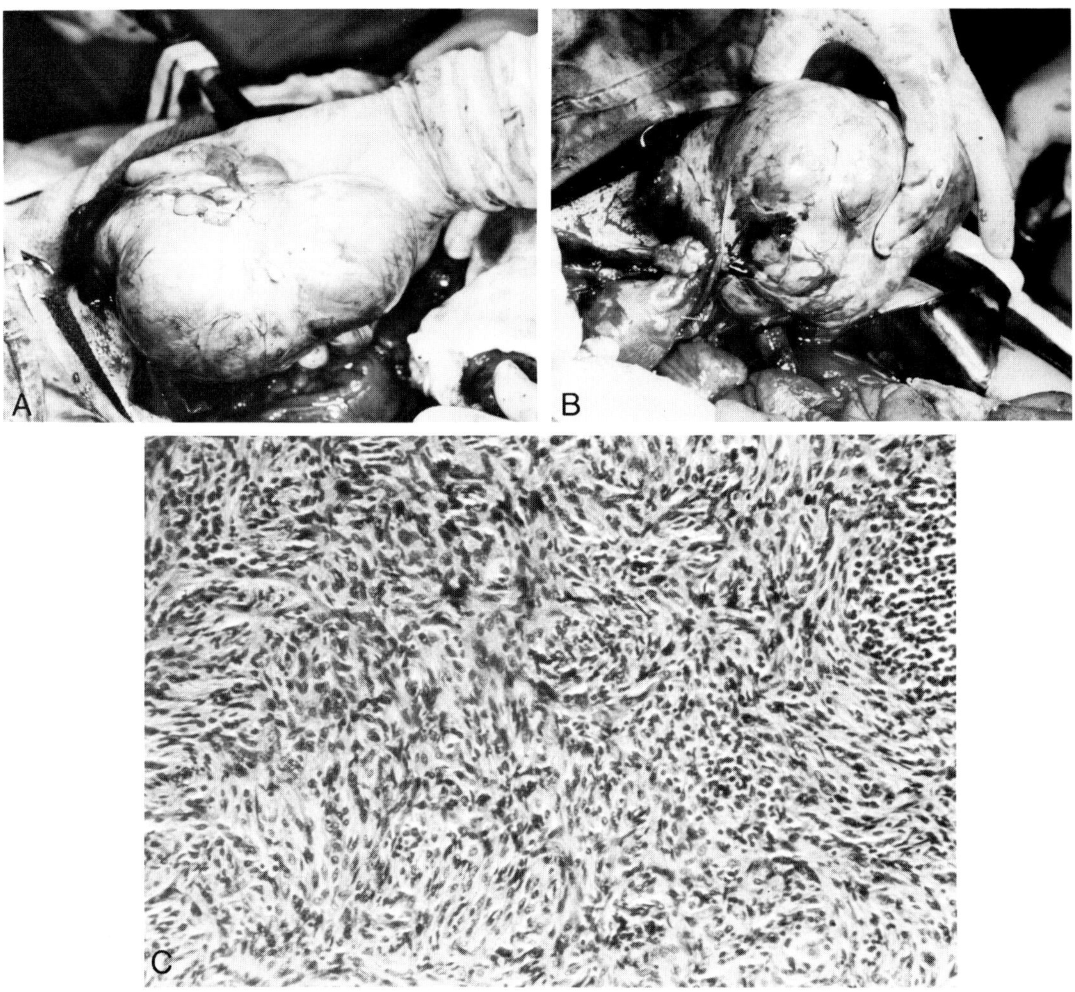

FIGURE 11–21. *A, Large infrarenal malignant fibrous histiocytoma. B, Mobilization of the tumor. C, Microscopic appearance of the malignant fibrous histiocytoma (× 100).*

21*A* and *B* shows a large infrarenal mass that obtained its blood supply from the retroperitoneal structures. The kidney appeared several centimeters above the primary lesion; it was not attached, and the tumor could be completely removed and the kidney left intact. Biopsy of this tumor proved it to be a malignant fibrous histiocytoma. Histologically the features included short fascicles of plump spindle cells arranged in a storiform pattern around slit-like blood vessels. Scattered giant cells, mitotic figures, and chronic inflammatory cells were also prominent (Fig. 11–21C). The patient was totally asymptomatic for the first year. At this time a CT scan was performed, revealing a large recurrent mass just inferior to the kidney and representing reappearance of this highly malignant tumor. No radiation therapy was offered postoperatively because of the failure of this particular type of tumor to respond. The patient was reexplored, at which time a radical nephrectomy en bloc with the tumor was performed. Kearney et al.[36] reported 15 malignant fibrous histiocytomas that were seen at the Mayo Clinic among 167 patients who had been operated on for retroperitoneal sarcoma. Approximately half of the patients at the time of surgery were diagnosed as having pleomorphic rhabdomyosarcoma. Symptoms were usually associated with fever, fatigue, loss of weight, or gastrointestinal symptoms. The tumor, on initial microscopic examination, was mainly pleomorphic with fibrogenic areas, clusters or sheets of histiocyte-like cells, foam cells, and benign and malignant giant cells. The tumors were subclassified into fibrous, giant cell, myxoid, and inflammatory variants. No difference in prognosis was found among the histologic subtypes. Of the 15 treated, only two were alive at the time of the report and both had pulmonary metastases. Pulmonary metastases were not a common finding for many of the patients since death was usually the result of failure to control local invasion.

Vascular Tumors

Vascular tumors most commonly occur in the retroperitoneum as hemangiopericytoma or hemangioendothelioma. Hemangiopericytomas are ubiquitous, appearing in all sites of the body. A malignant potential characterized by local recurrence and distant mestastases is present in 50% of the lesions. In the abdomen and retroperitoneum those tumors are most likely to behave in a malignant fashion. Regardless of their site of origin, they have a high rate of local recurrence. The treatment of choice is wide resection, when feasible. The extreme vascular nature of the tumors, especially in the pelvis, has made complete resection difficult. Arterial embolization should be considered preoperatively, based on angiographic findings. Binder et al.[8] reviewed the intra-abdominal lesions, adding 4 cases to the 54 already reported. Most exhibited direct local invasion, recurrence, or metastases. Angiographic studies have shown that the early arterial phase is characterized by displacement of the main arteries in the region of the tumor, with occasional feeding vessels forming a pedicle that branched into smaller spider-shaped vessels encircling the tumor. Numerous corkscrew-shaped vessels can be seen within the tumor, extending to larger encircling vessels. The early venous phase may suggest arteriovenous shunting.

In an attempt to control the vascular supply to the tumor before surgery, arterial embolization may be tried. This technique has been used to treat highly vascular renal lesions, gastrointestinal tract tumors, glomus and giant cell tumors, as well as metastatic vascular lesions to the liver. Numerous clot-forming materials, including Gelfoam, Ivalon, and Silastic spheres, have been utilized. When the tumor cannot be completely removed, debulking following embolization should be attempted, with postoperative radiation delivered to the remaining tumor.

Hemangioendotheliomas comprise the other large group of vascular neoplasms to be considered. Hansen[31] described such a lesion of the mesentery associated with thrombocytopenia. The hemangioendotheliomas are vascular lesions arising in a multitude of anatomic sites, with varying potential for local invasion and metastatic spread. A 7-month-old female infant was presented with an enlarging abdomen noted over a 2-month period. At laparotomy a large lobulated and vascular mass was found involving the base of the mesentery and surrounding the superior mesenteric artery. Biopsies were taken, and examination showed a complex arrangement of vascular spaces with marked cellularity. Lining cells showed occasional mitoses and atypia without malignant characteristics. A diagnosis of hemangioendothelioma was made. There was mild anemia and severe thrombocytopenia (5000), for which platelets were transfused prior to surgery. A dose of 1775 R was delivered to the tumor over a 40-day period. Prednisone was started after 30 days of radiation therapy. Five months after its first presentation, the tumor was only questionably palpable. Repeat aortography and selective superior mesenteric arteriography showed return to a normal appearance, with disappearance of the previously noted arterial displacement and encasement. The platelet count subsequently returned to normal.

While hemangioendotheliomas frequently behave as benignly as hemangiomas, they may suggest more aggressive behavior, requiring a more guarded prognosis. Sites of distant metastases that must be considered with this tumor are bone and liver, for which the prognosis may be grave.

Results of Surgical Resection

The experience in treating most retroperitoneal sarcomas has not been as favorable as for sarcomas found in other sites of the body.[5, 16, 20, 27] While aggressive resection can result in the removal of most retroperitoneal lesions, their highly malignant histologic characteristics and usual long-standing interval to diagnosis suggest invasion of adjacent structures followed by vascular dissemination. As a result, approximately 60% of tumors are reported to be unresectable. In our experience, however, this has not been true. Regardless of tumor size, we have usually been able to remove all gross tumor at the time of primary resection. This has held true for most cases so long as extensive liver involvement has not taken place. If an aggressive approach is employed and one anticipates that radical en-bloc resection will be required, one can assume that no more than 10 to 20% of the large primary sarcomas will be unresectable, depending on infiltration of structures such as the porta hepatis and superior mesenteric artery. What one does gain from an aggressive approach is prolongation of the interval to recurrence, since the survival for most of these tumors after 10 years rarely reaches 20 to 30%. This is especially true with bulky and, in particular, fully malignant sarcomas. Radiation therapy does not generally improve the overall statistics, and attempts at combined modality therapy have not been more successful. During the resection of large, bulky primary lesions, as well as recurrences, it is essential that the vascular supply to the neoplasm be controlled.

When the aorta is invaded by the tumor, the possibility of resection still exists.[17] Regardless of the size of the retroperitoneal tumor, direct invasion of major vascular structures is uncommon. This holds true even for the vena cava, where involvement intraluminally can be seen with renal or adrenal carcinoma. More frequently, investment of these vascular structures can occur with liposarcoma. Such tumors tend to encompass major visceral vascular structures, such as the renal vessels, which are easily sacrificed as part of the operative procedure. That major vessel involvement can occur has been documented clearly by Pack and Tabah.[48] They noted that 39% of their patients had this problem at the time of surgery. Two cases of homograft replacement or retroperitoneal tumors were described by Crawford and DeBakey[17]: one a possible embryonal carcinoma invading the aorta, the second a retroperitoneal leiomyosarcoma, 12 cm in diameter, arising in the midline and surrounding the cava and aorta. Vascular resections were performed en-bloc with the tumor. The presence of the homograft did not preclude radiation therapy, which was employed in the first case.

The major difficulty in handling most of the very large tumors still resides in the control of vascular supply. Therefore, attempts at isolating the blood supply to the tumor following angiography is important. Another approach in controlling intraoperative bleeding is the use of vascular embolization. Smullens et al.[52] reported two cases of retroperitoneal hemangiopericytoma, in which surgery was aided by palliative debulking with Gelfoam embolization. Angiographic techniques have been used to control bleeding and pain and to decrease hormone output from some tumors. Various embolic materials—including autologous clot, Gelfoam, Ivalon sponge, and Silastic spears—have been used to accomplish vascular occlusion. Occlusion is usually performed 24 to 48 hours before surgery. McMaster et al.[43] reviewed the long-term follow-up of 60 patients with this disease.

At Memorial Sloan-Kettering Cancer Center, 71% of retroperitoneal tumors were found to involve at least one major organ. Thirty-nine percent involved major vessels.

Fortner et al.[28] described 32 patients who required multiorgan resections for complete tumor removal. Colon and kidney were the most frequent visceral structures to be included as part of an en-bloc resection.

Most retroperitoneal sarcomas are considered to be slow-growing, many having symptoms for 1 to 2 years before the diagnosis can be established. With large tumors that are resectable, metastases may eventually appear even when they are considered histologically low-grade. Most of the common types spread to liver (17%) and lung (15%). Aggressive reexploration for solitary metastasis should be contemplated. Kohno et al.[38] followed one patient who survived for 10 years after resection of liver metastasis for intestinal leiomyosarcoma. The patient had originally undergone resection of a distal small bowel lesion with adjacent nodular metastases. A 9-cm liver lesion had been noted at surgery and was not resected initially, but was treated with 20 mg of intra-arterial mitomycin C, followed by resection 73 days after the operation on the primary tumor. Barium enema 7 years after initial surgery showed an abdominal recurrence. Following its removal, the patient remained free of tumor. Surgery is considered the primary treatment for this type of tumor, with radiation therapy used adjunctively only if there is question of residual tumor in the retroperitoneum. Radiation therapy has been used therapeutically and may have beneficial results, especially when delivered by implantation to the site of tumor resection, using ^{125}I. When the biologic nature of the tumor suggests the host's inability to prevent diffuse dissemination, then aggressive extirpation of solitary metastases should be entertained. At times this will lead to prolongation of the interval to recurrence and improve the survival rate. At other times, recurrence develops rapidly and at shorter intervals each time, suggesting that the new lesion is more aggressive than the former one. This problem has been investigated in terms of malignant melanoma. It has been showed that a greater degree of membrane inhibitory material is present with each successive recurrence. This appears to result either from the development of more aggressive strains of tumor cell populations that begin to regrow or in the modulation of cell surface antigens of existing cell populations. This build-up of inhibitory material eventually leads to more virulent patterns of tumor growth, resulting in uncontrollable spread.

REFERENCES

1. Ackerman L. U.: Tumors of the Retroperitoneal Mesentery and Peritoneum. Atlas of Tumors. Pathology AFIP, 1954.
2. Armstrong J. R., Cohn I.: Primary malignant retroperitoneal tumors. Am. J. Surg. 110:937–943, 1965
3. Bailey R. V., Stribling J., Weitzner S., Hardy J. D.: Leiomyosarcoma of the inferior vena cava: Report of a case and review of the literature. Ann. Surg. 184:169–173, 1976
4. Beckwith J. B., Perrin E. V.: In-situ nephroblastomas: A contribution to the natural history of neural crest tumors. Am. J. Pathol. 43:1089, 1963
5. Bek V.: Primary retroperitoneal tumors. Neoplasma 17:253, 1970
6. Bengmark S., Hafstrom L., Jonsson P. E., et al.: Retroperitoneal sarcoma treated by surgery. J. Surg. Oncol. 14:307–314, 1980
7. Berg J. W.: Angiomyoliposarcoma in a case with solitary metastasis from bronchogenic carcinoma. Cancer 8:759, 1955
8. Binder S. C., Katz B., Sheridan B.: Retroperitoneal liposarcoma. Ann. Surg. 187:257–261, 1978
9. Bose B.: Primary malignant retroperitoneal tumors: Analysis of 30 cases. Can. J. Surg. 22:215–220, 1979
10. Bose B., Boake R. C.: Obstructive uropathy due to primary retroperitoneal tumor. Br. J. Surg. 63:934–940, 1976
11. Braasch J. W., Mon A. B.: Primary retroperitoneal tumors. Surg. Clin. North Am. 47:663–678, 1967
12. Brewster D. C., Athanasoulis C. A., Darling R. C.: Leiomyosarcoma of the inferior vena cava: Diagnosis and surgical management. Arch. Surg. 111:1001–1005, 1976
13. Bryant R. L., Stevenson D. R., Hunton D. W., et al.: Primary malignant retroperitoneal tumors. Am. J. Surg. 144:646–649, 1982
14. Caplan B. B., Halasz N. A., Bloomer W. E.: Resection and ligation of the suprarenal inferior vena cava. J. Urol. 92:25, 1966
15. Cody H. S., III, Turnbull A. D., Fortner J. G., Hajdu S. I.: The continuing challenge of retroperitoneal sarcomas. Cancer 47:2147–2152, 1981
16. Coran A. G., Crocker D. W., Wilson R. E.: A twenty-five year experience with soft tissue sarcoma. Am. J. Surg. 119:288–293, 1970
17. Crawford E. S., DeBakey M. E.: Wide excision including involved aorta and vena cava and replacement with aortic monograft for retroperitoneal malignant tumors: Report of two cases. Cancer 9:1085–1091, 1956
18. DeSantos L. A., Ginaldi S., Wallace S.: Computed tomography in liposarcoma. Cancer 47:46–54, 1981
19. DeWeerd K. H., Dockerty M. B.: Lipomatous retroperitoneal tumors. Am. J. Surg. 84:397–407, 1953
20. Donnelly B. A.: Primary retroperitoneal tumors. Surg. Gynecol. Obstet. 83:705–718, 1946
21. Edland R. E.: Liposarcoma—a retrospective study of 15 cases, a review of the literature and discussion of radiosensitivity. Am. J. Roentgenol. 103:778–791, 1968
22. Eglund N., Eklund F., Sako M., Persson B.: CT of

soft tissue tumors. Am. J. Roentgenol. 137:725–729, 1981
23. Enterline H. T., Culberson J. D.: Liposarcoma: A clinical and pathological study of 53 cases. Cancer 13:932–950, 1960
24. Evans A. E., D'Angio G. J., Koop C. E.: Diagnosis and treatment of neuroblastoma. Pediatr. Clin. North. Am. 23:161, 1976
25. Exelby P. R.: Management of embryonal rhabdomyosarcoma in children. Surg. Clin. North Am. 54:849, 1974
26. Farberman A. A.: Retroperitoneal fatty tumors. Arch. Surg. 60:343–362, 1950
27. Felix E. L., Wood D. K., Das Gupta T. K.: Tumors of the retroperitoneum. Curr. Probl. Cancer 6(1), 1981
28. Forther J. G., Margin S., Hajdu S., et al.: Sarcoma of the retroperitoneum. Semin. Oncol. 8:180–814, 1981
29. Galloway J. R., Priestly J. T.: Retroperitoneal cysts. J. Miss. State Med. Assoc. 9:359–361, 1968
30. Hall G. M., Morris D. M., Mason G. R.: Nonfunctioning retroperitoneal paragangliomas. Am. J. Surg. 139:257–261, 1980
31. Hansen R. C., Catellino R. A., Lazerson J., Probert J.: Mesenteric hemangioendothelioma with thrombocytopenia. Cancer 32:136–140, 1973
32. Jacobsen S., Juul-Jorgensen S.: Primary retroperitoneal tumors: A review of 26 cases. Acta Chir. Scand. 140:498–500, 1974
33. Justiniani F. R., Cohen G. H., Roen S. A., et al.: Budd-Chiari syndrome due to leiomyosarcoma of the inferior vena cava. Am. J. Dig. Dis. 18:337–346, 1973
34. Kahn P. C., Frates R. E.: The value of angiography of the small branches of the abdominal aorta. Am. J. Roentgenol. 102:404, 1968
35. Kays S., McNeill D. D.: Leiomyosarcoma of the retroperitoneum. Surg. Gynecol. Obstet. 129:285–288, 1969
36. Kearney M. M., Soule E. H., Ivins J. C.: Malignant fibrous histiocytoma: A retrospective study of 167 cases. Cancer 29:961–976, 1972
37. Kinne D. W., Chu F. C. H., Huvos A. S., et al.: Liposarcoma of primary and recurrent retroperitoneal liposarcoma: Twenty-five year experience at Memorial Hospital. Cancer 31:53, 1973
38. Kohno H., Naofumi N., Araki S., Kato T.: Ten-year survival after synchronous resection of liver metastasis from intestinal leiomyosarcoma. Cancer 47:1421–1423, 1981
39. Kreel L., Bydder G. M.: Evaluation of retroperitoneal liposarcoma with computed tomography. CT 5:111–116, 1981
40. Lowman R. M., Grujd V., Peck D., et al.: The angiographic patterns of the primary retroperitoneal tumors. Radiology 104:259–268, 1972
41. Lowman R. M., Peck D. R., Love L., Dubash D.: Lumbar angiography in the diagnosis of primary retroperitoneal tumors. Surg. Gynecol. Obstet. 132:597–602, 1971
42. McGrath P. C., Neifeld, J. P., Lawrence W., Jr., et al.: Improved survival following complete excision of retroperitoneal sarcomas. Ann. Surg. 200:200–204, 1984
43. McMaster M. J., Sould E. H., Ivins J. C.: Hemangiopericytoma: A clinicopathologic study and long-term follow-up of 60 patients. Cancer 36:2232–2244, 1975
44. McNeer G. P., Cantin J., Chu F., Nickson J.: Effectiveness of radiation therapy in the management of sarcoma of the soft somatic tissues. Cancer 22:391–397, 1968
45. Moore S. V., Aldrete J. S.: Primary retroperitoneal sarcomas: The role of surgical treatment. Am. J. Surg. 142:358–360, 1981
46. Moore S., Aldrete J.: Primary retroperitoneal sarcomas: The role of surgical treatment. Am. J. Surg. 142:358–361, 1981
47. Neifeld J. P., Walsh J. W., Lawrence W., Jr.: Computed tomography in the management of soft tissue tumors. Surg. Gynecol. Obstet. 155:535–540, 1982
48. Pack G. T., Tabah E. J.: Primary retroperitoneal tumors: A study of 120 cases. Surg. Gynecol. Obstet. 99:209–231, 1954
49. Procter C. D., Bivins B. A., Griffen W. O., Gibull M. L.: Primary retroperitoneal cysts. Arch. Surg. 117:1089–1093, 1982
50. Regan J. F., Juler G. L., Schmutzer K. J.: Retroperitoneal neurilemmoma. Am. J. Surg. 134:140–145, 1977
51. Smith B. M., Mulherin J. L., Sawyers J. L., et al.: Suprarenal vena caval occlusion: Principles of operative management. Ann. Surg. 199:656–668, 1984
52. Smullens S. N., Scotti D. J., Osterholm J. L., Weiss A. J.: Preoperative embolization of retroperitoneal Hemangiopericytomas as an aid in their removal. Cancer 50:1870–1875, 1982
53. Stephens D. W., Sheedy P. F., Hattery R. R., Williamson B.: Diagnosis and evaluation of retroperitoneal tumors by computerized tomography. Am. J. Radiol. 129:395–402, 1977
54. Storm F. K., Eilber F. R., Mira J., Morton D. L.: Retroperitoneal sarcomas: A re-appraisal of treatment. J. Surg. Oncol. 17:1–7, 1981
55. Tegtmeyer C. J., Busch A.: The angiographic diagnosis of leiomyosarcoma of the inferior vena cava. Radiology 122:613–615, 1977
56. Tidrick R. T., Goldstein M. S.: Surgical treatment of retroperitoneal tumors. Arch. Surg. 70:203–206, 1955
57. Turner A. R.: Leiomyosarcoma of the inferior vena cava. Clin. Oncol. 4:187–193, 1978
58. Vanek V. W., Phillips A. K.: Retroperitoneal, mesenteric and omental cysts. Arch. Surg. 119:838–842, 1984
59. Weiss S. W., Enzinger F. M.: Myxoid variant of malignant fibrous histiocytoma. Cancer 39:1672–1685, 1977
60. Wiley A. L., Wirtanen G. W., Joo P. et al.: Clinical and theoretical aspects of the treatment of surgically unresectable retroperitoneal malignancy with combined intra-arterial Act-D and radiotherapy. Cancer 36:107–122, 1975
61. Donnelly B. A.: Primary retroperitoneal tumors: A report of 95 cases and a review of the literature. Surg. Gynecol. Obstet. 83:705, 1946
62. Newman H. R., Pinck B. D.: Primary retroperitoneal tumors. Arch. Surg. 60:879, 1950
63. Mellikow M. M.: Primary tumors of the retroperitoneum. Int. Coll. Surg. 19:401, 1953
64. Pack G. T., Tabah E. I.: Collective review. Primary retroperitoneal tumors: A study of 120 cases. Surg. Gynecol. Obstet. 99:209, 1954
65. Johnson A. H., Searls H. H., Grimes O. F.: Primary retroperitoneal tumors. Am. J. Surg. 88:155, 1954
66. Donhauser J. L., Bigelow N. H.: Primary retroperitoneal tumors. Arch. Surg. 71:234, 1955
67. Braasch J. W., Mon A. B.: Primary retroperitoneal tumors. Surg. Clin. North Am. 47:663, 1967
68. Felix E. L., Wood D. K., Das Gupta T. K.: Tumors of retroperitoneum. Curr. Probl. Cancer 60, 1, 1981

CHAPTER

12

Sarcomas of the Pelvis

Sarcomatous lesions of the pelvis generally originate from visceral structures such as bladder, vagina, uterus and, on occasion, from the rectum. Other lesions may arise from neurovascular structures as well as the musculature of the pelvic wall. In this chapter we are primarily concerned with those lesions that arise within the nonvisceral structures of the pelvis; Chapter 15 covers the management of primary visceral lesions.

The high rate of local recurrence noted with the pelvic tumors frequently necessitates that we perform extensively debulking procedures that may involve all or part of midline visceral structures; this is especially true when the tumors are found to be of high-grade malignancy. Such a resection would include structures such as rectum, uterus, vagina, and bladder that have been infiltrated by tumor; this would be the so-called pelvic exenteration defined by Brunschwig.[4] Variations in the pelvic exenteration procedure include anterior, posterior, or total resection of the pelvic visceral contents. The procedure to be performed is usually defined as we attempt to encompass the tumor mass. Low-grade malignancies may be approached in a more conservative fashion.

Primary soft part sarcomas in themselves are rare in the pelvis but have been reported by several authors.[2, 8, 10, 23] Many of these tumors occur in the pediatric age group. We have encountered a fair number of such lesions, but not as many as in the retroperitoneum. In addition, the distribution of histologic types is different from that of retroperitoneal sarcomas. The pelvic group includes hemangiopericytoma, angiosarcoma, neurogenic tumors, embryonal rhabdomyosarcoma, and leiomyosarcoma. At times their clinical and, for the most part, uncommon presentation requires an innovative approach. For example, sarcomas arising from structures such as sciatic nerve roots are virtually impossible to expose from an abdominal approach since these tumors lie deep to the hypogastric veins and are surrounded by a large plexus of fine venous structures which, if injured, can cause uncontrollable bleeding.

ANTERIOR COCCYGEAL APPROACH TO THE PELVIC WALL

One of us (Arlen) has employed an anterior coccygeal approach to such tumors, which offers exposure of lateral pelvic wall tumors arising under major pelvic vessels as well as retrorectal lesions arising off wall of the sacrum. If a transabdominal procedure were to be used, identification of the tumor would require resection of the hypogastric artery and vein as part of the process of exposure. The method for exposing the pelvic wall that we have utilized is more direct, is easily accomplished, and has resulted in minimal blood loss. With the patient in the lithotomy position, an incision is made between anus and coccyx, extending from the left ischial tuberosity to the right ischial tuberosity, using a Bovie cutting current (Fig. 12–1*A*). The levators are detached posteriorly from the sacral wall using sharp dissection; the retrorectal space is then entered, allowing the rectum to be elevated toward the pubis with a Deaver retractor (Fig. 12–1*B*). Careful finger dissection laterally exposes the sacral nerve roots as they course from behind the iliac vessels in a superior direction toward the sciatic notch.

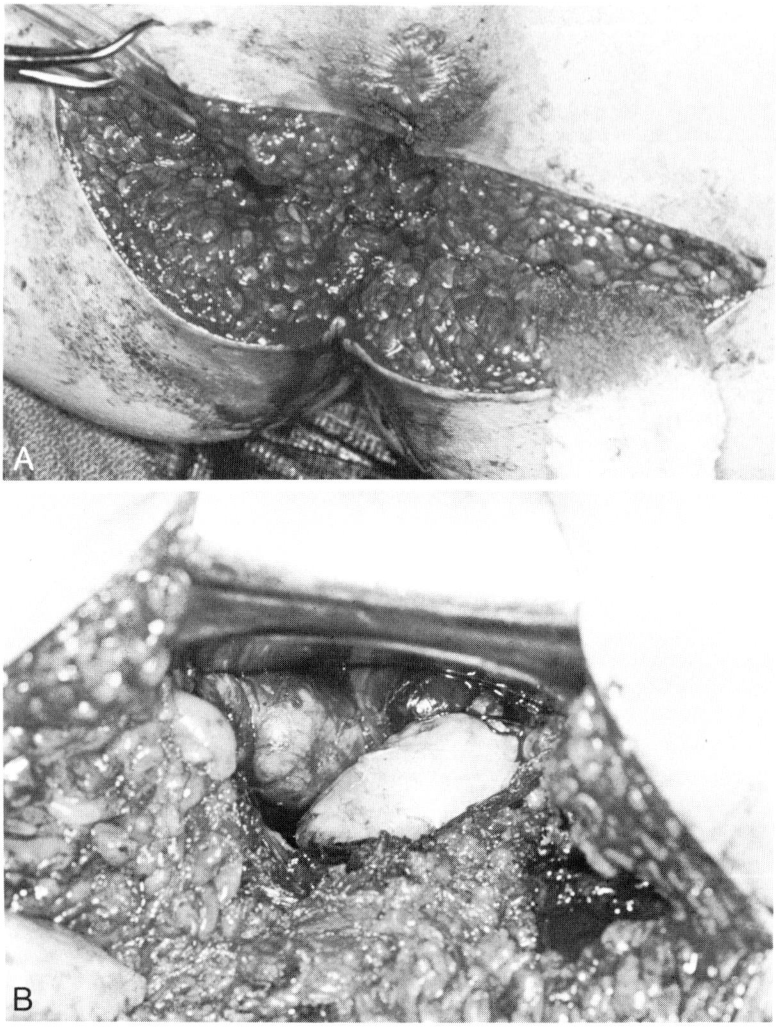

FIGURE 12–1. *A, Transcoccygeal (retroanal) approach to the retroperitoneum. B, Exposure of a schwannoma of the sciatic nerve. The rectum is being elevated superiorly using a Deaver Retractor.*

Tumors in this region are easily circumscribed; the vessels feeding them are identified and hemoclipped, and the tumors removed. Figure 12–2 shows the pelvic wall structures (muscular and ligamentous) that are encountered in any dissection in this region. The surgeon must be familiar with the relationship of these structures to the sciatic nerve roots and the iliac vessels.

TRANSABDOMINAL APPROACH TO THE PELVIS

We usually approach the pelvis through a midline incision beginning dissection, after exploration, on the pelvic wall vessels, such as common iliacs above the bifurcation of the hypogastrics. On rare occasions we use a strictly retroperitoneal approach, entering through the inguinal-type incision that allows retraction of the peritoneum above the iliac vessel bifurcation. After clearing node-bearing tissue from the iliacs we usually enter the obturator region along medial wall of the psoas muscle, where the obturator nerve and vessels are identified (see Fig. 13–2). At this point careful dissection along the obturator nerve in a retrograde fashion takes us to the sciatic nerve roots exiting from the sacrum as they form the main trunk of the nerve. This nerve, which is the largest in the body, is said to resemble a hand with outstretched fingers, the digits being its five roots (L4, 5 and S1, 2, 3). The sciatic nerve may now be traced to the sciatic notch, where it leaves the pelvis between the piriformis muscle and the ischial border of the

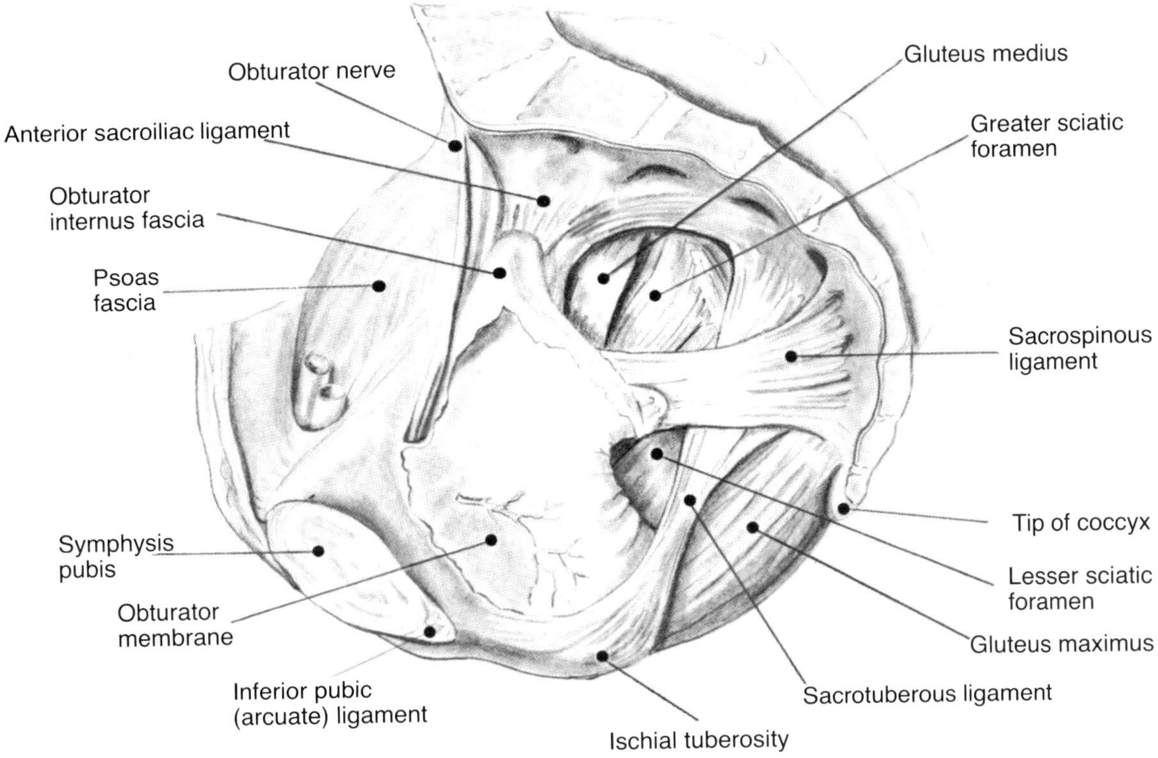

FIGURE 12–2. Structures of the pelvic wall showing muscles and ligaments.

greater sciatic notch. It is essential to be able to define such structures when surgically resecting tumors in this region. Typical of this situation is the finding of pelvic neurofibromas. A 40-year-old woman began complaining of pelvic pain, which was accentuated on pelvic examination. Multiple retrorectal and left lateral pelvic wall masses were palpated and thought to be consistent with what was found on scan (Fig. 12–3). Figure 12–4 shows that the tumor had extended out of the pelvis along the sciatic nerve to enter the posterior thigh. This tumor was approached by a transcoccygeal (retroanal) incision; the pelvic tumor was resected from the retrorectal region as well as from the left lateral pelvic wall and the sciatic nerve. Multiple nodules were removed during the surgery. The incision, which extended to the left ischial tuberosity, was then swung up into the left posterior thigh. The sciatic nerve was identified and traced from the sciatic notch toward the popliteal space. Multiple tumor nodules were removed in the thigh along the path of the sciatic nerve.

There are other approaches for resecting malignant tumors in the area of the lower retroperitoneum, the region of the iliopsoas muscle, or the external iliac vessels.[15] Karakousis[16] described a method for resecting tumors at these sites utilizing a midline incision from the umbilicus to the pubic symphysis. If the tumor was found to extend along the iliopsoas and removal of this muscle was considered important, then the incision was extended upward. Dissection was performed to mobilize and separate the ipsilateral ureter, wall of bladder, and rectosigmoid from the area of tumor. The lower portion of the abdominal wall and the ilioinguinal ligament were resected and replaced by an appropriate mesh when needed; grafts were used for vascular replacement when a locally resectable lesion infiltrated a major blood vessel. At the lower end of the dissection the incision on the abdominal wall was extended transversely in a lateral direction over the femoral canal, then continued in an inferior direction over the underlying vessels to the apex to the femoral triangle. This lower part of the incision is similar to what

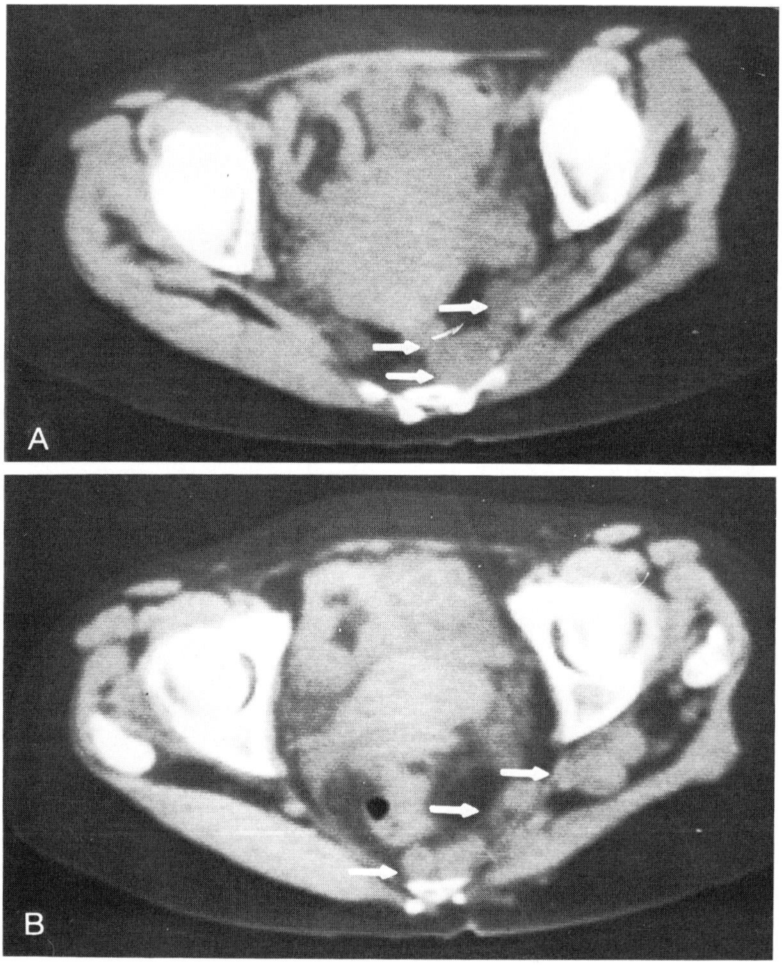

FIGURE 12–3. *A and B, Multiple neurofibromas (arrows) of the left pelvis.*

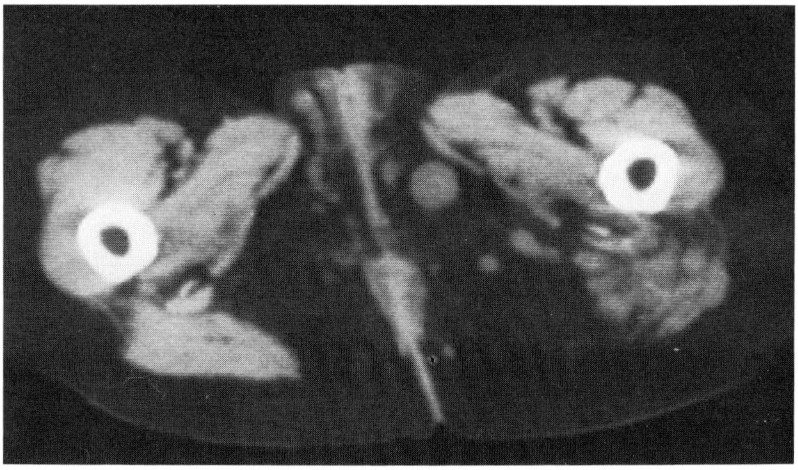

FIGURE 12–4. *Extension of neurofibromas into the left posterior thigh.*

is employed by many for use in the radical groin dissection. The rectus muscle and adjacent fascia were next divided as part of Karakousis' procedure. Removal of the inguinal nodes along the specimen was found to be easily accomplished. With only minimal dissection beneath the inguinal ligament lateral to the femoral artery, the entire lower abdominal wall could be retracted laterally to expose the iliopsoas muscle and iliac and common femoral vessels along their entire length. This technique was used on 10 patients with sarcomas of the lower pelvis and abdominal wall. Six of the patients with sarcomatous tumors had postoperative adjuvant radiation therapy; they have remained free of disease for 6 months to 3 years. Removal of the entire iliopsoas muscle in three patients caused no difficulties with hip flexion or walking. The lower portion of the abdominal wall and the inguinal ligament were replaced with appropriate mesh. Replacement or control of the iliofemoral vessels is easily accomplished with this approach. The technique is also useful for removing masses found in the obturator area.

PRESENTATION OF PELVIC TUMORS

The majority of tumors that we encounter in the pelvis can be defined on physical examination. On performing a rectal exam, one can usually palpate lateral pelvic wall masses indenting or displacing the rectum as well as the vagina in females. Retrorectal tumors such as chordomas displace the rectum anteriorly to abut the pubic symphysis. Should a pulsatile mass arising from sacral wall be palpated, a metastatic tumor such as renal cell carcinoma, thyroid carcinoma, or angiosarcoma is likely. Recently we encountered a large destructive sacral lesion with no evidence of a primary site. In order to define therapy, it was necessary to perform a biopsy. A posterior approach was used for exposure and on entering the area of the sacroiliac joint it was obvious that the tumor was pulsatile. A preoperative angiogram had not been performed. We had prepared two units of blood in the event that bleeding occurred. Both units of blood were administered because of the profuse bleeding that began as the incision was made. Biopsy suggested thyroid origin, even though no neck mass could be palpated. A thyroid scan revealed a small cold nodule. Appropriate therapy for the thyroid carcinoma was initiated with almost complete regression of the tumor of the pelvis.

Many pelvic tumors tend to displace bowel, as defined on barium enema. Figure 12–5 illustrates how pelvic tumors may present on x-ray studies. Such tumors are identified by mobilizing the left or right gutters of the bowel and tracing distally to the rectosigmoid, deep into the pelvis. With any of these dissections it is essential to identify and trace ureters and free them from the tumor mass. The ureters may be adherent to the pseudocapsule of the lesion and in the course of dissection must be traced into the trigone. Dissection is then carried over the aorta to its bifurcation, and the iliac artery is followed as it courses under the tumor mass. The descending colon is now divided and the mesentery taken to the root of aorta. The dissection proceeds to the bifurcation of iliacs and pelvic floor, staying under the tumor mass and constantly defining the dissected iliac vessels and ureter. If the tumor can be completely mobilized, transection of the distal rectum allows for complete removal of tumor and usually offers the opportunity for primary anastomosis of bowel should the distal segment be long enough. (We usually need 3 to 4 cm above the levators and a moderately wide pelvis.)

In the female patient, a pelvic/vaginal examination frequently defines the presence as well as the extent of the pelvic tumor. This examination is also important in evaluating various primary vaginal and bladder sarcomas. For example, vaginal bleeding may be found to arise from a primary lesion in the vaginal wall that is not of uterine origin. Primary tumors such as sarcoma botryoides (embryonal rhabdomyosarcoma) may be encountered in the young child, and tumors such as a primary leiomyosarcoma may be seen in the adult. In three such cases reported by Tobon et al.,[22] ultrastructural identification of the tumor cells was found to be valuable for the differential or confirmatory diagnosis of such soft tissue tumors of the female genital system.

Cystoscopy is also a necessary procedure for defining possible invasion of the bladder; however, invasion into the muscular layers alone may not be recognized. In many of our pelvic procedures we additionally perform a cystotomy at the time of laparotomy in order to palpate the trigone and define limits necessary for resection. When tumor that has invaded vagina also extends into the vesicovaginal septum, it is not uncommon

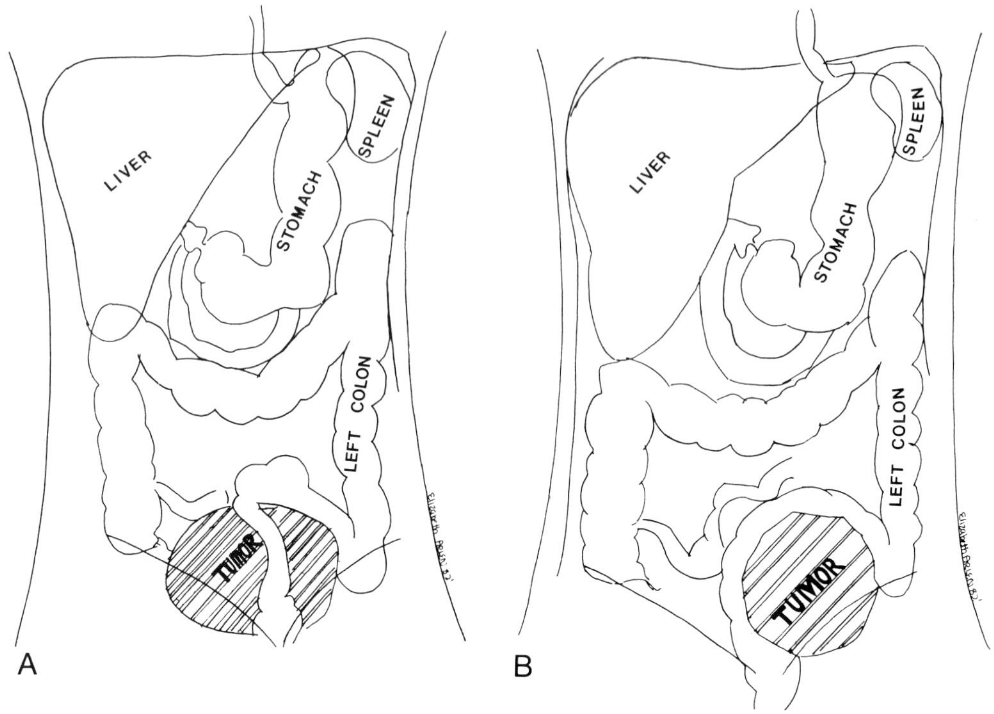

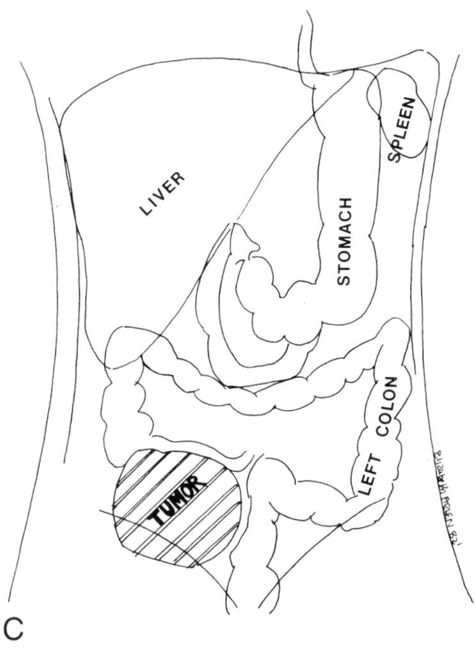

FIGURE 12–5. *Appearance of pelvic tumors. A, Pelvic tumor circumscribing the rectum. B, Pelvic tumor bulging into the sigmoid colon. C, Pelvic tumor off the right pelvic wall.*

for us to resect a portion of the trigone along with the specimen, bringing together both catheterized ureteral orifices in a midline "kissing" position. Should the trigone appear free on palpation through the open bladder, then separation of the vagina and vesicovaginal septum can best be accomplished through the cystotomy incision. Here the index finger is placed onto the trigone and the thumb is placed externally on the outside of the bladder wall between bladder and vagina. In this way the bladder can easily be dissected off the vagina, palpating the full thickness of the bladder wall that must be elevated. Using this maneuver the surgeon is prevented from cutting into tumor or into the floor of the bladder. It is important in many cases to know whether tumor from this region has extended above the pelvic brim and whether the abdominal wall has been involved. This would serve as a guide to entering the abdomen and pelvis.

Before an imaging technique such as CT scan or MRI is performed, it is important to evaluate any ureteral displacement by intravenous pyelography. At times there are difficulties in distinguishing between adenexal masses and pelvic soft part tumors. Gray-scale ultrasonography is useful in evaluating many tumors, especially the extent of existing cystic or vascular components.[24] Because skeletal structures limit ultrasonographic transmission, CT scanning and MRI may prove more useful. Figure 12–6 shows an extensive liposarcoma involving the pelvis, extending through the abdominal wall and above the pelvic brim. The tumor was debulked in preparation for radiation and chemotherapy and as an attempt to resolve the colonic obstruction that had occurred. Recently we have been employing MRI for pelvic lesions in order to obtain additional information. One of our patients had presented with a pelvic lesion that was thought to be a fibroid uterus. Because of pelvic pain and clinical evidence of uterine enlargement explorative surgery was performed on the gynecologic service. A large retroperitoneal mass was encountered, displacing the uterus. It was fixed to sacrum and felt to be unresectable. On reevaluation after the initial procedure, a CT scan (Fig. 12–7*A*) was performed and revealed a well-defined mass arising from sacrum and associated with a defect in the sacral wall. A rim of calcium was noted in the anterior capsule of the tumor. We requested MRI studies, which more clearly defined the relationship of the tumor to the sacrum and uterus on the sagittal and coronal views (Fig. 12–7*B* and *C*). A similar lesion arising from the sacrum was described by Wang et al.[24] Both their case and ours proved to be neurofibromas of sacral root origin.

Neurogenic Tumors

The benign lesions most frequently seen are those related to the pelvic fibromatosis and benign nerve tumors. The presence of a mass in the iliac fossa or lower pelvis in a female patient of 20 to 35 years of age may be a manifestation of pelvic fibromatosis, which can be confused with ovarian lesions. As these tumors enlarge they can encroach on the bladder, rectum, or vagina. Similar lesions have been found in the mesentery of the small bowel, omentum, or retroperitoneum. Many of these lesions reach a diameter of 15 cm or more. Wide resection is essentially curative.

Among the more common soft part tumors to be seen are the neural lesions either arising as primaries or those related to von Recklinghausen's disease, a disorder that was first described in 1882. This rare clinical condition is characterized by abnormal cutaneous pigmentation and numerous nodular skin lesions. At Memorial Hospital a review of 110 patients by Brasfield and Das Gupta[3] revealed that 41 of the patients (37%) died of complications related to their disease. The patients ranged in age from new-

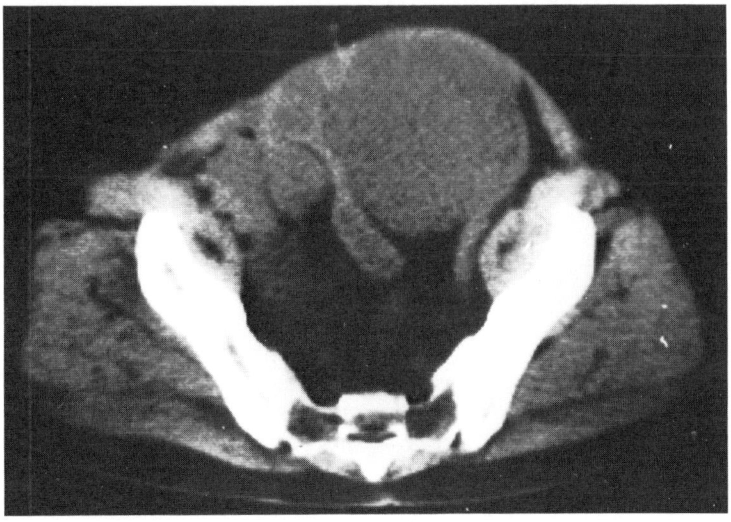

FIGURE 12–6. *CT scan of liposarcoma of the pelvis.*

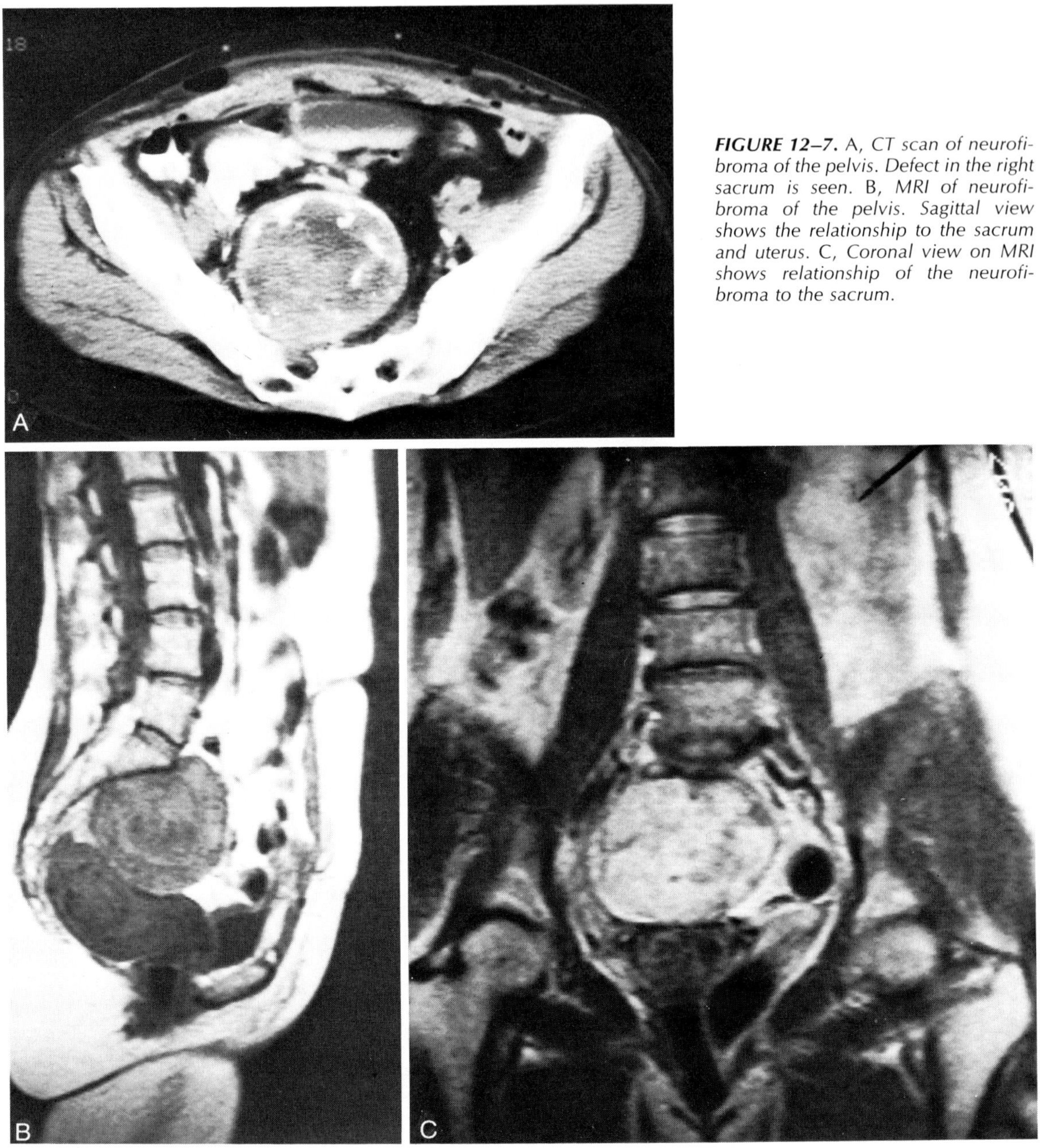

FIGURE 12–7. A, CT scan of neurofibroma of the pelvis. Defect in the right sacrum is seen. B, MRI of neurofibroma of the pelvis. Sagittal view shows the relationship to the sacrum and uterus. C, Coronal view on MRI shows relationship of the neurofibroma to the sacrum.

born to 50 years of age. Blacks composed 9% of the patients. In this series, 42% had familial disease, a statistic that coincided with that cited in other studies. Signs of disease first appeared in most of the patients with multiple lesions at the time of puberty. These patients also had a variety of endocrine-associated disorders, such as hyperthyroidism, pheochromocytoma, and thyroid enlargement. In one of our cases carcinoid of the pancreas developed.

Skin pigmentation appears here as a macular lesion and consists of abnormal melanin deposits in the basal layers (café-au-lait spots). Neural changes in the skin are characterized by an irregular overgrowth of Schwann cells, with an increase in reticulum and collagen. An endoneural origin of the collagen formation has been supported by electron-micrographic studies. The neural fibromas and schwannomas occur in all parts of the craniocerebral axis and peripheral nervous system. Most of the lesions remain discrete for several years, but others become sessile or pedunculated.

When large nerves are affected, irregular cylindrical enlargements can develop (plexiform neurofibromas), leading to local elephantiasis. One of the considerations in management of these neural tumors is their potential for malignant transformation. In the Memorial Hospital series, the incidence was reported to be 29%. In a review of published cases Hosi[14] reported an incidence of approximately 13%. It is also important to be aware that multifocal sites of neoplastic transformation occasionally occur. Eighteen per cent of the patients with von Recklinghausen's disease develop clinical manifestations before 1 year of age. Crowe[6] suggested that café-au-lait spots are pathognomonic for von Recklinghausen's disease when six or more of a diameter of at least 1.5 cm can be found. Brasfield and Das Gupta[3] noted that peripheral nerve tumors were one of the major neoplastic complications of this disease: 69% of children born with stigmata of von Recklinghausen's disease had one or more benign schwannomas by the age of 20, and 19% had malignant schwannoma by the age of 40. In this same group, there was osseous involvement in 54%, central nervous system disease in 19%, gastrointestinal involvement in 7.6%, and other forms of cancer in 15%.

Rare instances of synchronous leiomyomas, lipomas, and cranial nerve tumors have also been noted. Surgical extirpation of solitary schwannomas is not difficult, since they are usually encapsulated. When schwannomas are found in sites that are important to motor-sensory pathways, such as the brachial plexus or sciatic nerve plexus, essential nerve pathways should be kept intact by teasing out the nerve fibers under low magnification. Sarcomatous transformation in the solitary lesion is an exceedingly rare situation since most of the malignant tumors that have been noted occur in the patients with multiple neurofibromatosis.

Transformation has been most common in tumors of the back, neck, and axilla. The prognosis has been poor, with a 97% mortality for sarcomas originating in preexisting neurofibromas. For sarcomas unrelated to the neurofibromas of Recklinghausen's disease, the mortality rate is approximately 70%.

Histologically, the sarcomas that arise in association with neurofibromatosis are microscopically of the collagenous type, staining with trichrome stains; those tumors unassociated with von Recklinghausen's disease are almost all of the noncollagenous type. In the initial reviews of von Recklinghausen's disease at Memorial Hospital, among the 110 patients studied, 41 (37%) died of associated complications. Approximately half of these patients have relatives with the disease.

Analogous pathologic entities have been described in goldfish, turkeys, and cattle. Fish tend to present with ocular limbic lesions demonstrating accumulations of melanocytes.

The endocrine abnormalities known to occur in association with this disorder possibly result from congenital anomalies of the central nervous system in the region of the neuroendocrine axis. The café-au-lait spots that appear over the skin are essentially large freckles that contain melanin in basal layers. The neurofibromas themselves are characterized by an irregular overgrowth of Schwann cells associated with an increase of collagen and reticulum. When large nerves are affected, an irregular cylindrical enlargement called a "plexiform neurofibroma" can result. These structures can produce marked deformity of surrounding regions, leading to elephantiasis and at times severe facial distortion. Testing for the presence of cholinesterase in these tumors can be a useful method for differentiating neural from nonneural tumors. Malignant transformation in neurofibromas can usually be suspected by a rapid increase in size and shape as well as the sensation of pain in the lesions. The overall osseous involvement in these patients is approximately 47%. Benign schwannomas occur in 59% of the patients and malignant schwannomas in 29%; in approximately 14.5% the patients develop other malignancies such as melanoma, or carcinoma of the thyroid, breast, or lung. A review of cases of multiple neurofibromatosis treated at the Mayo Clinic[7] indicated that among 678 patients, 21 developed malignant neoplasms of the peripheral nerves or somatic tissue. Sarcomatous tissue adjacent to neurofibromatous tissue was seen in 12 patients. The findings of unclassified pleomorphic sarcoma, rhabdomyosarcoma, or liposarcoma in nine patients did not exclude the possibility of neurilemmal origin, since

Stout[20] and Russell and Rubenstein[19] had described a wide spectrum of metaplasia (fat, bone, cartilage, and striated muscle) attributed to the neurilemmal cell. The location of the sarcomas in this study had little bearing on the prognosis for this group of patients.

Pelvic Rhabdomyosarcoma

Among children and adolescents the presence of a mass in the pelvis may indicate that one is dealing with embryonal rhabdomyosarcoma.[5, 11, 12] Such tumors frequently arise within the cavity or lumen of pelvic viscera, taking on a pedunculated or grape-like appearance (sarcoma botryoides). With continued growth the tumor will invade the surrounding pelvic structures before metastasizing. In the vagina approximately half of the patients present with vaginal bleeding. In all cases there is a polypoid mass that will eventually protrude from the vagina.[8] In the urinary bladder the tumor grows near the trigone and usually involves the ureteral orifices.[9] A similar problem often arises with sarcomatous involvement of prostatic origin.[18] When pelvic structures are eventually invaded by these tumors, the bladder, vagina or prostate, and rectum frequently become involved at the same time. Radical surgery by exenteration may be needed to extirpate the disease[17]; however, attempts are being made to limit the extent of surgery by employing preoperative radiation and chemotherapy.[10]

In the female patient an attempt should be made to spare the rectum if tumor has not invaded bowel wall or entered the lumen but involves only the rectovaginal septum. Similarly, invasion of the vesicovaginal septum can be fairly well evaluated by cystoscopy and decisions made as to whether surgical resection is feasible. Trabeculation may indeed suggest that invasion of the bladder is taking place, but this must be confirmed by clinical examination and biopsy of the muscular wall of the bladder. When part of the rectum is superficially infiltrated the anterior wall can be removed and the rectum reconstructed by means of a two-layer anastomosis. If a suture line is necessary in the bladder and a second suture line exists in the rectum, then a diverting transverse colostomy will be necessary. The slightest drainage from the rectum into the pelvis, even when adequate drains are placed into the operative field, can cause disruption of the bladder suture line; a diverting colostomy here can be life-saving. One problem that must be recognized is that in the presence of partial cystectomy, a Foley catheter tip can occasionally erode through a bladder suture line. We have sometimes noted diminished Foley drainage at the time that suprapubic pelvic drainage (with a Jackson-Pratt catheter) increases. Such a finding suggests that urine is leaking through the suture line in the bladder and that a plugged Foley catheter must be changed or replaced by a catheter without a tip.

Occasionally unusual presentations may be recognized as a sign of early tumor development. Bennett[2] presented a case of a 13-year-old girl admitted for evaluation of right hip pain and a pelvic mass. The initial plain films of the pelvis showed periosteal reaction along the superior aspect of the right pubic ramus. On CT scan there was a large pelvic soft tissue mass extending from the level of the mid-portion of the right iliac bone to the acetabulum. A biopsy proved the presence of a neoplastic lesion with a moderate degree of necrosis. The cellular areas contained uniform small cells that were periodic acid–Schiff positive, thus ruling out lymphoma. The differential diagnosis included on Ewing's sarcoma, rhabdomyosarcoma, and neuroblastoma. Based on appearance under light microscopy, its location, and the lack of neurosecretory granules on electron microscopy, the tumor was treated as an embryonal rhabdomyosarcoma with disappearance of the pelvic mass following administration of chemotherapy. This type of histologic finding is frequently the only one to be defined, with a notable absence of cells showing cross-striations or eosinophilic cytoplasm of the large rhabdomyoblast (Fig. 12–8). Here sheets of densely packed round to oval hyperchromatic nuclei with scanty cytoplasm characterize the rhabdomyosarcomatous tumor. In this patient, symptoms of arthritis could have occurred because of the tendency of rhabdomyosarcoma to affect the growing skeleton, producing destructive bone lesions. An additional causative factor may have been the response to the presence of contiguous periarticular or periosseous tumor rather than due to actual bone invasion.

Fleming et al.[10] reviewed the experience in the management of pelvic rhabdomyosar-

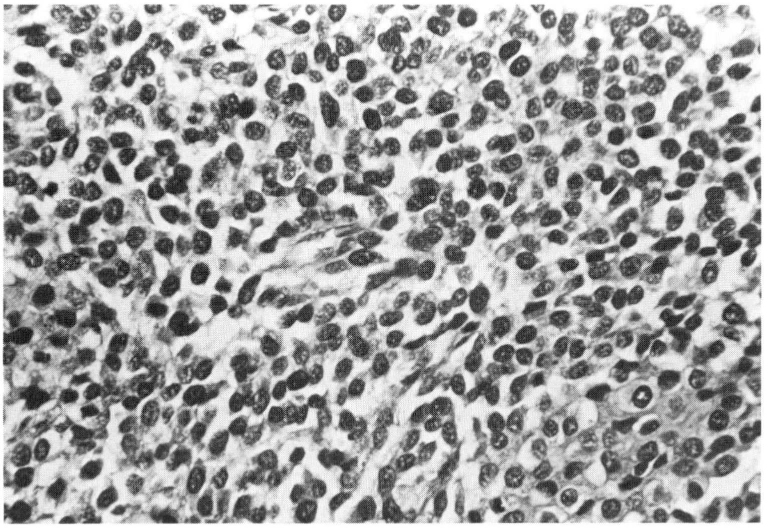

FIGURE 12–8. *Typical pattern seen with rhabdomyosarcoma (× 100).*

coma at St. Jude's Hospital. Ten children presented with cervical-vaginal tumors; various combinations of therapy were offered, depending on the primary lesion. Hysterectomy-vaginectomy was employed for eight of the patients and pelvic exenteration for one. Twelve children presented with bladder and prostate tumors, which were resected with segmental cystectomy in four, biopsy in five, and pelvic exenteration in three. Combination therapy was used postoperatively in eight of the ten in the vaginal group, surviving for 1 to 14 years, and in six of the twelve in the bladder-prostate group, surviving for 6 months to 16 years. Four different rhabdomyosarcoma protocols have been employed since 1968.

RMS I (1968): Surgery + dactinomycin, vincristine, and cyclophosphamide + radiation therapy

RMS II (1973): Surgery + dactinomycin, vincristine, cyclophosphamide, and Adriamycin + radiation therapy

RMS III (1977): Surgery + dactinomycin, vincristine, cyclophosphamide, and Adriamycin + (?)radiation therapy + (?)surgery

RMS IV (1981): Surgery + Adriamycin, DTIC-Dome, dactinomycin, vincristine, cyclophosphamide + (?)surgery + (?)radiation therapy + (?)surgery

In the past, patients with rhabdomyosarcoma have had a relatively poor prognosis. The 5-year survival rate that had been achieved was approximately 25% with a median of 10 months. With combination therapy protocols that included surgery, the prognosis markedly improved so that 2-year survival rates without relapse have now been reported at 71% for patients with local or regional disease and 28% for those with distant metastasis. Lesser surgery and improved adjuvant therapy has virtually become the rule in treating primary rhabdomyosarcomas.

Exploring the Pelvic Wall

The approach to the pelvic retroperitoneum for exploration and resection of pelvic sarcomas is via the iliac vessels. By creating a peritoneal opening in the paracolic gutter over the iliac vessels, the retroperitoneum in the pelvic region can be easily defined. The cecum is mobilized to create a right-sided window in the peritoneum; on the left the sigmoid is similarly dissected along the peritoneal reflection to create its respective window. In the female patient a similar approach can be used by dividing the round ligament against the lateral pelvic wall on each side. This creates similar exposure of the retroperitoneum on each side. With careful finger dissection the adventitia within the window is mobilized; the retroperitoneum is entered and the psoas defined, with the ureter identified and mobilized medially into the peritoneal fold of each respective window that has been created. The iliac vessels are noted at this point. A Richardson retractor is placed into the inferior aspect of the window, retracting inferiorly over the vessels to the femoral canal. The peritoneal opening is then extended superiorly toward the aortic bifurcation. A separate incision is made over the aorta from the ligament of Treitz to aortic bifurcation inferiorly so that complete dissection of the nodes can be performed if necessary. The ureters are isolated early in the dissection, looped for retraction with fine tapes, then traced toward the trigone to be assured that they are free from the site of dissection. It is essential that the bladder have a Foley catheter in place during the procedure and that it be kept in for at least 1 week after surgery to prevent the ureters from floating off the retroperitoneum while they are being secondarily revascularized from the bed on which they are lying. Without a catheter in the bladder the ureters would move up and down as the bladder filled with urine.

After external iliac artery dissection, the hypogastric nodes are dissected; at times the hypogastric artery is ligated at its junction with the common iliac artery as a means of controlling any pelvic bleeding that may occur. The ilioinguinal nerve is left intact on the psoas. The iliac vessels are now carefully dissected away from the psoas and retracted medially. With finger dissection the obturator space is entered by mobilizing the node containing fat pad off the deep medial psoas muscle, vessels still being retracted medially. One then palpates for the obturator nerve. Finger dissection is the primary method we use for identifying the obturator nerve, since Metzenbaum dissection here may inadvertently result in nerve damage. The nodes are freed medially off the nerve and displaced under the external iliac vein, at which time they are removed. Figure 12–9*A* shows the appearance of the left hemipelvis on completion of vascular

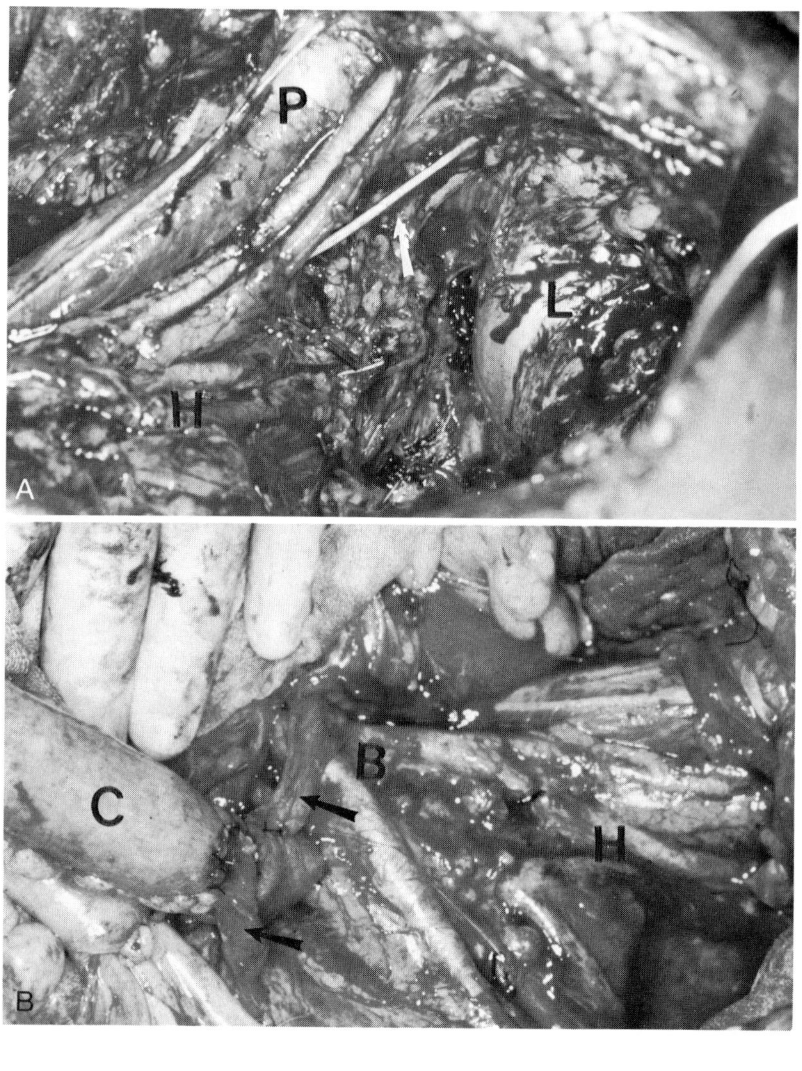

FIGURE 12–9. A, *Appearance of the pelvic wall on completion of dissection of the sarcoma. The psoas muscle (P) is seen with the ilioinguinal nerve crossing over it. H marks the bifurcation of the iliac artery into the hypogastric vessel. L is the bulging levator ani muscle, and the arrow points to the dissected obturator nerve.* B, *Appearance of the pelvis on completion of a total exenteration. H marks the position of the hypogastric vessels, B the bifurcation of aorta, and C the ileal conduit. The arrows point to the implanted ureters in the conduit.*

and obturator space dissection. This patient had undergone total pelvic exenteration; the levators, however, were left intact and can be seen bulging at the base of the operative field. For many of the sarcomatous lesions invading bladder and rectum, it is not necessary to complete the resection with an abdominoperineal resection, as may be necessary with advanced or recurrent gynecologic tumors.

The ureters in this case were mobilized and divided at the trigone as part of a pelvic exenteration. They have been implanted into the base of an ileal conduit (Fig. 12–9*B*), and the left ureter can be seen crossing the bifurcation of the aorta into the left and right common iliac vessels. The left hypogastric artery is also noted as it comes off the left common iliac artery.

Finger dissection of the obturator membrane defines the lower limit of the node dissection adjacent to the obturator membrane. With careful dissection the obturator nerve can be traced superiorly to the sacral foramina, at which point the roots of the sciatic nerve can be identified and followed to the sciatic notch. Fine branches of the hypogastric vein can be seen extending to the lateral pelvic wall and between roots of the sciatic nerve. These can be controlled by vascular clips. Should bleeding be encountered, the safest way for achieving vascular control is with pelvic packing, which can be brought out suprapubically. This packing can then be removed 48 hours later.

Hemangiopericytoma

Another lesion that is seen as a primary tumor in the pelvis, the hemangiopericytoma often presents as a large pelvic mass. This particular tumor is considered to arise from the pericytes of Zimmerman, which are found spiraling around the outside of blood capillaries and postcapillary venules. There has been some question of the relationship to glomus tumors, which arise from neuromyoarterial glomera and present as a caricature of that body to form a characteristically small tumor that causes typical paroxysmal attacks of pain. The glomus tumor is always benign but may recur locally, whereas the hemangiopericytoma, which shows no relationship with the glomera, is generally a large tumor and frequently exhibits a malignant clinical course. Since the pericyte is found in capillaries and venules of all types of tissue, hemangiopericytomas have been reported to arise in bone, CNS, viscera, and somatic soft tissue.

In 1970 Bachwinkel and Diddams[1] reviewed 247 cases; 103 of the lesions were located in the musculoskeletal system or skin. Fifty-two tumors recurred after treatment, 16 of which recurred 5 years after original treatment. Among 276 cases reported by Hollmann et al. (1971)[13] 65 were children. The overall malignancy rate was 41% for adults and 50% for the children in the series. In a review of those cases seen at the Mayo Clinic,[19] 60 patients with disease involving soft tissue were treated between 1915 and 1972. All had tumors histologically confirmed by the criteria of Stout and Murray.[21] Twelve tumors were classified as benign, 16 as borderline malignant, and 32 as histologically malignant. The commonest radiographic finding was a soft tissue density; there was evidence of some speckled calcification in five and erosion of adjacent bone structures in seven. Ten patients were found to have pulmonary metastasis. Of the 16 with borderline malignancy, six had local recurrence and three further metastasis to distant sites. Among 32 with malignant lesions 23 died of metastatic disease. Review of histologic material has suggested that a malignant course may be prediced in tumors exhibiting a few mitotic figures in association with moderate cellular anaplasia or moderate numbers of mitotic figures in association with slight cellular anaplasia. Foci of necrosis within a given tumor strongly indicate malignant potential.

Angiosarcoma as a primary tumor of the pelvis is less frequently encountered than hemangiopericytoma. Many of these tumors are not readily resectable because of invasion of pelvic wall structures. Figure 12–10*A* shows the application of cryosurgery with a toothed tumor probe (Brymill) placed into the obturator membrane adjacent to the iliac vessels. A zone of freezing was allowed to develop until it encroached on the iliac vessels (Fig. 12–10*B*). A Richardson retractor is always placed on the external iliac artery, with retraction in the direction of the femoral canal to expose the vessels that are needed for proper dissection. Sarcomas of the thigh situated close to the inguinal ligament may have a tendency to spread by extending through the lymphatics or fascial planes of the obturator membrane. Such spread usually manifests itself with the appearance of a pelvic mass bulging from the hypogastric fossa (Fig. 12–11*A*). Initial dissection showed the mass filling the region

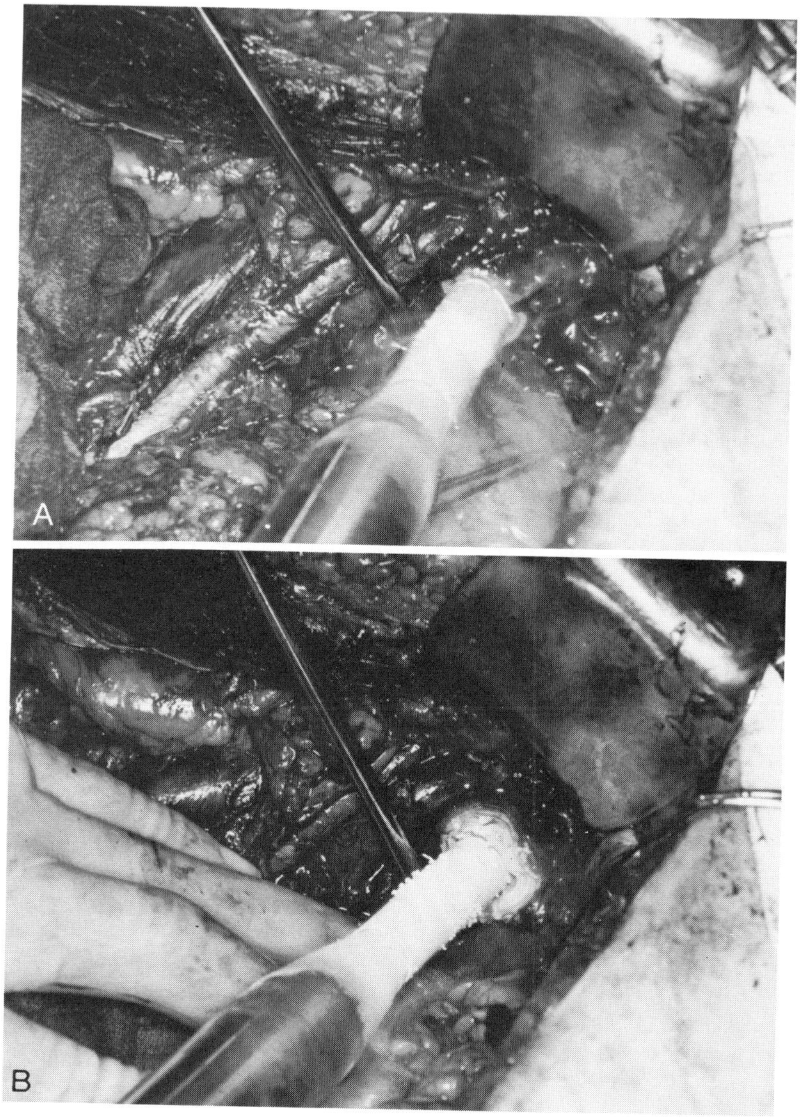

FIGURE 12–10. A, Cryosurgery of a pelvic tumor in the obturator muscle. A loop retractor is seen around the external iliac vein. B, Extension of the freezing process around the cryosurgical probe.

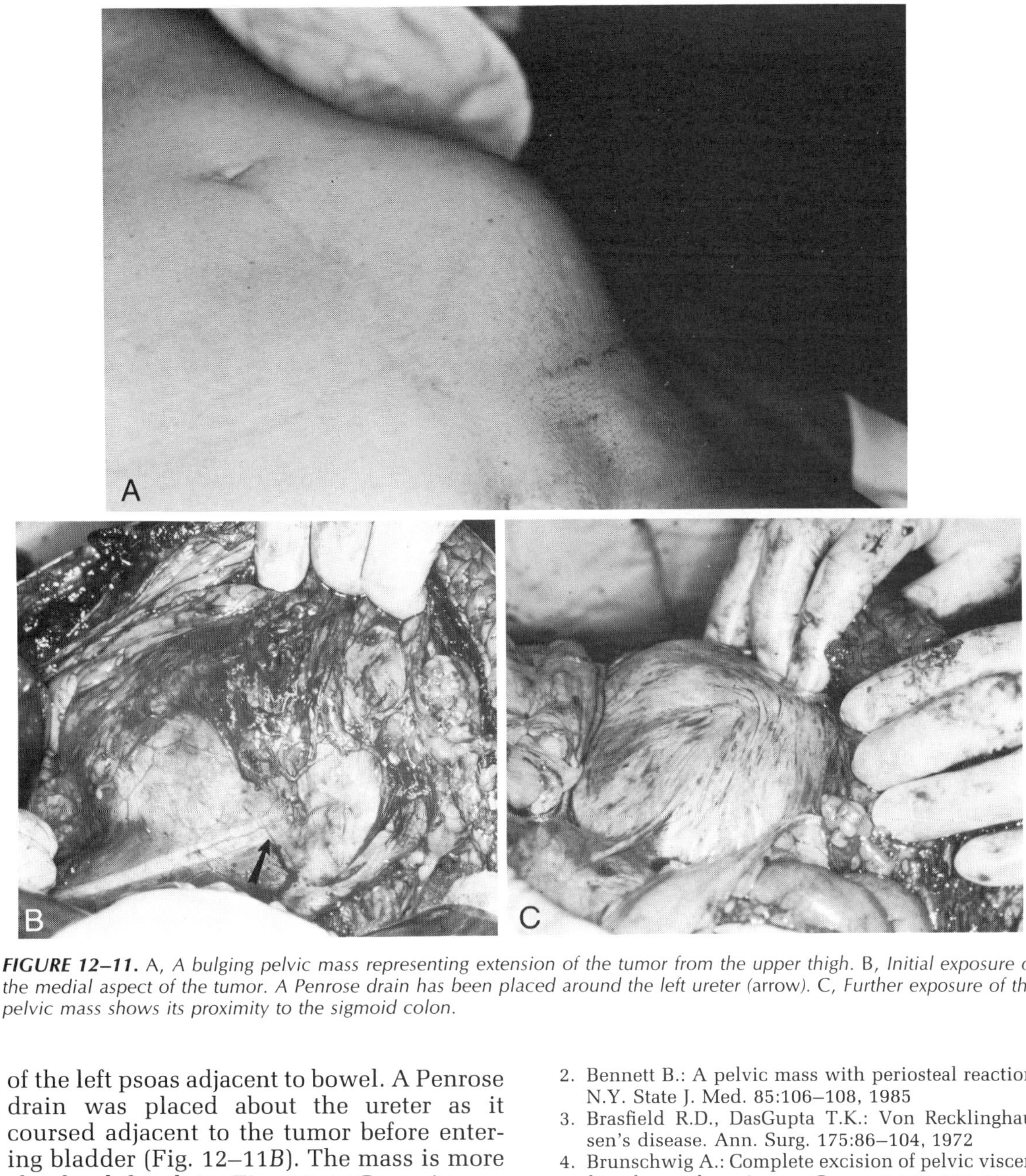

FIGURE 12–11. *A, A bulging pelvic mass representing extension of the tumor from the upper thigh. B, Initial exposure of the medial aspect of the tumor. A Penrose drain has been placed around the left ureter (arrow). C, Further exposure of the pelvic mass shows its proximity to the sigmoid colon.*

of the left psoas adjacent to bowel. A Penrose drain was placed about the ureter as it coursed adjacent to the tumor before entering bladder (Fig. 12–11*B*). The mass is more clearly defined in Fig. 12–11*C*, as it was being dissected away from distal sigmoid colon. Such tumors are rarely cured by local resection. After debulking, radiation therapy may be offered. Hemipelvectomy is an alternative in the attempt to totally control local recurrent disease.

REFERENCES

1. Bachwinkel K.D., Diddams J.A.: Hemangiopericytoma: Report of a case and review of the literature. Cancer 25:896, 1970
2. Bennett B.: A pelvic mass with periosteal reaction. N.Y. State J. Med. 85:106–108, 1985
3. Brasfield R.D., DasGupta T.K.: Von Recklinghausen's disease. Ann. Surg. 175:86–104, 1972
4. Brunschwig A.: Complete excision of pelvic viscera for advanced carcinoma. Cancer 1:177–183, 1948
5. Burrington J.D.: Rhabdomyosarcoma of the paratesticular tissues in children: Report of 8 cases. J. Pediatr. Surg. 4: 503–510, 1969
6. Crowe F.W., Schull W.J., Neel J.V.: A Clinical, Pathological and Genetic Study of Multiple Neurofibromatosis. Springfield, IL, Charles C Thomas, 1956
7. D'Agostino A.N., Soule E.H., Miller R.H.: Sarcomas of peripheral nerves and soft somatic tissues associated with multiple neurofibromatosis. Cancer 16:1015, 1963.
8. Daniel W.W., Koss L.G., Brunschwig A.: Sarcoma botryoides of the vagina. Cancer 12:74–84, 1959
9. Fleischman J., Perinette E.P., Catalona W.J.: Embryonal rhabdomyosarcoma of the genitourinary organs. J. Urol. 126:389–391, 1981

10. Fleming I.D., Etcubanas E., Patterson R., et al.: The role of surgical resection when combined with chemotherapy and radiation in the management of pelvic rhabdomyosarcoma. Ann. Surg. 199:509–514, 1984
11. Grosfeld J.L., Smith J.P., Clatworthy H.W., Jr.: Pelvic rhabdomyosarcoma in infants and children. J. Urol. 107:673–675, 1972
12. Hayes D.M., Raney R.B., Lawence W., Jr.: Rhabdomyosarcoma of the female urogenital tract. J. Pediatr. Surg. 16:828–834, 1981
13. Hollmann G., Hopner F., Daum R., et al.: Beitrag zur Klinik des Hemangiopericytoms. Langenbecks Arch. Chir. 330:128–139, 1971
14. Hosi K.: Multiple neurofibromatosis (von Recklinghausen's disease) with special reference to malignant transformation. Arch. Surg. 22:258, 1931
15. Kang-Ming H., Kahn A., Smith N.L.: Bilateral pelvic lymphadenectomy from a lower abdominal transverse skin incision and pararectal approach. Surg. Gynecol. Obstet. 156:443–448, 1983
16. Karakousis C.P.: Exposure and Reconstruction in the lower portions of the retroperitoneum and abdominal wall. Arch. Surg. 117:840–844, 1982
17. Kumar M., Wrenn E.L., Jr., Fleming I.D.: Combined therapy to prevent complete pelvic exenteration for rhabdomyosarcoma of the vagina. Cancer 37:118–122, 1976
18. McDougal W.S., Pesskey L.: Rhabdomyosarcoma of the bladder and prostate in children. J. Urol. 124:882–885, 1980
19. Russell D.S., Rubenstein L.J.: Pathology of Tumors of the Nervous System. London, E. Arnold Ltd., 1959
20. Stout A.P.: Tumors of the Peripheral Nervous System: Atlas of Tumor Pathology, Sect.2, Fascicle 6. Armed Forces Institute of Pathology, 1949
21. Stout A.P., Murray M.: Hemangiopericytoma—a vascular tumor featuring Zimmermann's pericytes. Ann. Surg. 116:26–33, 1942
22. Tobon H, Murphy A.I., Salazar H.: Primary leiomyosarcoma of the vagina. Cancer 32:450–457, 1973
23. Wang A, Blickman J.G., Rauktis F.F., et al: A 23-year-old woman with a pelvic mass studied by ultrasound and computed tomography. JAMA 249:2075–2076, 1983

CHAPTER

13

The Role of Regional Node Dissection in Sarcoma Surgery

Regional node dissection concerns the removal of major node-bearing areas in proximity to tumors that have a propensity for lymphatic spread and lymph node invasion. When performed, such dissections require removal of all visible lymph node–bearing tissue, sharply dissected from the major venous structure found in the region of surgery. Anatomically lymph node drainage occurs along the major venous structures at all sites in the body except for the colon, where patterns of nodal spread follow the inferior mesenteric artery. For the sarcomas the following patterns predominate: (1) head and neck region, (2) axillary region, (3) retroperitoneum, and (4) groin. An understanding of the anatomy of these node-bearing areas as well as of the techniques for performing such dissections (en-bloc tumor removal) is essential for proper patient management. Because many sarcomas arise in proximity to the major neurovascular structures near the nodal regions, it is important to carry out the dissection properly for the purposes of (1) isolating and separating vessels from surrounding tumor to prevent neurovascular injury, and (2) performing lymph node dissection for therapeutic and staging purposes. In essence, while each area is different and depends on the node-bearing tissue involved, certain characteristics are common to these regions; that is, a major nerve, artery, and vein constitute the neurovascular bundle in relation to a prominent muscular structure. In the head and neck, this includes the carotid artery, jugular vein, and vagus nerve in proximity to the sternomastoid muscle. In the axillary region it is the axillary artery, axillary vein, and brachial plexus in relationship to the pectoralis major and minor. In the retroperitoneal node region, the aorta, vena cava, and lumbar nerves are in proximity to the psoas muscle. In the groin, the femoral artery, femoral vein, and femoral nerve are in proximity to the sartorius muscle and those structures that form the femoral triangle.

The characteristics of each area are defined by the incision to be employed and the landmarks that define the areas of dissection. In the neck, the landmarks to be identified for dissection are the clavicle inferiorly, the digastric muscle superiorly, the larynx in the midline with its strap muscles anteriorly, and the trapezius muscle posteriorly. In the axillary region the margins of the pectoralis major form superior borders. Medially and inferiorly, the serratus muscles border the chest wall; the latissimus dorsi is found laterally and inferiorly. In the retroperitoneum, the sigmoid colon mesentery with the inferior mesenteric vein is laterally placed; the ligament of Treitz and the left renal vein are found superiorly and the bifurcation of the aorta is defined inferiorly. In the groin, the inguinal ligament occurs superiorly, the sartorius muscle is laterally placed, and the adductors are situated medially.

RADICAL GROIN DISSECTION

Radical groin dissection represents en-bloc removal of lymph nodes from the femoral triangle of the leg along the saphenous vein and the deep femoral vein, and usually includes retroperitoneal nodes as part of the dissection, extending from the femoral canal up the iliac vessels to the bifurcation of the hypogastric vessels. This operation is employed prophylactically for those extremity tumors with a high incidence of local spread, or in the face of palpable groin disease. One might elect to limit the dissection to the femoral triangle alone when no nodal involvement can be defined as part of the prophylactic dissection. It is important to explore and dissect the retroperitoneum when palpable groin nodes are present. On occasion, palpable tumor nodes can be noted above the inguinal ligament. At the time of dissection, however, these nodes are actually found to be wrapped around the saphenofemoral junction, below the inguinal ligament. With palpable disease it is important that a CT scan be performed in order to rule out the presence or absence of retroperitoneal nodal involvement. One may find extensive retroperitoneal disease not discernible clinically, and this might obviate the use of any surgical approach in treating the condition.

The radical groin dissection is begun using an S-shaped incision beginning near the anterosuperior iliac spine and continuing inferiorly toward the inguinal ligament. The incision then parallels the underside of the inguinal ligament and is extended to the region of the femoral canal, where it is then curved gently in an inferior direction for approximately 8 to 10 cm, reaching the apex of the femoral triangle. In those patients with negative nodes, Lahey clamps are placed on the skin edges and a relatively thick flap can be raised medially and laterally to expose the underlying femoral triangle. With palpable disease, thinner flaps should be raised with the possible subsequent development of wound necrosis. The tensor fasciae latae and the adductor group of muscles are exposed by the skin flaps. Sharp dissection is carried from a lateral to a medial direction after incision of fascia over the sartorius.

Medially, the dissection encompasses fascia over the adductor group of muscles. Both lateral and medial incisions meet at the apex of the femoral triangle, where the saphenous vein is identified, doubly clamped, divided, and ligated. Retraction of the flaps superiorly allows exposure of the external oblique fascia above the inguinal ligament, which represents the upper part of the dissection. Areolar tissue over the fascia is mobilized inferiorly by sharp scalpel dissection to the inguinal ligament, which is now carefully defined.

Sharp scalpel dissection is next performed to separate nodes from deep vessels by first defining the medial wall of the femoral vein. Kocher clamps are placed along the medial aspect of the node-bearing tissue situated on the deep vein, with the overlying tissue retracted in a lateral direction. A gauze sponge is used to tighten adventitial planes along the medial aspect of the wall of the vein, allowing it to be sharply incised from a superior to an inferior direction. This allows node-bearing tissue to be mobilized off the vessels with the saphenofemoral junction as the limiting point of dissection. Most involved nodes appear to be identified in this particular region. Arterial dissection is now begun from a lateral direction over the femoral nerves, again dissecting and isolating the saphenofemoral junction. This venous junction is then cross-clamped without tenting the femoral vein, and transection of the saphenofemoral junction is performed, allowing the node mass to be removed. Figure 13–1 shows the appearance of the dissected superficial groin. The boundaries of the femoral canal are clearly defined, with the lateral side formed by the medial border of the sartorius muscle and the medial side by the medial border of the adductor longus, the flattened tendon of which arises from the pubis. The base or upper margin of the triangle is the inguinal ligament. The vessels exit the triangle through the subsartorial or Hunter's canal.

When indicated, retroperitoneal dissection is now performed separately from the superficial groin dissection discontinuously. An incision is made in the external oblique fascia paralleling the inguinal ligament approximately 3 cm above it. This incision is then deepened by carrying it across the interal oblique muscle, transecting and ligating the inferior epigastric vessels. The transversalis fascia is now opened and the retroperitoneum entered. The peritoneal sac is retracted superiorly over the iliac vessels to the point at which the hypogastric bifurcation is noted. A folded moist laparotomy pad is inserted over the vessels, and with a Deaver retractor the peritoneal cavity is held up over the bifurcation of the iliac vessels. We usually find it advantageous to place a second retractor inferomedially to displace the bladder, the latter having been catheterized at the beginning of the procedure. At

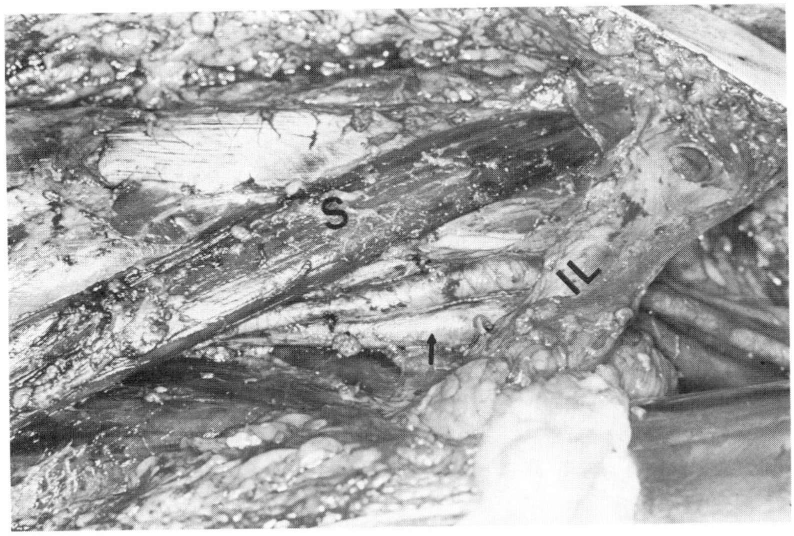

FIGURE 13–1. Superficial groin dissection. S shows the sartorius muscle, IL the inguinal ligament, and the arrow points to the femoral vessels.

this point the ureter in the retroperitoneal position should be identified near the base of the bladder as it enters the trigone.

Dissection is now carried over the iliac vessels to the hypogastrics, with the nodes of the hypogastric artery removed separately. Careful dissection of the adventitia and node-bearing tissue in the region of the psoas muscle and external iliac arteries is performed inferior to the femoral canal. The external iliac vessels nodes are taken as a separate specimen. The obturator space is now entered by separating the femoral vessels, retracting them medially from the psoas muscle. Dissection at this point is carried out bluntly, using the index finger without any instrumentation in the obturator fossa. The obturator nerve can easily be identified by finger dissection of the areolar tissue over the obturator nerve and vessels. These structures are found approximately 3 cm deep to the more superficial iliac vessels. The iliac vessels are next retracted over the psoas muscle in a lateral position, and the obturator nodes are pulled out medially from the deep pelvic structures, where they were adherent to obturator artery and nerve (Fig. 13–2). Hemoclips can be used to achieve hemostasis in this region. Cloquet's nodes are next cleared from the femoral canal, and a laparotomy pad is inserted temporarily into the retroperitoneal space for hemostasis. On completion of the node dissection the fascia is approximated with Dexon or prolene sutures and the wound closed. If there is a question of skin viability because of possible devascularization secondary to dissection of the femoral artery, then the edges of the wound should be trimmed. The femoral triangle is drained with a Hemovac or Jackson-Pratt catheter. An approach to bilateral simultaneous pelvic lymphadenectomy has been described by Kang-Ming et al.[13]

If loss of viability of part of the skin flap is noted postoperatively, debridement should not be performed immediately. Rather, the wound is painted daily with tincture of Merthiolate or Zephiran, converting the area of skin necrosis to a thick eschar that holds the wound edges together. If debridement is carried out early, the wound may separate apart widely, requiring several weeks for granulation tissue to fill the defect; skin grafting is performed to complete the successful healing of the wound.

Occasionally, as previously noted, a mass palpated in the region above the inguinal ligament may be considered to be metastatic nodal disease. Exploration usually reveals that these nodes are situated in the saphenofemoral junction and that there has been a misinterpretation of position of the actual nodes. With exposure of the vessels the opportunity arises for delivery of intra-arterial chemotherapeutic agents, when there is the potential for microscopic disease remaining in an extremity. A variety of drugs is available for slowing the rate of tumor growth. These drugs are injected into the femoral artery with an Intracath after cross-clamping of the vessels with vascular bulldog clamps. HN-2, methotrexate DTIC-Dome, Adriamycin, and vincristine have all been employed. After slow injection of the

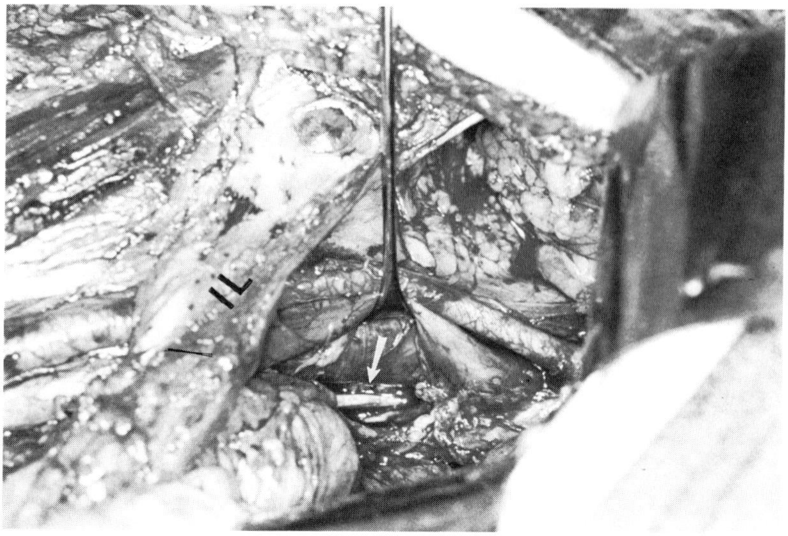

FIGURE 13–2. *The deep groin extension is illustrated, with IL representing the inguinal ligament and the arrow pointing to the obturator nerve. The iliac vessels are being retracted laterally.*

drugs, the arterial supply is opened and blood allowed to circulate against a cross-clamped femoral vein for approximately 5 minutes. At that time the vein is unclamped, allowing circulation to resume. For tumors in thigh or upper arm, a tourniquet can be applied to exclude the lower part of the extremity.

Several reports of various techniques used in performing groin dissections have been published, and most are similar to what we have described above. Harris et al.[9] reported on 95 dissections, 88 used for melanoma and 7 for squamous cell carcinoma and leiomyosarcoma. Das Gupta[4] defined his procedures as extending along the iliac vessels to the bifurcation of the aorta. Most other variations have been based on extensions of routine incisions.[21] Ariel[1] employed an elongated incision reaching down to the popliteal space. Such extended incisions are not too useful since complete lymphatic dissections of subcutaneous planes in the legs are not practical, and for low-lying primary tumors situated below the knee, discontinuous dissection and arterial infusion are probably as useful, if not more practical, in terms of the long-term results achieved. Hovnanian[11] described osteotomizing the anterosuperior iliac spine and retracting the inguinal ligament and its attached muscles for entry in the retroperitoneum. Most surgeons will agree, however, that the discontinuous dissection of retroperitoneal nodes above the femoral canal is not any less successful in controlling metastatic nodal disease, i.e., when disease is found along the iliac vessels, obturator fossa, or femoral canal. Bulky hypogastric and obturator disease found on CT scan should, however, be approached transabdominally.

AXILLARY NODE DISSECTION

Axillary node dissection is probably utilized more frequently for variations on the theme than is groin dissection, as it encompasses lesions arising on the back and chest wall, which are drained by this particular group of nodes, as well as lesions primarily arising in the upper extremity. It may also be employed as part of the four-quarter amputation or the Tikhoff-Lindberg dissection. As with other node-bearing areas, the primary anatomic structures to be dissected here are the axillary artery and vein as well as the brachial plexus. In comparison, the techniques to be employed for dissection are similar to what is used for the groin and neck. Nodes are dissected en-bloc from the femoral vein and artery, femoral nerve, or from corresponding carotid artery, jugular vein, and vagus nerve. By sharp scalpel dissection, occasionally using scissor dissection, fine vessels are clipped with 4-mm hemoclips and divided, as they course into lymph node–bearing tissue.

Two standard approaches have been used to enter the axilla and perform dissection of the lymph node–bearing area, either prophylactically or in the face of clinical disease. These approaches are employed either en-bloc (when the incision of the primary lesion is within 10 cm of the node-bearing area) or discontinuously (when the primary tumor is distant or has previously been resected). There are instances when axillary node dissection is accomplished as part of a Tikhoff-Lindberg or four-quarter amputation as noted above. The axillary incisions either parallel the pectoralis major fold or extend transversely across the axillary hollow from the lateral margin of the pectoralis to the anterior margin of the latissimus dorsi. We prefer the latter incision, originally described by Chretien,[3] since healing is most cosmetic and scar contracture does not develop as when the incision parallels the pectoralis. Either incision may be extended for greater exposure, the former by creating a T-limb from the mid-pectoralis incision across the chest wall to the mid-clavicle. In either instance, the pectoralis and the clavicular heads of the pectoralis major are split and the pectoral head is transected proximal at its tendinous insertion into the bicipital groove. The remainder of the two heads are then separated at the chest wall by dividing them between clamps; this allows adequate visualization for dissection of level I and, to some degree, level II nodes adjacent to the axillary vein. A fat pad adjacent to the lateral aspect of the head of the pectoralis minor is easily noted. This fat pad (Treves's) can be mobilized with a sponge on the index finger, sweeping it inferiorly off the axillary vein, which then allows for finger dissection between the vein and pectoralis minor. The pectoralis minor can now easily be mobilized and its head divided with a coagulating current at the coracoid process.

As mentioned, we prefer to use a transverse axillary incision for cosmetic as well as functional purposes. Skin flaps are raised superiorly over the lateral edge of the pectoralis, axillary hollow, and lateral margin of the latissimus. A posterior flap is then elevated in an inferior direction at the inferior edge of the pectoralis and the latissimus. The latissimus is defined and traced to its tendinous portion, which passes under the axillary vein, and sets the limit wherein all of the lower axillary dissection is carried out within its medial border. Nodes in the subscapular fossa are mobilized medially away from the latissimus. Dissection is carried at the level of the serratus against the chest wall and between the pectoral fold and the latissimus dorsi, just below the insertion of the subscapular nerve and its accompanying vein into the latissimus dorsi. The edge of the pectoralis is now elevated with a large right angle retractor, and with blunt dissection the fatty tissue is swept off the axillary vein to define its inferior margin. At this point the two heads of the pectoralis major can now easily be defined and divided to the chest wall. The remaining pectoral (clavicular) head retains the shape of the pectoral fold while the division of the other pectoral head exposes the clavipectoral fascia, which is incised to define the upper margin of the pectoralis minor. Treves's fat pad is mobilized inferiorly away from the vein, and the pectoralis minor tendon is identified and divided; with sharp scalpel dissection the fascia over the axillary vein is carefully incised and mobilized inferior to the vein. With fine clamp dissection the small branches off the axillary vein, artery, and nerves coursing into the node-bearing area can be identified, clipped, and transected. All node-bearing tissue is swept off levels II and III of the vein, and the subscapularis muscle is now identified with the thoracodorsal and long thoracic nerves being preserved. Harris[10] and Yonomoto[23] have described this technique primarily for melanoma dissection, preserving the pectoralis by resuturing the divided tendons for exposure if needed. Should there be a question of residual microscopic disease in the arm, the axillary vein can be cross-clamped with vascular bulldog clamps and the arterial region injected with the chemotherapeutic agent. The venous clamp is then removed approximately 5 minutes after drugs have been infused (Fig. 13–3).

RETROPERITONEAL PARA-AORTIC NODE DISSECTION

This dissection is usually carried out as part of the en-bloc resection of retroperitoneal sarcomas. For all large sarcomas it is necessary to have the aorta and vena cava exposed and dissected, removing node-bearing tissue along with tumor. For laterally placed lesions the small bowel is eviscerated and lapped from the field. The transverse colon is elevated superiorly to expose the retroperitoneal aorta-cava. For right-sided lesions the incision, a vertical one, is begun over the aorta, dissecting all tissue to the right. Left-sided tumors require dissection beginning over the cava and mobilization

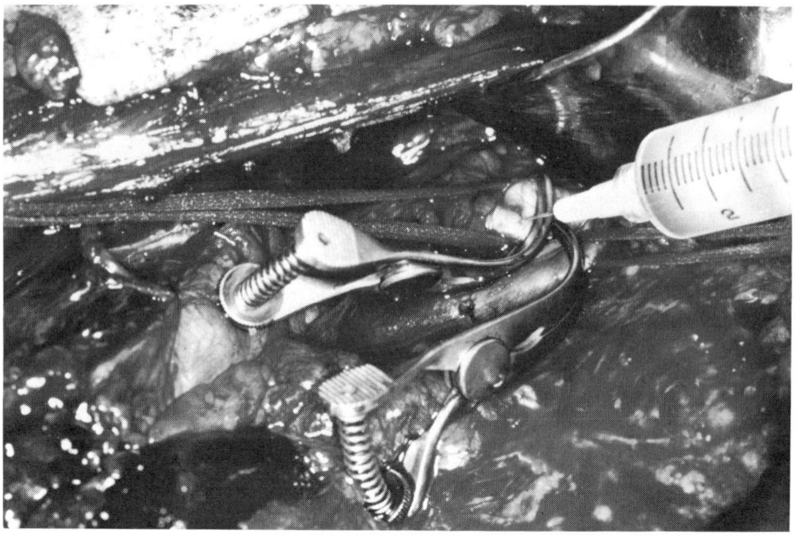

FIGURE 13–3. Axillary perfusion. Two bulldog clamps are placed across the vein and the artery. Chemotherapy is being injected into the artery.

carried to the aorta. The dissection extends from the ligament of Treitz to the bifurcation of the aorta and inferiorly to the respective hypogastric artery. Jejunum at the ligament of Treitz is elevated and dissection carried to the left renal veins. All nodes are mobilized off the vessels and swept to the tumor mass, defining the medial aspect of the surgical field. Lateral dissection of the tumor is then begun. For midline tumors, it is important to define the lateral margins of the cava and aorta, to dissect along the vessels, and to mobilize tumor off the aorta and cava. If the tumor is too large to approach, its pseudocapsule can be entered (provided that the tumor is relatively avascular, the tumor debulked, and the entire tumor then resected).

NECK DISSECTION FOR SARCOMAS OR WHEN APPROACHING BENIGN NERVE TUMORS

Dissection of the anatomic structures in the neck are carried out in a somewhat modified fashion since sarcomas and nerve tumors rarely require the need for suprahyoid neck dissection in the digastric triangle; a thyroid-type incision can be carried posteriorly to the mid-trapezius muscle, then curved upward to the mastoid process. With this incision, a large flap can be raised to expose the lesion to be dissected. At times, we have seen tumors extending into the region of the digastric triangle, in which case the incision can be extended superiorly to afford greater exposure. This can be accomplished by using a preauricular parotid-type incision, which is carried inferiorly behind the ear to join the mastoid extension of the neck incision. The large skin flap is then raised over the mandible, exposing the entire tumor that needs further dissection. The dissection can be carried anteriorly over the midline trachea and larynx. The sternomastoid muscle is then divided just above the clavicle to expose the jugular vein. Posterior node dissection is begun anterior to the trapezius muscle and is carried over the levator scapulae muscle to identify the jugular vein. The carotid sheath, if necessary, should be opened, and further dissection is carried up the jugular vein and carotid artery to the carotid bifurcation, separating the vagus nerve from tumor mass. The jugular vein may or may not have to be sacrificed and included with tumor mass, depending on the position of the tumor and the extent of its involvement. Dissection ends where the hypoglossal nerve crosses the carotid division. Figure 13–4 shows the dissected neck field with the carotid artery and vagus nerve intact on completion of the dissection. The hypoglossal nerve has a silk marker around it and can be seen passing up behind the posterior digastric muscle to enter the floor of the mouth and then innervate the tongue. The superior laryngeal nerve can also be seen as it comes from behind the carotid artery to enter the larynx between the wing of thyroid and the hyoid bones.

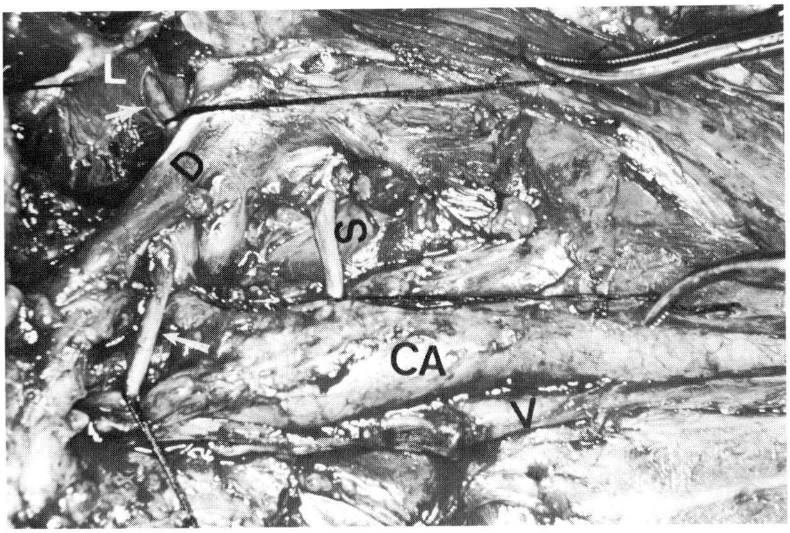

FIGURE 13–4. Radical neck dissection. CA represents the carotid artery. The jugular vein has been resected and the vagus nerve (V) is seen adjacent to the artery. Three nerves are identified: S shows the superior laryngeal nerve coursing under the carotid artery bifurcation to enter the larynx. L in the upper field represents the lingual nerve, and the arrows point to the hypoglossal nerve passing over the carotid artery to enter the floor of the mouth. The nerve is seen going under the digastric muscle (D) to reach its destination.

EXTREMITY EDEMA AS A COMPLICATION OF NODE DISSECTION

Occasionally extremity edema results either from axillary dissection or as a complication of radical groin dissection. When retroperitoneal sarcomas are resected en-bloc with the vena cava, edema of both legs is seen. Frequent lymphedema may be seen with groin dissection but rarely noted as a consequence of axillary dissection alone, unless radiation therapy has been delivered to the operative field. It may be that excision of a primary leg lesion carried out en-bloc with regional nodes is more of a causative factor in producing such lymphedema than is a discontinuous dissection. This question was raised by Papachristou and Fortner,[19] who found measurable lymphedema in 64% of patients who had an en-bloc procedure and 69% in the discontinuous dissection group. Edema of more than 2 inches occurred in 23% and 36%, respectively. Wound complications occurred in 41% and 42%, respectively, but did not affect the incidence of edema. Support stockings were used by only 58% of patients in the en-bloc dissection group and 71% of the discontinuous dissection group. Lymphangiograms obtained after groin and axillary dissection showed various patterns of collateral lymph circulation, but no regeneration of excised ducts. Studies of cross-circulation failed to reveal anastomosis between the medial and lateral superficial lymphatics, which would suggest that with major disruption in one part of the lymphatic circulation, cross-circulation from the remaining area does not occur.

In general, lymphedema can be classified as primary or secondary.

- I. Primary or idiopathic lymphedema
  - A. Congenital: Present at birth or shortly thereafter
    - 1. Milroy's Disease: Hereditary congenital lymphedema. Milroy in 1892 reported 22 cases of a previously undescribed variety of lymphedema. This was updated by him in 1928.[18] He was able to trace the deformity through six generations that included 97 individuals of the same family.
  - B. Praecox: Usually appears between the ages of 15 and 35 and affects young females more often than males.
- II. Secondary lymphedema
  - A. Surgical removal of lymph nodes and lymphatics.
  - B. Neoplastic invasion of lymph nodes and lymphatics, either by primary or metastatic neoplasms.
  - C. Lymphadenitis following:
    - 1. X-ray treatment: Fibrosis and scarring enhanced by x-rays may cause obstruction of the lymphatics and result in edema.
    - 2. Pyogenic infection.
    - 3. Granulomas due to:
      - a. Filariasis
      - b. Lymphogranuloma venereum
      - c. Tuberculosis
      - d. Syphilis

D. Post-traumatic

In extremity lymphedema, regardless of which component of the lymphatic system is affected (whether the lymphatic capillary, lymphatic trunk or lymph node) and whether it is of primary or secondary origin, stagnation of lymph flow within the lymphatic channels occurs. As a result, the connective tissue fills with edema fluid and swells. The tension of the connective tissue fibers attached to the lymphatic capillaries causes their walls to be drawn apart and the vessels become dilated; the lymphatic valves are consequently made incompetent. In the absence of competent valves, the pull of gravity forces the column of lymph downward, creating increased distention and stasis of lymph flow in the lymphatic channel and in the tissue spaces. In a normal individual, as much as 50% of the total circulating protein escapes from the blood vessels in the course of a day. This extravascular protein and tissue fluid, which is used in part for cell nutrition, readily enters the lymphatic capillaries, along with foreign particles, if any are present. As a result of the obstruction of the lymphatic flow, the protein content of the lymph and interstitial fluid increases. Lymph is an excellent medium for fibroblasts, hence proliferation is accelerated and fibrosis sets in in the subcutaneous tissues, thus obstructing still further the flow of lymph. The subcutis becomes thickened and the overlying skin assumes a stretched brawny appearance, exposing it to infection and resultant inflammation and thrombosis of the lymphatic vessels. More stasis supervenes until finally an irreversible situation is obtained. In the entire process the underlying muscles are not affected, leading some surgeons to employ a surgical approach toward managing some of the more difficult cases.

In an attempt to control developing or mild lymphedema, conservative therapy with leg elevation and compression stockings and mechanical milking devices are most frequently employed. To control moderate edema, operative procedures occasionally have been performed in an attempt to improve intrinsic drainage in the involved extremity. Handley[8] attempted to bury silk threads in the subcutaneous tissue, to improve lymphatic drainage in cases of the edematous postmastectomy arm. Kondoleon[15] designed a procedure based on observing that deep muscle compartments were not involved by edema; he attempted drainage of subcutaneous edema by excising strips of muscle fascia to redirect the lymph flow. Rapid fascial regrowth locked in the lymph that drained but led Thompson to devise a procedure for burying dermal flaps to redirect lymph flow. More recently, Goldsmith[6] described a technique for transposing an omental pedicle to the involved site in the hope that the lymphatic-rich omentum would open new conduits for drainage. In some instances, a marked decrease in the amount of edema was noted at the site where the omentum was buried. This operation was performed (1) to excise (en-bloc) the excess skin and underlying edematous and fibrotic subcutaneous tissue as well as deep fascia which tends to hold tissue fluid and thus prevent lymphatic flow, and (2) to introduce additional normal functioning lymphatic channels as well as blood vessels to bridge the area of lymphatic insufficiency and thus increase the number of functioning lymphatic channels. The procedure as described consists of mobilization of the intact omentum together with its gastroepiploic arcade from the greater curvature of the stomach and the transverse colon. The omentum is then fashioned into a pedicle and is brought out through the femoral canal and laid over the bare muscles of the anteromedial aspect of the thigh. In the upper extremity the omentum is brought out from the abdominal cavity through a subcutaneous tunnel in the anterior chest and laid over the infraclavicular and axillary areas along the course of the nerves and vessels and distally along the bare muscles of the anteromedial aspect of the arm. Before mobilization of the omentum, the excess skin and underlying thickened, edematous, and fibrotic subcutaneous tissues of the affected extremity are removed. Hemovac drainage tubes are placed into the wound at the end of the operation.

When lymphedema can not be controlled by any drainage procedure that is attempted, various methods of surgical reduction may be tried. In the procedure introduced by Charles,[2] the entire superficial compartment of the extremity and overlying skin are excised, with split-thickness grafts applied to muscle. Four more moderate forms of excisional therapy, referred to as Kondoleon procedures, have been widely used, and excision could be carried out beneath skin flaps without the deformity of the Charles procedure. In order to objectively evaluate improvement in lymphatic flow in an extremity, the technique of Ju et al.[12] was employed by several investigators. They used the disappearance of labeled serum albumin from the site of subcutaneous injection as an index of lymphatic function. Gorman and Navarre[7] demonstrated a significant difference between patients with congenital lymphedema and normal subjects. Injected radioiodinated human serum albumin was cleared in 28% of the lymphedematous extremities compared with 75% of the normals. Miller et al.[17] reported good results in six patients in whom staged procedures were performed at 2-month intervals. All underlying fibroadipose tissue, including deep muscle fascia, was removed. The extremities were immobilized with subcutaneous drains for at least 2 weeks. After form-fitting elastic stockings were applied, the patients were ambulated. Postoperative evaluation using radioiodinated albumin clearance showed that 70% was removed, compared with 39% preoperatively in a 24-hour period. Most of our patients in whom we expect extensive lymphatic swelling secondary to major lymphatic drainage are kept at bed rest for approximately 4 to 5 days with their legs elevated. In addition, elastic stockings are applied and used by the patients for several months after surgery. A major complicating factor that can result in lymphedema is the failure of adequate skin healing with secondary fibrosis at the operative site. This can be obviated by trimming the skin and assuring that good suction drainage is applied so that skin flaps can be kept adherent to the underlying muscle and fascial planes for revascularization.

Karakousis et al.[14] reviewed the experience with lymphedema following groin dissection at Roswell Park. Seventy-seven patients had undergone groin dissection; 40 had elective superficial and 27 therapeutic radical (ilioinguinal) groin dissection. The radical procedure involved the removal of iliac and obturator nodes. Hemovac drainage was employed until lymph drainage was below 50 ml per 24 hours. We have noted that the extent of drainage is related to the degree of clinical involvement and the volume of the tumor mass blocking the lymphatic channels. Should mild edema be present prior to surgery, then following removal of the node mass, prolonged and extensive drainage from dilated lymphatics can be anticipated. Elevation of the legs and the use of compression stockings were advised postoperatively. Three patients (4.4%) had minor skin edge necrosis; four (6%) had persistent lymphorrhea treated by repeat aspirations.

Extensive lymphedema may be associated with severe morbidity. Figure 13–5 shows massive edema with virtually complete loss of hand and arm function. Since the cause of the edema was recurrent tumor around the upper humerus, disarticulation was necessary. Persistent chronic edema has also been associated with a virulent form of angiosarcoma (Stewart-Treves syndrome), which has been almost uniformly fatal.[20, 22] Epstein and Mendelsohn.[5] described a patient with congenital lymphedema of the leg in whom squamous cell carcinoma developed at the site of long-standing verrucous hyperplasia. A parallel is drawn between the development of angiosarcoma in a setting of atypical lymphangiomatous proliferation and the appearance of squamous cell carcinoma with condylomatous and spindle features in the presence of verrucous hyperplasia. A viral role in the induction of such changes in the setting of chronic lymphedema is possible.

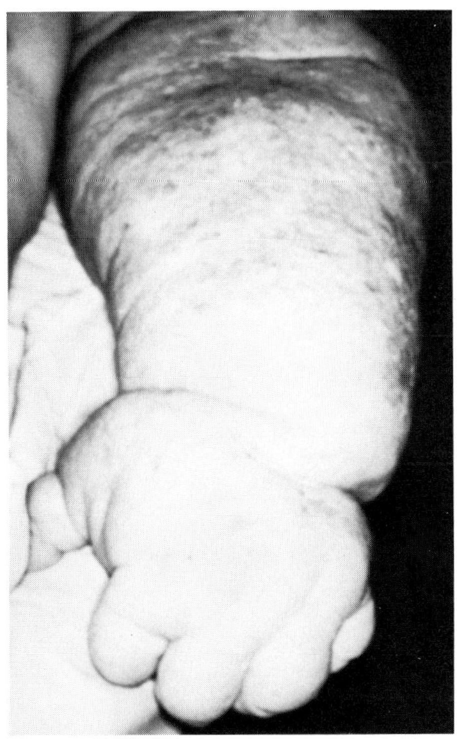

FIGURE 13–5. Extensive lymphedema of the left forearm.

REFERENCES

1. Ariel I.M.: The extended radical groin dissection for melanomas of the lower extremity. Surg. Gynecol. Obstet. 132:116, 1971
2. Charles R.H.: A System of Treatment. Volume 3. J.A. Churchill Ltd., 1912
3. Chretien P.B., Ketchum A.S., Hoye R.C., Sample F.: Axillary dissection with preservation of the pectoralis major muscle. Ann. Surg. 73:554, 1971
4. Das Gupta T.K.: Radical groin dissection. Surg. Gynecol. Obstet. 129:1275, 1969
5. Epstein J.I., Mendelsohn G.: Squamous carcinoma of the foot arising in association with long-standing verrucous hyperplasia in a patient with congenital lymphedema. Cancer 54:943–947, 1984
6. Goldsmith H.S., de Los Santos R.: Omental transposition in primary lymphedema. Surg. Gynecol. Obstet. 125:607–610, 1967
7. Gorman J.F., Navarre J.R.: Observations of lymphedema precox and its management with lymphangioplasty. Vasc. Dis. 2:1, 1965
8. Handley W.S.: Lymphangioplasty: A new method for the relief of the brawny arm of breast cancer and for similar conditions of lymphatic edema. Lancet 1:31, 1909
9. Harris M.H., Gumport S.L., Berman I.R., Bernard R.W.: Ilioinguinal lymph node dissection. Surg. Gynecol. Obstet. 136:33–39, 1973
10. Harris M.H., Gumport S.L., Maiwandi H.: Axillary dissection for melanoma. Surg. Gynecol. Obstet. 135:936–940, 1972
11. Hovnanian A.P.: Radical ilioinguinal lymphatic excision. Ann. Surg. 135:520, 1952
12. Ju D.M.C., Blakemore A., Stevenson T: A lymphatic function test. Surg. Forum, 1954
13. Kang-Ming H., Kahn A., Smith N.: Bilateral pelvic lymphadenectomy from a lower abdominal transverse skin incision and pararectal approach. Surg. Gynecol. Obstet. 156:443–448, 1983
14. Karakousis C.P., Heiser M.A., Moore R.H.: Lymphedema after groin dissection. Am. J. Surg. 145:205–208, 1983.
15. Kondoleon E.: Die operative Behandlung der elephantiastischen Oedema. Zentralbl. Chir. 39:1022, 1912
16. Miller T.A.: Charles procedure for lymphedema: A warning. Am. J. Surg. 139:290–292, 1980
17. Miller T.A., Harper J., Longmire W.P.: The management of lymphedema by staged subcutaneous excision. Surg. Gynecol. Obstet. 136:586–592, 1973
18. Milroy W.F.: Chronic hereditary edema: Millroy's disease. JAMA 91:1172, 1928
19. Papachristou D., Fortner J.G.: Comparison of lymphedema following incontinuity and discontinuity groin dissection. Ann. Surg. 185:13–16, 1977
20. Stewart F.W., Treves N.: Lymphangiosarcoma in postmastectomy lymphedema. Cancer 1:64, 1948
21. Wagner D.E., Rochlin D.B., Wilson A.P.: A new approach to radical retroperitoneal iliac and femoral node dissection. Arch. Surg. 103:681, 1971
22. Woodward A.H., Ivins J.C., Soule E.H.: Lymphangiosarcoma arising in chronic lymphedematous extremities. Cancer 30:562, 1972
23. Yonomoto R.H., Thompson W.C., Byron R.L., Riihimaki D.V.: Complete axillary node dissection with preservation of the pectoralis major muscle. Arch. Surg. 102:578, 1971

CHAPTER

14

Extraskeletal Osseous Tumors and Common Soft Part Lesions Presenting as Primary Lesions of Bone

An intriguing group of malignant sarcomas that we occasionally encounter comprises a subpopulation of common osseous tumors (osteosarcoma, chondrosarcoma, and Ewing's sarcoma) that are found to arise primarily within the soft tissues of the extremities, trunk and, in rarer instances, viscera. A second, somewhat parallel group of tumors with which we should be familiar comprises the more common soft part tumors (fibrosarcoma, malignant fibrous histiocytoma, angiosarcoma, and hemangiopericytoma) found to arise as primary tumors within bone. This latter group of tumors shows no evidence of any accompanying primary soft tissue components. Figure 14–1*A* shows a pretibial soft tissue mass that was clinically suspected to be a soft part sarcoma. When excised (Fig. 14-1*B*), the tumor appeared to have many of the characteristics of soft part lesions: It was well circumscribed, there was no evidence of extension to the bone, and it appeared to arise as a primary lesion within subcutaneous tissue or underlying fascia. Although this tumor occurred in the soft tissues of the pretibial region, it proved on histologic examination to be osteogenic sarcoma of extraskeletal origin.

EXTRASKELETAL OSTEOGENIC SARCOMA

While these tumors are exceedingly rare, more than 120 cases have been described to date.[1, 18, 27, 37, 39] By definition, it is essential that no osseous origin be identified in association with an extraskeletal lesion after careful clinical and radiologic evaluations have been performed. At times, a primary osteogenic sarcoma will have previously been resected and recurrence is now seen in the form of soft tissue metastasis. Such a soft tissue tumor is considered to be representative of a metastatic osteogenic sarcoma and cannot be considered to be an associated extraskeletal primary tumor. With the use of newer chemotherapy regimens it is not uncommon to see late metastatic tumors presenting with unusual patterns of recurrence in soft tissue such as liver, kidney, or pancreas. Figure 14–2 illustrates an unusual pattern of spread in a patient who had undergone previous amputation for tibial osteogenic sarcoma. Dissemination appeared as nodular masses within the soft tissues of the upper thigh as centripetal extension occurred toward the trunk.

In 1941 Wilson[37] described one of the first cases of extraskeletal osteogenic tumor, probably arising from the pericardium. The lesion was defined as a malignant bone-forming tumor arising from somatic soft tissue without connection to any osseous structure. In 1968 Das Gupta et al.[12] presented their experience in the management of nine such cases at Memorial Hospital. These tumors are usually found in the subcutaneous planes, occasionally ulcerating through skin. They vary in size from 1.5 to 20 cm and frequently are found to be cystic in their central portions. Occasionally, bone formation may be demonstrated. Microscopically

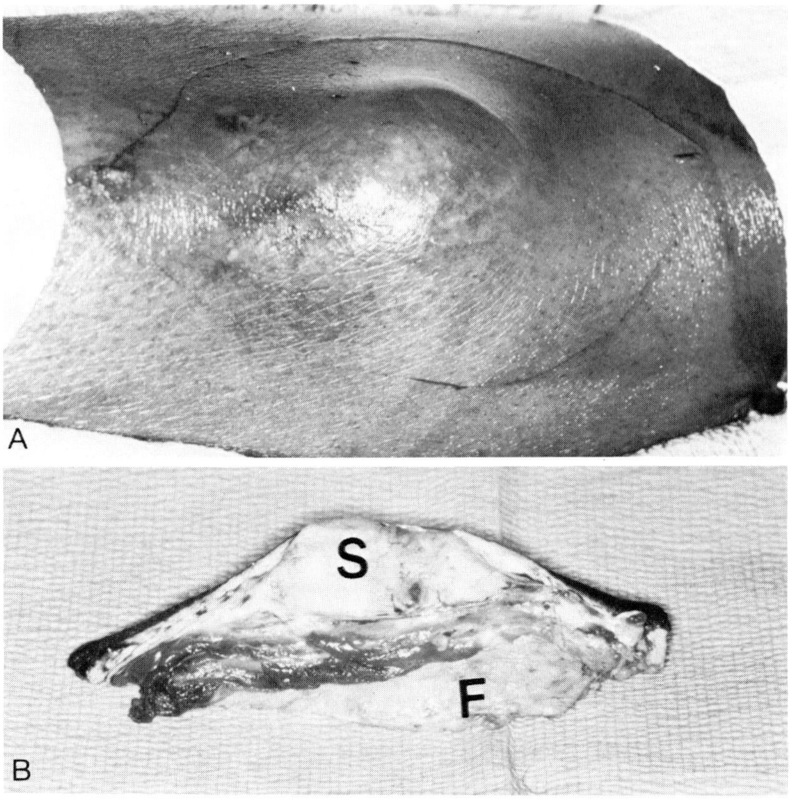

FIGURE 14–1. *A, Pretibial extraskeletal osteogenic sarcoma. B, Resected tumor showing sarcomatous lesion (S) situated in a subcutaneous position. F represents the pretibial fascia and periosteum.*

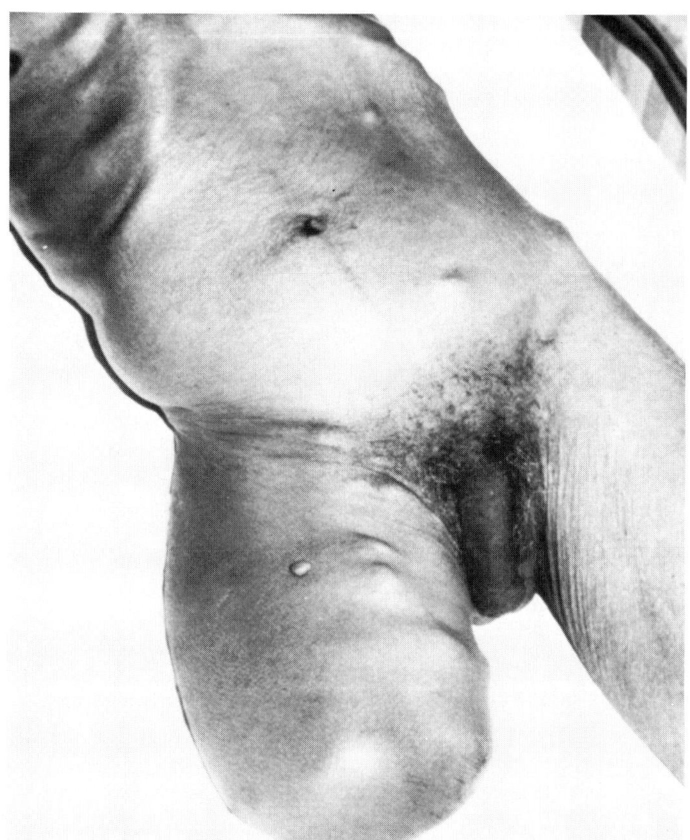

FIGURE 14–2. *Subcutaneous nodules of metastatic osteogenic sarcoma extending centripetally up the leg stump to the trunk.*

one usually finds a nodular arrangement of spindle cells with tumor giant cells, osteoblasts, and osteoid formation. In Das Gupta's series, five of the nine cases occurred within the thigh, and one each in the head and neck region, the buttock, chest wall, and arm. The only long-term survivor in this series was the patient with the primary tumor of head and neck origin arising in the region of the zygoma. Two of the patients were free of disease at the time of the report, but this represented a short interval from the time of surgery. Five of the nine patients had recurrence after multiple local excisions. Although wide resection has failed to improve survival in previously reported cases, amputation as a first line of therapy does not seem to be indicated in the initial treatment phase. Rather, en-bloc muscle group dissection with newer chemotherapeutic protocols directed toward the osteosarcoma is the approach we feel most comfortable with in the early stages of this disease.

In 1983 experience with extraskeletal osteosarcoma at the Memorial Sloan-Kettering Cancer Center was updated by Sordillo et al.[31] to include 48 patients. In this series, five lesions appeared in an area of prior radiation therapy;[2] six patients described a history of trauma to the area where their lesions later developed. This history of trauma appears suggestive of the concept that metaplasia developing in soft tissues acts to initiate onset of the tumor process. In experimental osteogenesis, where elevation in tissue carbon dioxide and a drop in pH to 6.8 to 7.2 has occurred, bone formation has been noted to result. Lee[23] described a patient who developed osteogenic sarcoma of soft tissue origin at the site of previous intramuscular injections. A number of cases have also been reported following the appearance of myositis ossificans.[30] The median age of the patients in Sordillo's series was 51 years (range, 6 to 80 years). This stands in contrast to the median age for primary osteogenic sarcoma arising in long bones, which is the teenage years. Twenty-nine of the cases in the Memorial series involved the buttock and lower extremity. Eleven patients had tumors arising in the upper extremity. Among those in the irradiated group, tumors have been noted to appear 13 to 21 years after treatment. One patient in this series, as with Shanoff's case,[30] had a biopsy-proven diagnosis of myositis ossificans at the site where the sarcoma appeared. In addition, tumors have been reported to develop following radiation damage to soft tissues as well as at sites of thorotrast extravasation.

In none of the cases considered to be an extraosseous primary did adherence of tumor to periosteum occur, nor did any lesion show evidence of intraosseous extension. There was no correlation between histologic appearance and survival. Many of the lesions that recurred after surgical resection appeared less differentiated and showed less osteoid than the primary tumor. Of the 45 patients 41 were followed for more than 1 year, 69% showed local recurrence and 8% had distant metastasis. Of the six treated initially with amputation, four eventually developed distant metastasis. Two patients treated initially with radiation therapy failed to respond. Chemotherapy using combinations with Adriamycin also failed to show a distinct beneficial response. Two of three patients who had a thorocotomy and resection of pulmonary metastasis followed by adjuvant chemotherapy remained free of disease.

VISCERAL OSTEOGENIC SARCOMA

Reports of approximately 120 cases of this lesion have appeared in the English literature to 1983. The extremities were the sites of 85% of these extraskeletal osteosarcomas. Axelrod[6] reported a case of a tumor of the kidney demonstrating ossified osteogenic sarcoma evenly distributed throughout that organ. The patient, a 48-year-old black man, had presented with abdominal distention, diarrhea, and a 60-lb weight loss. One year before, he had been found to have a primary inoperable retroperitoneal sarcoma. The patient died, and at autopsy 3 L of chylous fluid was present. The right kidney was replaced by a huge, bone-hard tumor that weighed 2200 gm. Microscopically, the renal tumor was composed of pleomorphic spindle cells which, in most areas, produced abundant osteoid and neoplastic bone. The histogenesis of such extraosseous osteogenic sarcomas has been speculative.

Primary osteosarcoma of the kidney was first described in 1936. Retroperitoneal osteosarcoma was described a decade later. The findings that aid in diagnosis include metastases with osteoblastic activity and a sunburst appearance radiographically. The metaplastic theory suggests that in certain circumstances connective tissue may revert to embryonic mesenchyme, then differentiate to produce osteoblasts with resultant new bone formation.

Belasco et al.,[7] in studying children with Wilms' tumor, noted that a large proportion of his patients had become long-term, disease-free survivors. A small percentage of these patients were later found to be at risk for developing second malignancies as a result of the therapeutic modalities employed. One of the patients in Belasco's series was a child with a stage I Wilms' tumor who developed bilateral pulmonary metastasis after failing on radiotherapy of 3600 R plus dactinomycin chemotherapy. Radiation therapy was again prescribed but with vincristine chemotherapy. Five years later, calcified nodules were noted in the left pleura. A thorocotomy revealed the lung to be encased in bone-like material. Biopsy showed sclerosing sites of osteosarcoma of the chest wall with no evidence of renal tumor. Work-up for metastatic renal disease outside the chest was negative. While bone formation can at times be found in renal neoplasms, there is no evidence that the origin of the chest lesion arose at the sight of nephrectomy. Rather, the new bone and osteoid that appeared in the chest metastasis of this patient seemed to represent a primary phenomenon of osteosarcoma developing within the pulmonary renal metastases. Valderama[34] described a case of an osseous sarcoma appearing in a hamartoma of thymus located in the left pleural cavity of an 11-year-old girl. The lesion was associated with a large left pleural effusion and displacement of the cardiac shadow to the right. CT scan of the chest revealed a homogeneous mass with dense clustered calcifications occupying the entire left lower hemithorax. Resection was performed and the patient was placed on chemotherapy. Sections from the tumor revealed thymic tissue interdigitated with abundant osseous tissue composed of mature lamellar bone. Areas containing poorly differentiated sarcoma were found with foci of cartilage and malignant osteoid. About half of the tumor was formed by hamartomatous thymus and half by osteosarcoma.

EXTRASKELETAL CHONDROSARCOMA

Another variant of an osseous neoplasm that may develop de novo within soft tissue is the chondrosarcoma.[16, 19, 26] Angervall[4] described a case of extraskeletal chondrosarcoma in which the lesion appeared to arise in the scrotum. The diagnosis of an extraosseous primary was suggested by histologic features as well as histochemical characterization. The tumor matrix was found to contain diastase-resistant, periodate-reactive material that showed metachromatic staining with toluidine blue at a pH of 4, susceptible to treatment with testicular hyaluronidase. Alcian-like staining with magnesium chloride showed a "critical electrolyte concentration" for dye-binding, approaching that of mast cells known to contain heparin. These studies indicated that the tumor matrix contained chrondroitin sulfate, or a related glycosaminoglycan characteristic for chondrosarcoma.[29, 38]

The existence of extraskeletal chondrosarcoma was originally established by Stout and Verner,[32] who found that mature chrondromatous tissue was a rare feature occurring within soft tissue tumors. Such lesions were found to behave in a less malignant fashion than those of skeletal origin in the adult; in children under 16 years of age, they have been found to behave as aggressive tumors. One of our patients, an 80-year-old diabetic, was seen with a draining paronychia of the first toe. On examination a mass was found near the head of the first metatarsal bone. Local resection of the first and second rays was performed to assure adequate margins. Figure 14–3*A* illustrates the appearance of this lesion, which proved to be a high-grade extraskeletal chondrosarcoma. A closer view of the lesion is seen in Figure 14–3*B*. Another patient presented with a soft tissue lesion near the upper end of the femur. Biopsy showed the tumor to be malignant. An en-bloc resection was performed. Initial examination (Fig. 14–4*A*) showed intrasynovial chondromatosis. Transection of the specimen showed a large soft tissue chondrosarcoma (Fig. 14–4*B*).

Chondrosarcoma arising in the lung has also been reported.[13] In 1972 Morgan and Salma[25] made a distinction between primary and secondary pulmonary chondrosarcomas. Primary chondrosarcomas arise de novo in the lung, whereas secondary ones are superimposed on a preexisting hamartoma. At the time of this report only eight cases had been reported that fulfilled the criteria of primary chondrosarcoma. Sun et al.[33] described an additional case in which intraoperative bleeding and aspiration were fatal complications and were attributed to

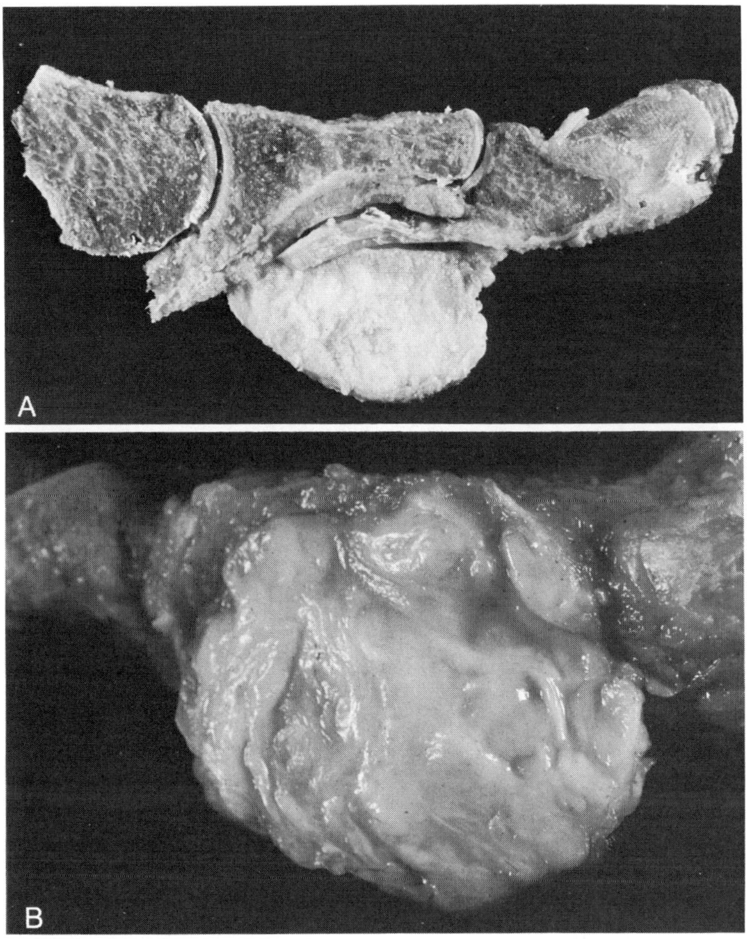

FIGURE 14–3. *A, Extraskeletal chondrosarcoma arising under the first metatarsal. B, Close-up view.*

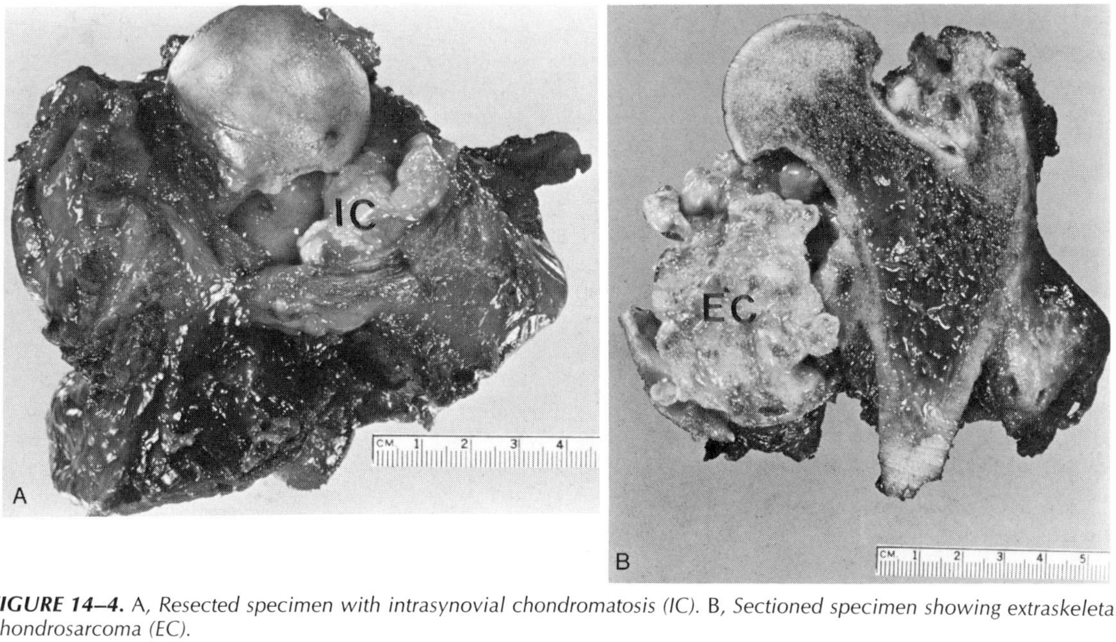

FIGURE 14–4. *A, Resected specimen with intrasynovial chondromatosis (IC). B, Sectioned specimen showing extraskeletal chondrosarcoma (EC).*

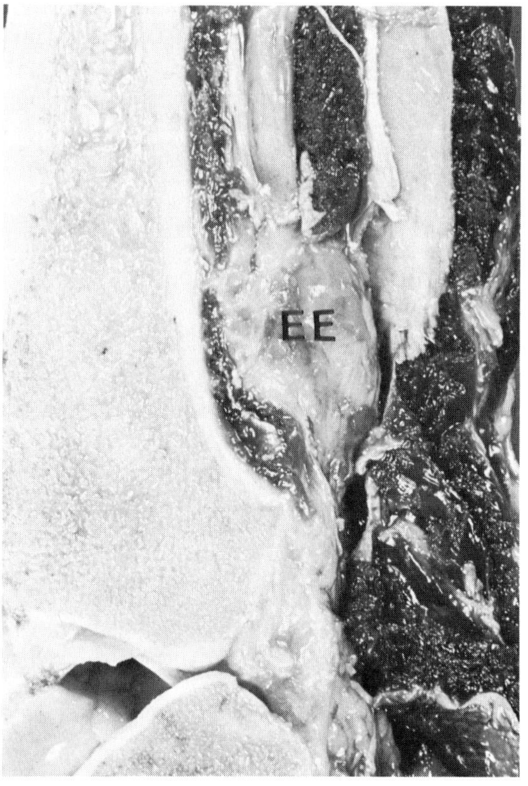

FIGURE 14–5. Extraskeletal Ewing's sarcoma (EE) adjacent to the distal tibia.

invasion of the pulmonary artery by the tumor. Tumorous involvement of multiple bronchi suggested either airborne or vascular intrapulmonary spread. Dyspnea and chest pain occur when there is bronchial obstruction or pleural involvement. The disease is best managed and can frequently be well controlled if the tumor is resected while localized.

Other variations in the types of extraskeletal cartilaginous lesions that may be encountered are seen in the rare cases of urogenital chondrosarcomas and the mesenchymal chondrosarcomas of soft tissue origin. The former group of tumors, especially when found arising in the uterus, fallopian tube and bladder, probably represent examples of one-sided development of so-called mixed mesodermal tumors. The mixed mesodermal tumor is basically a highly malignant sarcoma or carcinosarcoma, the bulk of which is made up of a multipotent cellular stroma of anaplastic appearance. This stroma often contains areas of rhabdomyoblastic,[20] chondroblastic, osteoblastic, and rarely lipoblastic differentiation. Mesenchymal chondrosarcoma refers to a recently described uncommon form of chondrosarcoma that, in general, has an unfavorable prognosis because of its aggressiveness. It can present in unusual osseous sites such as ribs, mandible and maxilla and frequently is seen to arise in soft tissues. Histologically the tumor is defined by its bimorphic growth pattern along with sheets of undifferentiated small round cells similar to those of Ewing's sarcoma and lobules of cartilage showing the characteristics of a low-grade chondrosarcoma.[8, 22]

Extraskeletal Ewing's sarcoma may also be found to occur as a soft tissue lesion.[5] Figure 14–5 shows the appearance of such a tumor in the lower extremity between the tibia and fibula.

COMMON SARCOMAS ARISING IN BONE

Fibrosarcoma of Bone

At times, various soft tissue tumors are found arising as primary bone lesions, e.g., fibrosarcoma,[19] malignant fibrous histiocytoma,[11, 21, 24] and leiomyosarcoma.[3] Fibrosarcomas, which represent one of the predominant lesions of soft part origin, also can be seen to appear within the medullary cavity of bone. When the latter breaks through cortical bone to invade surrounding soft tissue, the question of primary site of origin is raised. The nature of this variant of fibrosarcoma is of interest in terms of its behavior and response to therapy when compared with soft part fibrosarcoma and osteogenic sarcoma. Cunningham and Arlen[10] reviewed experience with handling this lesion at Memorial Hospital and found that it had its own characteristic behavior in terms of patterns of growth as well as response to therapy. This lesion was found to behave in a pattern intermediate between that of soft part fibrosarcoma and osteosarcoma. In a review of 28 cases the tumor was found to favor long bones, with approximately 77% occurring about the knee joint. Figure 14–6 shows a medullary fibrosarcoma of the distal femur. Whereas soft part fibrosarcomas can develop problems with regard to local control, the reappearance of medullary sarcomatous lesions is considered more ominous; local recurrence in the latter condition has not been noted to occur without the appearance of distant metastasis. The end result of surgery alone in terms of 5-year survival for

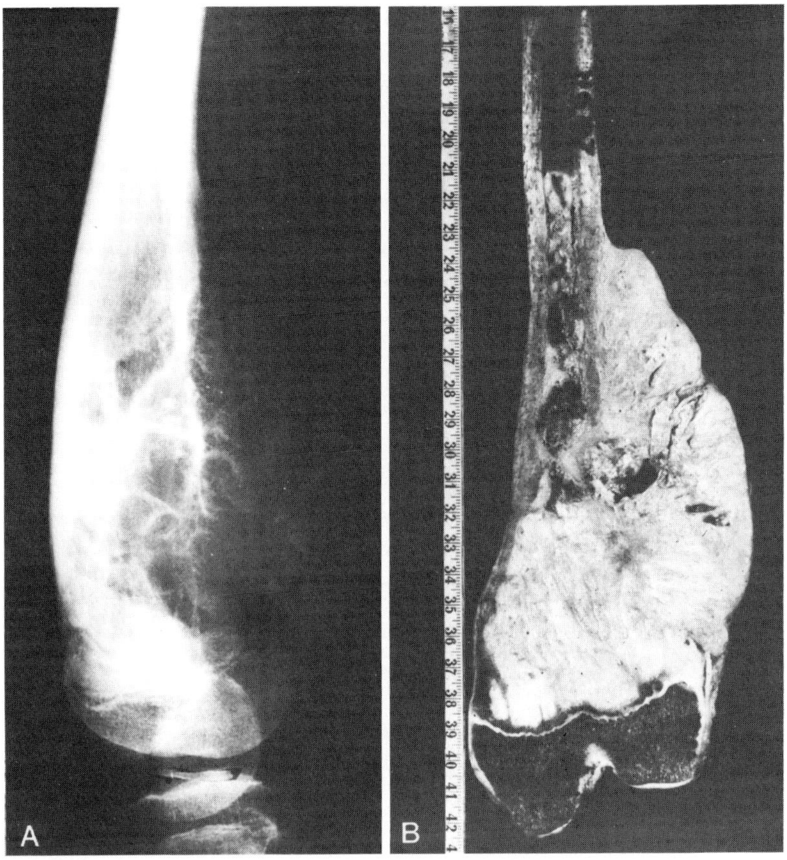

FIGURE 14–6. A, Medullary fibrosarcoma of bone. B, Resected specimen shows extent of soft tissue involvement of medullary fibrosarcoma.

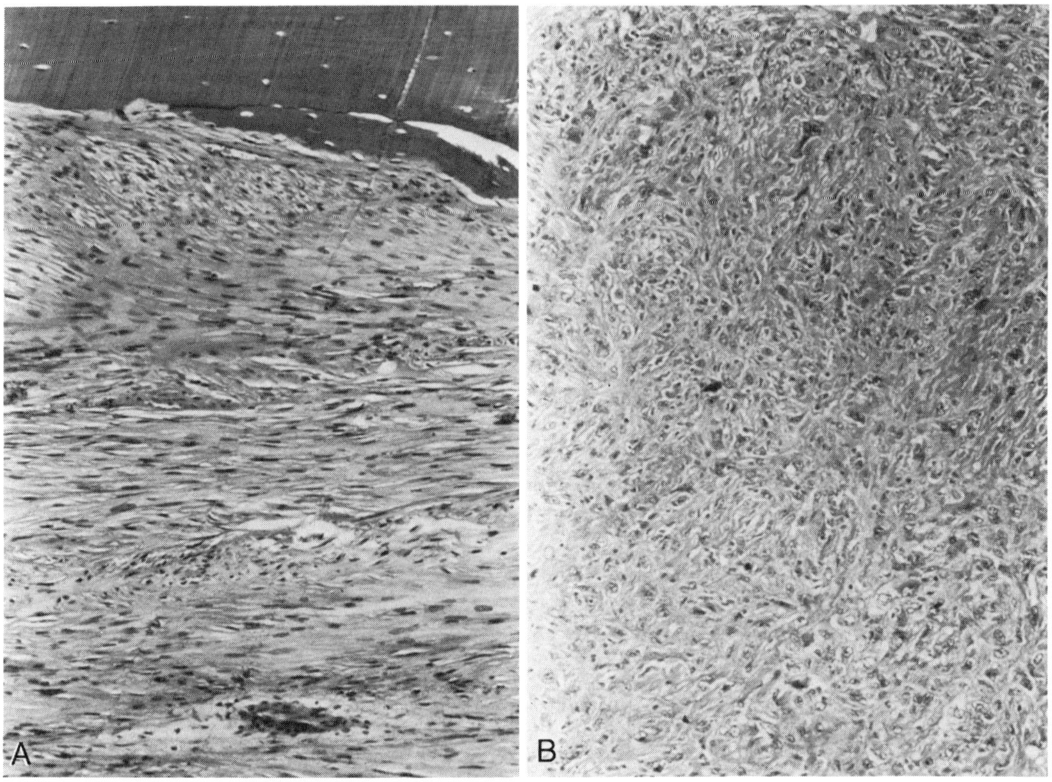

FIGURE 14–7. A, Low-grade medullary fibrosarcoma of bone. This well-defined spindle cell tumor has few, if any, mitotic figures. B, High-grade medullary fibrosarcoma shows marked pleomorphism and multiple mitotic figures.

the treatment of this tumor is approximately 30%, compared with 60% for primary soft part fibrosarcoma and 13% for osteogenic sarcoma (before newer chemotherapeutic procedures were available as part of the overall management of osteosarcoma). Low-grade tumors of medullary origin do exceptionally well regardless of the extent of invasion into soft tissue. In contrast, the more anaplastic lesions are almost uniformly fatal. Figure 14–7 shows the microscopic patterns of the low- and high-grade lesions of medullary fibrosarcoma which are useful in predicting clinical response to therapy.

Malignant Fibrous Histiocytoma of Bone

Malignant fibrous histiocytomas are well known among the tumors of the somatic soft tissues but recently have been recognized as primary in bone. Previously this lesion has been included in the osteosarcoma or fibrosarcoma groups. In the last few years, more than 170 cases have been reported in the literature. The minimum necessary histologic criteria for accepting a lesion as a malignant fibrous histiocytoma were as follows: (1) Three cell types are usually identified: spindle fibroblastic-fibrocytic cells, plump cells with histiocytic morphology and function, and both malignant and benign (reactive) giant cells. Both fibroblastic and histiocytic features are constantly present, but variation exists from case to case. This triphasic pattern is peculiar to malignant fibrous histiocytoma. (2) Osteoid should not be observed to be produced by the tumor cells. Osteoid production is considered to be an indication of osteosarcoma, which must be excluded. (3) The typical cartwheel or storiform patterns are present. This arrangement is prominent in the fibroblastic component more than in the histiocytic component. In a report of 90 cases by Capanna et al.[9] the lesions were noted to be purely osteolytic, some presenting as scattered small lytic areas that tended to merge (12%) but most as a single large lytic area (88%). The margins were most frequently ill defined and rarely had osteosclerotic margins. Tumor calcification and bone formation were not observed. Soft tissue invasion was demonstrated in 88% of the tumors and pathologic fractures occurred in 20%. The majority of cases appeared in long bones, especially around the knee. Overall survival rates were 34% at 5 years and 28% at 10 years. The recurrence rate after surgical treatment was high (31%) with significant differences after inadequate (64%), wide (19%), and radical (6.5%) surgical treatment.

Vascular Lesions of Bone

Angiosarcoma of bone, the so-called hemangiothelioma, arises in bone less fre-

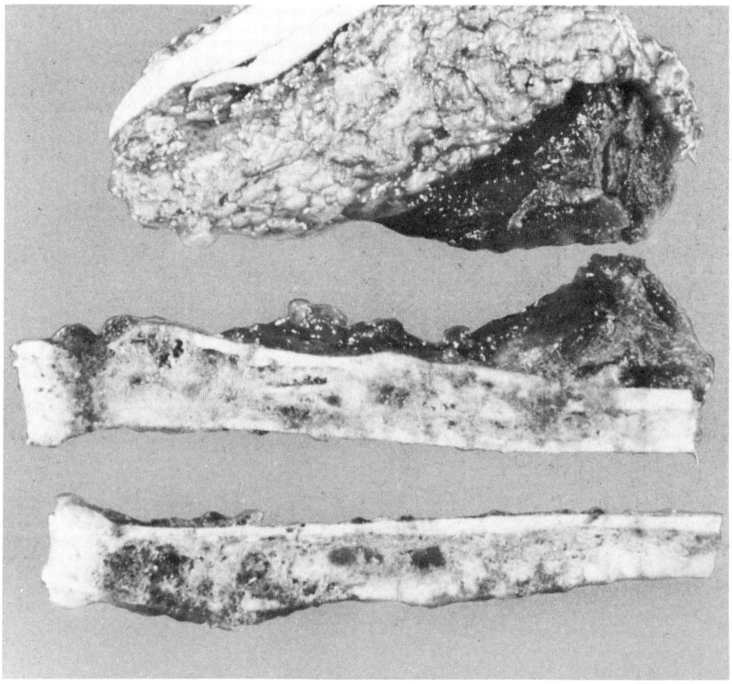

FIGURE 14–8. Angiosarcoma of the radius shows portion of the resected bone with site of invasion by the soft tissue lesion.

quently than other well-known soft tissue primary tumors. This lesion may be solitary or relatively solitary, being localized to one area of bone, as was found with one 16-year-old female patient (Fig. 14–8). It may, however, be found diffusely involving several bones within a limb bud (Fig. 14–9). The 16-year-old was referred to Memorial Hospital for management of a lesion of the forearm that bulged from the brachioradialis and appeared attached to underlying bone. On biopsy the mass proved to be an angiosarcoma arising in the mid-radial shaft and invading soft tissues of the forearm. She was referred to us for possible amputation. Because of the potential for this tumor to involve the limb bud, consideration was given to forequarter amputation; however, it was believed that an attempt at resection should be made. Muscle group dissection en-bloc with the radius, which would leave the patient with a one-bone forearm, was chosen (Fig. 14–10). She has remained clinically free of disease for over 10 years. In the 39 solitary cases evaluated at Memorial Hospital, the tibia, humerus, femur, and pelvic bones were the sites most frequently involved. En-bloc resection, with or without

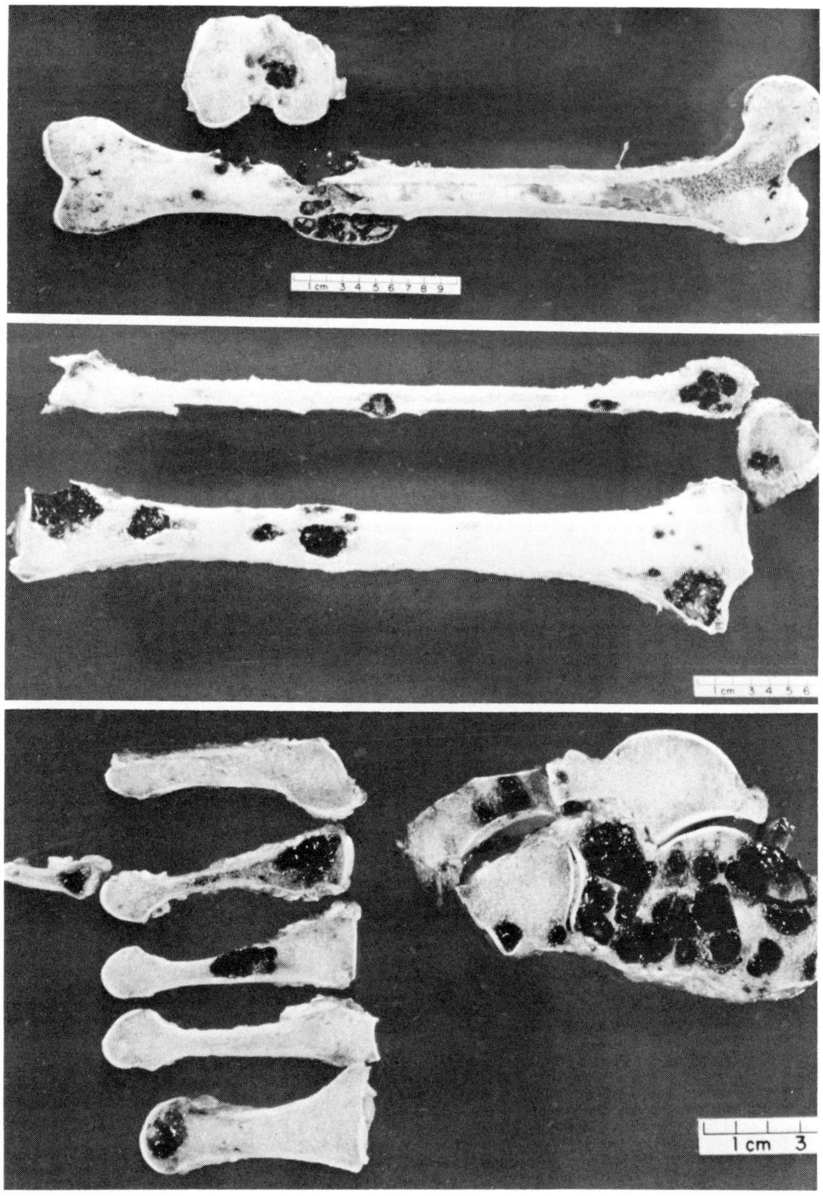

FIGURE 14–9. *Diffuse involvement of the limb bud is seen in this case of angiosarcoma of bone.*

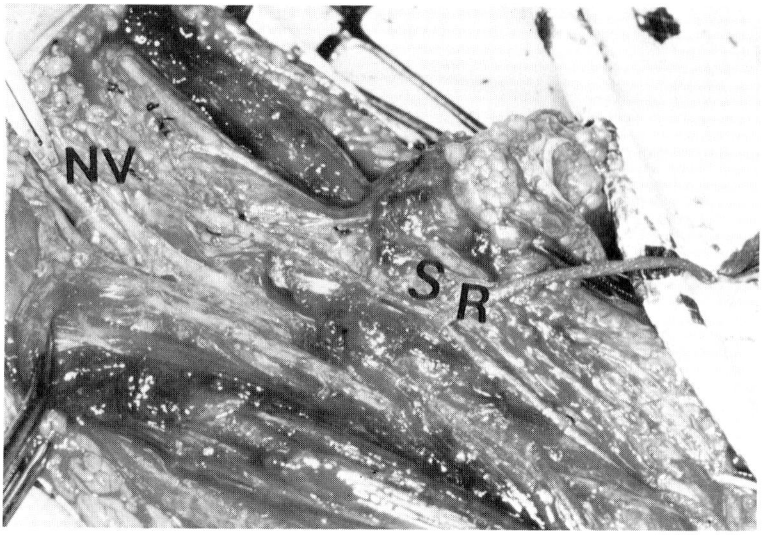

FIGURE 14–10. Operative field exposing the neurovascular pedicle (NV) containing the ulnar artery and the median nerve. The superficial radial nerve (SR) has been preserved.

endoprosthetic replacement, has been and remains the treatment of choice for the solitary form of the disease. When tumors are located in the vertebral body or skull, radiation therapy has been employed with some success. Where the sacrum, femur, tibia, and fibula were involved along with the limb bud (see Fig. 14–9), a hemipelvectomy provided long-term freedom from disease. Lymph nodes in the popliteal space of this patient eventually showed evidence of metastasis. Whether such tumors present in a solitary fashion or as multiple lesions within bone, it is important to evaluate whether the tumor is of low or high grade, as the latter may be extremely aggressive and metastasize rapidly. Differential diagnosis must include metastatic vascular tumors such as hypernephroma, thyroid carcinoma, and undifferentiated tumors from the lung and stomach. Even malignant synovioma may be misinterpreted because of the clefts within the tumor that may become filled with blood as a consequence of surgical trauma.

We have encountered one case of hemangiopericytoma arising primarily within bone. Two cases of this entity have been described by Dunlop.[15] Our patient presented with tumor within the scapula adjacent to the glenoid joint that had been present for at least 2 years prior to diagnosis. A routine x-ray film of the shoulder suggested the presence of a lesion in the glenoid region. Angiography revealed the highly vascular nature of this lesion, which proved on biopsy to be hemangiopericytoma. A Tikhoff-Lindberg resection was performed; the patient has remained free of disease for more than 5 years. Six patients with biopsy-proven hemangiopericytomas of bone have been treated at Memorial Hospital. Three of the patients died of widely disseminated disease following resection.

Leiomyosarcoma of Bone

Primary leiomyosarcoma of bone represents another rare lesion arising within bone, having the same characteristics of its soft part and visceral homologue. Two cases were first reported by Sanerkin[28] in 1965: one in the distal fibula of a 66-year-old man, and the other in the proximal tibia of a 61-year-old woman. Histologically there can be some difficulty in distinguishing this lesion from fibrosarcoma. The diagnosis depends on finding cytologic features that are not seen with fibrosarcoma, such as undue elongation and eosinophilia of cytoplasmic processes of the leiomyosarcoma cells. Histogenesis is believed to be related to the muscle structures within the blood vessels perforating the bone, although it is conceivable that the tumor could evolve through the development of myogenic metaplasia originating from the fibroblastic tissue. Von Hochstetter[35] more recently described a case of a 60-year-old man with a swelling anteromedially just below the knee. Plain films demonstrated osteolytic defects in the proximal tibial metaphysis without marginal sclerosis. A biopsy revealed a soft, grayish tumor in a subperiosteal location. The histopathologic diagnosis was leiomyosarcoma. This was the thirteenth documented case of primary leiomyosarcoma of bone outside the facial skeleton.[3, 17, 36]

At times, osseous lesions may occur in association with soft tissue pathology, especially in the presence of clinical disorders such as neurofibromatosis (von Recklinghausen's disease). In an attempt to evaluate the nature of osseous growths (malignant) that might appear in association with neurofibromatosis, Ducatman et al.[14] reviewed possible associations in approximately 4000 bone tumors seen at the Mayo Clinic. Three cases were found in patients with clinical manifestations of von Recklinghausen's disease. None were neurogenic tumors. One patient had a fibrosarcoma and two patients had malignant fibrous histiocytomas. No gross relationship to nerves was demonstrated. Primary neurogenic tumors of bone are uncommon. Confusion may arise in spindle cell lesions, especially if there is a suggestion of palisading or if the lesion approximates a nerve. Benign Schwann cell tumors may arise from intraosseous nerves, the most commonly reported one being the inferior alveolar nerve of the mandible. Malignant peripheral nerve sheath tumors may also occur in this location. The nerve sheath origin of an intraosseous neoplasm can be confirmed by demonstrating its association with an intraosseous nerve either grossly or by means of the Bodian staining technique for residual axons.

REFERENCES

1. Allan C. J., Soule E. H.: Osteogenic sarcoma of the somatic soft tissues. Cancer 27:1121–1133, 1971
2. Alpert L. S., Abaci I. F., Werthamer S.: Radiation-induced extraskeletal osteosarcoma. Cancer 31:1359–1363, 1973
3. Angervall L., Berlin O., Kindblom L. G., Stener B.: Primary leiomyosarcoma of bone: A study of 5 cases. Cancer 46:1270–1279, 1980
4. Angervall L., Enerback L., Knutsson H.: Chondrosarcoma of soft tissue origin. Cancer 32:507–513, 1973
5. Angervall L., Enzinger F. M.: Extraskeletal neoplasm resembling Ewing's sarcoma. Cancer 36:240–251, 1975
6. Axelrod R., Maidech H. J., Meyers J., Steinberg A.: Primary osteosarcoma of the kidney. Cancer 41:724–727, 1978
7. Belasco J. B., Meadows A. T., Chatten J., et al.: Extraskeletal osteogenic sarcoma after treatment for Wilms' tumor. Cancer 50:1894–1898, 1982
8. Bertoni F., Picci P., Bacchini P., et al.: Mesenchymal chondrosarcoma of bone and soft tissues. Cancer 52:533–541, 1983
9. Capanna R., Bertoni F., Bacchini P., et al.: Malignant fibrous histiocytoma of bone. Cancer 54:177–187, 1984
10. Cunningham M., Arlen M.: Medullary fibrosarcoma of bone. Cancer 21:31–37, 1969
11. Dahlin D. C., Unni K. K., Matsuno T.: Malignant (fibrous) histiocytoma of bone: Fact or fancy? Cancer 39:1508–1516, 1977
12. Das Gupta T. K., Hadju S. I., Foote F. W., Jr.: Extraosseous osteogenic sarcoma. Ann. Surg. 168:1011–1022, 1968
13. Daniels A. C., George H., Strans F. H.: Primary chondrosarcoma of the tracheobronchial tree. Arch. Pathol. 84:615, 1967
14. Ducatman B. S., Scheithauer B. W., Dahlin D. C.: Malignant bone tumors associated with neurofibromatosis. Mayo Clin. Proc. 58:578–582, 1983
15. Dunlop J.: Primary hemangiopericytoma of bone: Report of two cases. J. Bone Joint Surg. 55B:854–857, 1973
16. Enzinger F. M., Shiran M.: Extraskeletal myxoid chondrosarcoma; An analysis of 34 cases. Hum. Pathol. 3:421–435, 1972
17. Evans D. M. D., Sanerkin N. G.: Primary leiomyosarcoma of bone. J. Pathol. Bacteriol. 90:348–350, 1965
18. Fine G., Stout A. P.: Osteogenic sarcoma of the extraskeletal soft tissues. Cancer 9:1027–1043, 1956
19. Goldenberg R. R., Cohen P., Steinlauf P.: Chondrosarcoma of the extraskeletal soft tissues: A report of seven cases and review of the literature. J. Bone Joint Surg. 49A:1487–1507, 1967
20. Hiramoto R., Jurandowski J., Bernecky J., Pressman D.: Immunochemical differentiation of rhabdomyosarcomas. Cancer Res. 21:383–386, 1961
21. Huvos A. G.: Primary malignant fibrous histiocytoma of bone: Clinicopathologic study of 18 patients. N.Y. State J. Med. 76:552–559, 1976
22. Huvos A. G., Rosen G., Dabska M., Marcove R. C.: Mesenchymal chondrosarcoma: A clinicopathologic analysis of 35 patients with emphasis on treatment. Cancer 51:1230–1237, 1983
23. Lee J. H., Griffiths W. J., Bottomley R. H.: Extraosseous osteogenic sarcoma following an intramuscular injection. Cancer 40:3097–3101, 1977
24. McCarthy E. F., Matsuno T., Dorfman H. D.: Malignant fibrous histiocytoma of bone: Study of 35 cases. Hum. Pathol. 10:57–70, 1979
25. Morgan H. D., Salama F. D.: Primary chondrosarcoma of the lung. J. Thorac. Cardiovasc. Surg. 64:465, 1972
26. Pardo-Mindan F. J., Guillen F. J., Villas C., Vazquez J. J.: A comparative ultrastructural study of chondrosarcoma, chordoid chondrosarcoma and chordoma. Cancer 47:2611–2619, 1981
27. Rao V., Cheng A., Dildokar M. S.: Extraosseous osteosarcoma. Cancer 41:1488–1496, 1978
28. Sanerkin N. G.: Primary leiomyosarcoma of the bone and its comparison with fibrosarcoma. Cancer 44:1375–1387, 1979
29. Scott J. E., Dorling J.: Differential staining of acid glycosaminoglycans (mucopolysaccharides) by alcian blue in salt solutions. Histochemie 5:221–233, 1965

30. Shanoff L. B., Spira M., Hardy S. B.: Myositis ossificans, evolution to osteogenic sarcoma: A report of a histologically verified case. Am. J. Surg. 113:537–541, 1967
31. Sordillo P. D., Hajdu S. I., Magill G. B., Golbey R. B.: Extraosseous osteogenic sarcoma: A review of 48 patients. Cancer 51:727–734, 1983
32. Stout A. P., Verner E. W.: Chondrosarcoma of the extraskeletal soft tissues. Cancer 6:581–590, 1953
33. Sun C. C., Kroll M., Miller J. E.: Primary chondrosarcoma of the lung. Cancer 50:1864–1866, 1982
34. Valderama E., Kahn L. B., Wind E.: Extraskeletal osteosarcoma arising in an ectopic hamartomatous thymus. Cancer 51:1132–1137, 1983
35. Von Hochstetter A. R., Eberle H., Ruttner J. R.: Primary leiomyosarcoma of extragnathic bones. Cancer 53:2194–2200, 1984
36. Wang T., Erlandson R. A., Marcove R. C., Huvos A. G.: Primary leiomyosarcoma of bone. Arch. Pathol. Lab. Med. 104:100–104, 1980
37. Wilson H.: Extraskeletal ossifying tumors. Ann. Surg. 113:95, 1941
38. Winslow D. J., Enzinger F. H.: Hyaluronidase sensitive acid mucopolysaccharides in liposarcomas. Am. J. Pathol. 37:497–505, 1960
39. Wurlitzer F., Ayala A., Romsdahl M.: Extraosseous osteogenic sarcoma. Ann. Surg. 168:1011–1022, 1968

CHAPTER

15

Visceral Sarcomas

Because of the structural composition of the intraperitoneal viscera, a number of primary sarcomas can be found that are derived primarily from these organs. Clinically the tumors may appear as intra-abdominal masses and, because of size and position, may be difficult to distinguish from retroperitoneal sarcomas. At times they may mimic primary visceral adenocarcinomas. The gastrointestinal tract is a typical site for such sarcomatous transformation, beginning with benign smooth muscle neoplasms (leiomyoma) seen in the esophagus, stomach, and small bowel, and progressing to the leiomyoblastomas and leiomyosarcomas found throughout the entire gastrointestinal tract. The female genital system is also prone to the development of smooth muscle lesions (leiomyomas and leiomyosarcomas). Angiosarcomas, rhabdomyosarcomas, and mesodermal sarcomas are among the other sarcomatous tumors that arise primarily from visceral structures, but to a lesser extent than the smooth muscle tumors.

PRIMARY SMOOTH MUSCLE TUMORS OF ESOPHAGUS

High in the gastrointestinal tract the esophagus can become involved by the growth of primary smooth muscle lesions described above. Solomon et al.[64] reviewed nine cases of leiomyoma of the esophagus seen between 1960 and 1983. Four of these tumors occurred in men and five in women. The presenting symptoms included dysphagia in five and epigastric distress in three. In eight of the patients, a barium swallow was found to be diagnostic for defining the presence of the lesion. The tumors were also noted on upper endoscopy with the overlying mucosa of the esophagus described as being intact. One patient underwent an ultrasonic probe study of the esophagus during endoscopy, which revealed some of the structural details of the mass. The most common location for these tumors was in the mid-third of the esophagus. The lesions measured from 1 to 7 cm.

Seremetis et al.[59] found that almost one half of 838 patients with proven esophageal leiomyoma had dysphasia; 45% reported pain as the major complaint. Occasionally, the leiomyomas were found to enlarge to the point where manifestations of superior vena cava syndrome became apparent. Esophagrams were found to be helpful; the usual finding was a smooth, rounded filling defect with clearly defined edges. This was noted to be the classic appearance of essentially all of the tumors. In these cases the mucosa has essentially been described as being intact so that biopsies are usually of no value for defining histologic patterns. Other tumors, including cysts, granular cell tumors, duplication of the esophagus, mediastinal tumors, and aortic aneurysms, may mimic the primary esophageal leiomyoma. Takubo et al.[67] reported finding multiple leiomyomas in 7.9% of 342 individuals they studied. Among the rarer benign lesions to be found are the granular cell myoblastomas or Abrikossoff's tumor. Since it was first reported in 1926, fewer than 35 cases have been described.[12] Most pathologists believe that this lesion, which appears most commonly on the tongue and skin, has a neurogenic origin. In the majority of cases the lesion is picked up as an incidental finding. Barium swallow usually reveals a smooth, well-circumscribed, intramural filling defect that is first diagnosed as a leiomyoma, fibrous lipoma, neurofibroma, or duplication cyst.

When surgery is indicated because of symptoms produced by the presence of leiomyoma or any equivalent benign mass, enucleation has been found to be the best procedure, using either the left or right side of the chest, depending on the location of the lesion. When exposed, the esophageal muscle coat is split longitudinally during the procedure and the tumor can usually be enucleated without entering into the lumen of the esophagus. If the mucosa is violated, primary repair is usually performed with two-layer closure.

Among the malignant smooth muscle tumors of gastrointestinal tract origin, leiomyosarcoma is the most frequent tumor type; it appears most often in the mid-portion of the small bowel, stomach, esophagus, and occasionally the colorectal region. In 1965, 36 esophageal cases were reported.[55] Since then approximately 20 other cases have been reported.[23] It is therefore possible to review data on approximately 57 patients, 32 of whom were males and 25 females. The average age of these patients was 59 years (range, 57 to 78 years). Although dysphasia is the most common symptom (84%) with this tumor, it has not been universally present in all of these patients. In 70% of cases the lesion grew as an intraluminal polypoid mass with some preservation of the esophageal wall, allowing food to pass around the lesion. Substernal pain ranging from a vague burning sensation to a sharp crampy discomfort has been reported in 24% of the patients. Regurgitation from early luminal obstruction has been described in 11%; gastrointestinal bleeding is not common because mucosal erosion is a late manifestation of the growing lesion.

On routine chest x-ray films, patterns range from simple mediastinal widening to densely calcified masses. The esophagram usually demonstrates a large intraluminal polypoid filling defect which frequently leads to dilatation of the esophagus around the mass and which may be seen to move with peristalsis during fluoroscopy. Endoscopic biopsy may be unremarkable owing to the submucosal nature of the growing tumor, even in its malignant form. Thirty-nine of 57 tumors (69%) were found to be polypoid and noninvasive.[55] Eighteen of the 57 (31%) were noted to be infiltrating and to have invaded surrounding structures in the mediastinum. Metastatic disease has been relatively uncommon, even when the primary tumor is found to be large. Nine of 57 patients had spread of tumor to the liver, mediastinum, mediastinal nodes, and pericardium. Because these lesions tend to remain well localized, surgical resection is still considered to be the treatment of choice. Ten of 38 who underwent resection for cure survived 5 or more years.

MIXED ESOPHAGEAL TUMORS

Occasionally a lesion of the esophagus has been reported to have both sarcomatous and carcinomatous components. Squamous cell carcinoma and at times adenocarcinoma can be admixed with fibrosarcoma. Carcinomatous elements may also be seen in association with leiomyosarcoma, rhabdomyosarcoma, and chondrosarcoma. The majority of these mixed lesions (80%) tend to be polypoid and may become large. Symptoms due to encroachment on the lumen are dysphagia followed by weakness and weight loss. In 1949 Stout reviewed 19 such cases, with 28 more cases being reported by 1973. On barium swallow the pedunculated polypoid growth that is usually present is seen as an intraluminal filling defect. The infiltrative form produces esophageal constriction. In later stages of disease, infiltration extends into the mediastinum. Hyperalimentation followed by surgery is considered the treatment of choice.

In the stomach while adenocarcinoma is the most frequent tumor seen, noncarcinomatous tumors do occur and comprise approximately 2% of such gastric lesions. Clinically, these tumors can be bulky and may be associated with massive gastrointestinal bleeding. In spite of their usually large size, many of these tumors are resectable with a relatively favorable 5-year survival rate achieved when compared with the adenocarcinomas. The reason for the relative ease of resectability is that even in the presence of exophytic lesions, the tumor mass appears pseudoencapsulated and tends to be loosely adherent to the surrounding structures. We recently were referred a patient with vague gastrointestinal complaints and upper gastrointestinal bleeding in whom endoscopy revealed a lesion consistent with leiomyosarcoma. The classic superficial ulceration was identified, and biopsy was performed through the endoscope. Histologic sections revealed a pattern believed to be consistent

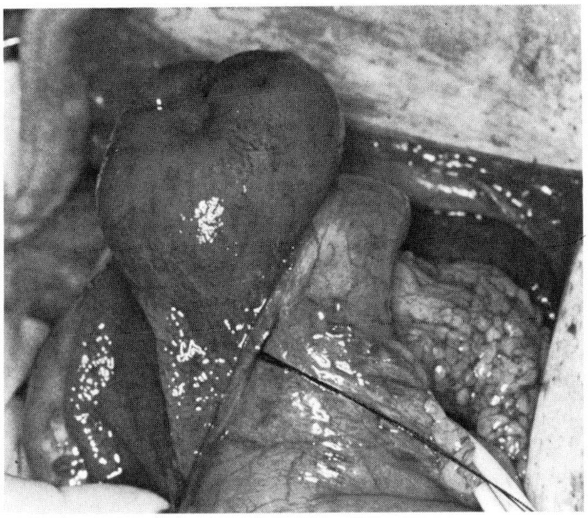

FIGURE 15–1. Polypoid intraluminal leiomyosarcoma of the stomach, visualized through a gastrotomy incision.

with leiomyosarcoma. CT scan did not reveal a clear separation of tumor from the pancreas. At exploration the mass was adherent to the pancreas, having infiltrated it as well as diaphragm. These structures were resected with the stomach. The lesion proved to be malignant histiocytic sarcoma (reticulum cell sarcoma).

GASTRIC LEIOMYOSARCOMA

Leiomyosarcomas arising primarily from the stomach appear to represent 0.1 to 3% of malignant tumors involving the stomach and 25 to 40% of gastric sarcomas. The tumors usually present intraluminally with a growth pattern that causes the lesion to become pedunculated (Fig. 15–1) or they

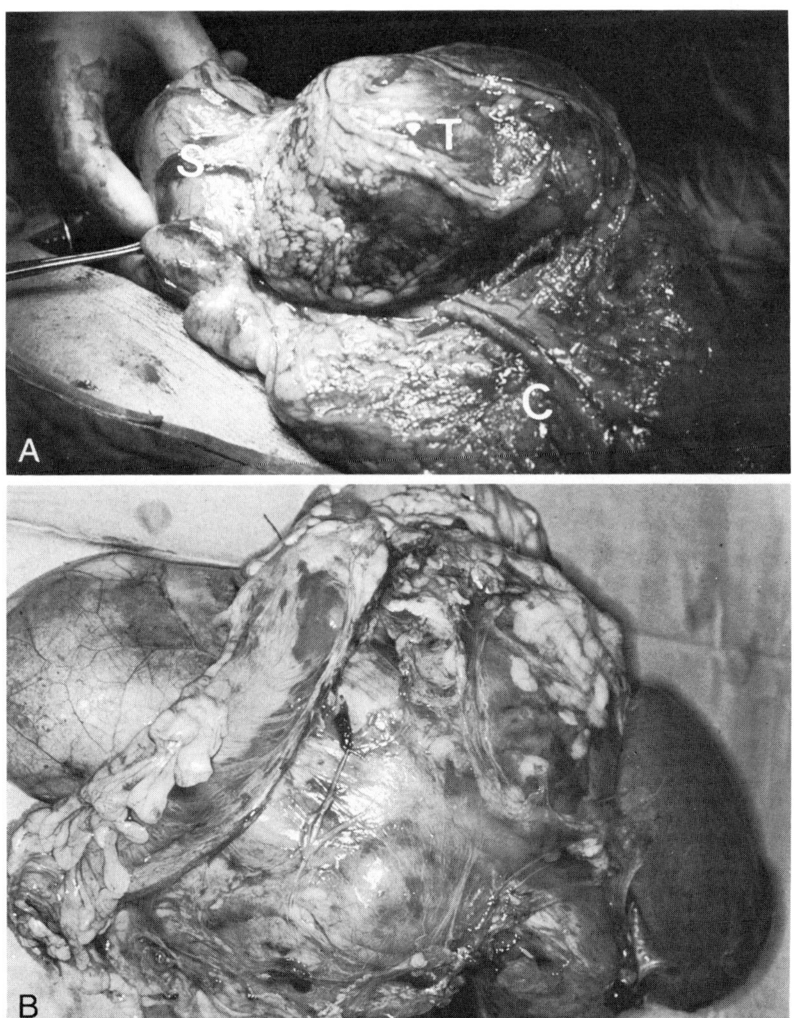

FIGURE 15–2. A, Large exophytic leiomyosarcoma of the stomach at laparotomy. The tumor is growing off the greater curvature of the stomach. B, Resected stomach with bulky leiomyosarcoma of the greater curvature with spleen adherent to the tumor mass.

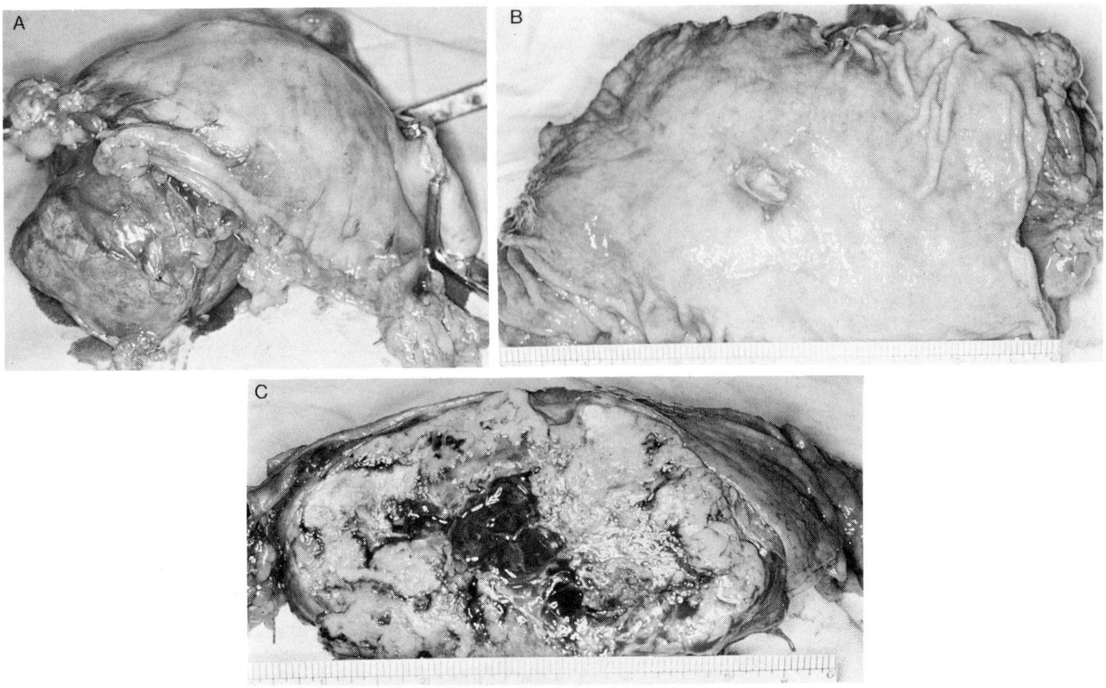

FIGURE 15–3. A, Resected stomach with bulky exophytic retrogastric leiomyosarcoma. B, Opened specimen shows the characteristic ulcer crater of this tumor which leads to bleeding. C, Transected stomach shows the relationship of the ulcer to the underlying lesion. The necrotic tumor that results in the bleeding is seen just under the ulcer crater.

may present extragastrically, intramurally, or both (Fig. 15–2). Any exophytic mass with ulceration or cavitation within the tumor usually proves to be a gastric leiomyosarcoma. Figure 15–3*A* shows a large exophytic retrogastric mass that had caused upper gastrointestinal bleeding. The open specimen shows the origin of the bleeding, an ulcerating mucosal lesion in the center of the tumor mass. A transverse cut through this region demonstrates the nature of the ulcer in relationship to the underlying necrotic tumor (Fig. 15–3*B* and *C*). Pseudodiverticula and fistula formation may be found in association with large tumors. This usually occurs secondary to the expression of necrotic debris into the gastric lumen and the appearance of a central tumor cavity. Barium may pass through the fistula into the central cavity with prolonged retention within the cavity. This phenomenon may occasionally be seen with adenocarcinoma of the stomach growing exophytically off the greater curvature of the stomach or perforating into the lesser sac. Necrosis may at times lead to evacuation of necrotic debris into the lumen of the stomach and the development of a sacular component, which on barium enema shows a cystic air-filled space within the lesser sac. While this is more likely to occur with a leiomyosarcomatous lesion, adenocarcinoma should enter into the differential diagnosis. We have encountered several such cases.

Gastroscopy may be of some value in evaluating the sarcomatous lesion; however, a biopsy showing benign disease does not exclude the presence of malignant tumor in the other foci of the mass. CT scan of the abdomen is a useful tool in defining the position and extent of the tumor that has been detected by other means such as a GI series. Figure 15–4*A* and *B* illustrates a large exophytic gastric mass arising from the greater curvature of the stomach to displace the spleen inferiorly as the tumor mass compresses the splenic hilum. The relationship of the tumor to the spleen is seen at the time the tumor was delivered into the operative field (Fig. 15–4C). Pedunculated intraluminal tumors can cause intermittent pyloric ball valve obstruction and the pylorus may, as a result, intusscept into the duodenum. Benign as well as malignant lesions may be multiple, and a large malignant tumor may be found to be surrounded by small leio-

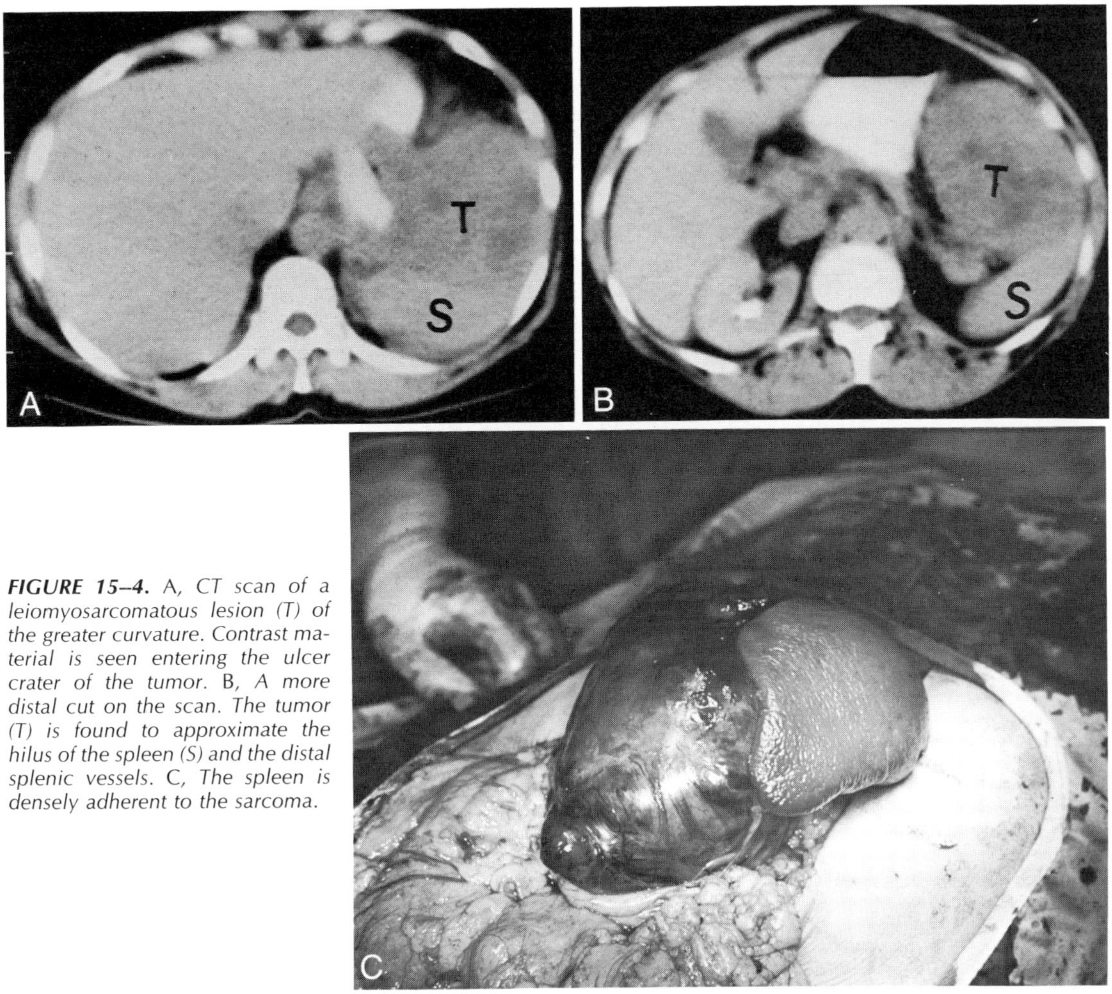

FIGURE 15–4. A, CT scan of a leiomyosarcomatous lesion (T) of the greater curvature. Contrast material is seen entering the ulcer crater of the tumor. B, A more distal cut on the scan. The tumor (T) is found to approximate the hilus of the spleen (S) and the distal splenic vessels. C, The spleen is densely adherent to the sarcoma.

myomas. The presence of calcification in the tumor suggests that it is benign.

Burgess et al.,[8] in reviewing the experience with gastric lesions at the Mayo Clinic between 1940 and 1965, found 270 patients (94 females and 176 males) with noncarcinomatous tumors arising from the stomach: 218 malignant lymphomas and 52 leiomyosarcomas. Fibrosarcoma and angiosarcoma were not noted among any of these patients, though in unusual circumstances they may be found arising from the stomach. For those lesions reported as leiomyosarcomas, 24 were in females and 28 in males. The age of diagnosis varied from 9 to 78 years of age (mean, 54 years). The duration of symptoms for the patients was approximately 10 months. Anorexia appeared in 11 and weight loss in 14 patients. These symptoms are not so common as one would find with lymphomas of the stomach, where anorexia and weight loss are usually the presenting complaints. Among the leiomyosarcoma patients, bleeding is noted to be a characteristic sign. Any epigastric distress that was reported by the patient was usually "slight." Abdominal tenderness was, in the series reviewed, a common complaint, with a palpable epigastric mass seen in 38 patients. Of 50 who had gastric fluid analysis, 35 were found to be achlorhydric. In 40 cases, a barium swallow had been performed. Review of the films showed carcinoma in 20 and benign leiomyoma in 20 of the 52 patients.

The lesions in this study were most frequently confined to the stomach itself, as noted in 37 of the patients in whom partial gastrectomy could be employed as the operative procedure. In 11 patients, a large tumor was found that had extended beyond the limits of the stomach by direct invasion into the surrounding structures. Five patients had metastatic liver disease. Follow-up examination revealed that 20 of the patients were alive and free of recurrent disease. When the tumor was confined to the stomach wall, a 5-year survival of 71% could be achieved. Extension to local nodes or to neighboring organs decreased survival to between 29 and 39%. Survival was also found to be related to the surgical procedure necessary to gain control of the disease process.

The experience in managing smooth muscle tumors of the stomach at Massachusetts General Hospital was reported by Welch.[75] During the years 1964 through 1974 40 patients in the series had gastric leiomyoma and 10 had leiomyosarcoma. In contrast to the mild complaints for most patients with benign lesions, those with malignant tumors had more bothersome side effects. Gastrointestinal bleeding was the most common symptom, with melena and anemia present in more than 50% of those studied. Two patients had abdominal masses, both with extensive liver and bone involvement. Most benign and malignant lesions were found in the fundus of the stomach. Tumor development was uncommon in the regions of the cardia and pylorus. Most of the benign tumors (85%) were less than 2 cm in diameter; the malignant lesions (81%) were greater than 4 cm. Mucosal ulceration was found in 60% of malignant tumors compared with 2.5% of benign lesions. The resectability rate for malignant tumors was 82%. Regional node metastasis appeared in two patients. All survivors had lesions that were well circumscribed or histologically found to be low-grade. The overall survival rate for the gastric sarcomas was 44%, a distinct improvement when compared with the adenocarcinomas.

Leiomyosarcomas usually spread by the hematogenous route. Regional nodes are rarely involved except by direct extension. Metastasis occurs late and is usually present in 12 to 25% of patients at initial exploration. Metastasis occurs most frequently with tumors that are exogastric or situated in the upper portion of the stomach. Spread usually occurs to the liver and peritoneal surfaces. Few mitoses are seen in benign lesions, whereas leiomyosarcomas show more frequent mitoses, nuclear pleomorphism, and local invasion. Differentiation of low-grade malignant disease from benign disease may be difficult to define even histologically. Only 25 to 30% of malignant smooth muscle tumors metastasize, and cases of benign-appearing lesions with liver metastasis have also been recorded.

Benign tumors are usually excised by wedge resection. In the malignant lesion, extension beyond the palpable margin can be expected and partial gastrectomy is required. When the lesion is exophytic it frequently infiltrates the lesser sac into the transverse mesocolon or pancreatic surface. In the former situation, en-bloc removal of involved colon is required. Should dissection off the surface of the pancreas be required, then the right colon and hepatic flexure should be mobilized and the entire duodenum dissected along its lateral margin (kocherization) to where superior mesenteric vessels are defined and protected prior to tumor dissection. At the Massachusetts General Hospital, 57% of patients being treated for gastric leiomyosarcoma have survived for 5 years.

Sarcomas of the stomach are almost always primary and rarely ever represent metastatic disease to the stomach.[57] Lesions other then leiomyosarcoma, such as schwannoma, angiosarcoma, liposarcoma, and chondrosarcoma, have been recorded. At Memorial Hospital, among the 1762 gastric tumors that were evaluated to define such tumors, 24 (13%) were described as leiomyosarcoma.[7] The commonest symptom in this series, as in other studies, was bleeding, followed by pain. The diagnosis was made radiologically in roughly 50% of the cases of intramural lesions. These tumors tended to be round and sharply demarcated and showed deep ulcers extending to the gastric luminal surface that were the source of bleeding. If the lesion was larger than 5 cm, it was more likely to be a leiomyosarcoma. The majority of the tumors were intramural but could also be found to be exophytic. When these tumors reach a size of 3 to 4 cm, ulcerations are usually seen. Wide resection is the indicated procedure, with en-bloc resection of surrounding organs required when the exophytic lesion has compressed the surrounding tissue. Total or even radical subtotal gastrectomy is not usually needed. The well-differentiated sarcomas may be difficult to distinguish from the benign leiomyoma and only when capsular or vascular invasion is seen can one suspect the true nature of the tumor. The finding of any anaplastic changes in small lesions suggests a relatively poor prognosis in contrast to a high degree of differentiation in larger tumors. Among the 52 patients reported by Burgess in 1971, 37 had tumors that were confined to the stomach. The accrued 5-year survival rate was 50% and the 10-year survival rate was 45%. When resection was performed, survival was 62% at 5 years and 45% at 10 years.

Shiu et al.[60] updated the Memorial statistics (1949 to 1973) and found that sarcomas represented approximately 1% of the primary malignant tumors of the stomach in that institution. Leiomyoblastoma also occurred in a number of patients included in this series. This lesion was first described by Martin et al. in 1960.[40] Malignant leiomyoblastomas arising in the stomach have been reported in other series[2, 37] and are characterized by a lobular arrangement of aggregates of a round polygonal or epithelioid cell pattern with larger perinuclear clear spaces due to extensive cytoplasmic vacuolization.

Among the 58 patients seen at Memorial Hospital with either gastric leiomyosarcoma or malignant leiomyoblastoma, 41 patients (17 males and 24 females) were suitable for study and were classified as having either high- or low-grade tumors. The age of the patients ranged from 27 to 89 years (median, 55 years). Sex and age had no distinct influence on survival. An abdominal mass and feeling of fullness were noted in 18 and, as with other series, was the most common complaint. Hematemesis, melena, or severe anemia was seen in 13. On x-ray examination, gross distortion of the shape and position of the stomach as well as pattern of gastric peristalsis resulted from the massive size of many of the lesions that were exogastric and produced marked compression on the body of the stomach. In others, a lesion with central ulceration was defined as part of the endogastric and intramural tumors. In 13 patients, the lesions presented in the cardiac region. In 12, tumors were found in the mid-portion of the stomach and in 4 in the distal one third. Seven of the tumors were intramural, 9 endogastric, and 22 exogastric. Three of the cases were not defined. Three of the exogastric tumors were pedunculated, while the majority were sessile. A disproportionately large number of exogastric tumors were massive and of high-grade malignancy. Mucosal ulcerations measuring from 0.2 cm to greater than 5 cm were present in more than half of the resected specimens. Direct invasion of adjacent organs occurred in 14. The liver was involved in five, the diaphragm in three, pancreas in four, and the colon in five of the patients. All died of their disease. Twenty-four of the tumors were classified as leiomyosarcomas and 17 as malignant leiomyoblastomas. Low-grade leiomyosarcomas showed abundant stroma with orderly interlacing fascicles of tumor cells. The cells had elongated nuclei with rounded ends and no distinct nucleoli. Cytoplasm was conspicuously eosinophilic. Mitotic figures ranged from one to nine per high-powered field. High-grade tumors had an irregular arrangement of fascicles of neoplastic cells, marked pleomorphism, and mitotic counts of greater than ten per high-power field.

Adjusted survival rates for 41 in the group were 56% at 5 years and 43% at 10 years, with no significant differences seen between leiomyosarcoma and leiomyoblastoma. Three patients died of disease at 12, 13½, and 19 years after resection; two of these patients had high-grade leiomysarcomas and one a low-grade malignant leiomyoblastoma. Eighty-one percent of the patients with low-grade tumors survived 5 or more years versus 32% with high-grade neoplasms. All of nine patients with small tumors (less than 5 cm) survived 5 years. Among the 41 patients, 32 underwent surgical resection for cure. Radiation therapy was used in six patients, with a partial response noted in two. No chemotherapeutic responses were seen.

Recurrence following surgical resection was noted anywhere from 3 months to 19 years (median, 24 months). The liver was the most common site for the appearance of metastatic tumor. Multiple peritoneal nodules were also common sites for recurrence, causing intractable ascites and intestinal obstruction. Metastasis to lymph nodes was found in three patients. Eleven of 27% developed additional (secondary) malignancies involving the breast and colon.

LEIOMYOBLASTOMA

Cornog[16] reported ten cases of gastric leiomyoblastoma, four of which were followed for periods longer than 5 years. It was believed that leiomyoblastoma could be evaluated reasonably for benign or malignant behavior by routine pathologic criteria that could be applied to smooth muscle tumors. This was especially true when using criteria such as growth rate, size, and frequency of mitosis. Because of the difficulty of prognosticating the behavior pattern for many of these tumors, however, the leiomyoblastomas (those suspected of being low-grade malignancies) have usually been treated by partial gastric resection rather than by simple enucleation. Electron-microscopic studies of leiomyoblastoma have demonstrated that the vacuolization described is not an adequate criterion for characterizing such a tumor and that similar artifacts can occasionally appear in leiomyomas and leiomyosarcomas.

Experimental models for gastric leiomyosarcoma have been reported. Cohen et al.,[15] in studying the effects of *N*-methyl-*N'*-nitro-*N*-nitrosoguanidine (MNNG) in the Buffalo rat, found that adenocarcinoma developed when the drug was employed singly, but that the large number of gastric leiomyosarcomas appeared with the combination of stress, aspirin, or sodium taurocholate.

GASTRIC CARCINOSARCOMAS

As we have seen, in rare instances, carcinosarcoma may involve the esophagus. It may also occasionally occur within the stomach.[68] Bansal et al.[6] described such a lesion in a 71-year-old patient with distinct adenocarcinomatous features associated with spindle cell components. The sarcomatous nature of the spindle cell lesion was confirmed by ultrastructural studies. These tumors are found more frequently in the uterus, ovary, breast, thyroid, esophagus, stomach, larynx, lung, and urinary tract, in descending order of frequency. Kitamura[33] divided the gastric carcinosarcomas into three types according to their gross presentation: (1) predominantly intramural infiltration, (2) extension of tumor beyond the serosa, and (3) predominantly intramural mass with cauliflower-like projections and/or a crater shape. Histologically the tumor itself has been categorized into three types: type 1—collision, in which there is a sharp interface between distinct histologic patterns with no or minimal mixing; type 2—combination, in which the two components mix completely without maintaining discrete stromal components; and type 3—composition, in which the two components mix but maintain recognizable stromal differentiating features. Metastasis may show either a carcinomatous or a sarcomatous pattern, or both. In general, it has been stated that metastases from carcinosarcoma occur later than those from carcinoma and are especially rare in collision tumors.

Carcinosarcomas have been reported in association with other lesions. Bansal et al.[6] described a case of carcinosarcoma of the stomach in association with a separate and distinct carcinoid tumor. Electron microscopy of the carcinoid region showed typical neurosecretory granules, and the lymph nodes contained only metastatic carcinoid tumor. This is consistent with the knowledge that carcinosarcoma is associated with a low incidence of metastasis but with a high rate of mortality. Additional soft tissue lesions may arise from the stomach. Burns et al.[9] described a primary melanocytic schwannoma arising in the stomach of a 51-year-old woman. She had been explored for a polypoid antral lesion which, on resection, extended through the muscularis propria of the gastric antrum to form a raised 5-cm mass. The overlying gastric mucosa was intact. After a Billroth I anastomosis the patient made an uneventful recovery. The lesion occurred in the absence of neurofibromatosis. Melanin pigmentation in nerve sheath tumors has usually been explained on the basis of phagocytosis of pigment by the tumor cells. More recently, evidence has emerged to suggest that neoplastic Schwann cells may function as "facultative melanocytes," a view first suggested by Masson. This melanogenic potential presumably reflects the common derivation of nerve sheath elements and melanocytes from the embryonic neural crest.

Tumors of neurogenic origin have also been reported to arise in the duodenum. Kheir and Halpern[32] described a case of duodenal paraganglioma in a patient with von Recklinghausen's disease. To date, 26 cases of duodenal paragangliomas have been reported, as well as related neurogenic tumors.[27, 38] The important features in identifying these paragangliomas histologically are the Zellballen pattern, best illustrated by reticulin stains; cytoplasmic argyrophilic granules shown by modified Pascual's argyrophil method; and ultrastructural evidence of dense-core membrane-bound neurosecretory granules. This tumor essentially occurs only in the duodenum, usually in the second portion. Epigastric pain and gastrointestinal bleeding are the predominant complaints. A gradation in histology from typical ganglioneuromas to pure paraganglioma has been reported. Recent findings suggest that such tumors may arise from multipotent cells that normally reside in the mucosal crypts, perhaps expressing the same cell line as that which gives origin to carcinoids of the foregut.

SMALL BOWEL SARCOMAS

As previously noted, leiomyosarcomas are found throughout the gastrointestinal tract and occasionally may be encountered within the small intestine.[29, 48, 56, 73, 74] When found, they comprise less than 20% of all malignant primary tumors of small bowel.[76] The tumors can arise from the smooth muscle of the wall of the bowel, the vascular smooth muscle, and the muscularis mucosa or propria. In general, these tumors are found to be extremely vascular. Because the bulk of the lesion is directed away from the lumen, it tends to become exophytic and produces symptoms late in the clinical course of disease. At this time mucosal invasion occurs and results in upper gastrointestinal bleeding. The benign smooth muscle variant, the leiomyoma, is a more common tumor, with 80% occurring equally in the jejunum and ileum and the remaining 20% in the duodenum. A small percentage of these tumors arise from the muscularis mucosa and tend to grow toward the lumen. More often this lesion has its origin in the subserosa and tends to grow away from the lumen. Various growth patterns take place as malignant degeneration occurs. Both benign and malignant variants are nonencapsulated. Rarely, benign lesions have been found to spread while malignant ones may remain confined to the site of origin. Wald[73] has described five patterns for malignant lesions: (1) exocentric, an exophytic subserosal lesion; (2) exocentric ulcerated; (3) exocentric with cavitation and/or fistula formation; (4) endocentric (submucosal) invaginating into the lumen; and (5) dumbbell, exocentric and endocentric. These tumors along with the rare fibrosarcomas and malignant schwannomas frequently metastasize to the liver. Seeding to lung, bone, and peritoneum is also possible.[49] One of the major complications possible is that when sarcomas, particularly leiomyosarcomas, metastasize to the liver, their highly vascular nature may account for part of the clinical symptomatology. It is not unheard of for a patient with metastatic disease to present with signs of hypovolemic shock secondary to extensive hemorrhage from spontaneous rupture of a metastatic tumor. In such an instance, angiographic demonstration followed by vascular catheter thrombosis can be useful; at times, surgical intervention may be necessary to stabilize the patient's clinical status. Figure 15–5*A* illustrates a metastatic small bowel leiomyosarcoma to the edge of the liver being prepared for resection. In the same patient, there is similar metastasis to the peritoneal surface of the urinary bladder (Fig. 15–5*B*). Both lesions were resected and the patient was placed on chemotherapy. Once dissemination occurs, surgical intervention is usually palliative. Kohno et al.[34] reported a case of intestinal leiomyosarcoma with metastases to the liver, peritoneum, and omentum which was successfully treated with four operations. The initial operation was performed for a primary intestinal leiomyosarcoma and intraperitoneal seeding. Three months later "shelling out" of a liver metastasis was carried out. This was followed by intra-arterial mitomycin C followed by reexploration and further liver tumor resection. Two years later a recurrent tumor was removed from the terminal ileum. The patient remains free of disease 10 years after the initial liver resection.

As these sarcomas grow, they may become sizable, accounting for the fact that among malignant tumors of small bowel, only 29% of the carcinomas may be palpable in contrast to 65% of the sarcomas which can be clinically identifiable on physical examination. At surgery 76% of lesions are found to be greater than 5 cm. In addition to hepatic spread, which is one of the common ways for dissemination, local infiltration, peritoneal implants, and invasion of adjacent nodes may occur.

Chiotasso[14] reviewed the experience with small bowel tumors at The Cleveland Clinic between 1950 and 1980; he classified the tumors as stage A, when they were confined to tissue of the intestinal wall; stage B, when they involved the peri-intestinal tissues; or stage C, when there was metastasis to lymph nodes, just as in the Duke's classification. Among the 176 primary malignant tumors seen at The Cleveland Clinic, 28 were leiomyosarcomas. During that same period, 12 benign leiomyomas of small intestine were

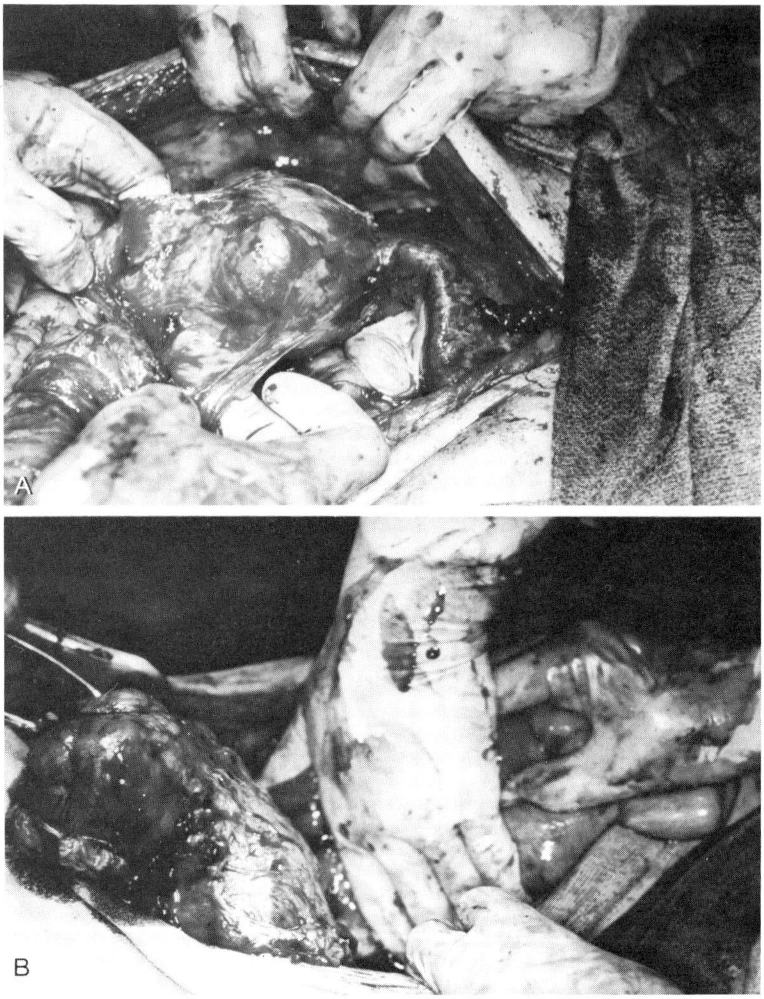

FIGURE 15–5. A, Exposed undersurface of the liver with metastatic leiomyosarcoma of the small bowel being prepared for resection. B, Leiomyosarcoma metastatic to the peritoneal surface of the urinary bladder.

found. The mean age of the patients was 53 years (range, 20 to 73 years). All of the patients in the series were symptomatic, with complaints ranging from approximately 23 months to 8.5 years. Thirteen patients presented with bleeding. The commonest sign was abdominal pain (in 20), followed by abdominal mass (10), obstruction (6), perforation (2), weakness (6), and weight loss (4). Of 14 patients who underwent a small bowel series, only four were positive. Arteriograms were employed in nine instances, with seven reported as positive. All patients underwent surgery; in 22 curative resection was attempted. Four tumors were considered to be stage A, 15 stage B, and 8 stage C. Five of those with stage C disease presented with distant visceral metastasis. Fifteen tumors occurred in the ileum; eight were in the jejunum, four in the duodenum, and one in Meckel's diverticulum. The average greatest diameter for any of the resected tumors was 7.7 cm (range, 2 to 30 cm). Four patients presented with an associated second malignancy, as has been noted with gastric leiomyosarcoma. There was no history of multicentricity with this particular tumor. Eight patients survived for 5 years; 13 died of metastatic leiomyosarcoma. Six patients were free of disease at 10 years.

Leiomyosarcoma of bowel is predominantly a disease of males and is commonly found during the fifth and sixth decades, but it may occasionally be seen in the young patient.[26] Seven patients have been described as having developed this disease in the second or third decades of life. One of the difficulties in defining this particular tumor is that the lesion may frequently grow outside the lumen of the small intestine without any significant mucosal changes, thus negating the value of small bowel series. Arteriograms seem to be more reliable in establishing the diagnosis. Leiomyosarcoma of the intestine appears hypervascularized and can frequently show up in an arterial blush. When seen in the liver this hypervascular pattern can be associated with spontaneous rupture and massive blood loss. Curative surgical treatment has resulted in a better prognosis than have palliative surgical procedures. It is a well-known fact that the larger such a tumor is at the time of resection, the worse the prognosis. This usually occurs in tumors with a diameter larger than 9 cm. In general, when symptoms last less than one year, when there is no metastasis, and when the tumor diameter is less than 9 cm, the best prognosis is achieved with proper therapy.

LEIOMYOSARCOMA OF THE LARGE BOWEL

Leiomyosarcoma can present in the distal colon and rectum.[3, 41] Nodal involvement is rare, but the colon should still be handled by left or right hemicolectomy as if one were approaching an adenocarcinoma of the large bowel. Figure 15–6*A* shows a segment of colon being mobilized from the pelvis with an umbilicated lesion representing partial intussusception of a polypoid leiomyosarcoma. The resected specimen is seen in Figure 15–6*B* and the opened, transected specimen in Figure 15–6*C*. It is apparent that the cut surface of the lesion is sarcomatous in nature and not characteristic of a mucin-producing adenocarcinoma of bowel. As with small bowel lesions, these tumors may arise in the muscularis mucosa, the circular and longitudinal muscle layers, and the walls of the blood vessels. Approximately 50% of the smooth muscle tumors of the rectum are malignant.[54] These tumors spread mainly via the bloodstream; the liver and lungs are most frequently involved, but metastases to brain, bones, and adjacent pelvic organs are possible. Because the distal

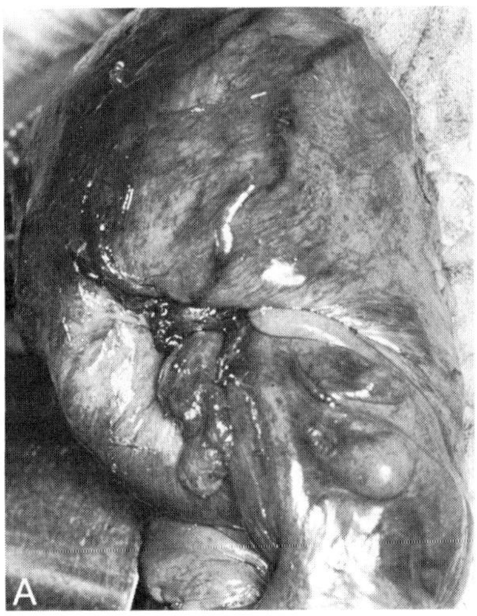

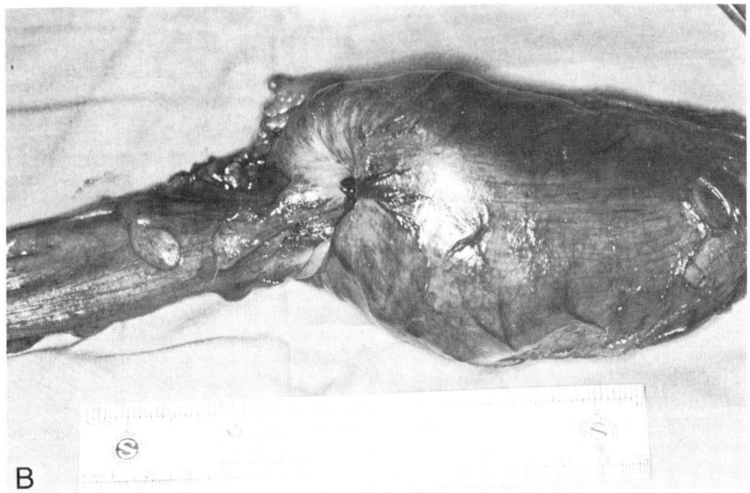

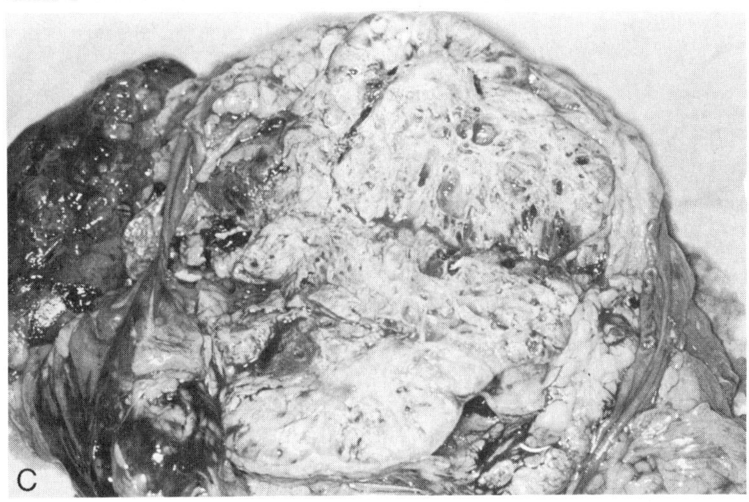

FIGURE 15–6. *A, Mobilization of the distal sigmoid with umbilicated leiomyosarcoma of the bowel. B, Resected leiomyosarcoma of the distal colon showing partial intussusception of the tumor mass. C, Transected specimen of leiomyosarcoma of the colon.*

colon and rectal lesions tend to obstruct the lumen of the bowel, crampy abdominal pain is common, as are melena and frank blood in the stools. Diagnosis is frequently made only after resection. There is the general impression that the rectal lesions do worse than those found in the colon.

Leiomyomatous lesions of the colon, when seen in childhood, can present with different symptoms than those in adults; there is a prolonged febrile response, anemia, and thrombocytosis. Witt et al.[77] described such a situation, where the tumor appeared primarily in omentum or gastrointestinal tract. In children, 85% of the colon lesions presented with gastrointestinal bleeding and/or anemia. A 21-month-old child was seen with fever, anemia, and thrombocytosis. Sonography of the abdomen revealed a 5-cm, solid, rounded mass just inferior to the liver. At surgery, a lobulated lesion was found arising from the wall of the right side of the transverse colon. The specimen measured 9 by 6 by 6 cm and weighed 98 gm. It originated from the muscularis of the colon and was considered to be a leiomyoma. Ultrastructural findings confirmed a well-differentiated leiomyoma which, on resection, resulted in resolution of all symptoms. Posen et al.[52] reported a case of leiomyosarcoma of the sigmoid in a 7-week-old infant presenting with signs of intestinal obstruction followed by colonic perforation and peritonitis. Such findings are typical of the few cases of this sarcoma that have been reported in childhood.

VASCULAR LESIONS OF SMALL BOWEL AND MESENTERY

Primary vascular lesions of the small bowel, such as angiosarcoma of the terminal ileum, have been described. Chen et al.[13] reported a case of a 66-year-old woman in whom the tumor developed 8 years after postoperative radiation for ovarian carcinoma. This case appeared to be the sixth in the literature of angiosarcoma arising at the site of therapeutic irradiation. While we have not seen angiosarcoma as a discrete entity of bowel, one of us (Arlen) was involved in the management of a patient who presented with diverticular disease and suddenly developed an acute abdomen, which was believed clinically to represent perforation of the disease process. At the time of exploratory laparotomy, massive blood loss was noted to be present in the free peritoneal cavity. The patient had rapidly lost blood volume and was in a state of hypotensive shock. Exploration of the abdomen showed a fragmented portion of the mesentery of mid-jejunum, with blood pouring from exposed vessels adjacent to the mesenteric edge of the bowel. This area was entirely resected. The lesion proved not to be a traumatic or inflammatory tear. Rather, Kaposi's sarcoma of the bowel invaded the mesentery and spontaneously ruptured. At the time of surgery, the patient was carefully checked for other sites of Kaposi's sarcoma. There appeared to be no other foci. In the abdomen all sites of visceral disease appeared to have been entirely resected at the time of surgery. Angiosarcomas have been known to involve visceral sites other than bowel. We had originally examined a patient with a pelvic mass adjacent to the bladder and uterus which was explored by one of our hospital's gynecologists. Biopsy had caused an almost fatal hemorrhage. Pelvic angiography suggested that a vascular lesion was present in the lower wall of the bladder adjacent to the vagina. Exploration revealed that this tumor was angiosarcoma, probably of bladder or vaginal origin. The tumor was treated primarily by hypogastric artery ligation and resection, leaving residual disease on the obturator membrane. This was followed by cryosurgery to the obturator region; the freezing was allowed to extend onto the iliac artery. This patient has remained clinically free of disease for more than 10 years following the single application of cryosurgery.

Mesenteric soft part tumors have been encountered at laparotomy. They are usually of smooth muscle or hemangioendothelial origin. The hemangioendotheliomas are vascular lesions arising in a multitude of anatomic sites and with varying potential for local invasiveness and metastatic spread. The abdomen of a 7-month-old female infant was found to enlarge for 2 months. At laparotomy a large lobulated vascular mass was noted to involve the base of the mesentery and surround the superior mesenteric artery. Biopsies were taken. Histologic sections showed a complex arrangement of vascular spaces with marked cellularity. Lining cells showed occasional mitosis and atypia without malignant characteristics. Hemangioendothelioma was diagnosed. Laboratory data revealed a mild anemia and severe thrombocytopenia (5000 per mm^3), for which platelets were transfused prior to surgery. Over a 40-day period, a dose of 1775 R was delivered to the tumor. A 20-day course of prednisone was started after 30 days of radiation. Five months after presentation the tumor was only questionably palpable. On repeat aortography and selective superior mesenteric arteriography the appearance was normal and the previously noted arterial displacement and encasement had resolved. The platelet count subsequently returned to normal. While hemangioendotheliomas frequently behave as benignly as hemangiomas, they may at times act in an unpredictable fashion, requiring a more guarded prognosis.

Shim[60] reviewed 74 children with vascular tumors that were associated with thrombocytopenia. Ten were hemangioendotheliomas. None of this group of 10 had any evidence of bony involvement. When multiple lesions involve the liver, the prognosis is considered grave.

When splenectomy has been offered for associated thrombocytopenia, it has proved to be ineffective and dangerous. A beneficial effect of steroids in hemangiomatous lesions with and without thrombocytopenia is well established. Complete surgical resection of the tumor is the obvious choice where feasible. Radiation therapy has been effective in selected cases and was chosen in this case because of the inoperability and local aggressiveness of the tumor.

SARCOMAS OF THE BILIARY TREE

Sarcomas may at times arise in uncommon locations within the gastrointestinal tract, such as the biliary tree. The first description of primary sarcoma of the gallbladder was by Sandsteiner in 1904. As of 1971, 93 cases were reported, with several more appearing in the literature since then.[11] The lesion is seen more often in females, and symptoms include acute cholecystitis and an upper abdominal mass. Jaundice and ascites are frequently present. Extended right hepatic resection with lymph node dissection and skeletonization of the biliary tree has been proposed, but in most instances the lesion is advanced and nonresectable at the time of identification. The biliary tree can be subject to malignant sarcomatous degeneration, especially portions of smooth muscle that may be present. Since there is a cavity in which the tumor may proliferate, the occasional rhabdomyosarcoma that arises may attain the grape-like pattern seen in the vagina and paranasal sinuses, the so-called sarcoma botryoides. This lesion, which is reported primarily in infants and children, involves other sites such as the bladder, orbit, middle ear, and nasopharynx. Stout has stated that these neoplasms may assume a rhabdomyosarcomatous, myxomatous, or mixed mesodermal form. Two cases involving the biliary duct have been reported: one each in a 5- and a 6-year-old child.[21] Early clinical symptoms were similar to those seen in infectious hepatitis. The tumor is locally invasive and rapidly infiltrates surrounding structures. Metastasis occurs infrequently. Sarcoma botryoides should be diagnosed in the presence of any polypoid lesion of the biliary tree where the subepithelial or cambium layer of the polyp contains neoplastic cells and a myxomatous stroma.

PELVIC RHABDOMYOSARCOMA

Rhabdomyosarcoma is essentially a ubiquitous tumor and in the pelvis arises in such structures as the prostate, bladder, and vagina. In young children a mass growing from these structures is embryonal rhabdomyosarcoma until proven otherwise. Mostofi and Morse[42] reported 10 cases of polypoid rhabdomyosarcoma (botryoides) in the bladder of infants. These tumors caused death by local infiltration rather than distant metastasis. Marshall[39] presented a case of a 7-month-old girl who was noted to have an ecchymotic, edematous mass at the urinary meatus. The lesion had been resected 4 months before, at which time embryonal rhabdomyosarcoma had been diagnosed. Total pelvic exenteration was performed. Whether this extensive procedure is still necessary in the presence of the newer radiation-chemotherapy protocols must be evaluated on an individual basis. Other sarcomas that have been encountered are the leiomyosarcomas[36] and the benign neural tumors,[70] which require modified resections short of cystectomy and depending on the extent to which they involve the bladder.

OVARIAN SARCOMA

Ovarian sarcomas are becoming more frequently recognized;[30] 43 cases were evaluated by Azoury and Woodruff in 1971.[4] Mixed mesodermal sarcomas have been reviewed by Carlson et al.[10] and Orchard.[47] Twenty patients with mixed mesodermal tumors treated at M.D. Anderson Hospital had postoperative therapy that included radiation therapy and combination chemotherapy with vincristine, dactinomycin, and cyclophosphamide (VAC); compared with previous reports, the combination postoperative therapy appears to give more satisfactory results. Carcinosarcomas as a separate group have been evaluated by Fenn et al.[22] Pratt and Scully[53] described the clinical features of 17 cases of obviously malignant as well as cellular fibromatous tumors of primary ovarian origin. The fibromas, which account for approximately 4% of ovarian neoplasms, are considered to originate from specialized ovarian stromal cells, as evidenced by the almost imperceptible merging of their morphologic features with those of the sarcomas. The active tumors fell into two categories distinguishable mainly by their degree of mitotic activity similar to other fibrous and smooth muscle tumors. A form that behaved benignly was defined by the presence of one to three mitotic figures per high-power field and designated as cellular fibroma; the more aggressive lesion had four or more mitotic figures and was considered to be fibrosarcoma. Because of the typically benign behavior of the cellular fibromas, salpingo-oophorectomy with preservation of the uterus can be considered in the younger patient. Patients with ruptured tumors should be followed carefully because of the possibility of intra-abdominal recurrence. The fully malignant fibrosarcomas are more aggressive and tend to metastasize within the pelvis and to liver. Their typically rapid course suggests that adjuvant chemotherapy should be considered after hysterectomy. Radiation therapy may be of additional value if local disease remains postoperatively.

The development of sarcomatous lesions in the uterus is well known. Eight cases of angiosarcoma of the uterus and two of ovary have been reported.[46] A 70-year-old woman was examined 25 years after menopause; she presented with a 12-lb weight loss and enlargement of the uterus. No adnexal masses were noted. At the time of laparotomy the uterus was large and distorted by a solid-appearing 12-cm mass arising from the corpus. A total hysterectomy was performed, and the pathology report stated the diagnosis as angiosarcoma of the uterus. Five months later she was readmitted for recurrence of disease confined to the pelvis; radiation therapy was employed. In another case, a 77-year-old woman presented with weight loss and a right adenexal mass. At laparotomy a large cystic mass was noted on the right side with adhesions to the cecum. Mucinous cystadenoma with angiosarcoma of the right ovary was diagnosed. Regional and distant metastases with ascites were defined. The patient died of peritonitis postoperatively.

UTERINE SARCOMAS

In terms of the frequent malignant tumors involving uterus, sarcomas can be found to be among the more aggressive ones encountered. They have a poorer prognosis than the adenocarcinomas. Roughly they comprise 4% of the uterine tumors and have been classified as follows:

1. Pure sarcomas
   a. Pure homologous
      1) Leiomyosarcoma
      2) Endometrial stromal sarcoma
      3) Fibrosarcoma
   b. Pure heterologous
      1) Rhabdomyosarcoma
      2) Osteosarcoma
2. Mixed sarcomas
   a. Mixed homologous
   b. Mixed heterologous

The homologous tumors contain only those cellular elements normally found in the uterus, whereas the heterologous lesions are composed of elements foreign to the normal uterus. In a review of these lesions 68% were found to be leiomyosarcomas and 32% mesenchymal endometrial sarcomas of the homologous, heterologous, and mixed varieties.[31, 44, 45, 58] At present the clinical data appearing in the literature suggest that leiomyosarcomas represent 40% of the uterine sarcomatous lesions, mixed mesodermal tumors an additional 40%, and endometrial stromal sarcomas 10%. The leiomyosarcomas are believed to represent a process of malignant degeneration taking place in previously benign leiomyomas. As with many spindle cell neoplasms, the point of transition may be difficult to judge, with over-interpretation or under-interpretation on histologic grounds. Unfortunately there are rare instances where benign neoplasms can enter the vascular system; those cells that escape can be implanted in organs such as lung, necessitating the use of terms such as benign metastasizing leiomyoma of the uterus.[66] Obviously the histologic picture of such metastatic tumors would be consistent with the benign primaries from which they arise. In a series of 28 uterine tumors classified as malignant leiomyosarcomas, 13 were downgraded to cellular myomas based on low mitotic index (less than three mitoses per high-power field), lack of nuclear atypia, and a uniformly benign course.

A variant of the smooth muscle tumors found in the uterus is the lesion known as intravenous leiomyomatosis. The tumor presents as nodular masses growing within veins. These intravascular growths take the form of worm-like projections extending variable distances into the uterine and hypogastric veins with direct extension occurring as far as the inferior vena cava. In a study of this disorder by Norris and Parmley,[43] who reviewed data from the AFIP, growths were found to extend beyond the uterus in 10 of 14 cases. The origin of these tumors appears two-fold in that they may arise from the wall of veins within the myometrium or result from extensive vascular invasion from a leiomyoma. A variety of other tumors may be confused with intravenous leiomyomatosis and include endometrial stromal sarcoma, leiomyosarcoma, and leiomyomatosis peritonealis disseminata.[50] The stromal sarcomas demonstrate infiltration of the myometrium as well as extension into veins and lymphatics. Leiomyosarcoma differs not only in the presence of atypical cells but by the presence of increased mitotic figures (Fig. 15–7). In leiomyomatosis peritonealis, multiple superficial sites on the peritoneum are involved by nodular implants, and intramural and intravascular growths are absent.

Leiomyosarcoma tends to occur at a somewhat earlier age than other uterine sarcomas, with an average of 50 compared with 60 years for the other neoplasms. Abnormal uterine bleeding is the primary complaint. The diagnosis is frequently established at dilatation and curettage. At other times rapid enlargement of a known myomatous mass may signify malignant transformation in a benign leiomyoma.[1, 62, 69, 71, 72] The presence of a polypoid endocervical mass associated with pain and bleeding typifies endometrial stromal sarcoma.

De Saia[18] found that among 28 patients with endometrial stromal sarcoma, 35% had pelvic node metastasis. In all cases the uterine tumor had invaded to the middle or outer third of the myometrium. For all histologic types, as holds true for most malignant sarcomas, the extent of disease is one of the most significant parameters for predicting outcome. Mitotic index may offer some help; those lesions with more than 10 mitoses per high-power field have a relatively poor prognosis, whereas those with fewer than five per high-power field generally have a better clinical course.

Among 80 cases reviewed by Salazar,[58] four major histologic variants were reviewed. The most common type was the mixed mesodermal sarcoma (44 cases), followed by leiomyosarcoma (20), endometrial stromal sarcoma (6), and a miscellaneous group of other sarcomas (3). The tumors

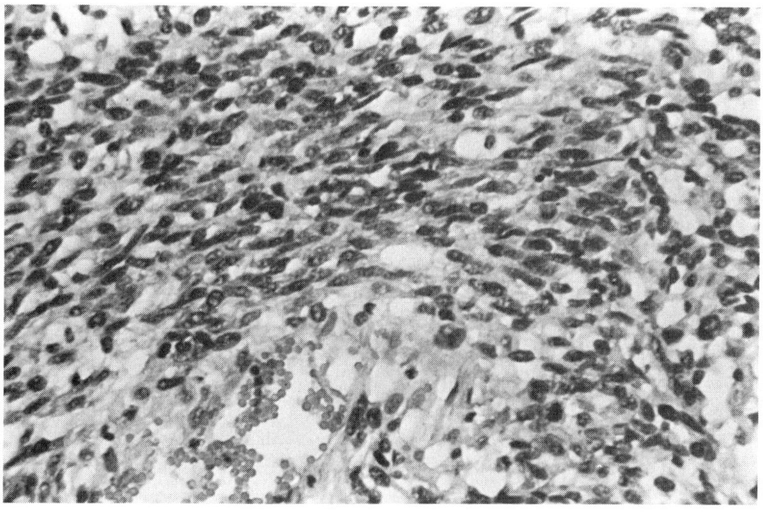

FIGURE 15–7. Microscopic appearance of leiomyosarcoma of the uterus (× 300).

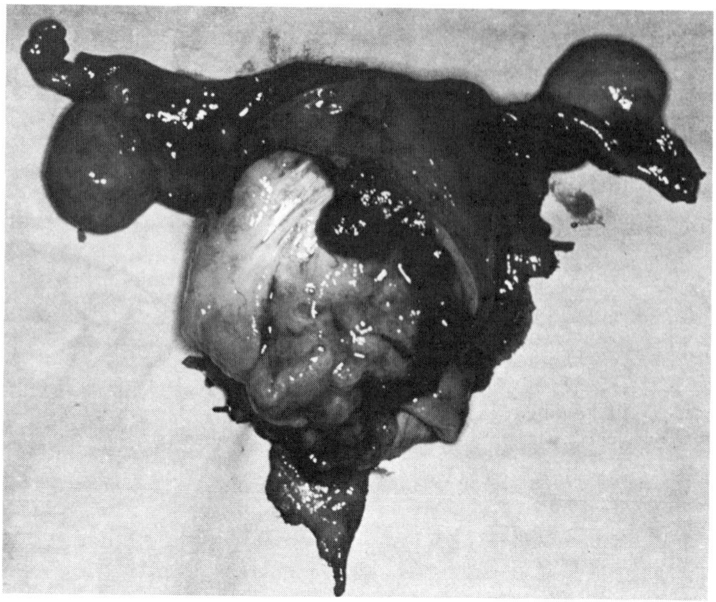

FIGURE 15–8. Opened uterine cavity showing bulky endometrial stromal sarcoma.

were staged by the FIOG classification for uterine tumors. Stage I disease (tumor confined to the uterine corpus) represented 56% of the cases, and stage II to stage IV, with tumor extension beyond the uterus, 44%. Surgery alone was employed in 33 patients and surgery with radiation in 31. The most common symptom for the sarcomas in general was vaginal bleeding in 86%, pain in 19%, and a mass in 15%. For stage I disease a better prognosis could be anticipated; the overall survival rate at 5 years was 49% compared with 16% for the more advanced stages. Though the sarcomas that have recurred have usually been widespread, we have encountered several patients where the recurrence was localized to the pelvis and surgical extirpation was accomplished by various modifications of the exenteration procedure. Almost 90% of Salazar's patients who failed on the initial approach toward management died during the first 2 years. The presence of metastatic pulmonary disease in a patient who underwent hysterectomy does not always suggest that an aggressive uterine sarcoma was present. It is essential that the pathology be reviewed especially if a fibroid uterus were to be diagnosed. Pulmonary metastasis from benign-appearing smooth muscle tumors of the uterus is a well-known entity and has been reviewed by Bachman and Wolff.[5]

With the endometrial sarcomas,[35, 79] node dissection is probably indicated. These tumors tend to fill the entire uterine cavity when defined and spread rapidly through the myometrial wall (Fig. 15–8). On completion of surgery, adjuvant radiation to the pelvis may be of value especially for large sarcomatous lesions confined to this region.[63]

REFERENCES

1. Aaro L. A., Dockerty M. B.: Leiomyosarcoma of the uterus. Am. J. Obstet. Gynecol. 77:1187–1198, 1959
2. Abramson D. J.: Leiomyoblastoma of the stomach. Surg. Gynecol. Obstet. 136:118–125, 1973
3. Akwaru I. F., Dozois R. R., Weiland L. H., Beahrs O.H.: Leiomyosarcoma of the small and large bowel. Cancer 42:1375–1384, 1978
4. Azoury R. S., Woodruff J. D.: Primary ovarian sarcomas: Report of 43 cases from the Emil Novak ovarian tumor registry. Obstet. Gynecol. 37:920–941, 1973
5. Bachman D., Wolff M.: Pulmonary metastasis from benign-appearing smooth muscle tumors of the uterus. Am. J. Roentgenol. 127:441–446, 1976
6. Bansal M., Kaneko M., Gordon R. E.: Carcinosarcoma and separate carcinoid tumor of the stomach. Cancer 50:1876–1881, 1982
7. Berg J., McNeer G.: Leiomyosarcoma of the stomach. Cancer 13:25–33, 1960
8. Burgess J. N., Dockerty M. B., ReMine W. H.: Sarcomatous lesions of the stomach. Ann. Surg. 173:758–765, 1971
9. Burns D. K., Silva F. G., Forde K. A., et al.: Primary melanocytic schwannoma of the stomach. Cancer 52:1432–1441, 1983
10. Carlson J. A., Edwards C., Wharton T.: Mixed mesodermal sarcoma of the ovary: Treatment with combination radiation therapy and chemotherapy. Cancer 52:1473–1477, 1983

11. Carpenter Y., Lambilliotte J. P.: Primary sarcoma of the gallbladder. Cancer 32:493–496, 1973
12. Chawala K., Adler L., Sobo S., Alexander L. L.: Granular cell tumor of the esophagus. N.Y. State J. Med. 84:107, 1984
13. Chen K. T. K., Hoffman K. D., Hendricks E. J.: Angiosarcoma following therapeutic irradiation. Cancer 44:2044–2048, 1979
14. Chiotasso P. J. P., Fazio V. W.: Prognostic factors of 28 leiomyosarcomas of the small intestine. Surg. Gynecol. Obstet. 155:197–201, 1982
15. Cohen A., Geller S. A., Horowitz I., et al.: Experimental models for gastric leiomyosarcoma. Cancer 53:1088–1092, 1984
16. Cornog J. L., Jr.: Gastric leiomyoblastoma: A clinical and ultrastructural study. Cancer 34:711–719, 1974
17. Corscaden J. A., Singh B. P.: Leiomyosarcoma of the uterus. Am. J. Obstet. Gynecol. 75:149–155, 1958
18. De Saia D. J.: Endometrial sarcoma: Lymphatic spread pattern. Am. J. Obstet. Gynecol. 130:104–105, 1975
19. Dinh T. V., Woodruff J. D.: Leiomyosarcoma of the uterus. Am. J. Obstet. Gynecol. 144:817–823, 1982
20. Drake E. T., Dobben G. D.: Leiomyosarcoma of the uterus with unusual metastasis. J.A.M.A. 179:1294–1298, 1959
21. Farinacci C. J., Fairchild J. P., Sulak M. H., Gilpatrick C. W.: Sarcoma botryoides (a form of embryonal rhabdomyosarcoma) of the common bile duct. Cancer 8:408–417, 1955
22. Fenn M. E., Abell M. R.: Carcinosarcoma of the ovary. Am. J. Obstet. Gynecol. 110:1066–1074, 1971
23. Franklin G. O., Antler A. S., Thelmo W. L., Rosenthal W. S.: Esophageal leiomyosarcoma. N.Y. State J. Med. 82:1100–1103, 1982
24. Friedell G. H.: Long survival with metastatic uterine leiomyosarcoma. Am. J. Obstet. Gynecol. 83:1579–1581, 1962
25. Gilbert H. A.: The value of radiation therapy in uterine sarcomas. Obstet. Gynecol. 45:84–88, 1975
26. Golden R., Stout A. P.: Smooth muscle tumors of the gastrointestinal tract and retroperitoneal tissues. Surg. Gynecol. Obstet. 73:784–810, 1941
27. Goldman R.: Ganglioneuroma of the duodenum: Relationship to nonchromaffin paraganglioma of the duodenum. Am. J. Surg. 115:716–719, 1968
28. Hannigan E. V., Gomez L. G.: Uterine leiomyosarcoma: A review of the prognostic clinical and pathologic features. Am. J. Obstet. Gynecol. 134:557–564, 1979
29. Herbsman H., Wetstein L., Rosen Y.: Tumors of the small intestine. Curr. Probl. Surg. 18:123–183, 1980
30. Istre B.: Sarcoma of the ovary. J. Oslo City Hosp. 1:231–237, 1951
31. Kempson R. L., Beri W.: Uterine sarcomas: Classification, diagnosis and prognosis. Hum. Pathol. 1:331–349, 1970
32. Kheir S. M., Halpern N. B.: Paraganglioma of the duodenum in association with congenital neurofibromatosis. Cancer 53:2491–2495, 1984
33. Kitamura S.: Study of carcinosarcoma of the stomach. Gann 41:15–25, 1950
34. Kohno H., Naofumi N., Araki S., Kato E.: Ten-year survival after synchronous resection of liver metastasis from intestinal leiomyosarcoma. Cancer 47:1421–1423, 1981
35. Koss L. G., Spiro R. H., Brunschwig A.: Endometrial stromal sarcoma. Surg. Gynecol. Obstet. 121:531–537, 1965
36. Kretschmer H. L., Doehring P.: Leiomyosarcoma of the urinary bladder. Arch. Surg. 38:274–286, 1939
37. Lavin P., Hajdu S. I., Foote F. W., Jr.: Gastric and extragastric leiomyoblastomas: Clinicopathologic study of 44 cases. Cancer 29:305–311, 1972
38. Lukash W. M., Hyams V. J., Nielson O. F.: Neurogenic neoplasms of the small bowel: Benign nonchromaffin paraganglioma of the duodenum. Am. J. Dig. Dis. 11:575–579, 1966
39. Marshall V. F.: Pelvic exenteration for polypoid myosarcoma (sarcoma botryoides) of the urinary bladder of an infant. Cancer 9:620–621, 1956
40. Martin J. F., Bazin P., Feroldi J., Cabanne F.: Tumeurs myoides intra-murales des l'estomac-considerations microscopiques a propos de 6 cas. Ann. Anat. Pathol. 13:25–33, 1960
41. Meszaros W. T.: Leiomyosarcoma of the colon. Am. J. Roentgenol. 89:766–770, 1963
42. Mostofi F. K., Morse W. H.: Polypoid rhabdomyosarcoma of bladder in children. J. Urol. 67:681–687, 1952
43. Norris H. J., Parmley T.: Mesenchymal tumors of the uterus: Intravenous leiomyomatosis. Cancer 36:2165–2178, 1975
44. Ober W. B.: Uterine sarcoma: Histogenesis and taxonomy. Ann. N.Y. Acad. Sci. 75:568–585, 1959
45. Ober W. B., Tovell H. M.: Mesenchymal sarcoma of the uterus. Am. J. Obstet. Gynecol. 77:246, 1959
46. Ongkasuwan C., Taylor J. E., Tang C. K., Prempree T.: Angiosarcomas of the uterus and ovary. Cancer 49:1469–1475, 1982
47. Orchard N. P.: Mixed mesodermal tumors of the ovary. Med. J. Aust. 2:151–155, 1972
48. Pagtalunan R. J. G., Mayo C. W., Dockerty M. B.: Primary malignant tumors of the small intestine. Am. J. Surg. 108:13–18, 1964
49. Patanaphan V., Hafiz M. A., Salazar O. M.: Metastatic leiomyosarcoma of iliac bone. N.Y. State J. Med. 85:220–222, 1985
50. Pearce P. N.: Leiomyomatosis peritonealis disseminata. Am. J. Obstet. Gynecol. 144:133–134, 1982
51. Peters W. A., Kunmar N. B., Fleming W. P., Morley, G. W.: Prognostic features of sarcomas and mixed tumors of the endometrium. Obstet. Gynecol. 63:550–556, 1984
52. Posen J. A., Sa F., Bar-Maor J. A.: Leiomyosarcoma of the colon in an infant. Cancer 52:1458–1461, 1983
53. Prat J, Scully R. E.: Cellular fibromas and fibrosarcomas of the ovary. Cancer 47:2663–2670, 1981
54. Quan S. H. G.: Leiomyoma and leiomyosarcoma of the rectum. Dis. Col. Rectum 5:415–425, 1962
55. Rainer W. G., Brus R.: Leiomyosarcoma of the esophagus: Review of the literature and report of three cases. Surgery 58:343–350, 1965
56. Ranchod M., Kempson R. L.: Smooth muscle tumors of the gastrointestinal tract and retroperitoneum: A pathologic analysis of 100 cases. Cancer 39:255–262, 1977
57. Remine W. H.: Gastric sarcomas. Am. J. Surg. 120:320–323, 1970
58. Salazar O. M., Bonfiglio T. A., Patten S. F., et al.: Uterine sarcomas: Natural history, treatment and prognosis. Cancer 42:1152–1160, 1978
59. Seremetis M. G., Lyons W. S., DeGuzman V. C., Peabody J. W.: Leiomyomata of the esophagus. Cancer 38:2166–2175, 1976
60. Shim W. K. T.: Hemangiomas of infancy complicated by thrombocytopenia. Am. J. Surg. 116:896–906, 1969

61. Shiu M. H., Farr G. H., Papachristou D. N., Hajdu S. I.: Myosarcomas of the stomach: Natural history, prognostic factors and management. Cancer 49:177–187, 1982
62. Silverberg S. G.: Leiomyosarcoma of the uterus. Obstet. Gynecol. 38:613–627, 1971
63. Smith J. P., et al.: Combined irradiation and chemotherapy for sarcomas of the pelvis in females. Am. J. Roentgenol. 123:571–576, 1975
64. Solomon M. P., Rosenblum H., Rosato F. E.: Leiomyoma of the esophagus. Ann. Surg. 199:246–248, 1984
65. Spiro R. H., Koss L. P.: Myosarcoma of the uterus: A clinicopathologic study. Cancer 18:571–588, 1965
66. Spiro R. H., McPeak C. J.: On the so-called metastasizing leiomyoma. Cancer 19:544–548, 1966
67. Takubo K., Nakagawa H., Tsuchiya S., et al.: Seeding leiomyoma of the esophagus and esophagogastric junction zone. Hum. Pathol. 12:1006–1010, 1981
68. Tanimura H., Furuta M.: Carcinosarcoma of the stomach. Am. J. Surg. 113:702–709, 1967
69. Taylor H. B., Norris H. J.: Mesenchymal tumors of the uterus. Arch. Pathol. 82:40–44, 1966
70. Thompson G. J., McDonald J. R.: Benign tumors of the urinary bladder: Report of a case of neurofibroma. J. Urol. 43:831–835, 1940
71. Vardi J. R., Tovell H. M.: Leiomyosarcoma of the uterus: A clinico-pathologic study. Obstet. Gynecol. 56:428–434, 1980
72. Vongtama V., Karlen J. R., Piver S. M., et al.: Treatment results and prognostic factors in stage I and II sarcomas of the corpus uteri. Am. J. Roentgenol. 126:139–147, 1976
73. Wald M.: Leiomyosarcoma of the jejunum. Aust. N.Z. J. Surg. 33:147–154, 1963
74. Weinstein M., Roberts M.: Leiomyosarcoma of the duodenum. Arch. Surg. 66:318–328, 1953
75. Welch J. P.: Smooth muscle tumors of the stomach. Am. J. Surg. 130:279–285, 1975
76. Wilson J. M., Melvin D. B., Gray G. F., Thorbjarnarson B.: Primary malignancies of the small bowel: A report of 96 cases and review of the literature. Ann. Surg. 1980:175–179, 1979
77. Witt J. H., Marks M. I., Smith E. I., et al.: Leiomyoma presenting as prolonged fever, anemia and thrombocytopenia. Cancer 52:2359–2362, 1983
78. Wood W. G., Burch T. K., Thomas C. Y., Jr.: Multiple leiomyosarcomas. South. Med. J. 70:381–383, 1977
79. Yoonessi M., Hart W. P.: Endometrial stromal sarcomas. Cancer 40:898, 1977

CHAPTER 16

Sarcoma Metastasis

Most sarcomas and, in particular, the fully malignant soft part sarcomas have a propensity for local recurrence as well as distant metastasis. In the past, such patterns for recurrence were believed to represent random selection by the escaping tumor cells. More recently it has been recognized that the pattern of metastasis is a phenomenon of tumor heterogeneity and that the organ or tissue of implantation is selected by cell populations migrating to a specific milieu. We began to realize this during immunotherapy trials employing melanoma tumor-associated antigen (TAA) that began in 1975. It was noted that when certain sites of metastasis resolved from what were believed to be the effects of immunotherapy, other nonrelated foci eventually became involved, even though the original metastatic site remained free. This prompted one of us (Arlen) to suggest that polyclonal antigens would probably be necessary to control metastasis since each metastatic focus probably represented a cell type with different surface antigenic expression. Studies by Wilson et al.[51] of the effect of chemotherapeutic agents on soft tissue sarcomas also suggested tumor heterogeneity. Their report documents that within a population of high-grade lesions treated with chemoradiotherapy or chemotherapy alone, the surgically resected residual or recurrent tumors were found to be low-grade histologically. Fidler[14, 42] made similar observations as to the heterogeneity of tumors in animal systems. It now appears that variations in the protein-glycoprotein make-up of the cell membrane determine the site of implantation to be selected and thus the milieu to which the tumor cells travel and implant. In many instances contrary to what Wilson had found, the heterogeneity manifests itself by the reappearance of more aggressive populations of cells.

Organ-specific adherence of metastatic tumor cells has been recently evaluated by Netland and Zetter.[38] As noted above, other investigators have also shown that certain tumors tend to metastasize preferentially to one or more specific organs. Binding of tumor cells to cryostat sections of host organs was studied using BI6-F10 melanoma and reticulum cell sarcoma cells. This work demonstrated the existence of organ specificity for cell binding 25 days after intravenous injection of the tumor line. The ability to bind to cryostat sections of mouse lung was greatly reduced by Pronase or a combination of neuraminidase and B-galactosidase. Treatment of BI6-F10 cells with the antibiotic tunicamycin, an inhibitor of glycoprotein synthesis, also reduced binding capacity. These findings were consistent with those of Irimura et al.,[26] who described an adhesive glycoprotein on the surface of the tumor cells that probably plays an important role in defining the site or sites of predilection for implantation of those cells escaping into the vascular system.

For the sarcomas, the lung is one of the more common sites for metastatic deposits to take hold; as such, work-up for any sarcoma patient, especially when amputation is being considered, requires careful evaluation of the lung fields, as well as evaluation of liver and retroperitoneum. While routine posteroanterior and lateral films of the chest may reveal most metastatic foci, CT scan can be important in picking up hidden or multiple lesions that may have been overlooked on the routine studies. There are, however, occasional problems in interpreting the results that one can obtain from lung CT scans.

Chang et al.[6] had the opportunity of comparing whole lung tomography with CT scan in evaluating the parenchyma of the lung. While the sensitivity of the scan was greater, specificity was somewhat less, possibly as a result of subpleural granulomas and lymph nodes that are found in the adult lung fields. Accordingly, suspected nodules noted in adults on CT scan should further be evaluated with conventional tomograms prior to possible thoracotomy or when deciding that a certain approach to the management of the primary tumor would not be warranted because of lung metastasis.

LIVER METASTASIS

Other sites of preference for implantation are the liver, which must always be considered whenever there is a primary retroperitoneal or visceral lesion, and the lymph nodes, which are least often evaluated as metastatic sites. Leiomyosarcomas are among those sarcomatous tumors most frequently found to metastasize to the liver, especially when they arise in the bowel.[31] When a follow-up CT scan reveals the presence of a solitary recurrence in the liver and there is no evidence of recurrence in the peritoneal cavity, then resection of the hepatic lesion should be considered. A great deal of experience has been obtained with liver resections, especially in the face of metastatic colon carcinoma. The feasibility of such surgery has now been well defined and may be employed even when it is necessary to do a trisegmentectomy.[26] We prefer segmental or wedge resections for the small metastatic tumors but do approach the porta hepatis for biliary tree and vascular isolation when more formidable resections are needed. The presence of metastatic leiomyosarcoma to the liver is frequently associated with the existence of multiple hepatic lesions. Owing to the vascularity of this tumor and, of course, the friability of its metastatic foci, hemorrhage can be a major complication. Under such circumstances control of bleeding resulting from liver involvement can be achieved by intra-arterial thrombosis via catheterization of the hepatic artery.

Intrahepatic artery catheterization can also be employed for delivery of specific chemotherapeutic agents directly into the liver to control metastatic foci. Interruption of arterial supply to the liver has also been used in an attempt to induce necrosis of tumor in both laboratory and clinical studies. In experiments performed by Hafstrom and Carlsson,[18] animals with transplanted hepatic lesions were found to show evidence of prolongation of survival as well as a statistically significant increase in body weight.

ASCITES FROM METASTATIC TUMOR

In association with liver involvement by metastatic tumor one can find ascites developing either as a result of secondary portal hypertension or carcinomatous seeding of the peritoneal cavity. Ascitic fluid appears secondary to tumor growth as a result of lymphatic permeability of the tumor implants and the pattern of lymphatic drainage from the peritoneal cavity. The peritoneal surfaces of the abdominal cavity are predominantly drained by the right thoracic duct. Viscera are predominantly drained by the left duct system. The right thoracic duct has been shown to account for 80% of the clearance from the peritoneal cavity in animals. The generation of malignant ascites by tumor seems to be due to a combination of subdiaphragmatic lymphatic obstruction and increased production of intraperitoneal fluid, especially from peritoneal surfaces, even those free of tumor. Hepatic metastasis may also result in malignant ascites as a result of outflow obstruction and hepatic dysfunction causing hypoalbuminemia. Management should begin with abdominal paracentesis for both diagnosis and therapy. Radiocolloids have been used with limited benefit. P-32 (in doses of 100 to 200 mc) has resulted in the decreased reformation of ascites in better than 80% of cases. Intracavitary chemotherapy has been disappointing. The therapeutic effect is related to obliteration of the potential space for fluid accumulation. In 1974 LeVeen[34] introduced the peritoneovenous shunt with a pressure-sensitive valve. This silicone strut valve used a critical opening pressure of 3 to 5 cm of water to prevent blood from regurgitating into the silicone tubing. Management with such shunts has been described by others.[32] We have found such a shunting procedure especially effective with ascites resulting from liver metastasis.

NODAL SPREAD OF TUMOR

While the sarcomas are essentially a group of neoplastic lesions that metastasize predominantly via the bloodstream, their spread along lymph channels has long been recognized. Andree, in 1874, described a sarcomatous lesion of the pelvis that had extension along iliac and hypogastric vessels presumably passing through the pelvic lymphatic channels. Zohner (1890) described a sarcoma of the thigh with massive extension along the femoral and iliac veins with associated pulmonary metastasis. Kaufman later described invasion of the inferior vena cava by retroperitoneal sarcoma. In such instances, pulmonary embolization by invading tumor has been well known and may even be expected. The possibility of using anticoagulation under these circumstances is to be considered, especially when venous invasion or thrombosis within the pelvic veins can be identified. This is especially true should extremity edema be noted. Clipping of the vena cava may be an important alternative during dissection of the para-aortic vena cava nodes, especially when there is a potential for embolization.

Lymph node metastasis, although more common with rhabdomyosarcoma, may also be seen in other lesions such as leiomyosarcoma. Synoviomas may also present with nodal involvement (5 to 20%) so that extremity lesions approximating the groin or axilla may best be handled by en-bloc node resection. Historically, Prym (1930) described a papillary tumor of the knee joint (probably synovioma) with involvement of nodes in the groin. Wright (1952) reported that among 47 synoviomas studied, regional lymphatic involvement was demonstrated in nine. In a review of the epithelioid sarcomas at Memorial Hospital, 42% of the cases studied had lymph node metastasis. In other studies the incidence has been as high as 62%. It is our belief that if studies of the synovioma group culled out their epithelioid sarcomas, then the aforementioned incidence for nodal metastasis with synovioma would be reduced. In terms of evaluating such lymph node involvement, lymphangiograms may be helpful. One of the benefits of such studies is that the dye used remains present for years, enabling follow-up studies (including flat film and lateral views of the abdomen) to detect late shifting or enlargement of the lymph node pattern, suggesting reappearance or reactivation of disease. CT scan and MRI studies can aid in follow-up evaluation of the lymph node patterns.

Because of the potential for lymph node involvement, nodal disease patterns should be considered in the initial management of a number of tumors such as rhabdomyosarcoma, synovioma, epithelioid sarcoma, and malignant fibrous histiocytoma.[51] Where the lesion is in proximity to the regional node–bearing area, the nodes should be removed prophylactically; this is especially true when there is a high degree of clinical suspicion of nodal involvement. Therapeutic dissection here is essential. Since embryonal rhabdomyosarcomas are known to involve regional nodes in up to 20% of cases it is essential that node dissection be included as part of the operative treatment for this disease.[33] When local resection alone was the treatment of choice for rhabdomyosarcoma of the spermatic cord, essentially few, if any, survivors were recorded. The addition of retroperitoneal node dissection made a significant difference in the results obtained; when chemotherapy was added, a major curative program could be outlined. We have recommended and employed similar prophylactic node resections for many cases of embryonal rhabdomyosarcomas seen in the head and neck. Other tumors such as neuroblastoma may spread to regional as well as distant nodal sites. A case of neuroblastoma arising in an immature teratoma of the ovary was reported by Block et al.[4] Metastasis to retroperitoneal, mediastinal, and supraclavicular nodes as well as to bone was diagnosed and treated effectively with chemotherapy in this patient. Knowledge of the patterns of metastasis can be important in determining what regional sites might be necessary for inclusion in en-bloc resection and how sites of distant metastasis should be handled.

The vascular system is still a predominant pathway for spread of sarcoma; however, regional spread along local lymphatic or tissue planes must be taken into account when tumors recur within the operative field.[5] Figure 16–1 shows an exenteration specimen with leiomyosarcoma of uterus recurring in the vagina 1 year after hysterectomy for malignant degeneration of a fibroid tumor. This type of approach may be effective when there is an interval of more than 1 year from the time of primary surgery and when work-up fails to show any site of distant recurrence. Benign smooth muscle tumors of the uterus have been known on rare occasions to metastasize distantly via the bloodstream. Benign metastasizing leiomyoma is such a tumor, arising in uterus as the classic fibroid does, but with the potential for spreading to lung.[2, 20] We suspect that with the newer techniques of cell-

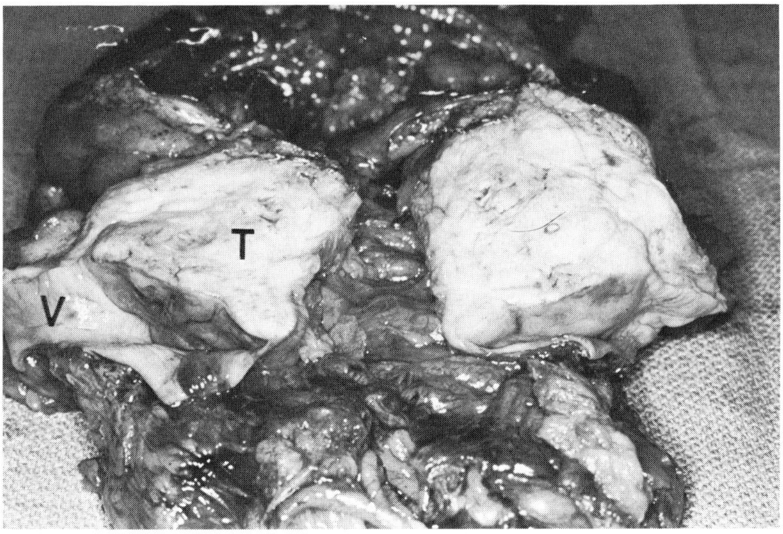

FIGURE 16–1. Recurrent leiomyosarcoma of the uterus in exenteration specimen. T shows the position of the tumor mass in the vagina (V).

flow cytometry, a differential in DNA content between this tumor and its nonmetastasizing counterpart will be found. Keasby[29] did report a case of another lesion considered to be benign, fibroma of the thumb, found to be associated with a pulmonary lesion that proved to be metastatic when the resected lung lesion was compared with the primary tumor. In some instances, the vascular spread may be entirely mechanical—for instance, the appearance of fat in the lung following trauma or the appearance of metastatic giant cell tumor in the lung after curettage of benign giant cell tumor of bone. In contrast to this phenomenon, however, the appearance of metastatic sarcoma in the lung or other sites as a result of vascular dissemination usually results in progressive growth of the implanted foci with the potential of the metastases to disseminate further.

One of the unusual areas of involvement by metastatic sarcoma is the retrobulbar space.[1] Normally with clinical evidence of proptosis of the orbit, a primary retrobulbar tumor should be considered. One of the more common tumors to have associated metastasis to the retrobulbar space is carcinoma of the breast. Sarcomas, except for those developing in the paranasal sinuses, rarely involve the orbit. Recently we examined a 46-year-old man who had undergone local resection for liposarcoma of the right lower leg. We were asked to evaluate him for more definitive therapy. CT scan of the leg was normal. On exploration of the surgical site of the leg we encountered residual tumor. The patient remained well for 6

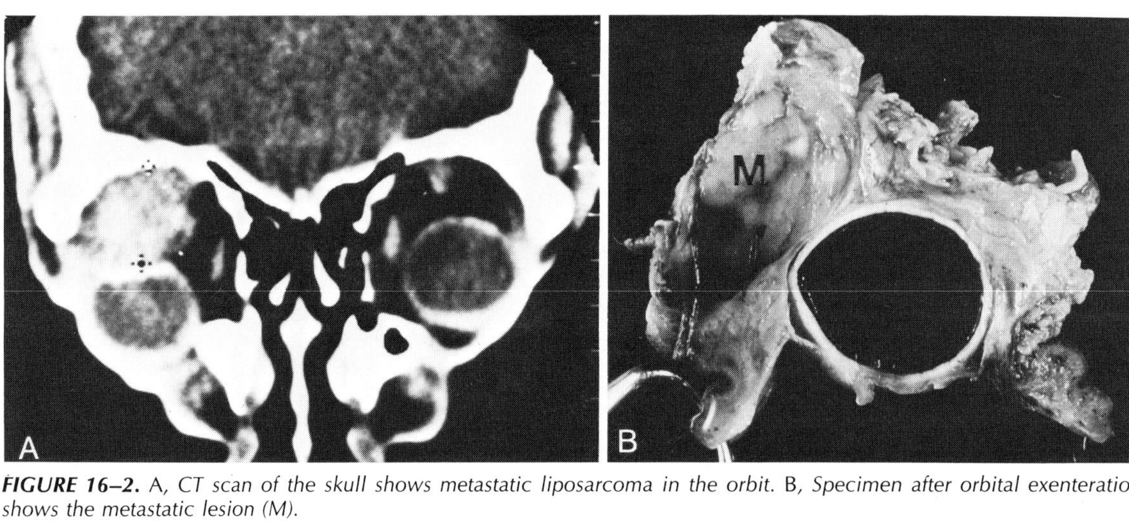

FIGURE 16–2. A, CT scan of the skull shows metastatic liposarcoma in the orbit. B, Specimen after orbital exenteration shows the metastatic lesion (M).

months in that he was clinically free of recurrent local tumor. He returned suddenly to our office with orbital pain and early evidence of proptosis. Within 2 weeks it was obvious that we were dealing with retrobulbar tumor. A CT scan taken at this time demonstrated a well-defined mass sitting above the globe (Fig. 16–2*A*). We were hoping to initiate radiotherapy to the orbit in an attempt to control the lesion locally; then we would attempt to resect the tumor while saving the globe. The growth of this tumor was so rapid, however, that orbital exenteration was needed. Figure 16–2*B* shows sections taken through the globe and the surrounding orbital contents demonstrating the tumor mass. Following this, recurrent tumor in both legs was found. All biopsy specimens showed liposarcoma.

PULMONARY AND CHEST METASTASIS

When chest metastasis is found during work-up it is necessary to define whether the lesion is solitary or multiple and what the dimension of the lesion is at the time; if previous films showing tumor are available, it is advantageous to estimate doubling time.[8, 27] Such determinations have helped in predicting behavioral response. It is also important to know whether the metastatic tumor is in lung parenchyma or in the mediastinal nodes. We examined a young male patient who had recently undergone forequarter amputation for a sarcoma of the axilla. Knowing that he had von Recklinghausen's disease, we presumed that the amputation had been performed for neurogenic sarcoma. When pulmonary metastasis was suspected, we believed we were dealing with a classic pattern of spread for this tumor. The findings of the chest films, however, revealed the presence of mediastinal involvement, suggesting that nodal rather than parenchymal spread had taken place. This pattern is far from characteristic for the spread of neurogenic sarcoma. We therefore began to think of more unusual lesions that might involve this site in the chest. A variant of neurogenic sarcoma, the clear cell schwannoma, is known to behave like melanoma, spreading to mediastinal nodes when it involves the upper extremity. Biopsy of the chest lesion confirmed that our impression was correct.

Review of biopsies taken from the primary site are always important since the original sections may have been misinterpreted and review may offer better insight into the true nature of the primary. Comparison with biopsies from the metastatic site may also show it to be a completely different tumor, suggesting the presence of two separate primaries.

One of the complications of pulmonary involvement by metastatic tumor is progressive compromise of effective alveolar space, resulting in progressive respiratory distress. However, we have seen patients with extensive bilateral cannonball lesions who show little evidence of dyspnea except on marked exertion. Another complication is the development of pleural effusion representing an additional mechanism resulting in respiratory symptoms. This finding usually necessitates drainage and the addition of agents such as talc or tetracycline to the pleural space in an attempt to minimize reaccumulation of the fluid. When pulmonary metastases invade the pleural surfaces of the lung, they can rupture at the surface like emphysematous blebs, resulting in pneumothorax, which would necessitate emergency tube thoracotomy. Similar leakage of air into the pleural space can occur as a result of an excellent chemotherapeutic response in which tumor has disappeared from the surface of the lung, leaving only the leaking bronchiolar defect.

A secondary phenomenon of pulmonary metastasis appears as a sequela in the skeletal system. Gibbs (1960)[17] reported osteoarthropathy accompanying the development of large pulmonary metastasis from a uterine leiomyosarcoma that had been removed 4 years before. Resection of such pulmonary lesions can occasionally result in disappearance of the osteoarthropathy. This phenomenon, known as secondary pulmonary osteoarthropathy, usually results from metastatic pulmonary disease. We mention this because we saw a case of giant cell tumor of the posterior rib associated with osteoarthropathy devoid of pulmonary metastasis. Successful treatment of the local disease resulted in complete reversal of the osteoarthropathy. Others have described similar osteoarthropathy secondary to renal or hepatic disease. It is important to know that there is a primary form of this disease that presents with clubbing of the fingers, inflamed swollen joints, and tender long bones with periosteal new bone formation which is not secondary to existing pulmonary disease. The diagnostic clue to this primary condition is the presence of a peculiar thickening of the skin above the eyelids (so-called bulldog scalp). Another manifestation of pulmonary involvement can be an attack of secondary gout. Here the patient may have a classic attack of gout which may be peculiar in that the usual medications prescribed do not help. Intravenous cortisone provides only temporary relief of pain from the red, hot, swollen joint. Such resistant gout should alert the physician to look for an irritating primary cause such as malignancy of lung. On x-ray examination the offending lesion may appear incredibly small and therefore highly curable by surgery. Following removal of this lesion the gout usually subsides.

NEURAL SPREAD

Neural spread of sarcoma along the peripheral nerve trunks has been described as another pathway for sarcoma metastasis.[3] In 1905 Ernst reported that neural spaces served as channels for tumor metastases. In some cases he noted that invading tumor had a degenerating effect on the medullary sheath of the involved nerve. In 1936 Myerding reported that pain, either local or radiating, was a prominent feature in 36% of the fibrosarcomas they removed. They found that referred pain, numbness, and partial or complete palsy were indicative of peripheral neuritis, which resulted from invasion by infiltrating sarcoma. In the performance of en-bloc muscle group dissection it is essential that the tumor be resected with adjacent nerve structures as long as the lesion is fully malignant. We have adapted this principle when dealing with low-grade sarcomas in close approximation to such structures as the brachial plexus and sciatic nerve. At times we have used cryosurgery in proximity to the nerves, since the chance of permanent damage to the nerve trunks is minimal and regeneration in function has usually been seen. Eilber[11] has recommended a somewhat similar conservative approach but for higher grades of sarcoma. His group employs intra-arterial Adriamycin given preoperatively. He has reported not only a significant decrease in the need for amputation but also a local recurrence rate of less than 10%.

SKELETAL INVOLVEMENT

Soft tissue sarcomas may occasionally produce skeletal metastasis. Such findings are common with childhood neuroblastoma but may be noted with adult angiosarcomas in particular. One of our patients with Kaposi's sarcoma presented with a pattern showing so many punched-out skull lesions that the film was initially thought to represent a case of multiple myeloma. Bone biopsy finally confirmed the diagnosis of metastatic tumor. Bone marrow involvement is an additional manifestation of osseous disease occurring in children and adolescents with rhabdomyosarcoma; 30 patients in an intergroup study had involvement of bone at the time of entrance in the study.[46] In general, the patients were older and frequently had primary tumors of the extremity. Eleven received vincristine, dactinomycin, and cyclophosphamide (VAC) and 19 VAC plus Adriamycin. A complete response rate of 60% was seen. The median disease-free times were 17 weeks with VAC and 32 weeks with VAC plus Adriamycin. A higher incidence of marrow disease was seen with alveolar patterns consistent with the hypothesis that this disease variant represents a more aggressive lesion than other forms of embryonal rhabdomyosarcoma. Bone marrow aspirate from the iliac crest appears to be the site to sample when looking for disease. In one instance we encountered a solitary metastatic focus of liposarcoma to the skull, with cure achieved after resection and radiation.

Laboratory results that may suggest marrow involvement are positive bone scan, lactic dehydrogenase >500 IU/L, anemia, and elevated uric acid. The association of anemia and thrombocytopenia should raise suspicion for the possible appearance of disseminated intravascular coagulation (DIC). A review of the peripheral smear, coupled with a prothrombin time, partial thromboplastin time, fibrinogen and fibrin-split product assay is indicated in the patient at risk for DIC. Tumor cell embolization with destruction of endothelium with tumor invasion has been suggested as a possible mechanism for DIC in malignancies. Thromboelastograms have been used in the past to determine the earliest phases of DIC. Here, heparin has frequently been found to abort the problem. In the rhabdomyosarcoma series, central nervous system metastasis by hematogenous spread was the most common reason for failure.

While osseous involvement is a poor prognostic indicator, therapy can be advantageous in a number of instances. Patanaphan et al.[40] described a case of prolonged survival following radiation therapy for metastatic uterine leiomyosarcoma to the iliac bone. Soft tissue disease had developed 2 years after excision of a regional leiomyosarcoma, with involvement of the iliac bone 5 years later. Following therapy to the osseous lesion this patient has remained free of disease 10 years after initial diagnosis. For the most part, leiomyosarcoma rarely metastasizes to bone and is more frequently associated with widespread metastatic disease, which portends poor survival.[20] Results in the evaluation of any unusual pattern of behavior for the smooth muscle tumors should take biologic activity into account.[10, 19] Kempson and Bari[30] have suggested using mitotic counts to differentiate tumors (primary as well as metastatic) into truly malignant and lower-grade variants. Such differentiation may explain variations in the results of treatment. In VAC chemotherapy trials of patients, survival time is significantly prolonged (median, 19.3 months) compared with mixed mesodermal sarcoma (median, 9.27 months). If patients with low-grade leiomyosarcoma are not included, then the survival between the two groups is no longer statistically significant.

As osseous lesions expand, their destructive lytic process can eventually result in the appearance of a pathologic fracture. This is especially true in weightbearing bones.[16] Among 19 fractures treated by Takita and Watne,[49] 16 were in the femur; 11 of these had arisen in the hip. All had or were receiving some type of treatment for their primary disease, either chemotherapeutic hormone manipulation or radiation therapy. The criterion used in patient selection for surgery was the ability to withstand the procedure rather than the patient's prognosis. Surgery was intended to provide relief from pain and secondarily to permit resumption of ambulation. A Lorenzo screw and plate were used in 11 patients. Seven were able to walk postoperatively with the aid of crutches or a walker.

One of the larger studies by Higinbotham and Marcove[21] reviewed surgical intervention in 150 patients with pathologic fractures treated at Memorial Hospital between 1931 and 1965. The most common operation used the Smith-Petersen nail alone or with McLaughlin bar for intertrochanteric and subtrochanteric pathologic fractures. Excision of the femoral head was carried out 57 times and 48 Küntscher rods were inserted. Rush pins were employed in 17 instances: 11 in the femur, 5 in the humerus, and 1 in a radius. Approximately one third of the patients lived 1 or more years after fracture. The rapid relief of pain, decrease in narcotic requirements, ease of nursing care, and improved mobility suggested that surgery was more advantageous in selected patients than were closed reduction techniques. At the time of internal fixation, local control of disease, especially with cryosurgery, has been attempted.[36]

BRAIN INVOLVEMENT

Brain metastasis, when suspected, should be evaluated in terms of whether the lesion is solitary or multiple. Recent reports comparing various treatments for a single lesion seem to suggest an overall survival advantage for those undergoing craniotomy. Among 125 patients undergoing surgery with or without postoperative radiation, 8% were from soft part sarcoma primary tumors.[47] In the overall series, 83 patients (66%) were neurologically improved. The overall median survival was 12 months, and eight patients (12%) were alive at 5 years.

As newer chemotherapeutic modalities become more effective, it becomes apparent that many tumors are composed of heterogeneous clones destroyed to a great part by the therapeutic modalities initially employed. Where one is later able to resect an isolated pulmonary lesion, unusual populations of cell growth not previously noted may appear even later. In one instance, soft tissue metastasis from an osteosarcoma appeared in the pancreatic bed. A pulmonary metastasis had been resected 3 years before, for a primary tumor of the femur that had been initially treated at age 15 (5 years prior to the retroperitoneal lesion). Such findings will probably be noted more frequently in the future as chemotherapeutic protocols control the major clones comprising a tumor mass but fail to eliminate small residual subpopulations of resistant cells that usually never appear in the normal natural history of the lesion.

SURGICAL RESECTION OF PULMONARY METASTASIS

The resection of sarcomatous metastasis to lung has been well defined, beginning with Marcove's original studies of metastatic osteosarcoma to lung.[35] The information gained in these studies allowed the pursuit of more aggressive attempts in handling metastasis from other sites such as bowel, kidney, and the sarcomas. At Memorial Hospital pulmonary nodules have been resected after definitive amputation for extremity sarcoma, regardless of their being solitary or multiple, provided that no other foci of disease were present.[37]

It was found that after primary amputation, among those patients who developed pulmonary metastasis and were untreated, only 5% would be alive after 3 years. In those who had aggressive multiple thoracotomies and multiple, yet minimal, wedge resections, 45% were alive at 3 years. At 5 years 31% were still alive. The development of metastatic disease at sites other than lung appeared to be the largest single factor causing failure of multiple pulmonary resections in this disease. The largest number of pulmonary nodules excised in a surviving patient was 11; however, one patient who had had 21 nodules removed died of a pulmonary embolus; at autopsy no residual disease was found. The principle of searching for pulmonary metastasis after primary treatment is based on Marcove's use of monthly follow-up x-ray films. The reason for such an initial approach when treating aggressive extremity lesions is that a small overlooked nodule is more likely to be detected at the second month of growth. Follow-up x-ray films taken every 2 months would detect a similar lesion after 4 months of growth but the lesion would then be inoperable.

Some surgeons advocate pulmonary resection only in the patient with solitary metastasis confined to one lung after a prolonged disease-free interval. Others have noted that the results of surgical resection with multiple metastases are frequently as favorable as those in patients with a solitary lesion.[13, 22, 24, 44, 45, 48]

Doubling time for evaluating potential growth patterns in tumors has been described by Collins[8] using serial x-ray measurements. Within the limits of a 7 to 10% error in measurement, it is believed that a 1-cm nodule with 10^9 cells has undergone 30 doubling periods. In general, multiple metastases tend to grow at a fixed rate. When varying growth patterns are noted, the prognosis is based on the lesion with the quickest doubling time. When there is a long disease-free interval between treatment of the primary and detection of metastasis, then there is usually a longer span between tumor doubling. It has been found that intervals to recurrence decrease as metastases are treated and appear related to inhibitory material on the cell surface membrane. Thus a low level of inhibitory material is found in the first recurrence at 5 years after primary therapy. Should a second recurrence appear, it may occur 1 year later, when the tumor has a markedly increased level. Should a third recurrence appear, it would be in a matter of months and inhibitory material would be further increased, suggesting constant cell surface modulation as the tumor grows.

Tumor doubling has been used by Joseph and Morton[27] to predict response to pulmonary resection for metastasis. For those lesions with a doubling time of more than 40 days there was approximately a 60% 5-year survival with surgery compared with a poor survival with nonoperative therapy. For those tumors with doubling times under 20 days, resection proved to be of no value. However, if one waited for an evaluation of doubling characteristics prospectively, it is uncertain whether in some instances a patient would be converted from an operable to an inoperable situation. When synchronous metastases were found to be present in other viscera, surgery did not appear to offer a good prognosis.

Tumors such as osteosarcoma, fibrosarcoma, and other soft tissue neoplasms tend to spread primarily to lung and are good candidates for surgical extirpation, especially when the interval of freedom of disease is greater than 3 years. The survival of patients with lung metastasis is directly related to resectability, with nonsurgical results extremely poor. From 1952 to 1979, 234 patients underwent resection of a wide array of metastatic lung lesions at Memorial Hospital. There were 112 solitary and 42 unilateral but multiple lesions; 80 lesions were bilateral. Among the types of lesions that were resected, there were 59 sarcomas, 102 genitourinary/gynecologic tumors, 21 gastrointestinal tumors, 20 head and neck tumors, 17 melanomas, 10 breast tumors, and 5 others.

Preoperative work-up included tomography (CT scan), doubling time, skeletal survey, bone scan and, when indicated, arteriography. No matter how extensive the pulmonary lesions were in size and number, if preservation of a sufficient amount of lung tissue could be anticipated, then surgical resection was considered, especially if the primary disease was controllable. In the past 10 years of the study, 16 patients (76%) with bilateral lung disease underwent resection through a median sternotomy rather than bilateral thoracotomy. Lesions of the lung were excised with 0.5 to 1 cm of surrounding normal lung tissue. Blood vessels and small bronchi were controlled by hemostatic clips. Local excision was used in 146 patients, lobectomy in 52, pneumonectomy in 20, and local resection plus lobectomy in 16.

The number of lesions visualized on x-ray examination averaged 2.2, but on thoracotomy was found to be 5. Among 212 patients who underwent complete resection, the median survival time was 24.4 months. The group with a doubling time of 45 days or less had a worse survival (17.2 months) compared with the group with a doubling time greater than 45 days (median survival, 37 months).

The first major series reporting the natural history of metastatic lesions to the lung was the study by Farrell in 1935.[12] He documented 78 patients that went untreated but had been followed. Death occurred within 6 months in 44.8%; only 8.9% survived for more than 2 years. When resection was offered as a modality of therapy to carefully selected patients, it became apparent that the pattern of behavior could be altered in selected instances. At Roswell Park 55 patients were studied between 1956 and 1977.[23] Seventeen patients underwent resection for solitary metastatic sarcoma; 33 had resection of multiple pulmonary metastases. Eighteen of the lesions represented metastases from soft part sarcomas of the extremity; six were from trunk lesions. Visceral lesions and osteosarcomas comprised the remaining primary tumors. The most common procedure for the lung lesions was wedge resection. Median sternotomy was used to approach bilateral synchronous disease. Lobectomy was necessary in six patients and pneumonectomy in four. In two patients the involved mediastinal nodes were removed. The disease-free interval from surgery of the primary to demonstrable lung metastasis ranged from 0 to 88 months. Twenty-three of the patients presented with their lung lesions within 12 months of the primary tumor resection. Tumor doubling time ranged from 13 to 98 days. The estimated median survival was 22.2 months. The group with the doubling time of more than 40 days had a better survival rate. When the length of duration (less than or greater than 3 months) was considered in defining the lesion, the results of survival for the two groups were identical, indicating that the time needed for careful preoperative evaluation did not jeopardize the outcome. In addition, no statistical significance was found when patients had undergone resection of solitary or multiple lesions in the same lung. Clagett et al. demonstrated a 23% 5-year survival following excision of metastatic lung lesions in a group of 41 diverse sarcoma patients treated at the Mayo Clinic between 1941 and 1962. A further analysis of 112 patients treated between 1950 and 1976 was made by Creagan et al.;[9] the 5-year post-thoracotomy survival was 29% (median, 18 months). Regal et al.,[43] in reviewing 131 patients at Roswell Park, found that aggressive management of primary tumors and their metastatic manifestations is associated with improved survival. In this study median sternotomy was preferred to unilateral or staged bilateral thoracotomies since it provided simultaneous access to both hemithoraces, resulted in lowered morbidity, and allowed earlier resumption of systemic therapy.

REFERENCES

1. Abdalla M. L., Ghaly A. F., Nosni F.: Liposarcoma with orbital metastasis. Br. J. Ophthalmol. 50:426–428, 1966
2. Bachman D., Wolff M.: Pulmonary metastasis from benign-appearing, smooth muscle tumors of the uterus. Am. J. Roentgenol. 127:441–446, 1976
3. Barber J. R., Coventry M. D., McDonald J. R.: The spread of soft tissue sarcomas of the extremities along peripheral nerve trunks. J. Bone Joint Surg. 39:534–540, 1957
4. Block M., Gilbert E., Davis C.: Neuroblastoma arising in an immature teratoma of ovary. Cancer 54:590–595, 1984
5. Cantin J., McNeer G. P., Chu F. C., Booher R. J.: The problem of local recurrence after treatment of soft tissue sarcoma. Ann. Surg. 168:47–53, 1968
6. Chang A. E., Schaner E. G., Conkle D. M., et al.: Evaluation of computed tomography in the detection of pulmonary metastasis: A prospective study. Cancer 43:913–916, 1979
7. Cheung D. K., Rafe J. H.: Selection of patients with malignant ascites for a peritoneocutaneous shunt. Cancer 50:1204–1209, 1982
8. Collins V. P., Loeffler R. K., Tivey H.: Observations

on growth rates of human tumors. Am. J. Roentgenol. 76:988–1000, 1956
9. Creagan E. T., Fleming T. R., Edmonson J. H., Pariolero P. C.: Pulmonary resection for metastatic sarcoma. Cancer 44:1908–1912, 1979
10. Drake E. T., Dobben G. D.: Leiomyosarcoma of the uterus with unusual metastases. J.A.M.A. 170:1294–1298, 1959
11. Eilber F. R., Morton D. L.: Soft tissue sarcoma. Contemp. Surg. 22:17–25, 1983
12. Farrell J. T., Jr.: Pulmonary metastasis. Radiology 24:444–451, 1935
13. Feldman P. S., Kyriakos M.: Pulmonary resection for metastatic sarcoma. J. Thorac. Cardiovasc. Surg. 64:784–799, 1972
14. Fidler I. J.: Tumor heterogeneity and the biology of cancer invasion and metastasis. Cancer Res. 38:2651–2660, 1978
15. Fisher E. R., Hellstrom H. R.: Dermatofibrosarcoma with metastasis simulating Hodgkin's disease and reticulum cell sarcoma. Cancer 19:1165, 1966
16. Frances K.: Treatment of metastatic fractures with internal fixation. Am. J. Surg. 97:484, 1959
17. Gibbs: Pulmonary osteoarthropathy from metastatic leiomyosarcoma. Lancet 1:623–625, 1960
18. Hafstrom L., Carlsson G.: Influence of hepatic artery ligation on survival. Am. J. Surg. 147:688–691, 1984
19. Hannigan E. V.: Long-term survival with metastatic uterine sarcoma. N.Y. State J. Med. 85:195, 1985
20. Hannigan E. V., Gomez L. G.: Uterine leiomyosarcoma: A review of prognostic clinical and pathologic features. Am. J. Obstet. Gynecol. 134:557–564, 1979
21. Higinbotham N. L., Marcove R. C.: The management of pathologic fractures. J. Trauma 5:792–798, 1965
22. Holmes E. C., Ranning K. P., Eilber F. R., Morton D. L.: The surgical management of pulmonary metastasis. Semin. Oncol. 4:65–69, 1977
23. Huang M. M., Ederton F., Takita H., et al.: Lung resection for metastatic sarcoma. Am. J. Surg. 135:804–806, 1978
24. Huth J. F., Holmes E. C., Vernon S. E., et al.: Pulmonary resection for metastatic sarcoma. Am. J. Surg. 140:9–16, 1980
25. Irimura T., Gonzalez R., Nicolson G. L.: Effects of tunicamycin on B16 metastatic melanoma cell surface glycoproteins and blood-borne arrest and survival properties. Cancer Res. 41:3411, 1981
26. Iwatsuki S., Shaw B. W., Jr., Starzl T.: Experience with 150 liver resections. Ann. Surg. 197:247–253, 1983
27. Joseph W. L., Morton D. L., Adkins P. C.: Variation in tumor doubling time in patients with pulmonary metastatic disease. J. Surg. Oncol. 3:143–149, 1971
28. Kearney M. M., Soule E. H., Ivins J. C.: Malignant fibrous histiocytoma: A retrospective study of 167 cases. Cancer 45:167–178, 1980
29. Keasby L. E.: Juvenile aponeurotic fibroma (calcifying fibroma). Cancer 6:338–346, 1953
30. Kempson R. L., Bari W.: Uterine sarcomas: classification, diagnosis and prognosis. Hum. Pathol. 1:331–349, 1971
31. Kohno H., Nagasue N., Araki S., Tetsuo K.: Ten-year survival after synchronous resection of liver metastasis from intestinal leiomyosarcoma. Cancer 47:1421–1423, 1981
32. Lacy J. H., Wieman T. J., Shively E. H.: Management ascites for a peritoneocutaneous shunt. Cancer 50:1204–1209, 1982
33. Lawrence W., Jr., Hays D. M., Moon T. E.: Lymphatic metastasis with childhood rhabdomyosarcoma. Cancer 39:556–559, 1977
34. LeVeen H. H., Christoudia G.: Peritoneocutaneous shunting for ascites. Ann. Surg. 180:580–591, 1974
35. Marcove R. C., Martini N., Rosen G.: The treatment of pulmonary metastasis in osteogenic sarcoma. Clin. Orthop. 3:65–70, 1975
36. Marcove R., Sadrieh J., Huvos A. G., Grabstald H.: Cryosurgery in the treatment of solitary or multiple bone metastases from renal cell carcinoma. J. Urol. 108:540–547, 1972
37. McCormack P., Martini N.: The changing role in surgery for pulmonary metastasis. Ann. Thorac. Surg. 23:139–145, 1979
38. Netland P. A., Zetter B. R.: Organ-specific adhesion of metastatic tumor cells in vitro. Science 224:1113–1114, 1984
39. Nicolson G. L.: . Biochim. Biophys. Acta 695:113, 1982
40. Patanaphan V., Hafiz M. A., Salazar O. M.: Metastatic leiomyosarcoma of iliac bone. N.Y. State J. Med. 85:220–221, 1985
41. Penner R. W.: Metastasizing dermatofibrosarcoma protuberans. Cancer 4:1083, 1951
42. Poste G., Fidler I. J.: The pathogenesis of cancer metastasis. Nature 283:139, 1980
43. Regal A. M., Reese P., Antkowiak J., et al.: Median sternotomy for metastatic lung lesions in 131 patients. Cancer 55:1334–1339, 1985
44. Rogers B. M., Talbert J. L., Alexander J. A.: Pulmonary metastases in childhood sarcoma. Ann. Thorac. Surg. 28:139–145, 1979
45. Roth J. A., Putnam J. B., Jr., Welsey M. N., Rosenberg S. A.: Differing determinants of prognosis following resection of pulmonary metastasis from osteogenic and soft tissue sarcoma patients. Cancer 55:1361–1366, 1985
46. Ruymann F. B., Newton W. A., Jr., Abdelsalam H. R., et al.: Bone marrow metastases at diagnosis in children and adolescents with rhabdomyosarcoma. Cancer 53:368–373, 1984
47. Sundaresan N., Galicich J.: Surgical treatment of brain metastasis. Cancer 55:1382–1388, 1985
48. Takita H., Edgerton F., Karakousis C., et al.: Surgical management of metastases to the lung. Surg. Gynecol. Obstet. 152:191–194, 1981
49. Takita H., Watne A. L.: Operative treatment of pathologic fractures. Surg. Gynecol. Obstet. 116: 683–692, 1963
50. Weingrad D. N., Rosenberg S. A.: Early lymphatic spread of osteogenic and soft tissue sarcomas. Surgery 84:231–240, 1978
51. Wilson R. E., Antman K. H., Brodsky G., Greenberger J. S.: Tumor-cell heterogeneity in soft tissue sarcomas as defined by chemotherapy. Cancer 53:1420–1425, 1984

CHAPTER

17

The Chemotherapy of Soft Tissue Sarcomas

PATRICIA A. JOHNSON
JULES E. HARRIS

Chemotherapy plays several roles in the management of the soft tissue sarcomas. The most obvious of these is systemic therapy for patients with unresectable or metastatic disease. In a large series, the 5-year survival for patients with stage IV soft tissue sarcomas was only 7%.[96] This group made up 110 of 702, or 16%, cases reviewed. Because sarcomas are relatively uncommon, comprising only 1% of all cancers, various investigators reporting cytotoxic therapy for soft tissue sarcomas usually group together tumors of various histologies. Even when the stages are identical, the survival rate may vary with histology (e.g., from 0% for stage IV rhabdomyosarcoma and liposarcoma, to 40% for synovial sarcoma in Russell's series). Furthermore, some reports group together adult patients with soft tissue sarcomas, bone sarcomas, mesotheliomas, and even pediatric sarcoma patients for purposes of describing the results of chemotherapy. The histologic heterogeneity of the sarcoma series reported from different institutions makes comparison of response rates and survival figures hazardous. The literature of this topic must, therefore, be interpreted cautiously.

The second role of chemotherapy in the soft tissue sarcomas is currently quite controversial. Since most patients will have recurrence with distant disease even after adequate local therapy, systemic adjuvant chemotherapy would be highly desirable and appears theoretically possible given the variety of chemotherapeutic agents active in disseminated disease. However, this area of investigation is still in its infancy and is marked by studies that rely on historical controls rather than concomitantly treated patients randomly assigned to receive local therapy only versus others receiving additional systemic chemotherapy. Prospective randomized studies now in progress should shed some light on this topic in the next few years.

The third way in which cytotoxic agents are employed in the management of soft tissue sarcomas is by local perfusion. Often used in combination with radiation therapy, this technique can cause sufficient tumor regression to allow conservative surgery in place of amputation. It has also been used preoperatively to decrease the rate of local recurrence in patients undergoing wide excision.

SYSTEMIC CHEMOTHERAPY FOR ADVANCED DISEASE

The drug used most frequently as a single agent for advanced soft tissue sarcomas is the anthracycline Adriamycin (doxorubicin), a glycoside antibiotic originally isolated as a fermentation product of the fungus *Streptomyces peucetius* var. *caesius*.[11] While this agent is usually given in a dose of 60 to 75 mg per M^2 intravenously every 3 to 4 weeks,[4, 46, 77, 78, 89, 100, 112] Bonadonna (1975)[14] developed a regimen consisting of an induction course followed by weekly administra-

TABLE 17–1. Adriamycin as a Single Agent in Advanced Soft Tissue Sarcomas

Reference	Number of Patients	PR	CR	PR + CR
Savlov, 1981	88			14
Beretta, 1976	52			12
Omura, 1978	51			15
Bonadonna, 1975	50	11	0	11
O'Bryan, 1973	45			13
Mitts, 1979	43	13	5	18
Weiss, 1976	42	14	4	18
Gottlieb, 1975	42	14	1	15
Cruz, 1979	41	6	1	7
Rosenbaum, 1977	39	8	3	11
Gottlieb, 1975	34	9	1	10
Benjamin, 1975	25	4	6	10
Piver, 1979	17	1	0	1
Benjamin, 1974	17	7	0	7
Van Dyk, 1976	11	3	2	5
Barlow, 1973	7	5	0	5
TOTAL	604			172 (28%)

PR, partial remission
CR, complete remission

tion of smaller doses of Adriamycin which has been used, with some modification, by various investigators in soft tissue sarcomas.[33, 70, 115] Dose-limiting toxicities include myelosuppression, stomatitis, nausea, and vomiting; alopecia occurs in nearly all patients, and cardiac damage becomes a significant problem at cumulative doses above 550 mg per M^2.[11]

The results of sixteen trials of Adriamycin in soft tissue sarcomas are presented in Table 17–1. (In this and all other tables in this chapter, attempts have been made to exclude those patients with bony sarcomas and pediatric sarcomas from the reported series.) There were a total of 172 objective responses among the 604 patients, for a collective response rate of 28%. However, there is considerable variation in the response rate from series to series; even among the largest series of 40 or more patients, the fraction of objective responders varies from 16%[100] to 36%,[46] and the lower dose/frequent administration regimens similarly yield responses ranging from 17%[33] to 43%.[115] The variation in response rate from series to series may be a reflection of the histologic heterogeneity of the different groups of patients. However, the EORTC has analyzed its data regarding factors predicting response to combination chemotherapy in soft tissue sarcomas and has discovered that the most important factor predicting response is the pretreatment performance status of the patients.[20] It is very likely that the same is true for Adriamycin response and that the variation in the response to Adriamycin from group to group is best explained by variation in the general condition of the patients prior to treatment. Adriamycin given by continuous infusion plus radiotherapy is effective in advanced localized soft tissue sarcoma, perhaps through a radiosensitizing effect.[94]

Median response durations for the Adriamycin studies range from 12 to 36 weeks.[6, 7, 14, 78, 100] Several investigators have noted that the Adriamycin-responders survive longer than the nonresponders.[7, 46, 115]

Many other drugs have been evaluated for activity in adult soft tissue sarcomas, although none has been studied as extensively as Adriamycin. The activity of some of these other cytotoxic agents is summarized in Table 17–2.

The chemotherapeutic agent 5-(3,3-dimethyl-1-triazeno) imidazole-4-carboxamide, or DTIC, is a triazene whose major toxicities are gastrointestinal and hematologic.[62] The use of DTIC as a single agent in the treatment of soft tissue sarcomas has been reviewed by Gottlieb (1976);[48] from the data presented in Table 17–2, it is apparent that the response rate is approximately 18%. The major role of DTIC in sarcoma chemotherapy has been as a part of combination chemotherapy rather than as a single agent.

Ifosfamide has been recently introduced as an agent active in soft tissue sarcoma.[25, 65, 75] It will produce significant complete and partial remissions of disease with median response durations upwards of 11 months. An advantage to this agent is its apparent lack of cross-resistance to cyclophosphamide and perhaps, too, its therapeutic advantage over cyclophosphamide. It may replace cyclophosphamide in combination regimens with Adriamycin.[21]

Various nitrosoureas, whose dose-limiting toxicities are mainly hematologic, have been used as single agents in patients with advanced soft tissue sarcomas who have failed other therapy. Collected series are reported in Table 17–2. Chlorozotocin appears to be an inactive agent,[73, 102] and methyl CCNU also has minimal activity.[27, 32, 87] CCNU has a response rate of approximately 11%.

Methotrexate in low doses has a response rate of approximately 37% in previously untreated patients.[106] Because high-dose methotrexate with leucovorin rescue has been reported as useful in the adjuvant therapy of bony sarcomas,[42] Karakousis treated a series of soft tissue sarcomas with this regimen. His patients had been previously treated with combination chemotherapy; in this group of patients, the effectiveness of high-dose methotrexate with leucovorin rescue was minimal.[57]

There has been considerable interest in cisplatin in soft tissue sarcomas, particularly as salvage therapy. However, six studies[18, 29, 51, 55, 99, 107] that have evaluated the effectiveness of this drug given systemically in sarcoma patients have not been encouraging: the overall response rate is only 7%.

Of the other cytotoxic agents tested in large groups of sarcoma patients, only

TABLE 17–2. Other Single Agents in Advanced Soft Tissue Sarcomas

Drug	*Number of Patients*	*PR*	*CR*	*PR + CR*	*Reference*
DTIC	134	21	4	25	Gottlieb, 1976; Luce, 1970
	53	8	1	9	Gottlieb, 1976
	187			34 (18%)	TOTAL
Methotrexate	41	9	6	15	Subramanian, 1978
	18	0	1	1	Karakousis, 1980
	59			16 (27%)	TOTAL
Cisplatin	50	3	1	4	Samson, 1979
	17	0	0	0	Bramwell, 1979
	13	1	2	3	Karakousis, 1979
	8	0	0	0	Tekuzman, 1976
	5	0	0	0	Hayes, 1977
	3	0	0	0	Corder, 1977
	96			7 (7%)	TOTAL
MAMSA	26	1	0	1	Yap, 1981
	2	1	0	1	Woodcock, 1980
	23	1	0	1	Sordillo, 1980
	51			3 (6%)	TOTAL
Carminomycin	48	13	0	13 (27%)	Perevodchekova, 1977
Vindesine	46	3	0	3 (7%)	Sordillo, 1981
Metoprine	46	2	2	4 (9%)	Magill, 1981
Prednimustine	25	2	1	3 (12%)	Karakousis, 1982
ICRF 159	34	1	0	1 (3%)	Borden, 1980
Methyl CCNU	20	1	0	1	Chang, 1976
	11*	0	0	0	Creagan, 1976
	31			1 (3%)	TOTAL
CCNU	26	5	0	5	Mitts, 1979
	55			4	Rivkin, 1981
	81			9 (11%)	TOTAL
Chlorozotocin	22	0	0	0	Mouridsen, 1981
	27	0	0	0	Sordillo, 1981
	49			0 (0%)	TOTAL
Cycloleucine	9	0	0	0	Mitts, 1979
	89			8	Savlov, 1981
	11	0	0	0	Baker, 1981
	109			8 (7%)	TOTAL
Hexamethylmelamine	40	3	0	3 (8%)	Borden, 1977
VP-16-213	5	2	0	2 (40%)	Nissen, 1975

TABLE 17–3. Inactive Single Agents in Soft Tissue Sarcomas

Baker's antifol (Thigpen, 1977)
Azotomycin (Chang, 1977)
Pyrazofurin (Cormier, 1980; Gralla, 1978)
Dianhydrogalactitol (Thigpen, 1979)
5-Azacytidine (Mitts, 1979)
Anguidine (Thigpen, 1981)
Dibromodulcitol (Borden, 1980)
Maytansine (Wasserman, 1981; Borden, 1980)
Gallium nitrate (Sacki, 1981)
Diglycoaldehyde (Vosika, 1981)
Piperazinedione (Presant, 1982)
Vinblastine (Yap, 1983)
Etoposide (Welt, 1983)
Mitoxantrone (Smith, 1983)
Aziridinylbenzoquinone-AZQ (Zidar, 1985)

carminomycin[80] and prednimustine[54] have response rates over 10%. It must be remembered that most of the patients who have received these drugs have been heavily pretreated with other forms of chemotherapy; this may in part explain the low response rates. Adriamycin was found to be superior to carminomycin when the drugs were compared in a randomized EORTC clinical trial.[19] Epirubicin appears to be as effective as Adriamycin given in the same dose schedule.[74] This was true for both response rate and survival. Gastrointestinal and hematologic toxicity with epirubicin was less than for Adriamycin. A list of agents that showed no activity in series of more than ten soft tissue sarcoma patients is given in Table 17–3.

In an effort to increase the response rate and lengthen the remissions obtained in soft tissue sarcomas, various combination chemotherapeutic regimens have been developed (see Tables 17–4 to 17–7). Unfortunately, the VAC (vincristine, Actinomycin D, cyclophosphamide) regimen, which is quite effective in childhood sarcomas,[67] proved much less useful in the treatment of sarcomas in adults,[32, 53, 89] so other combinations were investigated.

Based on clinical studies showing the activity of Adriamycin and DTIC used separately, and laboratory evidence for synergy between the two drugs in rodents, Gottlieb (1972) developed a combination regimen using these two agents as follows: Adriamycin (60 mg per M^2) intravenously on day 1 and DTIC (250 mg per M^2) intravenously on days 1 through 5, with the cycle repeating every 21 days. The overall response for the initial series of 78 soft tissue sarcomas was 42%,

TABLE 17–4. Adriamycin Plus DTIC in Advanced Soft Tissue Sarcomas

Reference	Number of Patients	PR	CR	PR + CR
Baker, 1979	81			18
Gottlieb, 1972; Gottlieb, 1975	171	56	22	78
Omura, 1978	40			11
Foley, 1975	27	7	3	10
Beretta, 1976	21	8	4	12
Bonadonna, 1975	18			9
Saiki, 1982	93	13	6	19
TOTAL	451			157 (35%)

PR, partial response
CR, complete response

with 6% of the patients achieving complete remissions.[47] This response rate is not unlike that produced by Adriamycin alone, in the series from several institutions;[6, 7, 70, 112, 115] the issue was therefore raised as to whether the added nausea, vomiting, and myelosuppression (especially thrombocytopenia) from DTIC could be justified.

Sarcoma patients at the M.D. Anderson Hospital and in the Southwest Oncology Group (SWOG) continued to be treated with the Adriamycin-DTIC combination, and the results of these trials were analyzed in 1976. Gottlieb compared the response rates, duration of remission, and survival of patients treated with Adriamycin as a single agent with the results of the Adriamycin-DTIC combination. Because the addition of vincristine to Adriamycin and DTIC in another SWOG study did not change the survival or response rate compared with the two drug regimens, he added those patients' data to the Adriamycin-DTIC group. The response rate of the patients treated with Adriamycin alone was approximately 31%; that of the patients who received DTIC in addition to Adriamycin was 42%. The median survival of the Adriamycin group was 6 months and

TABLE 17–5. CYVADIC in Soft Tissue Sarcomas

Reference	Number of Patients	PR	CR	PR + CR
Bernard, 1982	13	0	1	1
Yap, 1980	125	42	21	63
Bodey, 1981	43	19	11	30
Pinedo, 1982	84	18	14	32
Giuliano, 1978	20	1	2	3
Pinedo, 1982*	78	7	4	11
TOTAL	363	87 (24%)	53 (15%)	140 (39%)

*Cycling regimen

TABLE 17–6. Other Adriamycin-Containing Combination Regimens for Soft Tissue Sarcomas

Regimen	Number of Patients	PR	CR	PR + CR	Reference
Adriamycin, DTIC, vincristine	31	2	1	3	Creagan, 1976
	86	32	8	40	Gottlieb, 1975
	117			43 (37%)	TOTAL
Adriamycin, cylophosphamide, vincristine	38	4	1	5 (13%)	Rosenbaum, 1977
Adriamycin, cisplatin	3	1	0	1 (33%)	Higby, 1977
Adriamycin, cyclophosphamide	6	1	0	1 (17%)	Higby, 1977
Cyclophosphamide, Adriamycin, cisplatin	20	4	1	5 (25%)	Cormier, 1980
CYVADACT	175	47	21	68 (39%)*	Benjamin, 1976
Adriamycin, cyclophosphamide, actinomycin D, DTIC	20	4		4	Daley, 1981
	29	6		6	Creagan, 1978
	49			10 (20%)	TOTAL
Adriamycin, methotrexate, DTIC	22	6	3	9 (41%)	Subramanian, 1978
Adriamycin, vincristine, methotrexate	14	2	1	3	Kaufman, 1977
	13	4	1	5	Biano, 1974
	27			8 (30%)	TOTAL
Adriamycin, vincristine, methotrexate, DTIC	5	2	0	2 (40%)	Kaufman, 1977
Adriamycin, vincristine, actinomycin D, methotrexate, leucovorin	34			15 (44%)	Magill, 1977
Vincristine, methotrexate, leucovorin, Adriamycin, actinomycin D, DTIC, chlorambucil	33			9 (27%)	Magill, 1977
Adriamycin, actinomycin D	19	4	2	6 (32%)	Brenner, 1981
Adriamycin, vincristine, methyl CCNU	42			11 (26%)	Magill, 1977
Adriamycin, methotrexate	67			11 (16%)	Bull, 1976
Adriamycin, cyclophosphamide, DTIC	23	9	4	13 (56%)	Blum, 1980
Adriamycin, bleomycin	3	1	0	1 (33%)	Barlow, 1973
Adriamycin, vincristine, cyclophosphamide, methotrexate, actinomycin D	37	3	2	5 (14%)	Bryant, 1980
Adriamycin, cyclophosphamide, vincristine, actinomycin D	18			8 (44%)	Matejovsky, 1980
Adriamycin, vindesine, cyclophosphamide	23	6	5	11 (48%)	Brenner, 1983
Adriamycin, cyclophosphamide, methotrexate	100			36 (36%)	Lowenbraun, 1977
Adriamycin, methyl CCNU	50	19	4	23 (46%)	Rivkin, 1980
Adriamycin, cyclophosphamide, cisplatin	15	0	6	6 (33.5%)	Edmonson, 1983

TABLE 17–7. Combinations Without Adriamycin for Soft Tissue Sarcomas

Regimen	*Number of Patients*	*PR*	*CR*	*PR + CR*	*Reference*
Actinomycin D, LPAM	25	1		1 (4%)	Cruz, 1979
Actinomycin D, LPAM, vincristine	26			0 (0%)	Cruz, 1979
Actinomycin D, LPAM, NSC 1026	25			0 (%)	Cruz, 1979
Vincristine, actinomycin D, cyclophosphamide, mithramycin	2	1		1 (50%)	Jacobs, 1970
Methyl CCNU, actinomycin D	28	3	1	4 (14%)	Yap, 1981
Cyclophosphamide, vincristine, methotrexate	28	1	3	4	Beretta, 1976
	19			2	Bonadonna, 1976
	47			6 (13%)	TOTAL
5-FU, methotrexate, vincristine, cyclophosphamide	6	1	1	2	Mitts, 1979
	10	0	0	0	Gerner, 1973
	16			2 (13%)	TOTAL
5-FU, methotrexate, vincristine, cyclophosphamide, prednisone	27	10	0	10 (37%)	Mitts, 1979
Cyclophosphamide, 5-FU, vincristine, actinomycin D, methotrexate	12	5	3	8 (67%)	Subramanian, 1978
Cyclophosphamide, actinomycin D, vincristine	38	1	1	2	Rosenbaum, 1977
	61	4	1	5	Creagan, 1976
	13	6	1	7	Jacobs, 1980
	112			14 (13%)	TOTAL

PR, partial response
CR, complete response

that of the group who also received DTIC was 10 months ($p < 0.001$). The median duration of remission for the Adriamycin group (4 months) was also inferior to that of the DTIC group (5.5+ months). From this analysis, Gottlieb concluded that DTIC enhances the response rate compared with that seen with Adriamycin alone, and more importantly, prolongs remission duration and survival.[48]

However, Gottlieb's conclusions were drawn from a comparison of the Adriamycin-DTIC group with a historical control group treated with the single agent Adriamycin. Given the wide variation in response rate (16% to 43%) and remission duration (12 to 36 weeks) in the larger Adriamycin series cited in Table 17–1, the validity of Gottlieb's comparisons must be suspect. In a randomized series that compared Adriamycin to the two-drug combination Adriamycin-DTIC in a group of patients with uterine sarcomas; the response to Adriamycin was not significantly different from that of Adriamycin plus DTIC; the progression-free intervals were similar and survival figures did not differ significantly. The addition of DTIC increased the incidence of major gastrointestial toxicity and the frequency of major hematologic toxicity.[79] There was, therefore, no advantage found for the two-drug combination over Adriamycin alone.

From the data in Table 17–4, it is clear that the Adriamycin plus DTIC regimen is active, and indeed the collective response rate for the 451 patients (35%) is higher than the 28% collective response to Adriamycin alone (Table 17–1). The Eastern Cooperative Oncology Group has demonstrated a modest improvement in overall response with the two-drug regimen over Adriamycin alone, but median survival and frequency of complete remission were not significantly enhanced.[17] As in the Omura study, gastrointestinal and hematologic toxicity were more frequent with the two-drug combination.

The best-studied combination after Adriamycin-DTIC is the CYVADIC regimen developed at the M.D. Anderson Hospital. It consists of cyclophosphamide (500 mg per M^2) and Adriamycin (50 mg per M^2) intravenously on day 1, DTIC (250 mg per M^2) intravenously on days 1 through 5, and vincristine (1.5 mg per M^2) intravenously on days 1 and 5.[118] CYVADIC has yielded response rates from 30 to 70%, with median duration of response from 18 to 63 weeks.[9, 13, 20, 44, 118] Experience with this combination in soft tissue sarcomas is summarized in Table 17–5, which includes some variations on the original regimen, including a "one-day" version developed at the M.D. Anderson Hospital by Bernard (1982), which resulted in a lower response rate than the previous schedule.[9] Bodey (1981) developed a schedule of dose escalations that required a protected environment and prophylactic antibiotics;[13] dose escalation was rewarded by a higher complete remission rate (33% versus 15%) but a similar overall response rate (71% versus 67%) compared with the standard regimen.[13] The EORTC compared the standard CYVADIC schedule to a cycling regimen that consisted of cyclophosphamide (1200 mg per M^2) and vincristine (1.4 mg per M^2) intravenously on day 1 alternated with Adriamycin (50 mg per M^2) intravenously on day 1 and DTIC (250 mg per M^2) intravenously on days 1 through 5, with the cycles given every 4 weeks.[82, 83] The standard regimen produced more complete remissions (17% versus 5%) and more objective responses (38% versus 14%) than the cycling regimen.[20]

Even if the EORTC cycling regimen is excluded from consideration, it is clear that the response rates achieved by the M.D. Anderson Hospital and the SWOG (94 of 181, or 52%)[9, 13, 118] exceed those observed elsewhere; the collective response rate for the EORTC and UCLA is 35 of 104, or 34%.[20, 44] There are a few possible explanations for this difference. Bramwell concluded from analysis of the EORTC data that pretreatment performance status was the most important predictor of response to CYVADIC; the response rate for patients with a Karnofsky score of 90 to 100 was 41%, while the response rate for those with a score of 50 to 80 was only 14%.[20] If the SWOG and M.D. Anderson patients had higher performance scores than the UCLA and EORTC patients, the differences in response rates would in part be explained. Further, Bodey demonstrated that higher doses resulting in leukopenia resulted in higher complete response rates,[13] and Bramwell showed that dose reductions for elderly patients were associated with lower complete response rates.[20] It is possible that there may have been dose reductions to avoid leukopenia in the EORTC and UCLA studies that lowered the response rates. It becomes important to know the true response rate to CYVADIC when one realizes that the effectiveness of this regimen in the EORTC and at UCLA falls within the range achievable by Adriamycin alone, at the expense of considerably more toxicity. However, the impressive complete response rate from the M.D. Anderson studies and the fact that some complete responders remain free of disease for extended periods (median, 37+ months)[122] make the CYVADIC regimen quite attractive. More recent studies by other groups have reported a 23% overall response rate for CYVADIC in sarcomas of the female genital tract, most patients previously treated with chemotherapy,[81] and a response rate of 34% for patients with advanced soft tissue sarcoma not previously treated.[85]

Many other combination regimens have been devised and are summarized in Tables 17–6 and 17–7. CYVADACT, in which actinomycin D was substituted for cyclophosphamide in the CYVADIC combination, was shown in randomized study to be slightly inferior to CYVADIC for soft tissue sarcomas. The methyl CCNU and Adriamycin combination (MAD) developed by SWOG yielded a relatively high response rate of 46% in 50 patients with soft tissue sarcomas and was more convenient for patients than CYVADIC because it required fewer clinic visits and fewer injections.[88]

A comparison of Table 17–6 and Table 17–7 suggests that the Adriamycin-containing combinations are much more effective than combinations that lack this drug. Despite the large number of combinations and single drugs tested in soft tissue sarcoma patients, it is clear that Adriamycin is still the most important cytotoxic agent in this disease. Moreover, randomized studies comparing Adriamycin alone versus Adriamycin-containing regimens have not shown any consistently convincing advantage for combination chemotherapy over Adriamycin alone. Studies to the contrary have been almost without exception retrospective or prospective but not randomized.

ADJUVANT SYSTEMIC CHEMOTHERAPY

Because of the relatively high rate of distant metastases in patients with soft tissue sarcomas treated locally, several investigators have used systemic chemotherapy after local excision and/or radiation therapy. Two early randomized studies showed no benefit for adjuvant systemic therapy in adults with soft tissue sarcomas. The first study, done at the M.D. Anderson Hospital,[60] included adult patients with extremity and trunk soft tissue sarcomas thought to be at high risk for recurrence (i.e., with lesions 5 cm or larger and grade 2 or 3). These patients were randomly assigned to adjuvant chemotherapy or not, after local surgery and radiation. The 19-month VACAR chemotherapeutic regimen was as follows: vincristine (1.5 mg per M^2 up to 2 mg) intravenously on day 1 and weekly for 9 weeks, then on day 1 of each cycle; Adriamycin (60 mg per M^2) intravenously on day 2 and every 4 weeks for seven doses (cumulative dose limit, 420 mg per M^2); cyclosphosphamide (200 mg per M^2) orally on days 3, 4, and 5 every 4 weeks with Adriamycin and then every 8 weeks with actinomycin D; actinomycin D (0.3 mg per M^2; top dose, 0.5 mg) intravenously on days 1 through 5 of each cycle every 8 weeks for six courses over one year, after the allowed cumulative Adriamycin dose was reached. Twenty patients were randomized to the control group and 27 to the adjuvant chemotherapy group. With a follow-up of 9 to 34 months, 17 of 20 control patients and 18 of 27 chemotherapy patients were free of disease. The incidence of distant metastases was 9 of 27 in the chemotherapy group and 3 of 20 in the control group. Signs of toxicity of the VACAR regimen included nausea, vomiting, and alopecia in nearly 100%, augmented skin reactions within the radiated field, leukopenia, and three episodes of congestive heart failure, of which two may have been Adriamycin-related. Cyclophosphamide-induced hemorrhagic cystitis developed in one patient. These results were disturbing to the investigators, since the incidence of distant metastases in the adjuvant chemotherapy group was more than twice that of the control group, with substantial toxicity leading to no discernible benefit.

The other randomized study that showed no benefit for adjuvant chemotherapy in sarcomas included 12 patients with early uterine sarcomas treated surgically who were randomly assigned to a control group or an Adriamycin regimen (60 to 75 mg per M^2 every 4 weeks for 6 months). Distant metastases developed in two of the six patients in the Adriamycin group and life-threatening congestive heart failure in two. Distant metastases developed in two of the six women in the control group. Again, substantial toxicity was incurred with no reduction in the frequency of distant metastases. Omura et al. also failed to demonstrate benefit for Adriamycin versus no adjuvant chemotherapy in a randomized trial involving 159 patients with uterine sarcomas.[78]

At least four nonrandomized studies, however, have suggested some benefit from adjuvant chemotherapy, compared with historical controls treated with surgery alone. Rosenberg's studies at the National Cancer Institute treated all patients with adjuvant chemotherapy plus or minus *C. parvum*, after they had been randomly assigned to amputation or limb-sparing local therapy.[90–93] The chemotherapy included Adriamycin (50 to 70 mg per M^2) intravenously and cyclophosphamide (500 to 700 mg per M^2) intravenously on day 1 every 3 weeks; after a cumulative Adriamycin dosage of 530 mg per M^2 was reached (usually after 8 to 9 months), monthly methotrexate (250 mg per kg) with leucovorin rescue was substituted for the Adriamycin and cyclophosphamide, for a total of six doses. In addition, the immunotherapy group received intravenous *C. parvum*, 5 mg per M^2 on day 21, and subcutaneous *C. parvum*, 1.5 mg per M^2 on days 23, 25, and 27. By 1977 it was clear that there was no difference between the chemoimmunotherapy and chemotherapy groups, and they were subsequently analyzed together. With a minimum 3-year follow-up, the 5-year disease-free survival for the patients treated with adjuvant systemic therapy is 74%, compared with 41% for historical controls treated only with surgery. Overall survival in the chemotherapy group is 84% at 3 years, compared with 53% in the historical control group. Both of these differences are statistically significant ($p < 0.001$).[93]

Townsend (1976)[111] reported that postoperative adjuvant chemotherapy with Adriamycin plus high-dose methotrexate with leucovorin rescue lowered the rate of recurrence from 14 of 19 (77%) in a concomitant control group to 5 of 16 (32%) in the chemotherapy group. This was not a randomized study, however.

Sordillo (1978)[105] reported a six-drug combination known as ALOMAD (vincristine, methotrexate with leucovorin rescue, DTIC, chlorambucil, actinomycin D, and Adriamycin) used in the adjuvant setting. Of 19 patients treated after primary surgery, 18 were free of disease 3 to 34 months later. Six of eight patients treated with ALOMAD after surgery for local recurrence were disease-free 4 to 33 months later. The investigators concluded that ALOMAD prolonged disease-free survival after surgery, although their study does not include controls treated with surgery alone.

Das Gupta (1982)[35] designed a nonrandomized prospective study in which chemotherapy was used as an adjuvant to surgery in the initial treatment of adults with primary soft tissue sarcomas; the results are compared with those of a group of patients with similar histologic types treated with surgery alone. Chemotherapy included Adriamycin (60 mg per M^2) intravenously on day 1 and DTIC (250 mg per M^2) intravenously on days 1 through 5, repeated every 22 days. Adriamycin was given to a total cumulative dose of 500 mg per M^2 and the DTIC was continued for a total of 1 year. In the adjuvant group, 87 of 133 (77%) were disease-free at 2 years, compared with 85 of 144 (59%) of the control group. Of the patients eligible for 5-year survival analysis, 74% were disease-free in the chemotherapy group compared with 50% of the control group.

A randomized study conducted at the Mayo Clinic showed a decrease in the frequency of hematogenous metastases in a group of sarcoma patients given adjuvant chemotherapy. The regimen used is as follows: vincristine, cyclophosphamide, and actinomycin D, alternated with vincristine, Adriamycin, and DTIC at 6-week intervals. At 2 years, hematogenous metastases had occurred in only 1 of 30 patients who received chemotherapy but in 7 of 31 who were treated with surgery alone.[38] There was no increase, however, in the frequency of local recurrence in the chemotherapy group (30%) compared with the controls treated only locally (32%). At 4 years, 92% of the adjuvant therapy group and 82% of the controls survived. The exceptionally good survival in both groups points up the need for randomized prospective studies with untreated controls to evaluate the effectiveness of adjuvant chemotherapy in the adult soft tissue sarcomas[39] rather than relying on historical controls.

Sarcoma patients treated with limb-sparing resection together with adjuvant radiation therapy appear to have the same disease-free and overall survival rates as patients treated with amputation alone when both groups are given adjuvant chemotherapy consisting of Adriamycin, cyclophosphamide, and high-dose methotrexate.[93] The Rosenberg study conducted at the National Cancer Institute was a randomized clinical trial and by itself provides strong support for the position that adult patients with soft tissue sarcoma of the extremity should receive adjuvant chemotherapy. There was, however, a relatively high incidence of cardiomyopathy associated with the therapy given, which included doxorubicin.[37] This should prompt caution in the use of adjuvant chemotherapy for soft tissue sarcomas. A role for adjuvant chemotherapy in soft tissue sarcoma, even of the extremity, will not be established until multi-institutional studies are conducted with large numbers of randomized patients (with randomization to include a nontreated control group) and longer median times for follow-up. At the present time, adjuvant chemotherapy cannot be recommended as the standard or conventional treatment for resected soft tissue sarcomas.

Chemotherapy with an Adriamycin-containing regimen followed by surgery alone and additional chemotherapy may be more effective than chemotherapy alone in prolonging time to progression and overall survival.[95, 123] This form of "neo-adjuvant" therapy requires further clinical evaluation.

REGIONAL CHEMOTHERAPY OF SOFT TISSUE SARCOMAS

Another approach to the chemotherapy of soft tissue sarcomas has been local perfusion, either via an extracorporeal isolation-perfusion system,[69] or infusion via the artery supplying the affected limb, e.g., the femoral artery.[26, 40, 45, 50, 59, 71, 72] This regional chemotherapy is often combined with other treatment modalities; the aim is often to permit limb-sparing surgery or to convert an inoperable tumor to one of a size that will permit surgery.

McBride reported a series of 89 perfusions in 85 patients with soft tissue sarcomas, mostly using Alkeran or actinomycin D.[69] Canine studies at Roswell Park[36] have shown that the highest tissue levels of infused drug are obtained by the isolation-perfusion technique as used by McBride, as compared with systemic chemotherapy or femoral artery infusion. In McBride's series, patients received preoperative regional chemotherapy in order to decrease the magnitude of the surgery to be performed. For the 72 patients with at least 5-year follow-up, there was a regional recurrence rate of 20%, and systemic metastases were found in 18%. Complications of perfusion for the 85 patients included one death from pulmonary embolus, four with edema of the limb, one major skin slough, one major wound infection, and nine who required subsequent amputation.

Intra-arterial Adriamycin produced an objective response in four of seven sarcoma patients at UCLA.[50] This lead has been studied further by several investigators. Morton and Eilber have used intra-arterial Adriamycin infusion and radiation therapy in order to permit limb-sparing surgery in patients who would otherwise require amputation.[40, 71, 72]

Krementz treated 17 patients with preoperative regional infusions of melphalan, nitrogen mustard, actinomycin D, or combinations of these drugs; 6 of 17 had tumor regressions of greater than 50%. Two of eight stage I lesions and seven of eight stage II lesions had tumor reductions sufficient to permit conservative surgery; one stage III tumor had a response permitting a hemipelvectomy. Complications included wound infection, thrombophlebitis, neuropathy, and pulmonary embolus. In a group of 73 patients in whom regional chemotherapy was given as an adjunct to surgery in order to decrease the local recurrence rate, the 5-year disease-free survival for 49 stage I lesions was 66%, and for 24 stage II lesions, 59%. Use of regional chemotherapy without surgery for 39 patients resulted in eight partial and four complete responses.

Giuliano reports that a group of 16 patients given preoperative radiation and intra-arterial Adriamycin were then able to undergo limb-salvage procedures. After resection, there have been no local recurrences; the length of follow-up is unclear from this report, however.[44] Intra-arterial doxorubicin given preoperatively has been shown to produce extensive areas of necrosis in limb sarcomas.

Cisplatin has been administered regionally in at least two groups of sarcoma patients. Mavligit gave intra-arterial cisplatin to a group of 23 patients with inoperable bone and soft tissue sarcomas, and assessed response both radiographically and histopathologically (by grading tumor necrosis). The overall response rate was 53% (two complete and seven partial responses); four patients were rendered suitable for limb-sparing surgery, and one was able to undergo a hemipelvectomy.[68] Calvo treated a group of ten bone sarcoma and soft tissue sarcoma patients with intra-arterial cisplatin, and achieved three partial and one complete response.[26]

All of the reports regarding regional chemotherapy are somewhat difficult to interpret. Other treatment modalities are combined with local chemotherapy to varying degrees, and there is of necessity a considerable amount of judgment required in the selection of appropriate patients for such procedures. Nevertheless, it appears that regional perfusion, particularly with Adriamycin, may make conservative surgery possible in a number of cases without sacrificing local control.

REFERENCES

1. Azzarelli A., Quagliuolo V., Audisio R. A., et al.: Intra-arterial Adriamycin followed by surgery for limb sarcomas: Preliminary report. Eur. J. Cancer Clin. Oncol. 19:885–890, 1983
2. Baker L., Benjamin R., Fine G., et al.: Combination chemotherapy in the management of disseminated soft tissue sarcomas: A Southwest Oncology Group (SWOG) study. Proc. Am. Soc. Clin. Oncol. 20:378, 1979
3. Baker L. H., Fraile J., Samson K., Cummings G.: Phase II evaluation of cycloleucine in the treatment of patients with disseminated sarcomas. Cancer Treat. Rep. 65:358–359, 1981
4. Barlow J. J., Piver M. S., Chuang J. T., et al.: Adriamycin and bleomycin alone and in combination in gynecologic cancers. Cancer 32:735–743, 1973
5. Benjamin R. S., Gottlieb J. A., Baker L. O., Sinkovics J. G.: CYVADIC vs CYVADACT—A randomized trial of cyclophosphamide (CY), vincristine (V), and Adriamycin (A), plus dacarbazine (DIC), or actinomycin-D (DACT) in metastatic sarcomas. Proc. Am. Soc. Clin. Oncol. 17:256, 1976
6. Benjamin R. S., Wiernik P. H., Bachur N. R.: Adriamycin chemotherapy—Efficacy, safety, and pharmacologic basis of an intermittent single high-dose schedule. Cancer 33:19–27, 1974
7. Benjamin R. S., Wiernik P. H., Bachur N. R.: Adriamycin: A new effective agent in the therapy of disseminated sarcomas. Med. Pediatr. Oncol. 1:63–76, 1975

8. Beretta G., Bonadonna G., Bajetta E., et al.: Combination chemotherapy with DTIC (NSC 45388) in advanced malignant melanoma, soft tissue sarcomas, and Hodgkin's disease. Cancer Treat. Rep. 60:205–211, 1976
9. Bernard S. A., Capizzi R. L., Rudnick S. A., et al.: A one-day combination chemotherapy (CYVADIC) regimen in soft tissue sarcomas. Proc. Am. Soc. Clin. Oncol. 1:170, 1982
10. Biano G., Lokich J. J., Frei E., III: Combined vincristine, Adriamycin, and methotrexate (VAM) therapy in soft tissue sarcomas (STS). Proc. Am. Soc. Clin. Oncol. 15:189, 1974
11. Blum R. H., Carter S. K.: Adriamycin: A new anticancer drug with significant clinical activity. Ann. Intern. Med. 80:249–259, 1974
12. Blum R. H., Corson J. M., Wilson R. E., et al.: Successful treatment of metastatic sarcomas with cyclophosphamide, Adriamycin, and DTIC (CAD). Cancer 46:1722–1726, 1980
13. Bodey G. P., Rodriguez V., Murphy W. K., et al.: Protected environment-prophylactic antibiotic program for malignant sarcomas: Randomized trial during remission induction chemotherapy. Cancer 47:2422–2429, 1981
14. Bonadonna G., Beretta G., Tancini G., et al.: III. Adriamycin (NSC 123127) studies at the Instituto Nazionale Tumori, Milan. Cancer Chemother. Rep. 6:231–245, 1975
15. Borden E. C., Larson P., Ansfield F. J., et al.: Hexamethylmelamine treatment of sarcomas and lymphomas. Med. Pediatr. Oncol. 3:401–406, 1977
16. Borden E., Ash A., Rosenbaum C., Lerner H.: Phase II evaluation of dibromoduicitol (DBD), ICRF159, and maytansine in sarcomas and mesotheliomas. Proc. Am. Soc. Clin. Oncol. 21:481, 1980
17. Borden E. C., Amato D., Enterline H. T., et al.: Randomized comparison of Adriamycin regimens for treatment of metastatic soft tissue sarcomas. Proc. Am. Soc. Clin. Oncol. 2:231, 1983
18. Bramwell V. H. C., Brugarolas A., Mouridsen H. T., et al.: E.O.R.T.C. Phase II study of cisplatin in CYVADIC resistant soft tissue sarcoma. Eur. J. Cancer 15:1511–1513, 1979
19. Bramwell V. H., Mouridsen H. T., Mulder J. H., et al.: Carminomycin vs Adriamycin in advanced soft tissue sarcomas: An EORTC randomized phase II study. Eur. J. Cancer Clin. Oncol. 19:1097–1104, 1983
20. Bramwell V. H. C., Mouridsen H. T., Somers R., et al.: EORTC: The influence of scheduling and performance status (PS) on chemotherapy of advanced soft tissue sarcoma with cyclophosphamide (CY), vincristine (V), Adriamycin (A), and DTIC (DIC). Proc. Am. Soc. Clin. Oncol. 1:23, 1982
21. Bramwell V., Mouridsen H. T., Santoro A., et al.: Cyclophosphamide (CP) vs Ifosfamide (IF): A randomized phase II trial in adult soft tissue sarcomas (STS): Preliminary report of EORTC soft tissue and bone sarcoma group. Proc. Am. Soc. Clin. Oncol. 4:143, 1985
22. Brenner J., Magill G. B., Wissel P., and Sordillo P. P.: Chemotherapy of patients with advanced soft tissue sarcoma with use of DVA (vindesine sulfate), Adriamycin and cyclophosphamide (DAC). Cancer 52:1142–1145, 1983
23. Bryant B. M., Wiltshaw E.: Results of the Royal Marsden Hospital Second Soft Tissue Sarcoma Schedule (STS II) chemotherapy regimen in the management of advanced sarcoma. Cancer Treat. Rep. 64:689–692, 1980
24. Bull F. E., Irwin L. E., Pugh R. P., Bateman J. R.: Phase I study of Adriamycin-methotrexate combination in sarcomas. Proc. Am. Soc. Clin. Oncol. 17:249, 1976
25. Burkert H.: Ifosfamide: European perspective. Semin. Oncol. 9:28–35, 1983
26. Calvo D. B., III, Batt Y. Z., Wallace S., et al.: Phase I-II trial for percutaneous intraarterial cisdiamminedichloroplatinum (II) for regionally confined malignancy. Cancer 45:1278–1283, 1980
27. Chang P., Levine M. A., Wiernik P. H., Walker M. D.: A phase II study of intravenously administered methyl CCNU in the treatment of advanced sarcomas. Cancer 27:615–619, 1976
28. Chang P., Wiernik P. H.: Phase II study of azotomycin in sarcomas. Cancer Treat. Rep. 61:1719–1720, 1977
29. Corder M. P., Maguire L. C., Witte D. L., et al.: Weekly outpatient cisplatinum (II) diamminedichloride (CPDD) and diuresis with dose-limiting myelosuppression. Proc. Am. Soc. Clin. Oncol. 18:344, 1977
30. Cormier W. J., Hahn R. G., Edmonson J. H., Eagan R. T.: Phase II study in advanced sarcoma: Randomized trial of pyrazofurin versus combination cyclophosphamide, doxorubicin, and cis-diammine platinum (II) (CAP). Cancer Treat. Rep. 64:655–658, 1980
31. Creagan E. T., Edmonson J. H., Hahn R. G., et al.: A preliminary study of cyclophosphamide (NCS-26271), Adriamycin (NSC-123127), imidazole carboxamide (NSC-45388), and actinomycin D (NSC-3053) with or without MER-BCG in patients with advanced sarcomas. Med. Pediatr. Oncol. 4:85–96, 1978
32. Creagan E. T., Hahn R. G., Ahmann D. L., et al.: A comparative clinical trial evaluating the combination of Adriamycin, DTIC, and vincristine, the combination of actinomycin D, cyclophosphamide, and vincristine, and a single agent, methyl CCNU, in advanced sarcomas. Cancer Treat. Rep. 60:1385–1387, 1976
33. Cruz A. B., Thames E. A., Jr., Aust J. B., et al.: Combination chemotherapy for soft tissue sarcomas: A phase III study. J. Surg. Oncol. 11:313–323, 1979
34. Dalley D. N., Levi J. A., Nesbitt R. A., et al.: Cyclical combination chemotherapeutic regimen in adult soft tissue sarcoma. Cancer Clin. Trials 4:163–165, 1981
35. Das Gupta T. K., Patel M. K., Chaudhuri P. K., Briele H. A.: The role of chemotherapy as an adjuvant to surgery in the initial treatment of primary soft tissue sarcomas in adults. J. Surg. Oncol. 19:139–144, 1982
36. Didolkar M. S., Kanter P. M., Baffi R. R.: Comparison of regional versus systemic chemotherapy with Adriamycin. Ann. Surg. 187:332–336, 1978
37. Dresdale A., Bonow R. O., Wesley R., et al.: Prospective evaluation of doxorubicin-induced cardiomyopathy resulting from postsurgical adjuvant treatment of patients with soft tissue sarcomas. Cancer 52:51–60, 1983
38. Edmonson J. H., Fleming T. R., Ivins J. C., et al.: Reduced hematogenous metastasis in patients who receive systemic chemotherapy following excision of soft tissue sarcomas: Preliminary report. Proc. Am. Soc. Clin. Oncol. 21:193, 1980

39. Edmonson J. H., Hahn R. G., Schutt A. J., et al.: Cyclophosphamide, doxorubicin and cisplatin combined in the treatment of advanced sarcomas. Med. Pediatr. Oncol. 11:319–321, 1983
40. Eilber F. R.: Soft tissue sarcomas of the extremity. Curr. Probl. Cancer 8:29–31, 1984
41. Foley J. F., Kessinger A., Lemon H. M.: Prolonging the use of Adriamycin in the chemotherapy of sarcomas. Proc. Am. Soc. Clin. Oncol. 16:259, 1975
42. Frei E., III, Jaffe N., Tattersall M. H. N., et al.: New approaches to cancer chemotherapy with methotrexate. N. Engl. J. Med. 292:846–851, 1975
43. Gerner R. E., Moore, G. E.: Multiple-drug therapy for malignant solid tumors in adults. Cancer Chemother. Rep. 57:237–239, 1973
44. Giuliano A. E., Eilber F. R., Morton D. L.: Failure of combination chemotherapy (CYVADIC) in metastatic soft tissue sarcomas: Implications for adjuvant studies. Proc. Am. Soc. Clin. Oncol. 19:359, 1978
45. Golomb F. M., Postel A. H., Hall A. B., et al.: Chemotherapy of human cancer by regional perfusion: Report of 52 perfusions. Cancer 15:828–845, 1962
46. Gottlieb J. A., Baker L. H., O'Bryan R. M.: Adriamycin (NSC 123127) used alone and in combination for soft tissue and bony sarcomas. Cancer Chemother. Rep. 6:271–282, 1975
47. Gottlieb J. A., Baker L. H., Quagliana J. M., et al.: Chemotherapy of sarcomas with a combination of Adriamycin and dimethyl triazeno imidazole carboxamide. Cancer 30:1632–1683, 1972
48. Gottlieb J. A., Benjamin R. S., Baker L. H., et al.: Role of DTIC (NSC-45388) in the chemotherapy of sarcomas. Cancer Treat. Rep. 60:199–203, 1976
49. Gralla R. J., Sordillo P. P., Magill G. B.: Phase II evaluation of pyrazofurin in patients with metastatic sarcoma. Cancer Treat. Rep. 62:1573–1574, 1978
50. Haskell C. M., Eilber F. R., Moon D. L.: Adriamycin (NSC-123127) by arterial infusion. Cancer Chemother. Rep. 6:187–189, 1975
51. Hayes D. M., Cvitkovic E., Golbey R. B., et al.: High dose cisplatin diammine dichloride: Amelioration of renal toxicity by mannitol diuresis. Cancer 39:1372–1381, 1977
52. Higby D. J., Wilber D., Wallace H. J., Jr., et al.: Adriamycin-cyclophosphamide and Adriamycin-cis-dichlorodiammine platinum (II) combination chemotherapy in patients with advanced cancer. Cancer Treat. Rep. 61:869–873, 1977
53. Jacobs E.M.: Combination chemotherapy of metastatic testicular germinal cell tumors and soft part sarcomas. Cancer 25:324–332, 1970
54. Karakousis C. P., Didolkar J. L., Ambrus J. L., Holyoke E. D.: Prednimustine in advanced soft tissue sarcoma. Cancer Treat. Rep. 66:201–202, 1982
55. Karakousis C. P., Holtermann C. A., Holyoke E. D.: Cis-dichlorodiammine platinum (II) in metastatic soft tissue sarcomas. Cancer Treat. Rep. 63:2071–2075, 1979
56. Karakousis C. P., Lopez R., Catane R., et al.: Intraarterial Adriamycin in the treatment of soft tissue sarcomas. J. Surg. Oncol. 13:21–27, 1980
57. Karakousis C. P., Rao U., Carlson M.: High-dose methotrexate as secondary chemotherapy in metastatic soft tissue sarcoma. Cancer 46:1345–1348, 1980
58. Kaufman J. H., Catane R., Douglass H. O., Jr.: Combined Adriamycin, vincristine, and methotrexate. N.Y. State J. Med. 77:742–743, 1977
59. Krementz E. T., Carter R. D., Sutherland C. M., Hutton I.: Chemotherapy of sarcomas of the limbs by regional perfusion. Ann. Surg. 185:555–564, 1977
60. Lindberg R. D., Murphy W. K., Benjamin R. S., et al.: Adjuvant chemotherapy in the treatment of soft tissue sarcomas: A preliminary report. *In* M.D. Anderson Hospital and Tumor Institute (ed.): Management of Primary and Soft Tissue Tumors. Chicago, Year Book Publishers, 1977
61. Lowenbraun S., Moffitt S., Smalley R., Presant C.: Combination chemotherapy with Adriamycin, cyclophosphamide and methotrexate (ACM) in metastatic sarcoma. Proc. Am. Soc. Clin. Oncol. 18:286, 1977
62. Luce J. K., Thurman W. G., Isaacs B. L., Talley R. W.: Clinical trials with the antitumor agent 5-(3,3-dimethyl-1-triazeno) imidazole-4-carboxamide (NSC-45388). Cancer Chemother. Rep. 54:119–124, 1970
63. Magill G. B., Brenner J., Sordillo P. P., et al.: Phase II trials of metoprine (DDMP) in pretreated adults with advanced soft tissue sarcomas. Proc. Am. Soc. Clin. Oncol. 1:22, 1982
64. Magill G. B., Golbey R. B., Krakoff I. H.: Chemotherapy combinations in adult sarcomas. Proc. Am. Soc. Clin. Oncol. 18:332, 1977
65. Magrath I. T., Sandlund J. T., Rayner A., et al.: Treatment of recurrent sarcomas with Ifosfamide (IF). Proc. Am. Soc. Clin. Oncol. 4:136, 1985
66. Matejovsky Z.: Chemotherapy in complex treatmont of bonc and soft tissue sarcomas. Oncology 37:97–103, 1980
67. Maurer H. M.: The intergroup rhabdomyosarcoma study: Update. November 1978. Natl. Cancer Inst. Monogr. 56:61–68, 1981
68. Mavligit G. M., Benjamin R., Patt Y. Z., et al.: Intraarterial cisplatin for patients with inoperable skeletal tumors. Cancer 48:1–4, 1981
69. McBride C. M.: Regional chemotherapy for soft tissue sarcomas. *In* M.D. Anderson Hospital and Tumor Institute (ed.): Management of Primary and Soft Tissue Tumors. Chicago, Year Book Publishers, 1977
70. Mitts D. L., Gerhardt H., Armstrong D., et al.: Chemotherapy for advanced soft tissue sarcomas: Results of Phase I and II cooperative studies. Tex. Med. 75:43–47, 1979
71. Morton D. L., Eilber F. R., Townsend C. M., Jr., et al.: Limb salvage from a multidisciplinary treatment approach for skeletal and soft tissue sarcomas of the extremity. Ann. Surg. 184:268–278, 1976
72. Morton D. L., Eilber F. R., Weisenburger, T. H., et al.: Limb salvage using preoperative intraarterial Adriamycin and radiation therapy for extremity soft tissue sarcomas. Aust. N.Z. J. Surg. 48:56–59, 1978
73. Mouridsen H. T., Bramwell V. H. C., Lacave J., et al.: Treatment of advanced soft tissue sarcomas with chlorozotocin: A Phase II trial of the EORTC soft tissue and bone sarcoma group. Cancer Treat. Rep. 65:509–511, 1981
74. Mouridsen H. T., Somers R., Santoro A., et al.: Adriamycin vs 4′-epi-adriamycin in advanced soft tissue sarcomas: A randomized EORTC study. *In* Proceedings of the Fourth NCI-EORTC Sympo-

sium on New Drugs in Cancer Therapy. Brussels, 1983

75. Niederle N., Scheulen M. E., Cremer M., et al.: Ifosfamide in combination chemotherapy for sarcomas and testicular carcinomas. Cancer Treat. Rep. 10(A):129, 1983
76. Nissen N. I., Hansen H. H., Pedersen H., et al.: Clinical trial of the oral form of a new podophyllotoxin derivative, VP-16-213 (NSC-141540), in patients with advanced disease. Cancer Chemother. Rep. 59:1027–1029, 1975
77. O'Bryan R. M., Luce J. K., Talley R. W., et al.: Phase II evaluation of Adriamycin in human neoplasia. Cancer 32:1–8, 1973
78. Omura G. A., Blessing J. A., Major F., Sedlacek T. V.: A randomized trial of Adriamycin versus no adjuvant chemotherapy in stage I and stage II uterine sarcoma. J. Clin. Oncol., 3:1240–1245, 1985.
79. Omura G. A., Major F. J., Blessing J. A., et al.: A randomized study of Adriamycin with and without dimethyl triazenoimidazole carboxamide in advanced uterine sarcomas. Cancer 52:626–632, 1983
80. Perevodchikova N. I., Lichinitser M. R., Gorbunova V. A.: Phase I clinical study of carminomycin: Its activity against soft tissue sarcomas. Cancer Treat. Rep. 61:1705–1707, 1977
81. Pfeffer M. R., Sulkes A., Biran S.: Modified CYVADIC chemotherapy for soft tissue sarcomas (STS). *In* Proceedings of the 2nd European Conference on Clinical Oncology and Cancer Nursing, Pergamon Press, 1985.
82. Pinedo H. M., Vendrik C. P., Bramwell V. H. C., et al.: EORTC soft tissue and bone sarcoma group: Re-evaluation of the CYVADIC regimen for metastatic soft tissue sarcoma. Proc. Am. Soc. Clin. Oncol. 20:346, 1979
83. Pinedo H. M., Vendrik C. P. J., Bramwell V. H. C., et al.: Evaluation of adjuvant therapy in soft tissue sarcoma: A collaborative multidisciplinary approach. Eur. J. Cancer 15:811–820, 1979
84. Piver M. S., Barlow J. J., Lele S. B., Yazigi R.: Adriamycin in localized and metastatic uterine sarcomas. J. Surg. Oncol. 12:263–265, 1979
85. Piver M. S., DeEulis T. G., Lele S. B., Barlow J. J.: Cyclophosphamide, vincristine, adriamycin and dimethyl-triazeno imidazole carboxamide (CYVADIC) for sarcomas of the female genital tract. Gynecol. Oncol. 14:319–323, 1982
86. Presant C. A., Bartolucci A. A.: Phase II trial of piperazinedione in metastatic sarcoma. Am. J. Clin. Oncol. 5:185–187, 1982
87. Rivkin S. E.: Clinical trials of nitrosourea in metastatic sarcoma. *In* Prestayko A. W., Baker L. H., Crooke S. T., et al. (eds.): Nitrosoureas: Current Status and New Developments. New York, Academic Press, 1981
88. Rivkin S. E., Gottlieb J. A., Thigpen T., et al.: Methyl CCNU and Adriamycin for patients with metastatic sarcomas: A Southwest Oncology Group Study. Cancer 46:446–451, 1980
89. Rosenbaum C., Schoenfeld D.: Treatment of advanced soft tissue sarcoma. Proc. Am. Soc. Clin. Oncol. 18:287, 1977
90. Rosenberg S. A.: Treatment of soft tissue and bone sarcomas: Review of studies at the National Cancer Institute. Natl. Cancer Inst. Monogr. 56:241–244, 1981
91. Rosenberg S. A., Glatstein E. J.: Perspectives of the role of surgery and radiation therapy in the treatment of soft tissue sarcomas of the extremities. Semin. Oncol. 8:190–200, 1981
92. Rosenberg S. A., Kent H., Costa J., et al.: Prospective randomized evaluation of the role of limb sparing surgery, radiation therapy and adjuvant chemoimmunotherapy in the treatment of adult soft tissue sarcomas. Surgery 84:62–69, 1978
93. Rosenberg S. A., Tepper J., Glatstein E., et al.: The treatment of soft tissue sarcomas of the extremities: Prospective randomized evaluations of (1) limb sparing surgery plus radiation therapy compared with amputation and (2) the role of adjuvant chemotherapy. Ann. Surg. 196:305–315, 1982
94. Rosenthal C. J., Park H. S., Choi K., et al.: Effective therapy for advanced localized soft tissue sarcomas (STS): Adriamycin (ADR) by continuous infusion (CI) and concomitant radiation therapy (RT). Proc. Am. Soc. Clin. Oncol. 4:145, 1985
95. Rouesse J., Le Chevalier T., Contesso G., et al.: Chimiotherapie premiere dans les sarcomes des parties molles consideres comme inoperable. Sem. Hop. Paris 59:1441–1444, 1983
96. Russell W. O., Cohen J., Edmonson J. H., et al.: Staging system for soft tissue sarcoma. Semin. Oncol. 8:156–159, 1981
97. Saiki J. H., Rivkin S. E., Baker L. H., et al.: Adriamycin and single dose DTIC in soft tissue and bone sarcomas: A Southwest Oncology Group Study. Proc. Am. Soc. Clin. Oncol. 1:181, 1982
98. Saiki J. H., Stephens R., Fabian C., et al.: Phase II evaluation of gallium nitrate (NSC 15200) in soft tissue and bone sarcomas. Proc. Am. Soc. Clin. Oncol. 22:525, 1981
99. Samson M. K., Baker L. H., Benjamin R. S., et al.: Cis-dichlorodiammine-platinum (II) in advanced soft tissue and bone sarcomas: A Southwest Oncology Group Study. Cancer Treat. Rep. 63:2027–2029, 1979
100. Savlov E. D., MacIntyre J. M., Knight E., Wolter J.: Comparison of doxorubicin with cycloleucine in the treatment of sarcomas. Cancer Treat. Rep. 65:21–27, 1981
101. Smith I. E.: Mitoxantrone (novantrone): A review of experimental and early clinical studies. Cancer Treat. Rev. 10:103–115, 1983
102. Sordillo P. P., Magill G. B., Gralla R. J.: Chlorozotocin: Phase II evaluation in patients with advanced sarcomas. Cancer Treat. Rep. 65:513–514, 1981
103. Sordillo P. P., Magill G. B., Gralla R. J.: Phase II evaluation of vindesine sulfate in patients with advanced sarcomas. Cancer Treat. Rep. 65:515–516, 1981
104. Sordillo P. P., Magill G. B., Gralla R. J., Golbey R. B.: Phase II evaluation of 4'-(9-acridinylamino)-methanesulfon-m-anisidide (AMSA) in patients with advanced sarcoma. Cancer Treat. Rep. 64:1129–1130, 1980
105. Sordillo P. P., Magill G. B., Howard J., Golbey R. B.: Adjuvant chemotherapy in adult soft part sarcomas with "ALOMAD." Proc. Am. Soc. Clin. Oncol. 19:353, 1978
106. Subramanian S., Wiltshaw E.: Chemotherapy of sarcoma: Comparison of three regimens. Lancet 1:683–686, 1978
107. Tekuzman G., Kucuksu N., Ruacan S., et al.: Treatment of solid tumors, soft tissue sarcomas and

lymphomas with cisplatin diamminedichloride (NSC 119875): A phase II study. Cancer 6:17–27, 1976

108. Thigpen J. T., O'Bryan R. M., Benjamin R. S., Coltman C. A., Jr.: Phase II trial of Bakers antifol in metastatic sarcoma. Cancer Treat. Rep. 61:1485–1487, 1977
109. Thigpen J. T., Sampson M. K.: Phase II trial of dianhydrogalactitol in advanced soft tissue and bone sarcomas: A Southwest Oncology Group Study. Cancer Treat. Rep. 63:553–555, 1979
110. Thigpen J. T., Vaughan C., Stuckey W. J.: Phase II trial of anguidine in patients ith sarcomas unresponsive to prior chemotherapy: A Southwest Oncology Group Study. Cancer Treat. Rep. 65:881–882, 1981
111. Townsend C. M., Jr., Eilber F. R., Morton D. L.: Skeletal and soft tissue sarcomas: Results of surgical adjuvant chemotherapy. Proc. Am. Soc. Clin. Oncol. 17:265, 1976
112. Van Dyk J. J., Van der Merve A. M., Falkson H. C., Falkson G.: Adriamycin in the treatment of cancer. S. Afr. Med. J. 50:61–66, 1976
113. Vosika G. J., Bruscoe K., Parey R. W., et al.: Phase II study of diglycoaldehyde in malignant melanomas and soft tissue sarcomas. Cancer Treat. Rep. 65:823–825, 1981
114. Wasserman P.: Maytansine in advanced sarcoma. Proc. Am. Soc. Clin. Oncol. 22:524, 1981
115. Weiss A. J., Metter B. E., Fletcher W. S., et al.: Studies on Adriamycin using a weekly regimen demonstrating its clinical effectiveness and lack of cardiac toxicity. Cancer Treat. Rep. 60:813–822, 1976
116. Welt S., Magil G. P., Sordillo P. P., et al.: Phase II trial of VP-16-213 in adults with soft tissue sarcomas. Proc. Am. Soc. Clin. Oncol. 2:234, 1983
117. Woodcock T. M., Schneider R. J., Young C. W.: Phase I evaluation of 4′-(9-acridinyl-amino) methanesulfon-m-aniside (AMSA) by a weekly intravenous dose schedule. Cancer Treat. Rep. 64:53–55, 1980
118. Yap B.-S., Baker L. H., Sinkovics J. G., et al.: Cyclophosphamide, vincristine, Adriamycin, and DTIC (CYVADIC) combination chemotherapy for the treatment of advanced sarcomas. Cancer Treat. Rep. 64:93–98, 1980
119. Yap B.-S., Benjamin R. S., Burgess M. A., et al.: A phase II evaluation of methyl CCNU and actinomycin D in the treatment of advanced sarcomas in adults. Cancer 47:2807–2809, 1981
120. Yap B.-S., Benjamin R. S., Plager C., et al.: A randomized study of continuous infusion vindesine versus vinblastine in adults with refractory metastatic sarcomas. Am. J. Clin. Oncol. 6:235–238, 1983
121. Yap B.-S., Plager C., Benjamin R. S., et al.: A phase II evaluation of AMSA in adult sarcomas. Cancer Treat. Rep. 65:341–342, 1981
122. Yap B.-S., Sinkovics J. G., Benjamin R. S., Bodey G. P.: Survival and relapse patterns of complete responders in adults with advanced soft tissue sarcomas. Proc. Am. Soc. Clin. Oncol. 20:352, 1979
123. Yap B.-S., Sinkovics J. G., Burgess M. A., et al.: The curability of advanced soft tissue sarcoma in adults with chemotherapy. Proc. Am. Soc. Clin. Oncol. 2:238, 1983
124. Zidar B., Baker L., Rivkin S., et al.: A phase II study of aziridinylbenzoquinone (AZQ) in advanced soft tissue and bone sarcoma: A Southwest Oncology Group (SWOG) study. Proc. Am. Soc. Clin. Oncol. 4:130, 1985

CHAPTER

18

Radiotherapy of Soft Tissue Sarcomas

S. RAFLA
H. SELIM
E. YOUSSEF
K. PARIKH

The controversy surrounding the role of radiotherapy in soft tissue sarcoma management is almost as old as radiotherapy itself. Under the effect of low voltage and orthovoltage radiation, these tumors were believed to be radioresistant. However, some inoperable or recurrent lesions did show a surprisingly good response. Despaigna and del Regatto in 1930 reported a case of recurrent myxosarcoma that was controlled for many years with radiation therapy. Leucutia and Ewing reported in 1935 about the noted radiosensitivity of liposarcomas, which was confirmed by later reports published by Stout. Response of other types of soft tissue sarcomas was claimed by Viets and Witenborg in 1945. Pack et al. reported few long-term survivals among 15 patients treated with radiation therapy after surgery for synovial sarcoma. The flurry of recent activity in exploring the role of radiation therapy while linked to this historical progress has been brought into focus by the development of new radiation beams, the revival of old techniques (e.g., intraoperative brachytherapy), and a more aggressive approach to the treatment of cancer in general and sarcoma management in particular.

In order to better understand the role of radiotherapy in the treatment of soft tissue sarcomas it is important to appreciate the *biologic effect of radiation on soft tissue sarcomas and the factors modifying it*. These tumors are not highly radiosensitive, as measured by their clinical response to radiation; histologic changes afterward may be minimal and indeed the ability of radiation alone to exercise an effective degree of local disease control is questionable. Table 18–1 offers a partial list of authors who reported on local failure after radiotherapy, which amounted to an average of about 60% when this form of treatment was applied alone. Reports of histologic changes in irradiated tumors are rather sparse, even in those series that reported a large number of preoperatively irradiated cases. Changes occurring after high-dose irradiation include formation of excess fibrous tissue within the stroma of the tumor as well as that surrounding the lesion, resulting in the formation of a false capsule. There is also evidence of destruction of tumor cells of various degrees of intensity. However, viable residual tumors can be present in the overwhelming number of specimens. Mansson reported on histologic changes in 21 cases in which substantially increased interstitial fibrosis and foci of massive sclerosis were noted. Mantravadi reported on 32 cases treated with intra-arterial Adriamycin and a modest radiation dose (2500 Cgy in 10 treatments) with 27% complete histologic regression. There was variation in response according to cell type: 50% in synovial sarcomas, 22% in malignant fibrous histiocytoma, and 28% in rhabdomyosarcoma. McNeer claimed histologic sterilization in one third of a small group of cases irradiated to a fairly high dose. Several *factors* were claimed as *influential in determining the degree of radiation sensitivity*; some have stood the test of time and others

TABLE 18–1. Local Recurrence of Soft Tissue Sarcomas After Radiation

Reference	Number of Cases	Clinical Response	Local Failure Rate (%)	Remarks
Cade, 1951[7]	22	—	72	—
Perry et al., 1962[30]	227	74%*	—	—
Windeyer et al., 1966[51]	11	72%	—	Tumors were fibrosarcoma
McNeer et al., 1968[22]	7	—	57	Spindle and giant cell
	4	—	25	Liposarcoma
	3	—	66	Rhabdomyosarcoma
	5	—	60	Synovioma
	2	—	50	Embryonal rhabdomyosarcoma
Lindberg, 1973[21]	—	—	66	—
Suit et al., 1981[41]	2	—	50	Pediatric tumors other than rhabdomyosarcoma
Leibel, 1982[17]	5	—	100	—
Suit et al., 1982[43]	3	—	66	—
Mansson et al., 1983[24]	23	2/23†	—	Patients treated preoperatively to 4000 R but two received higher doses
Shiu et al., 1984[36]	31	—	19	All patients were treated with brachytherapy after incomplete resection
Bramwell et al., 1985[5]	10	—	80	Tumors were inoperable
Tepper et al., 1985[48]	13	—	85	Dose given >100 TDF. Patients received varying doses
	36	—	56	>105 TDF
Ornitz et al., 1980[27]	10	—	50	Patients treated with 15 MEV neutrons
Salinas et al., 1980[34]	29	—	31	Treated with neutrons or combination with photons
Batterman et al., 1981[4]	13	—	38	Treated with neutrons

*Clinical response in 227 incidences of treatment.
†One complete and one partial 20 patients (of 23) showed marked histologic changes after irradiation.

became less important as more experience has been gained. Among the most important factors are the dose delivered and the volume of tumor burden irradiated. McNeer analyzed the response to modest doses of radiation (about 4000 Cgy) in a group of 58 patients and found that the majority of tumor had regressed only by about 25% of their presenting size. Using an objective response for recurrent and metastatic lesions as a parameter of effectiveness, Perry et al. indicated that doses above 3000 Cgy are necessary for a minimal response. Tepper et al. reported on 49 patients treated by radiation only where the local control rate amounted to 15% when the dose was less than 100 TDF (time-dose fractionation) as calculated according to the formulation of Orton and Ellis. This compared with 56% when the dose exceeded 105 TDF. Even in combination with surgery, the dose delivered seemed to play an important role in local disease control, as reported by Suit, who indicated that tumor recurred in sites that received doses of 4000 Cgy, more than in areas of higher dose. The role of fractionation of the dose delivered is beset by uncertainty since almost all series employed a standard fraction size of about 200 Cgy delivered once daily.

The effect of hyperfraction (i.e., the use of more than one daily fraction) is under investigation at several centers. Recently Bryant (1985) reported on a group of patients who were treated with a combination of limb-salvage surgery and mostly preoperative radiation delivered twice daily at a dose of 180 Cgy fraction. Lesions were high-grade and tended to be large (average, 1475 cc). Postoperative booster radiation was given to most patients. Morbidity that accompanied hyperfractionation was noticeably more than in patients treated by standard fractionation. More than half were able to complete the full therapy course. However, the locoregional disease control was impressive, about 95%.

An equally important factor is the tumor burden. There is an almost unanimous agreement that smaller tumors respond better and for longer periods of time. Tepper et al. reported a local failure rate of 12% when tumors were less than 5 cm as compared with 70% in tumors greater than 10 cm in diameter. Even when combined with surgery, the size of tumors seems to exercise an effect on local control. Suit et al., reporting on 52 patients treated by preoperative radiation, showed that the local recurrence rate in tumors staged I and II was 3% as compared with 23% in stages IIIA and IIIB. A local recurrence rate of 12.5% was reported when the tumor volume was less than 150 mm, as compared with 35% when the volume was larger regardless of the sequence of treatment. The impact of local control as an implication of ultimate cure is repeatedly demonstrated and here again tumor burden seems to exercise a substantial influence. Total disease control can reach over 90% when the tumor is less than 25 mm, compared with 42% for tumors of 100 to 150 mm and 26% for larger tumors. The effect of optimal selection combining high-dose radiation with small tumor burden was demonstrated by Shiu et al.

Other factors that have a less definitive effect on radiation response include tumor cell type and tumor cell differentiation: several claims have been made as to the differing radiosensitivity of sarcomas, dependent on their cell types. As recently as 1968, McNeer claimed that this is an important element, with liposarcoma being most sensitive with a local failure rate of 25% after treatment by radiation only. Others have also contributed to this theory, claiming that malignant synovioma and adult rhabdomyosarcoma are the least sensitive, whereas spindle cell sarcoma and malignant fibrous histiocytoma occupy a middle position. However, recent publications seem to veer from this path, stressing only the primary factors discussed earlier. Another question that remains unanswered is the relation between radiosensitivity and cell differentiation. While there is a general agreement that poorly differentiated tumors bear a significantly poorer prognosis than well-differentiated ones, failures seem to be related more to metastatic disease than to locoregional recurrences, implying that no link exists between the degree of differentiation and radiosensitivity. Lindberg claimed that a higher dose is necessary for control of a high-grade tumor. Earlier claims that anaplastic tumors display a certain degree of increased radiation response had not been borne out by recent studies.

The role played by modifiers of radiation response in soft tissue sarcomas has been under investigation in the last few years. Chemical radiation sensitizers such as misonidazole and various cytotoxic agents were explored. Misonidazole given at therapeutically tolerated doses did not seem to improve the response to radiation. Zhang claimed that addition of agent AT1727 to standard radiotherapy has resulted in an objective remission rate of 60% in patients with advanced lesions. Other sensitizers such as IUDR and BUDR showed promise in phase I trials. The addition of certain cytotoxic agents such as doxorubicin in adequate doses seems to improve responses, especially in extremity lesions. This is reflected in a significantly improved locoregional control and disease-free survival. The degree of enhancement is still too uncertain to be quantified. However, Mantravadi reported on 32 cases in which tumors were completely eradicated in one fourth of the patients after a combination of intra-arterial Adriamycin and radiation and reduced to a minimum in an additional 41% of patients.

Physical modifiers of radiation response, especially hyperthermia, seem to be effective only at a temperature of 42°C or higher when applied for a period of about 1 hour following radiation. The use of neutrons, while still experimental, seems to hold great potential. In a series of 10 patients who received neutron therapy using only a 15 MEV beam, local control was reported in half the cases. Other authors reported a local control rate of 60 to 70% in patients treated with either neutron therapy alone or a mixed beam of neutrons and photons. Lesions situated in sites abutting the central nervous system seemed to be particularly amenable to treatment by proton therapy, another form of heavy particle radiation under investigation.

RATIONALE FOR COMBINING SURGERY AND RADIATION

An awareness of the principles underlying the biologic effects of radiation on soft tissue sarcoma paves the way to an appreciation of the fact that radiotherapy has its best effect when used in combination with surgery. As early as 1951, Cade showed the beneficial effect of radiation in reducing the incidence of local recurrence even after relatively limited surgical excision. The rationale of combining the two modalities is linked to the improved effectiveness of radiation when applied to minimal tumor sizes. On the other hand, preoperative radiation helps in reducing the extent of surgery, and thereby reduces the cosmetic, anatomic, and functional loss. The addition of a complement of moderate radiation doses to conservative surgery would destroy the subclinical extension of tumor into the adjacent grossly normal tissues that are invariably invaded by microscopic fringes of the neoplastic process. Simple excision of tumor will almost universally be followed by regrowth. To eradicate subclinical disease by surgery alone requires a radical approach and is associated in most cases with a functional and anatomic deficit. The addition of adequate radiation, on the other hand, is highly capable of destroying microscopic disease, thus improving the chances of locoregional control while avoiding morbidity associated with radical surgery. The control rate after a combined approach by surgery, brachytherapy, and teletherapy was reported to be as high as 94% with good preservation of function.

Irradiation is delivered prior to surgery (preoperative), during surgery (intraoperative) using an electron beam or interstitial implant, or after surgery (post-operative).

Preoperative Radiation Therapy

Preoperative radiation followed by conservative surgery has several advantages, which are summarized as follows:

1. The surgical procedure will be of less magnitude after radiation, as the tumor may have regressed partially. Even a lesion previously considered inoperable may become accessible to surgery. Wound healing is expected to be rather uneventful following radiation dose levels of 5000 Cgy in 5 weeks at a rate of 200 Cgy per fraction.

2. The chances of autotransplantation of tumor cells into the surgical bed or production of metastases due to exfoliation of viable tumor cells into the vascular spaces are less likely to occur after preoperative radiation. Two reasons contribute to this result: (a) most of the tumor cells will be inactivated by preoperative radiation, and (b) the formation of a dense false capsule that completely isolates the growth from the surrounding tissue by the time surgery is performed.

3. When a tumor is treated preoperatively, the volume of tissues treated is planned only on the basis of a clinically and radiographically demonstrated lesion as well as the known and expected pattern of subclinical extension of the tumor. Such a volume will invariably be smaller than the one used for postoperative radiotherapy, which is usually delivered not only to the original tumor volume but to all the tissues handled surgically and the site of the drain wound as well. Since radiation morbidity is linked to the extent of volume irradiated, the acute and late radiation effects should be less severe in patients who receive preoperative radiotherapy as compared with postoperative radiation.

4. The multidisciplinary approach necessary for preoperative irradiation is usually carried through the whole course of therapy, thus optimizing the chances of the delivery of other booster therapy such as effective intraoperative radiation when necessary. Disadvantages of preoperative irradiation are primarily related to a delay in surgery, which may theoretically increase the chances of disease dissemination. However, in slow-growing lesions, the delay of a few weeks is unlikely to be of consequence and the natural history of tumors treated by preoperative radiation and surgery has not demonstrated such occurrences.

Results

As early as 1963 Atkinson and associates described local control in 14 out of 15 patients who were radiated preoperatively with doses of 4500 Cgy in 4 to 5 weeks followed by en-bloc dissection (median follow-up period, 41 months). Martin et al. reported no local recurrence among 10 patients who received doses of over 5000 Cgy. They confirmed that reduction of size and encapsulation of tumor made local excision easier to perform. Mansson et al. reported local control of 95% in 23 patients treated with 4000 Cgy preoperatively and followed for over 62 months. Delayed wound healing was observed in two cases. Tepper et al. reported results of 60 patients who have been treated by radiation followed by local surgical resection, with a 5-year actuarial local control rate of 84%. In addition to a preoperative dose of 50 to 60 Cgy (in 5 to 6 weeks) followed by conservative surgery, these patients received a booster dose of 10 to 15 Cgy given to the tumor bed either intraoperatively (by electrons or interstitially) or postoperatively by external beam technique with a small field. Twenty-four cases (of 60) were so locally advanced that they were considered unresectable at presentation and would have required amputation if surgery had been performed initially. Table 18–2 summarizes the results of preoperative radiation.

In conclusion, a high degreee of local control can be obtained with moderate doses of radiation delivered preoperatively followed by conservative surgery. Survival rates are at least equivalent to those obtained with radical surgery (e.g., amputation). Delay in wound healing does not pose a real hazard when doses of radiation are limited to 5000 Cgy in 5 weeks. In the vast majority of cases limb function is preserved at near normal.

POSTOPERATIVE RADIATION THERAPY

Conservative surgery followed by irradiation has the following advantages and disadvantages.

Advantages

1. Better control for subclinical disease after resection of the gross disease.
2. The entire specimen is examined for histologic grade, type, and tumor extension, enabling better planning of the whole course of management and other adjuvant therapies.
3. The extent of the tumor is assessed by direct visual and palpation examination. This is especially important when tumor outline is difficult to discover accurately during preoperative assessment, as in some limb lesions, even after detailed thin-section CT scanning.
4. The adoption of such a policy would encourage the surgeon to concern himself primarily with the gross tumor, thus preserving a functional limb.
5. No delay in starting surgery, which may represent to the patient the ultimate deliverance from cancer evils.

Disadvantages

1. Any delay in wound healing would delay starting irradiation, allowing tumor cells a better chance of continued growth

TABLE 18–2. Results of Preoperative Radiation and Surgery

Reference	Number of Cases	Locoregional Control (%)	Survival	Remarks
Suit, 1981[41]	21	100	71% 3-yr disease-free	Patients ≤ 21 yr
Mantravadi, 1984[23]	32	97	70% 3-yr actuarial disease-free	Preoperative intra-arterial chemotherapy + radiotherapy + surgery + radiotherapy
Mansson, 1983[24]	23	91	70% 5-yr	30% developed metastatic disease
Eilber, 1984[84]	183	97	76%	—
Atkinson, 1963[3]	122	—	45% 5-yr	All sites including uterus
Martin, 1977[25]	10	—	80% 1-yr	—
Suit, 1985[45]	60	90	62% 5-yr actuarial	—

and thus increasing the number of tumor cells that must be inactivated by the radiation. However, such chances ought to be minimal if proper techniques for surgical excision are followed.

2. The volume treated is, by necessity, large, since it will have to encompass the whole incision as well as drainage sites with adequate margin. This may jeopardize the delivery of an adequate dose.

Results

Lindberg reported on 300 patients who were treated with conservative surgery and postoperative radiation to a dose of 70 to 75 Gy (in about 7 weeks) with an absolute 2- and 5-year disease-free survival of 74% and 61%, respectively. Local control was achieved in 78% in the whole group. Some of the failures were salvaged by subsequent surgery. Of the patients with extremity lesions 84% maintained a functional limb.

Shiu et al. reported on the application of brachytherapy using iridium-192, following conservative surgery boosted with external radiation in large tumors. Local control was 100% in the previously untreated lesions and 62.5% in the previously treated and recurrent cases. Median follow-up was 36 months. However, one third of the patients developed problems with wound healing, sometimes necessitating amputation.

In a review of 110 patients, Suit et al. reported a local failure rate of 11%. Apart from a marginally increased failure rate among stages IIB and IIIB (22% and 18%, respectively), there was no impact of staging on local failures. However, patients with advanced stages suffered a noticeably high local failure rate when surgery was incomplete, 42% versus 17% after complete surgery. The completion of surgery did not seem to have an impact on local control rate in earlier stage tumors (88% after complete surgery versus 92% otherwise). Table 18–3 lists a summary of series of postoperative radiotherapy.

TABLE 18–3. Results of Postoperative Radiotherapy

Reference	Number of Cases	Locoregional Control (%)	Survival	Remarks
Shiu, 1984[36]	17	100	90% actuarial 5 yr	Previously untreated (Surgery + ^{192}Ir implant and limb-sparing surgery)
	16	52	60% actuarial 5 yr	Recurrent cases (Surgery + ^{192}Ir implant and limb-sparing surgery)
Rosenberg, 1982[31]	27	85	71% 5-yr disease-free	Limb-sparing surgery + radiotherapy + chemotherapy
Coe, 1981[11]	77	86	68% 5-yr; 80% 2 yr	Conservative surgery + radiotherapy All limb lesions
	109	62		Sarcomas in all sites
Mills, 1981[26]	17	94	—	Resection and brachytherapy + teletherapy
Lindberg, 1981[21]	300 (total)		61% 5-yr disease-free 74% 2-yr disease-free	Conservative surgery + radiotherapy
	108	84 (at least)	69% 5-year disease-free	Extremity lesions
	15		33% 5-yr disease-free	Abdominal lesions
Abatucci, 1984[1]	69	91 at 2-yr 83 at 5-yr	76% 5-yr	Some patients received preoperative radiotherapy also
Gunderson, 1984	47	53	—	All are abdominal tumors treated by surgery + intraoperative radiotherapy + postoperative radiotherapy
Leibel, 1982[17]	29	90	81% 5-yr 68% 5-yr disease-free	
Suit, 1985[44]	110	88	73% actuarial 5 yr	Primarily limb lesions

*Few patients followed-up.

RADIOTHERAPY COMBINED WITH CHEMOTHERAPY AS ADJUVANT TO CONSERVATIVE SURGERY

The benefit accrued by the addition of chemotherapy to the standard combination of radiotherapy and surgery is still far from clear. Mantravadi (1984) reported a local control rate of 97% in a group of 32 patients treated by preoperative radiation concomitant with intra-arterial infusion of Adriamycin followed by surgical excision and postoperative radiation boost. All suffered from high-grade tumors. Over one fourth of the lesions were completely sterilized by the preoperative therapy, and only minimal tumor was found in 41% of cases. On the other hand, a report by Eilber and his collegues, who treated 100 patients with a similar approach, did not confirm these findings. In addition, in the group of patients with grade III tumors no significant survival benefit was noted that could be attributed to adjuvant chemotherapy (80% with chemotherapy versus 70% without).

In a prospective randomized trial of adjuvant Adriamycin given after completion of adequate locoregional therapy (surgery and radiotherapy), the use of the chemotherapy seemed to have significantly improved continuous disease-free survival and overall survival in a group of 65 patients. All patients had high-grade tumors of extremities. No such benefit was demonstrated in cases of head and neck or retroperitoneal lesions. A study conducted by Cancer and Leukemia Group B confirmed the beneficial effect of adjuvant Adriamycin but only in high-grade tumors and when doses were pushed almost to the level of toxicity.

COMPLICATIONS OF RADIATION THERAPY

Delay of wound healing in patients receiving preoperative radiation is rare since the dose is limited to about 5000 Cgy. Most patients who receive postoperative irradiation exhibit some degree of clinically detectable fibrosis in the irradiated area. Significant complications develop in about 6% of cases, including soft tissue necrosis, bone fractures, fibrosis with limited motion of the extremity, nerve damage, vascular damage, and edema of the extremity below the irradiated field. Complications occur more often in the lower extremities than the upper ones, head and neck, or the torso. This is due mainly to the large size of the lesions in the lower extremities, the extent of surgery necessary for their resection, and subsequent large volume irradiation. The physiologic effect of the dependency of lower limbs, causing increased edema and subsequent soft tissue fibrosis, is well documented in other conditions, e.g., fractures in which radiation is not implicated. Most complications can be avoided by careful treatment planning.

RADIATION THERAPY ALONE FOR SOFT TISSUE SARCOMAS

There are few patients who are not candidates for surgery because of the anatomic location of their tumor, medical inoperability, or refusal of consent. There are relatively few data available on the efficacy of radiotherapy alone in sarcomas of soft tissue origin, but a review of Table 18–1 shows that local control can be expected in 20 to 50% of cases so treated, depending on the size of the primary tumor and cell type. The prognosis of patients treated with radiation alone for soft tissue sarcomas is not good, but long-term cures can be expected in some. Doses of 6600 Cgy are necessary for response evocation and maximization of local control.

THE PALLIATIVE ROLE OF RADIATION THERAPY

Radiation therapy has an effective role in the palliative management of soft tissue sarcomas. In unresectable lesions, radiation therapy helps in shrinking the tumor mass and thus reduces secondary mass effect such as edema and pain. This is invariably achieved by a modest dose of 4000 to 5000 Cgy delivered in 3 to 4 weeks.

RADIOTHERAPY TECHNIQUES

Although the treatment technique for each soft tissue sarcoma is heavily dependent on many variables, there are a number of basic principles common to all. Thorough knowledge of the anatomy of the involved tissues is essential in determining the volume to be irradiated. These tumors are known to spread locally along tissue compartments. Extension through the boundaries of individual compartments into adjacent compartments occurs only late in the course of the disease. CT scans can be helpful in delineating the tumor and outlining the boundaries of the involved compartment. These tumors can track along the sheath of surrounding blood vessels and nerves, and recurrences are known to occur at some distance from the primary. Although some tumors are surrounded by a pseudocapsule, true encapsulation is never present and one should assume some degree of contamination of the area surrounding the primary. Lymph nodes are rarely involved and do not have to be routinely included in the radiation field. An essential part of treatment planning is to review the operative and pathology reports to determine the extent of the resection, relation of the tumor to adjacent muscles, blood vessels, bones, and critical organs, as well as presence or absence of gross or microscopic residual disease. Metallic clips, which were considered very helpful in delineating the tumor bed and areas of residual disease, may, on the other hand, create numerous artifacts in subsequent CT scanning, and their use must be judiciously controlled. MRI scanning can now be substituted so that problems with clips left in the wound can be minimized. The surgeon must be aware of the limitations that the surgical procedure he selects places on subsequent radiotherapy, especially when dealing with tumors of the extremities, where preservation of function is of major importance. Ideally, the skin incision should be placed directly over the tumor mass and the amount of tissue handling should be kept to the minimum, compatible with adequate exploration. The larger the surgical field, the larger the radiation field required and the less will be the tolerance of the various tissues. Planning of both surgery and radiotherapy should be carried out by the same team if best results are to be obtained.

Generally, the initial radiation field should encompass the tissue compartment where the tumor arises including the entire surgical field. The skin incision is not always a good indicator of the extent of the tissues manipulated during surgery. This initial volume should receive a dose of 45 to 50 Gy over a period of 5 to 6 weeks (1.80 Gy per day). An additional 18 to 20 Gy should subsequently be given to a smaller volume, encompassing the site of the primary tumor with a 5 to 10 cm margin in all directions. The higher the histologic grade of the tumor, the wider should be the margin.

Individualized shielding blocks and tissue compensators should always be used to insure shielding of uninvolved tissues and optimal homogeneous dose distribution.

The cardinal principles to be followed for successful delivery of radiation are as follows:

1. The surgical wound must heal completely before radiation is started.
2. The entire length of the scar and the site of the drainage tube must be covered.
3. It is beneficial for limb lesions only if the surgeon marks the distal sites of the tumor margins with metallic clips.
4. Spare as much normal tissue as possible during irradiation to prevent edema.
5. The entire circumference of an extremity must not be irradiated.
6. Use shrinking field techniques.
7. Plan treatment carefully.

Head and Neck

Irradiation of a soft tissue sarcoma in the head and neck region is no different from irradiation of other malignant lesions. The only variance is the need to deliver a higher dose to a volume that includes the primary site along with generous margins. Generally, it is not necessary to treat nodal sites. Because cosmesis and preservation of function are of paramount importance in head and neck sites, the following aspects are mandatory: careful treatment planning, the use of beam directing devices, shaping of field to spare and protect surrounding vital structures, and individualization of approach.

Limbs

Preservation of good function is the main benefit from combining surgery with radiotherapy. Every effort should be made to minimize fibrosis, contractures, and loss of function. This starts with preplanned surgery; skin incisions should be placed longitudinally (along the direction of all the muscles in the limbs) in order to be able to spare a portion of the circumference of the extremity from irradiation. Circumferential irradiation can result in severe fibrosis, pain with distal edema, and loss of function. It is also preferable to avoid incisions over sites exposed to recurrent trauma (e.g., elbow, groin, patella, anterior tibia, and Achilles tendon) so that they could be spared irradiation.

A portion of the circumference of an uninvolved bone should be shielded to maintain the strength of the bone and minimize the possibility of future traumatic fractures.

Isocenteric treatment set-ups are superior to turning the patient over (to treat both sides), as the latter will invariably introduce some rotation along the long axis of the limb, creating a certain degree of inaccuracy. In order to be able to reproduce the same setup daily it is essential to use an immobilization device applied to the part treated to maintain a constant.

Opposing anteroposterior fields could be used; however, oblique fields with tissue compensators can avoid irradiating uninvolved tissue compartments while maintaining homogeneous dose distribution.

Thigh. The thigh is the commonest site for soft tissue sarcomas in the extremities. The proximity of the perineal region and the scrotum in the male complicates treatment in that area. Three major muscle groups are present: anterior, anteromedial, and posterior. For a small tumor in either the vastus medialis or lateralis, it is probably not necessary to treat the entire width of the quadriceps and the use of oblique fields could be adequate. Tumors of the rest of the quadriceps can be treated with slightly angled fields protecting the skin for the medial thigh, provided that an anterior incision was used. Fields do not need to extend beyond the femoral neck superiorly and the patella inferiorly.

For tumors in the anteromedial group, fields should extend from the pubic symphysis superomedially to the middle of the femur laterally except in situations in which the tumor was in contact with the bone, where the full width of the bone must be included.

The posterior group is best treated with the patient lying on his side with the thighs widely separated or prone with the other thigh positioned off the table.

Leg. The leg has three compartments: anterior, posterior, and lateral. The interosseous membrane acts as a natural barrier between the anterior and posterior groups.

The anterior group is best treated with oblique portals. Treatment fields do not need to be extended to cover the insertion of these muscles into the foot.

The posterior group has an attachment above the knee joint superiorly and blends with the Achilles tendon inferiorly. Using individually shaped lateral fields, a skin strip overlying the anterior tibia and the skin overlying the Achilles tendon can be shielded. A portion of the knee joint can be included in the initial large field and excluded from the cone-down boost unless the tumor overlies the joint and has to be included in the high-dose region.

Foot. The foot is rarely involved by soft tissue sarcomas. Complete removal of tumors in that region, leaving a functioning foot, is technically difficult. In treating tumors on the dorsum of the foot great care must be taken to spare the sole and a portion of the toes. Below-the-knee amputation for a foot sarcoma may yield a better functioning limb.

Arm. The arm has two groups of muscles: anterior and posterior. The best position for treatment is that where the arm is abducted 90° from the trunk. The treatment couch should be rotated by 90° to allow free angulation of the gantry.

Forearm. The forearm has two muscle compartments: anterior and posterior. The interosseous membrane forms a natural barrier between the two. For most tumors it is usually possible to avoid irradiating most of the elbow and the joints of the hand unless very close to the tumor or covered by an incision.

Retroperitoneal Sarcomas

Many of these tumors present at an advanced stage, and complete excision is not always possible. Accurate determination of the extent of the tumor growth prior to surgery is essential if all potential areas of tumor spread are to be covered by the radiation field. This can be achieved by a detailed review of the operative report as well as other pertinent reports (e.g., sonograms). Thin-section CT scans are essential. The use of metal clips at the time of surgery is rather controversial. While they may help delineate sites involved, their presence would so impair the quality of postoperative CT scans that it is preferable not to implant any metal during surgery. Radiotherapy planning is dependent primarily on CT scans and operative detail. Low tolerance of certain abdominal organs—e.g., liver, kidney, and bowels—would be a major limiting factor to the radiation dose that can be delivered.

Multi-field plans using wedge filters should be employed if the desired high dose of radiation is to be delivered safely. Intraoperative irradiation utilizing electron beam or interstitial implant is being used in several centers to augment the dose delivered to the tumor-bearing area while sparing normal tissues.

CONCLUSION

We believe that a combined preplanned approach to the treatment of soft tissue sarcomas is essential to achieve the highest level of cure consistent with optimal function and limb preservation. Radiotherapy must be delivered carefully and with a great degree of attention to meticulous detail if complications are to be minimized. It is expected that future development of radiation modifiers and new beams would further enhance the beneficial effect of radiation in the treatment of these tumors.

REFERENCES

1. Abbatucci J. S., Boulier N., de Ranieri, J., et al.: Radiotherapy as an integrated part of the treatment of soft tissue sarcomas. Radiother. Oncol. 2:115–121, 1984
2. Antman K., Suit H., Amato D., et al.: Preliminary results of a randomized trial of adjuvant doxorubicin for sarcomas, lack of apparent difference between treatment groups. J. Clin. Oncol. 2:601–608, 1984
3. Atkinson L., Garvan J. M., Newton N. C.: Behavior and management of soft connective tissue sarcomas. Cancer 1552–1562, 1963
4. Battermann J. J., Brewer K.: Fast neutron therapy for locally advanced sarcomas. Int. J. Radiat. Oncol. Biol. Phys. 1051–1053, 1981; Radiother. Oncol. 2:115–121, 1984
5. Bramwell V. H. C., Crowther D., Deakin D. P., et al.: Combined modality management of local and disseminated adult soft tissue sarcomas; a review of 257 cases seen over 10 years at the Christie Hospital and Holt Radium Institute, Manchester. Br. J. Cancer 51:301–318, 1985
6. Bryant M., Martinez A., Pritchard D., et al.: Soft tissue sarcomas of the extremities: Morbidity of combined radiation and limb salvage with special emphasis on twice a day fractionation. Int. J. Radiat. Oncol. Biol. Phys. 11(Suppl. 1):87, 1985
7. Cade S.: Soft tissue tumors: Their natural history and treatment. Proc. R. Soc. Med., vol. XLIV, 19–36, Jan. 1951
8. Cadman J., et al.: Synovial sarcoma: An analysis of 2x tumors. Cancer 18:613–627, 1965
9. Cantin J., et al.: The problem of local recurrence after treatment of soft tissue sarcoma. Ann. Surg. 168:47–53, 1968
10. Carabell S. C., Goodman R. L.: Radiation therapy for soft tissue sarcoma. Semin. Oncol. 8:201–206, 1981
11. Coe M. A., Madden J., Mould R. F.: The role of radiotherapy in the treatment of soft tissue sarcomas, a retrospective study 1958–1973. Clin. Radiol. 32:47–51, 1981
12. del Regato J. A.: Radiotherapy of soft tissue sarcomas. JAMA, July 20, 1963, 185–216
13. Eilber F. R., Morton D. L., Eckardt J., et al.: Limb salvage for skeletal and soft tissue sarcomas. Cancer 53:2579–2584, 1984
14. Ewing J.: Fascial sarcoma and intermuscular mymliposarcoma. Arch. Surg. 31:507–520, 1935
15. Friedman M., Egan J. W.: Irradiation of liposarcoma. Acta Radiol. (Stockholm) 54:225–238, 1960
16. Glatstein E., Kinsella T. J., Rosenberg S. A.: Phase I experience with intravenous sensitizers in the treatment of unresectable sarcomas. Int. J. Radiat. Oncol. Biol. Phys. 11(Suppl. 1):87, 1985
17. Leibel S. A., Tranbaugh R. F., Wassa W. M., et al.: Soft tissue sarcomas of the extremities. Cancer 50:1076–1083, 1982
18. Leucutia T.: Radiotherapy of sarcomas of soft parts. Radiology 25:403–415, 1935
19. Lindberg R. D.: The role of radiotherapy in the treatment of soft tissue sarcomas of adults. Proceedings Seventh National Cancer Conference, 883–888, 1973
20. Lindberg R. D., Martin R. G., Romsdahl M. M., et al.: Conservative surgery and radiation therapy for soft tissue sarcomas. *In* Management of Primary Bone and Soft Tissue Tumors. Chicago, Yearbook Medical Publishers, 1977
21. Lindberg R. D., Martin R. G., Romsdahl M. M., et al.: Conservative surgery and postoperative radiotherapy in 300 adults with soft tissue sarcomas. Cancer 47:2391–2397, 1981
22. McNeer G. P., Cantin J., Chu F., et al.: Effectiveness of radiation therapy in the management of sarcoma of the soft somatic tissues. Cancer 22:391–397, 1968
23. Mantravadi R. V., Trippon M. J., Patel M. K., et al.: Limb salvage in extremity soft tissue sarcoma: Combined modality therapy. Radiology 152:523–526, 1984
24. Mansson E., Williams J., Aparisi T., et al.: Preoperative radiation therapy of high malignancy grade soft tissue sarcoma. Acta Radiol. [Oncol.] 22:461–464, 1983
25. Martin R. G., Lindberg R. D., Russel W. O.: Preoperative radiotherapy and surgery in the management of soft tissue sarcoma. *In* Management of Primary Bone and Soft Tissue Tumors. Chicago, Yearbook Medical Publishers, 1977
26. Mills E. E., Hering E. R.: Management of soft tissue tumors by limited surgery combined with tumor bed irradiation using brachytherapy and supplementary teletherapy. Br. J. Radiol. 54:312–317, 1981
27. Ornitz R., Herkovic A., Shell M., et al.: Treatment experience: Locally advanced sarcomas with 15 MEV fast neutrons. Cancer 45:2712–2716, 1980

28. Orton C. G., Ellis F. A.: Simplification in the use of the NSD concept in practical radiotherapy. Br. J. Radiol. 46:529–537, 1973
29. Pack G. T., Pierson J. C.: Liposarcoma. Surgery 36:687–712, 1954
30. Perry H., Chu F. C. H.: Radiation management of soft tissue sarcomas. Cancer 15:179–183, 1962
31. Rosenberg S. A., Tepper J., Glatstein E., et al.: The treatment of soft tissue sarcomas of the extremities. Prospective randomized evaluations of (1) limb-sparing surgery plus radiation therapy compared with amputation and (2) the role of adjuvant chemotherapy. Ann. Surg. 196:305–315, 1982
32. Rosenberg S. A.: Prospective randomized trials demonstrating the efficiency of adjuvant chemotherapy in adult patients with soft tissue sarcomas. Cancer Treatment Reports 68:1067–1078, 1984
33. Russel N. O., Choen J., Enzinger F., et al.: Clinical and pathological staging systems for soft tissue sarcoma. Cancer 40:1562–1570, 1977
34. Salinas R., et al.: Experience with fast neutron therapy for locally advanced sarcomas. Int. J. Radiat. Oncol. Biol. Phys. 6:267–272, 1980
35. Shieber W., et al.: An experience with sarcoma of the soft tissues in adults. Surgery 52:295–298, 1962
36. Shiu M. H., et al.: Control of locally advanced extremity soft tissue sarcomas by function-servicing resection and brachytherapy. Cancer 53:1385–1392, 1984
37. Schmitt G., Passow J., Schnabel K., et al.: Radiotherapy of soft tissue sarcomas with neutrons or a neutron boost. Br. J. Radiol. 57:247–250, 1984
38. Simon M. A., et al.: Management of adult soft tissue sarcomas of the extremities. Ann. Surg. 11:363–402, 1979
39. Slater J. D., et al.: Radiation therapy for unresectable soft tissue sarcomas. Int. J. Radiat. Oncol. Biol. Phys. 10(Suppl. 2):Oct. 1984
40. Stout A. P.: Liposarcoma-malignant tumor of lipoblasts. Ann. Surg. 119:86–107, 1944
41. Suit H.: Soft tissue sarcomas (excluding rhabdomyosarcomas). National Cancer Institute Monograms (56):245–249, 1981
42. Suit H., Russel W. O., Martin R. G.: Sarcoma of soft tissue. Clinical and histopathologic parameters and response to treatment. Cancer 35:1478–1483, 1975
43. Suit H., Goitein M., Munzenreider J., et al.: Evaluation of clinical applicability of proton beam in definitive fractionated radiation therapy. Int. J. Radiat. Oncol. Biol. Phys. 8(12):2199–2205, 1982
44. Suit H. D., et al.: Preoperative, intraoperative and postoperative radiation in the treatment of primary soft tissue sarcoma. Cancer 55:2659–2667, 1985
45. Suit H. P., Tepper J. E.: Radiation therapy alone for sarcoma of soft tissue. Cancer 56:475–479, 1985
46. Tepper J., Rosenberg S., Glatstein E.: Radiation therapy technique in soft tissue sarcomas of the extremity. Int. J. Radiat. Oncol. Biol. Phys. 8:263–273.
47. Tepper J., Suit H.: Radiation therapy of retroperitoneal soft tissue sarcomas. Int. J. Radiat. Oncol. Biol. Phys. 10:825–830.
48. Tepper J. E., et al.: Radiation therapy of soft tissue sarcomas. Cancer 55:2273–2277, 1985
49. Weingrad D. W., Rosenberg S. A.: Early lymphatic spread of osteogenic and soft tissue sarcomas. Surgery 84:231–240, 1978
50. Viets H. R., Wittenborg M. H.: Rhabdomyosarcoma eroding spinal column and compression of spinal cord. Arch. Pathol. 40:179–181, 1985
51. Windeyer B., Dische S., Mansfield C. M.: The place of radiotherapy in the management of fibrosarcomas of the soft tissues. Clin. Radiol. 17:32–40, 1966
52. Zhang Z. Y., Liu T. F., Zhang X. F.: Preliminary report on AT1727 as a potential radiosensitizer. Int. J. Radiat. Oncol. Biol. Phys. 10:2305–2307, 1984
53. CALGB—Rose Ruth Ellison and Eng. Cortes, personal communication.

INDEX

Numbers in italics refer to figures; numbers followed by t refer to tables.